TI
DRUG USERS BIBLE

HARM REDUCTION, RISK MITIGATION, PERSONAL SAFETY

AN ANTIDOTE TO THE WAR ON DRUGS

DOMINIC MILTON TROTT

Published by
MxZero Publishing, 2019
publisher@u9.org

Neither the author nor the publisher accepts any legal responsibility or liability for any inaccuracies, errors or omissions. The information and text within is supplied without warranty, and is not presented as a service or as advice in any capacity. The contents merely reflect the author's experiences and personal observations.

First Edition

ISBN 978-0-9955936-8-8 (paperback)

www.DrugUsersBible.com

IMPORTANT NOTICES

Nothing in this book should be taken to imply that any chemical or botanical is safe to use. The usage of chemicals and botanicals represent a risk to your personal safety, and the information published is intended to help you to mitigate some of that risk. It represents a start point for your own research, should you choose to sample any psychoactive material.

No law was broken during the research process or the writing of this book. By definition, the legal highs were legal in the United Kingdom when the research was undertaken. The other materials were sampled in jurisdictions in which possession was not a criminal offence. The author does not endorse or encourage any unlawful activity whatsoever.

> *"If the words 'life, liberty, and the pursuit of happiness' don't include the right to experiment with your own consciousness, then the Declaration of Independence isn't worth the hemp it was written on."*
>
> ~ Terence McKenna

Dedicated to the victims of the *war on drugs*

Acknowledgements:
Thanks are due to *Spooks*, for the endless patience, positive feedback, and invaluable advice.
I am indebted to Frantastic, Bazzz, and CharlieH for proof reading all or part of the book.
Finally, thanks to the staff and members of the *UK Research Forum* for providing both inspiration and knowledge.

Table of Contents

3. BOTSCAPE: A BOTANICAL JOURNEY

PREFACE

Drugs. What image does this word conjure in your mind? What picture is painted for you by newspapers and broadcasters?

It is a word that has become so stigmatised and misappropriated that, in our society, rational discourse is almost impossible, and factual information is buried. The result, in terms of human misery, is everywhere to be seen.

This is the context against which I wrote this book.

My own introduction to drugs was not uncommon. I was always curious, but not enough to fully engage. I smoked cannabis a couple of times at university, and tripped on LSD once, in my twenties.

I then strayed from the script, albeit temporarily. I stumbled upon Adam Gottlieb's tiny book, *Legal Highs*, which introduced the world of botanicals. From this, foolishly, I sampled a couple of... nutmegs. These induced an experience which was so horrendous that I didn't touch another psychoactive for many years.

It was back exclusively to booze; the socially accepted but deadly intoxicant. Like many of us trapped in a certain culture, I drank too much. This wasn't habitual, or daily. It was just that when I did drink, I tended to binge somewhat. I could probably claim that I was perfectly normal.

It was a generation or so later that my curiosity and interest in the subject of this book was re-awakened by exposure to a series of loosely related topics.

The first of these was quantum physics. I had grasped that my original perception of life was flawed when I first encountered Einstein's *Theory of Relativity*. Quantum physics, however, with it's demonstrations of connectedness (*entanglement*) and the need for an observer to collapse potential into matter (*double-slit experiment*), obliterated all preconceptions, and at the same time appeared to place consciousness at the centre of the mandala.

On the back of this, courtesy of YouTube, I discovered the charismatic Terence McKenna. Some of his theories on the nature of reality were staggering, but plausible. Psychedelics were the name of the game; expanding consciousness and facilitating a sojourn from our limited static perspective. Of particular interest were his frequent references to shamanic rituals, embracing strange vision inducing cocktails. The most common of these brews was the famed *ayahuasca*, which almost came with a guarantee to open the door to the indescribable.

I was intrigued; so intrigued that I researched this field intensively, and in the fullness of time determined that I must travel to Peru to engage in the ritual. With the research for this expedition came my first home-based experiments, always cautious, always scientific, always with a clear objective.

Ayahuasca not only provided an unimaginably beautiful and beneficial experience, but bestowed the confidence to continue the quest for knowledge. The journey, at least as far as psychedelics were concerned, was underway.

It wasn't too long before I became interested in widening my field of exploration to at least embrace dissociatives, oneirogens and nootropics. In terms of safety I understood that in a comparative sense psychedelics tended to have an excellent profile, but it was increasingly obvious that other classes of drugs could also be navigated sanely and sensibly, if a methodical and scientific approach was used. I therefore proceeded, with what I considered to be due care.

I was soon to encounter a disturbing tendency. Whilst I perused forums and message boards I occasionally noticed that regular contributors had disappeared. Sometimes word would get back that they had made a mistake, and had died. This was horrific, more so as I understood that most of the deaths were completely avoidable.

People were dying, and they were dying because of ignorance. They were dying because they didn't know how to use their drug, because they were experimenting with insane doses, buying from dodgy sources and not testing, underestimating onset and double dosing, and taking crazy drug combinations.

They were dying because unremitting propaganda against psychoactives was denying them vital safety information. They were dying because legislators and the media were censoring the science, and ruthlessly pushing an ideological agenda instead. They were dying because the first casualty of war is truth, and the *war on drugs* is no different.

Prohibition kills people, education saves lives, yet the education provided broadly amounted to '*take drugs and you will die*'. This lie was so obvious that no-one took it seriously.

However, here, before me, was my own *modus operandi*, and a database of my own experiences. It included precisely the sort of risk mitigation and personal safety information that would surely be of value to others, and which might actually save some of those lives. This juxtaposition was so stark that the embryo of this book was quickly envisioned.

So my course was set. I would expand my initial mission, and embrace all commonly available chemicals and botanicals. I would document the journey directly and accurately, emphasizing and explaining the safety aspects throughout. I would seek to document the hidden truths, spanning the entire drugscape.

The undertaking was daunting, and at times I experienced anger and frustration at the blindness of a society which made it necessary. I overcame this and a myriad of other issues by reminding myself that if it saved a single life it would all be worth it.

After the best part of ten years, the book was finally published. I now hope on hope that the information within it reaches those who need it most.

Dominic Milton Trott

1

THE DRUGSCAPE

1. DRUGSCAPE: AN INTRODUCTION

Psychoactive substances are generally considered to be materials that alter perception, mood or consciousness. However, the context of their use far exceeds that of recreation. As entheogens, many are used for ritual, spiritual, or shamanic purposes, and are immersed in history. Others are used to explore new insights and engineer different perspectives, both for personal development, nootropic, and academic purposes.

This book embraces all of these dimensions. It charts and examines the entire drugscape, which was investigated and researched during a time of unparalleled access to psychoactive materials of all types and classes.

BACKGROUND & FORMAT

This was an unprecedented period of chemical discovery and innovation, which was fuelled by demand for *legal highs*. A substantial array of popular and emerging research chemicals was developed and brought to the market. These chemicals were systematically obtained and sampled, and are reported in the first half of the book.

Equally, full advantage was taken of the fact that the import of almost all psychotropic botanicals was entirely legal, enabling methodical desktop research to be undertaken without geographic restraint. Simultaneously, the world was traversed to experience as many as possible in an authentic setting. These are reported in the second half of the book.

Whilst the media distorted public perception, via the sort of misreporting and censorship which has been almost universally standard with respect to the grotesqueries of the *war on drugs*, a window of opportunity remained open: the opportunity to explore a new and developing frontier, rationally and relatively unhindered.

It was recognized from the outset that this situation wouldn't last. It would only be a matter of time before ideological legislation blindly closed many of the available avenues, making some of the materials almost impossible to acquire.

An intentional and sustained effort was therefore made to sample and research materials from across the entire canopy of the psychoactive landscape, within the time frame available. The approach was systematic and structured, purposely alternating between the different drug classifications, and where possible, between chemical and botanical forms.

The layout of each individual report is framed to introduce the named psychoactive via factual and objective data, followed by a narrative of subjective experience. The latter comprise a mixture of live *trip reports* (logs recorded during the experience itself) and experience summaries which were documented retrospectively.

Given that they were usually written whilst under the influence of a psychoactive, the live reports can be a little disjointed, and are sometimes less eloquent than they might be. However, to retain authenticity, only minimal editing has been applied. It should also be noted here that these are individual experiences, and that they can differ widely, from person to person. They are dependent upon personal physiology and psychology, and in many cases, upon set and setting.

For each substance or material, basic information is also quoted from a number of third party harm reduction sources. These offer important public services, and the references provide generic rather than individual experience data.

USA, CANADA, THE WORLD

The social-media drug scene is unsurprisingly dominated by the United States. However, the overlap of the particular drugs used in the United States and the rest of the English speaking world, including the UK, is huge. Even those chemicals and botanicals which are widely used in the United States but not elsewhere are globally available, courtesy of a little effort.

To make this book relevant to all, I therefore imported where possible, and travelled where necessary. Ensuring applicability and credibility across the international domain was a clear objective throughout.

Whilst references to the UK situation may be present in the first and final sections of the book, the major content is location neutral, and any such reference can be taken as illustrative of the situation in most other nations.

With respect to terminology, on those rare occasions on which a chemical or botanical has different common names between nations effort has been made to specify and explain all such nomenclature.

THE SAFETY IMPERATIVE

The contents are the product of a scientific pursuit, a quest for knowledge, and an adventure. They are the fruits of a journey of the mind, but one from which important lessons were drawn and recorded. The first and foremost of these was safety.

It is strongly recommended that *Section 1.1* is the first port of call for anyone who intends to embark upon a psychoactive experience. These measures, and those further elaborated throughout the book, should never be skipped or shortcut.

Finally, none of this information is intended to encourage the use of any legal or illegal compound. It comprises data and insight which is provided to support harm reduction, and a safer approach by anyone experimenting with any of the materials covered.

1.1 SAFETY FIRST

It should go without saying that safety is the paramount consideration when experimenting with any substance of this nature. You are exposing your mind and body to the unknown, and potentially, putting your life and welfare on the line. Risks include addiction, overdose, allergy, and even physical harm resulting from loss or impairment of normal mental or physical control.

With this reality comes a responsibility which too many people fail to uphold. This is the responsibility to mitigate, manage, and as much as possible, reduce exposure to these risks. The following step by step list may assist with respect to this.

1.1.1 The 10 Commandments Of Safer Drug Use

Always remember that your life is in your own hands. Should you choose to use a psychoactive substance, this framework may help you to take more measured and informed decisions.

1. Research, research, and research. Use the internet, consult books, ask those with experience, and take your time about it. There is no imperative to rush, but there is imperative to get it right. Know as much as is reasonably possible about the chemical or botanical you intend to use well before you do so.

2. Source carefully. How confident are you that the substance is exactly what you expect it to be? Is it likely to have been cut with something undesirable? Could it be something close to, but not exactly what you ordered? Could something have gone wrong during manufacture or transport? Does your source have any sort of reputation?

   When you have obtained the substance itself, the safety process has barely begun. Don't succumb to temptation to shortcut any of the following steps.

3. Test it. Reagent testing can be used to identify many popular chemicals, and this isn't rocket science to undertake. Test kits can be easily purchased online, and basic guides are abundant. See section 1.1.2 for a demonstration of use.

   An alternative is to use a third party service, such as WEDINOS, the *Welsh Emerging Drugs & Identification of Novel Substances Project*. With an online generated form, substances can be sent anonymously for free laboratory testing, with the results being published for your perusal on the WEDINOS website.

   Similar services are now provided by organisations in a number of nations, using a variety of operational models. Examples include *ecstasydata.org* and *energycontrol-international.org*. Many festivals also provide on-site testing services.

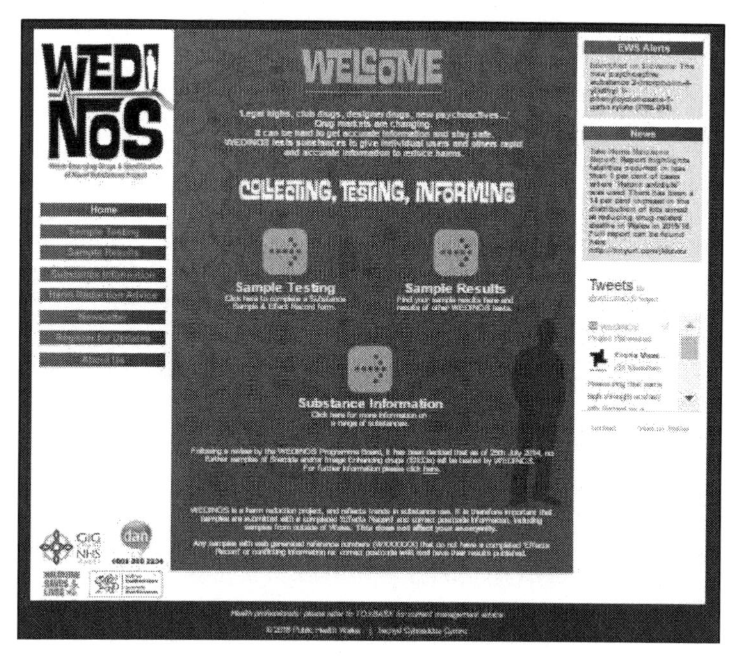

If you are less than 100% certain regarding the content or purity of your substance, testing it is an absolute must-do.

4. Invest in, and use, some milligram (0.001g) scales. It should be obvious that dosing is a central issue, and that many chemicals are extremely dose sensitive, including at low levels. Don't scrimp on or bypass this matter under any circumstances.

> A quick layman's guide on how to use your scales:
> - Take the pan off your scales and turn them on.
> - Place the pan back on the scales. It will show a weight, perhaps something like 2.671g.
> - Press the *tare* button, and then remove the pan.
> - The scale will now read -2.671, or whatever the weight of the pan was.
> - Place the substance in the pan, and place the pan back on the scales.
> - The scales will now show the weight of the substance.

Bear in mind here that most scales are not precise enough to weigh accurately at the individual milligram level, but do tend to be reasonable for perhaps units of 10mg. If the intended dose is in the single milligram range, you will need a set of high quality scales or a set of microgram scales.

For smaller doses, perhaps of less than 1mg, or in the low milligram range, an approach known as *volumetric dosing* is commonly used. This involves dissolving a known quantity of a compound into a liquid, and then measuring the dose by millilitre, via the mg/ml ratio created.

For substances that do not dissolve in water, liquids such as alcohol or propylene glycol are used. It is worth remembering that the lower the concentration of the substance in the liquid, the easier and safer it is to dose.

TripSit offers an excellent guide to volumetric dosing on its website: http://wiki.tripsit.me/wiki/Quick_Guide_to_Volumetric_Dosing

One last word on dosing: caution and concentration are vital. Take all sensible measures when handling chemicals, preferably using gloves and eye protection.

5. Properly and rationally consider the dose. Have regard for your circumstance, and all the information you have accumulated about the drug. If you are in a social setting, do not succumb to peer-pressure.

   Always remember that you can take more if you need to, but you cannot un-take what you have already taken. This is something I cannot emphasize enough.

   If this is the first time you have used this drug, you are introducing a new chemical into your body and you do not know how it will react. A low dose will usually reduce the risks to your personal safety and psychological well being, including the prospect of having an overdose or a bad experience.

   Take your time to explore, tread carefully, and don't make hasty decisions.

6. Perform allergy tests. The risk here may appear to be small, but in some cases the impact of a serious allergy could be fatal.

   Measure the smallest amount of the substance that you can. Then split it into smaller amounts. Place one part of this under or on to your tongue. If you experience any irritation, swelling or soreness, you could be allergic. Pending further tests and assurance, do not consume the substance in any way.

   Note that allergy testing can also help to verify that you haven't acquired something significantly more potent than you intended.

7. Ask yourself if you are feeling okay. It is a serious question. If you are unwell, sick, or in poor health, these conditions may be amplified during the experience, or may have serious implications with respect to body load. If in any doubt, don't proceed.

This also applies to mental health. Some drugs can intensify whatever mood, feeling or psychological space you are experiencing at present. They may take you higher or lower, in terms of your current mental state, and hold you there. This can extend for uncomfortable periods with respect to the latter. This potential manifestation applies equally to both popular and uncommon drugs.

Delay or abandon the experience if there are any doubts or concerns.

8. Plan the experience, and its parameters, so that you don't take rash decisions under the influence. Having taken whatever dose you have chosen, be patient, and don't jump to the conclusion that it didn't work, should onset not materialize. A common mistake is to double-dose, which can have dire consequences. Equally, unless you actually intend to redose at the outset, it is suggested that the rest of the material is placed out of immediate reach. If redosing is intended, perhaps place a maximum cap on this by having only a pre-determined total amount available to you.

   Carefully consider *set and setting*: the place and circumstances under which you are going to undertake the experience. For psychedelics this will often determine the nature of the trip, and it can sometimes induce a bad or damaging ordeal. Consider the use of a trip-sitter if you are not experienced with this particular class of drug.

   Have to hand water, food, or whatever other provisions or entertainment you are going to need.

   For all psychoactives, bear in mind that your judgement and functionality may be severely impaired, which could be a significant factor if you are likely to find yourself in a public place, or indeed, any location in which you may be subjected to risk or danger.

9. Have the contact details of help services to hand in case of urgent need. See Section 4 for some options. Write down what you are dosing and place the note in a prominent place on your person. In the worst scenario, this may assist the emergency services.

   If you are undertaking the experience with a group, seek to nominate an individual to abstain, in case help and objective rationality is needed.

10. Give your body plenty of time to recover and your mind due time to assimilate the experience. In other words, if you are a regular drug user, take a break between psychoactive sessions, and a long break between sessions using substances from the same class.

    The former helps to ensure that the experiences do not become more intrusive in your life than you want them to be, and the latter helps to manage tolerance and reduce the risk of addiction. Under no circumstances allow yourself to habitualise drug use (including alcohol).

Some people maintain a log to support this process. The example below demonstrates a simple spreadsheet approach, with the grey bands indicating drug free days.

◄ January **FEBRUARY** March ►

Sunday	Monday	Tuesday	Wednesday	Thursday	Friday	Saturday
			1 2C-B-Fly 1mg	2	3	4 Alcohol (5)
5	6	7 4F-MPH 12mg Etizolam 1mg	8	9	10 1P-LSD 150ug	11
12	13	14	15 Celastrus Panic	16	17 Alcohol (4)	18
19 Guayusa	20	21	22	23 HBWS	24	25
26	27	28 Yohimbe 3g	Notes:			

Finally, never skip any of the items in this list. Also bear in mind that familiarity breeds complacency, which breeds tragedy.

A NOTE ON COMBINATIONS

Taking two or more different drugs is not something I personally practice, at least in terms of recreational pursuit. I take the view that if I am to sample a compound, it should be rewarding enough in its own right. There are one or two exceptions, for instance regarding trip management, but broadly speaking I choose not to exacerbate risk for dubious return.

However, if you choose to take this path be aware that it is fraught with danger. Whilst many combinations are known to be extremely dangerous, some are less obvious. MAOIs require particular care, but in truth, there are too many variables and specific cases to list within a text.

Fortunately, a comprehensive and regularly maintained chart has been published, again by TripSit. This is particularly useful, and can be viewed on the following web page: http://wiki.tripsit.me/wiki/Drug_combinations

If you do intend to mix your drugs, it is recommended that you refer to this for initial awareness, and use it in conjunction with the information provided in this book, and alongside a significant personal research effort. Tread carefully. Tread very carefully.

A SAMPLE CHECKLIST
The following checklist can be applied against the measures listed on the previous pages. It can be photocopied and used freely. Only proceed if all checks are 100% positive and clear.

SAFETY CHECKS	DONE	NOTES
1. Research It Thoroughly		
2. Source It Carefully		
3. Test It		
4. Determine Dose		
5. Weigh It (Accurately)		
6. Allergy Test It		
7. Health Check		
8. Experience Plan		
9. Contact List (Help)		
10. Recovery Gap		

Think again before embarking: are you sure you wish to proceed and are you ready?

The following diagram represents an example of a completed checklist. Although it was used for LSD, which is a relatively benign chemical, it illustrates that there should be no complacency or short cuts.

Never short change or gamble with your life.

SAFETY CHECKS	DONE	NOTES
1. Research It Thoroughly	✔	No MJ with it. Eat/exercise well before. Think +ve. Set time. Oral RoA.
2. Source It Carefully	✔	Double checked. Same batch as Jane's. Rep established.
3. Test It	✔	Ehrlich/marquis/froehde tests ok. WEDINOS confirmed
4. Determine Dose	✔	75ug is right for me this time. Will not redose.
5. Weigh It (Accurately)	✔	It is actually 73ug.
6. Allergy Test It	✔	Tiny corner of tab tested last Tue. Clear.
7. Health Check	✔	Tip top physical and positive psych. All good.
8. Experience Plan	✔	Sitter (John). Stash emptied. Prepared entertainment. All day free. Secure.
9. Contact List (Help)	✔	Phone list created and placed in back pocket. 75ug of LSD noted on it.
10. Recovery Gap	✔	3 wks since 2-cb. Nothing this week.

1.1.2 How To Use A Drug Testing Kit

To the unfamiliar, the idea of identifying a drug by testing it yourself may sound like a difficult and daunting undertaking. It isn't. With a little knowledge it becomes trivial.

The science is simple enough. If you drop a chemically infused fluid on to a sample of your drug it will change colour. The colour it changes to will help you to identify the drug. No colour change is also information which will help you to identify it.

This chemically infused fluid is known as a *reagent.*

There are a number of different types of this fluid; different reagents. Each one tends to react differently to the drug in question, often creating a different colour.

The different reagents have different names. Amongst the most commonly used reagents are *Marquis, Mecke, Mandelin, Froehde, Liebermann* and *Eldrich.*

Why is it necessary to have different reagents? One reason is that certain reagents are particularly sensitive and useful for specific drugs, or classes of drugs.

Another is that with a single reagent, two different drugs may produce the same or almost the same colour. However, with a second specifically selected reagent they will produce different colours. Multiple reagent tests also increase the prospect of identifying the presence of an unwanted additive.

Generally, testing with more than one reagent will produce more accurate and precise results, which in turn reduces risk.

I mentioned at the start that this is not difficult. The next few pages will demonstrate an actual test using a single reagent kit. A more complex three reagent process will then be illustrated.

Firstly some common sense: reagents are toxic so treat them accordingly. Handle them with care (using gloves and lab equipment if possible) and avoid getting them on to your skin and in your eyes. Don't breathe the vapours and don't ingest. Also, dispose of them responsibly after testing. I am seeking to enhance safety here, not kill you in the process.

Note that the standard identification tests don't measure strength or purity: they simply provide an indication of the presence (or absence) of specific substances. Also, a positive result doesn't guarantee that the substance is safe or unadulterated: further assurance requires the use of testing labs, where methods such as chromatography and spectroscopy are available.

More information on this subject and on the general topic is available via a variety of websites, including: dancesafe.org, bunkpolice.com, reagent-base.net, reagent-tests.uk and safetest4.co.uk.

A SINGLE-REAGENT SPOT CHECK - DEMO

Single-reagent testing kits are readily available, from both retail outlets and via Internet websites. Whilst these kits have limitations (see the information on the previous page) they are certainly quick and easy to use.

Each kit targets a specific set of drugs, with the test returning a different colour for each. The drugs covered by a particular kit are identified on the packet or in the product literature.

The following steps illustrate the testing of two samples, which were sold as MDMA and amphetamine respectively.

1. Choose a kit that is applicable to the drug you wish to test.

For this demonstration I searched the internet using Google, seeking the simplest kit available. I then checked its efficacy via forum reviews.

I identified a popular kit which was branded under the name *eztest*. Its website indicated that this tested for MDMA, amphetamine, 2C-B/C/I, methylone/butylone, and DXM, and that it used the Marquis reagent. [https://en.wikipedia.org/wiki/Marquis_reagent]

I purchased two of these: one for the MDMA and one for the amphetamine.

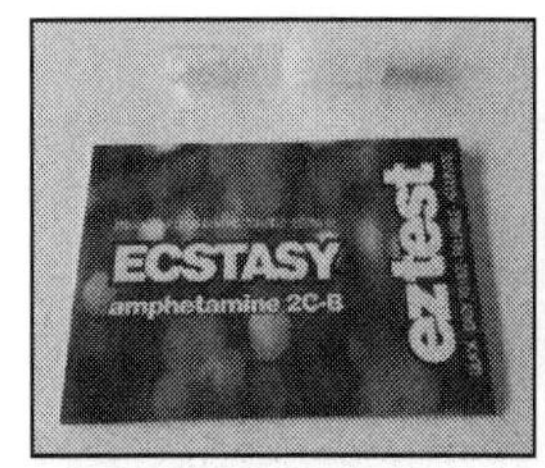

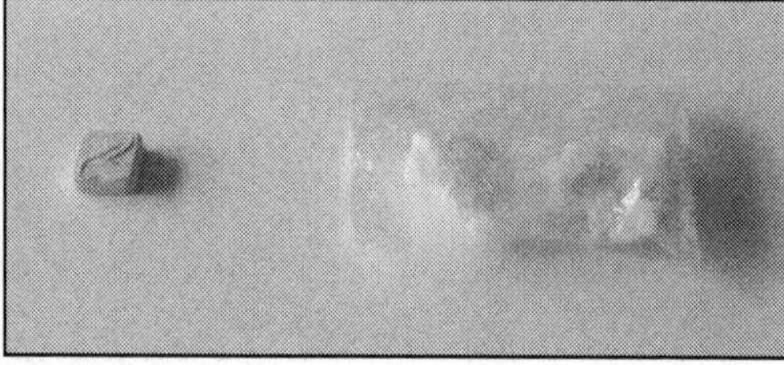

2. To test a specific drug, break the top off the glass ampoule.

A quick twist and turn and the top snapped off easily.

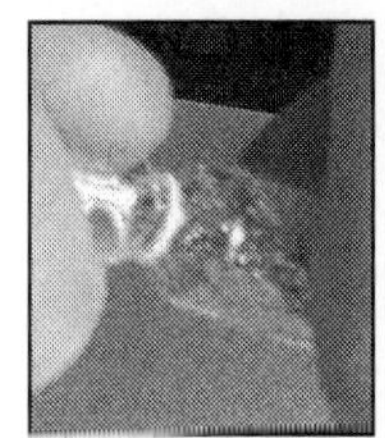

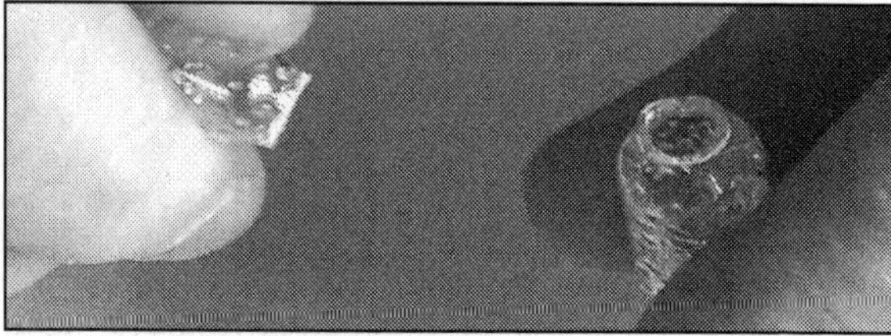

3. Insert a small sample of the drug into the ampoule.

Here, I scraped at the MDMA pill with a knife sufficiently to allow a couple of fragments to fall into its waiting glass ampoule.

For the amphetamine I used a pair of tweezers to drop a tiny dab of the powder into its ampoule.

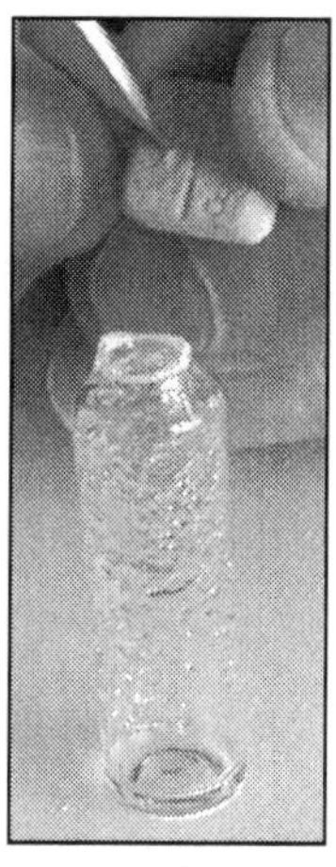

Ampoule 1
MDMA

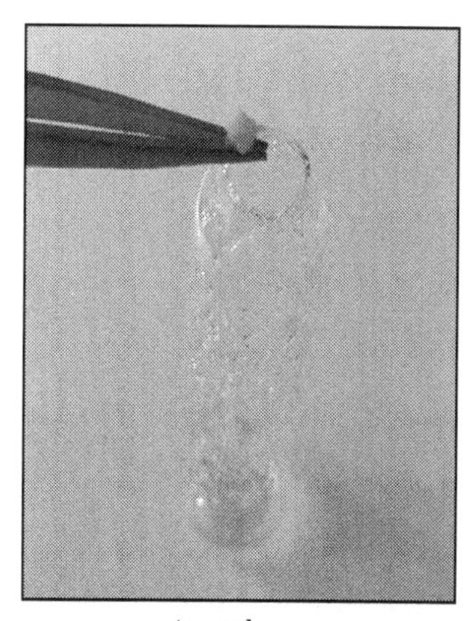

Ampoule 2
Amphetamine

3. Shake the ampoule gently.

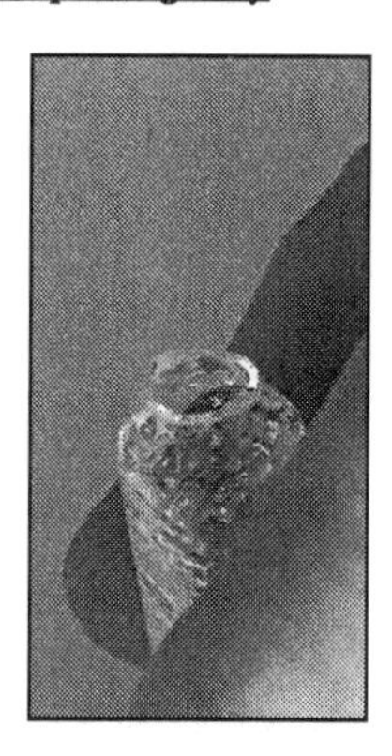

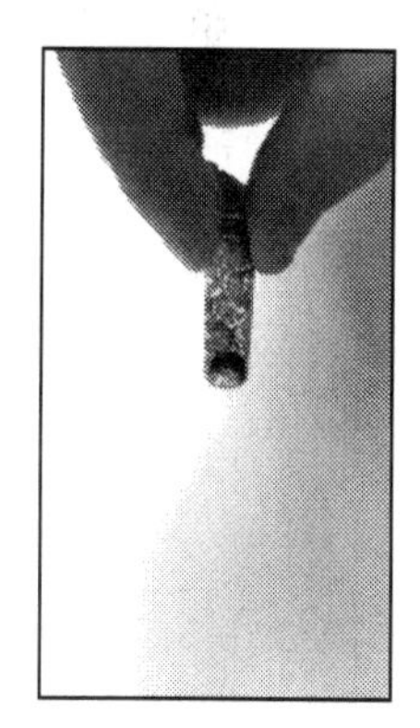

I lightly shook each of the two ampoules, whilst observing the colour change.

4. <u>A colour will emerge as the drug reacts in the ampoule. Compare this colour with the colour chart provided with the test kit instructions</u>.

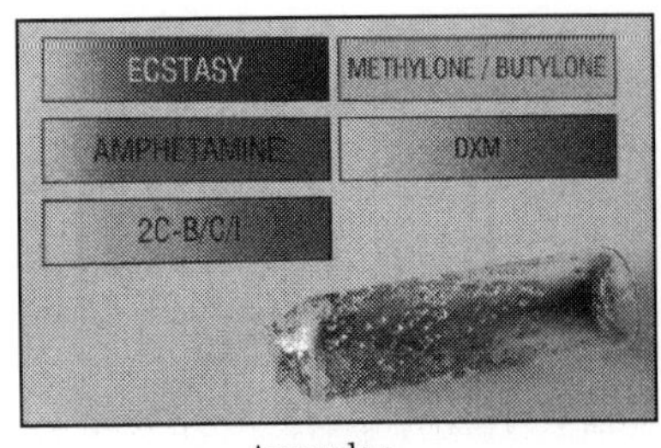

Ampoule 1
MDMA

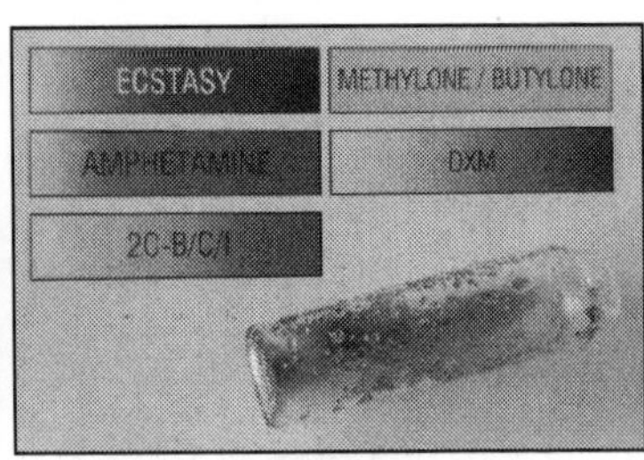

Ampoule 2
Amphetamine

As can be seen (far more clearly in the colour version of this book), there was a match between the colour in the ampoules and the colours specified for MDMA and amphetamine.

Wikipedia offered the following with respect to Marquis tests generally:

Substance	Colour	Notes
MDMA or MDA	Purple to black	May have dark purple tint
Amphetamine	Orange to brown	May have a brown tint
2CB	Yellow to green	Colour may change from initial result
DXM	Grey to Black	Initially no change; takes much longer to reach black than MDMA

On completion of the test I safely disposed of the ampoules and their contents.

Having tested a sample, if there is no match, or no colour at all, or if you are unsure, do not use the drug.

Always heed this advice: *if in doubt, chuck it out.*

Finally it should be noted that product disclaimers tend to present the kits as "*for entertainment only*", and state that they do not provide a 100% guarantee. In other words, their use is at your own risk. With this in mind, exercise appropriate care and caution.

If the sample tested positively, this information can be used in conjunction with both your own research and the safety measures documented in Section 1.1.1.

A MULTI-REAGENT TEST – DEMO

For this slightly more complex demonstration, I purchased three reagents from *Reagent Tests UK:* Marquis, Froehde and Mecke. These arrived as a kit, which also included an instruction card and a colour comparison chart.

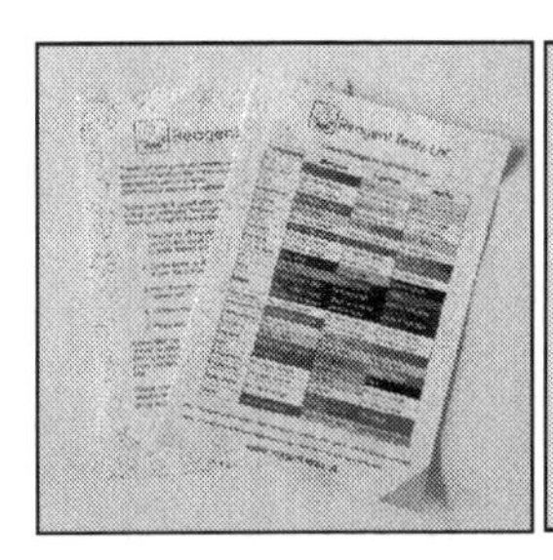

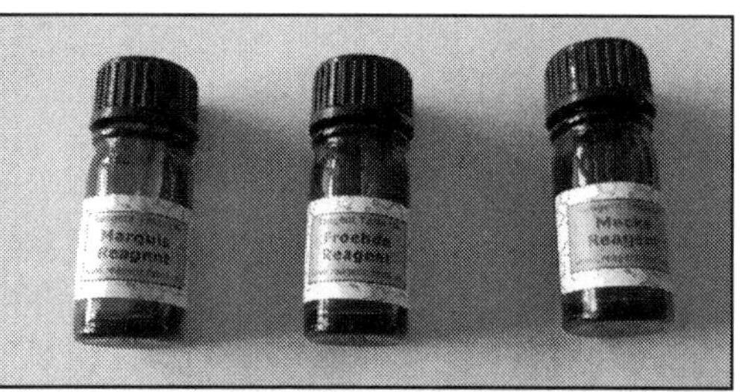

The following steps illustrate the testing of the same MDMA pill which was used for the single-reagent spot check.

1. Prepare your work space and surface

I chose a nice quiet area with plenty of natural light (my desk).

For the surface I grabbed a glazed ceramic white plate. Although some people use the bottom of a mug, I found that a plate offered a wider area, enabling steadier access to the surface itself.

2. Place the drug sample on the surface

Here I scraped a fragment of the pill on to the surface of the plate. Had I been testing a powder I would have placed a dab of the powder using tweezers, a micro spoon, or a similar implement.

The instructions supplied with the kit suggested that a sample of about 5mg is usually about right.

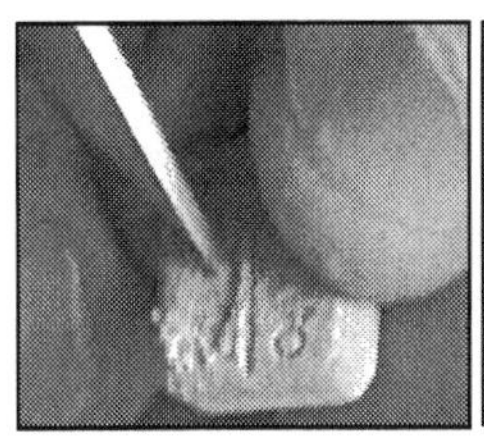

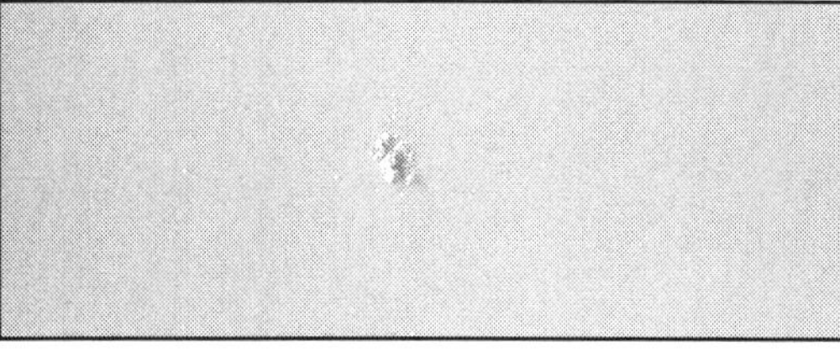

3. <u>Tip the bottle so that a drop of fluid falls on to the sample</u>

Choosing the Marquis reagent for the first test, I took the lid off the bottle. I gently tilted this over the sample and then rotated slowly. Patiently, I tilted and turned until a drop of the fluid finally emerged and fell.

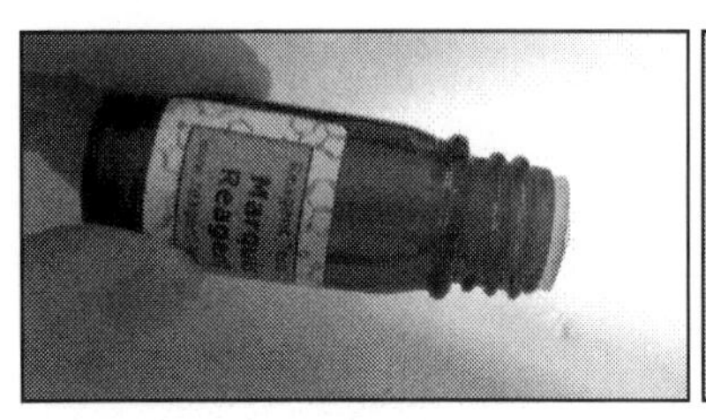

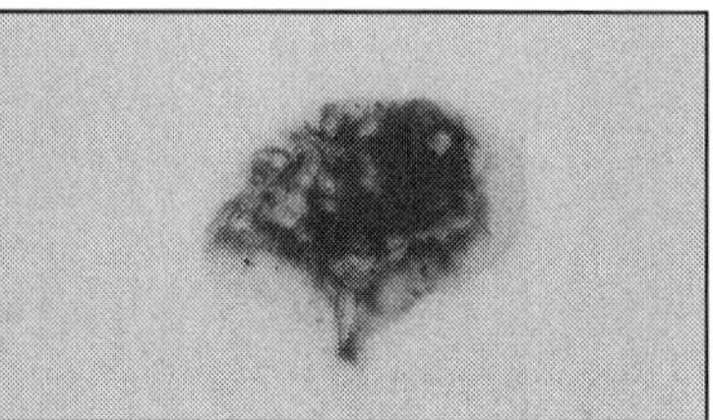

4. <u>A colour will emerge as the drug reacts with the reagent</u>

I watched the sample carefully, over about 30 seconds, as it gradually changed colour.

5. <u>Compare this colour with the colour chart provided with the instructions</u>

As can be seen (more clearly in the colour version of this book), the colour matched that specified for MDMA (purple-black) under Marquis.

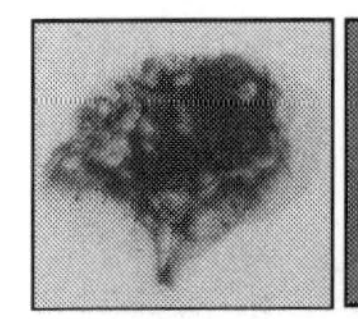

Compound	Marquis	Froehde	Mecke
MDMA	Blue > Violet > Black (Maybe hint of green)	Black with hints of greenish brown	Green > Dark Blue
[illegible]	No colour change	No colour change	No colour change

6. <u>Repeat the same steps (2-5) using the other reagents</u>

I rinsed and washed the plate, and then repeated steps 2, 3, 4 and 5 using the Froehde reagent. This time the sample turned black, which again matched MDMA on the chart.

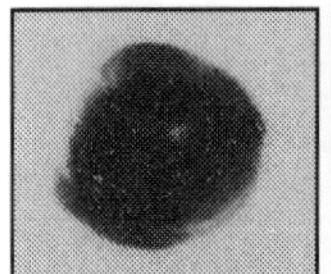

Compound	Marquis	Froehde	Mecke
MDMA	Blue > Violet > Black (Maybe hint of green)	Black with hints of greenish brown	Green > Dark Blue
[illegible]	No colour change	No colour change	No colour change

I then rinsed and washed the plate again, and repeated steps 2, 3, 4 and 5 using the Mecke reagent. The sample turned dark green-blue, which also matched MDMA on the chart.

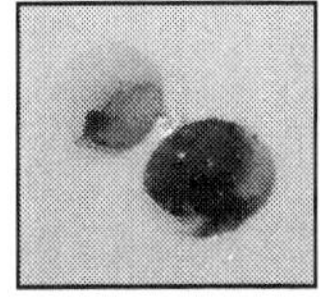

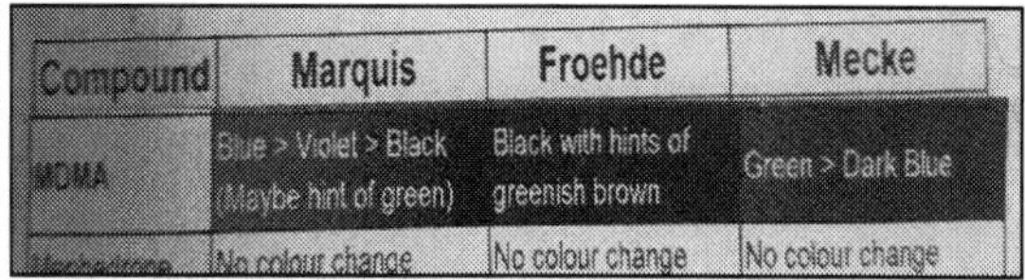

Compound	Marquis	Froehde	Mecke
MDMA	Blue > Violet > Black (Maybe hint of green)	Black with hints of greenish brown	Green > Dark Blue
[illegible]	No colour change	No colour change	No colour change

Being pedantic, I took photographs using my phone for a more considered comparison (and not just for the purposes of this book).

Carefully examining the chart and comparing the colours for all three tests, I had a clear match with MDMA.

I washed the plate properly for the final time, and stored the reagent bottles securely.

Having performed the reagent tests, I would again stress that if you are unsure do not use the drug. Remember the advice: *if in doubt chuck it out.*

Also bear in mind the disclaimers and warnings listed on the previous pages, and any printed within the test kit instructions.

If the sample tested positively, this information can be used in conjunction with both your own research and the other safety measures documented in Section 1.1.1.

COMPARISON CHARTS

Your test kit should include a comparison chart. If you purchased the reagents independently of a kit, a number of charts can be found online or directly via the websites referenced earlier.

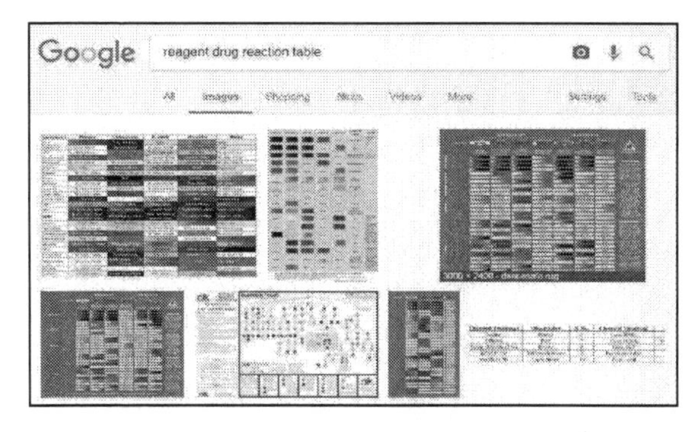

1.2 INTERPRETING THE REPORTS

1.2.1 Definition of Terms

The words and terms used to introduce each chemical or botanical are defined as follows:

COMMON NOMENCLATURE
This is the commonly used name for the particular substance, as opposed to the more formal less user-friendly systematic name.

ANTICIPATED DURATION
This is the expected duration of the trip or psychoactive experience. It is the time expended from reaching threshold to the point at which normality or baseline is broadly reached. This does not include after effects, such as tiredness, hangover, or simply the residue of a state or frame of mind, which can persist for a considerable time in some cases.

ANTICIPATED ONSET
This is the expected time it will take to reach the point at which the psychoactive experience has reached its threshold level. In other words, the length of time before the subject is aware that the effects of the chemical or botanical are active.

Safety warning: when using a compound, if there is no effect within the expected time scale, do not redose. Onset can vary considerably from person to person, and it can be influenced by a variety of factors (related to both the individual and the substance).

REFERENCE DOSES
These are figures published by the major psychoactive related communities, on the Internet. They are not scientific, in that they are generally produced from feedback, anecdotal material, and estimation. They should not form the basis to determine an individual's dose, but are commonly used as one of a variety of inputs for consideration. They do not indicate that a particular dose is safe for you.

The specific community sources used were: erowid.com, tripbot.tripsit.me, psychonautwiki.org, and drugs-forum.com. A point to bear in mind here is the possibility that a drug related community may have higher tolerance than ordinary members of the public.

Remember that inexperienced users should always start with a very low dose. Note also that where it is not specified or clear, the relevant RoA should be assumed to be oral.

STREET & REFERENCE NAMES
These are alternative names by which the chemical or botanical are known. They can range from slang or street names, to alternative forms of nomenclature framed by organisations or professional bodies.

MAXIMUM DOSE EXPERIENCED
This is the highest dose which I personally experienced. In some cases, this is represented in the form of an arithmetic addition (a+b+c). This represents an initial dose, and subsequent redosing, thus accumulating a total exposure to the psychoactive. Note that in some cases I dosed foolishly and recklessly.

As my personal attributes are relevant with respect to this, I declare these as: male; 5ft 10" (177cm); 12st (76kg).

PERSONAL RATING ON THE SHULGIN SCALE
This is the personal assessment of the author's own experience whilst testing a particular chemical or botanical, measured against the *Shulgin Scale*. Note that such measurement is not suitable for all experiences, but was adapted for use where possible.

FORM
This is the form in which the substance was used. Common forms include powder, fluid, plant matter, blotter and pill.

SOURCE / JURISDICTION
The source indicates from where the chemical was procured. The jurisdiction specifies where it was sampled.

ROUTE OF ADMINISTRATION (RoA)
This is the path by which the active molecules of the chemical or botanical are taken into the body. A variety of possibilities are available, which are discussed later in this section.

INDIGENOUS SOURCE
This specifies the region or country the botanical is native to or originates from.

BINOMIAL / BOTANICAL NAME
This is the formal name of the species, or the general name of the plant or fungi, which pertains to the botanical being researched.

MAJOR ACTIVE COMPOUND
This is the primary psychoactive chemical which is present and active within a botanical. Note that some botanicals can have a multitude of active chemicals, not all of which are listed.

For a general dictionary of drug-related terms and phrases see Section 4.8.

1.2.2 The Shulgin Rating Scale

The *Shulgin Rating Scale* is a simple reference scale for reporting the subjective effects of a psychedelic substance at a given dosage and time. It was developed by the legendry biochemist, Alexander Shulgin, and published in the remarkable book, *PiHKAL: A Chemical Love Story*.

The scale:

> MINUS, n. (-) On the quantitative potency scale (-, ±, +, ++, +++), there were no effects observed.
>
> PLUS/MINUS, n. (±) The level of effectiveness of a drug that indicates a threshold action. If a higher dosage produces a greater response, then the plus/minus (±) was valid. If a higher dosage produces nothing, then this was a false positive.
>
> PLUS ONE, n. (+) The drug is quite certainly active. The chronology can be determined with some accuracy, but the nature of the drug's effects are not yet apparent.
>
> PLUS TWO, n. (++) Both the chronology and the nature of the action of a drug are unmistakably apparent. But you still have some choice as to whether you will accept the adventure; or rather just continue with your ordinary day's plans (if you are an experienced researcher, that is). The effects can be allowed a predominant role, or they may be repressible and made secondary to other chosen activities.
>
> PLUS THREE, n. (+++) Not only are the chronology and the nature of a drug's action quite clear, but ignoring its action is no longer an option. The subject is totally engaged in the experience, for better or worse.
>
> PLUS FOUR, n. (++++) A rare and precious transcendental state, which has been called a "*peak experience*," a "*religious experience*," "*divine transformation*," a "*state of Samadhi*" and many other names in other cultures. It is not connected to the +1, +2, and +3 of the measuring of a drug's intensity. It is a state of bliss, a participation mystique, a connectedness with both the interior and exterior universes, which has come about after the ingestion of a psychedelic drug, but which is not necessarily repeatable with a subsequent ingestion of that same drug. If a drug (or technique or process) were ever to be discovered which would consistently produce a plus four experience in all human beings, it is conceivable that it would signal the ultimate evolution, and perhaps the end, of the human experiment.

This scale is referred to throughout the book. Its use has been extended well beyond psychedelics, and indeed, it has been employed as a measure across most categories and classifications. Note that in a number of cases I have also added an asterisk to the + indicator to denote a slightly strengthened response.

1.2.3 Classification

The chemicals and botanicals have been categorized in terms of their primary effect. This broadly reflects the approach taken by *Erowid*, and other online authorities.

The specific groupings are as follows:

PSYCHEDELICS
This is a substance which alters perception and cognition, creating an experience which is different to ordinary consciousness, often significantly so.

The *psychedelic state* is often related to forms such as meditation, dreaming, yoga, near-death or out-of-body experiences, and access to other realms or dimensions of reality.

STIMULANTS
Stimulants, or *stims*, enhance or improve mental and/or physical capability or function. Manifestations of this can include alertness, wakefulness, focus, and apparent increased energy. As a consequence, stimulants are sometimes referred to as *uppers*.

DISSOCIATIVES
A dissociative produces a sense of detachment from normal sights, sounds and experiences of self. This dissociation from environment is often classified as a hallucinogenic experience.

INTOXICATING DEPRESSANTS
Depressants induce depression of the central nervous system (CNS), which reduces arousal or stimulation. This slows down the activity of the brain and nervous system, with the physical and psychoactive effects often dependent upon dose. Intoxicants excite or stupefy to the point where physical and mental control is diminished.

Intoxicating depressants tend to combine these experiences, with their effects transforming and morphing towards the former, as the duration unfolds.

CANNABINOIDS
Cannabinoids are synthetic substances which act upon cannabinoid receptors, creating effects which can be perceived as similar to the cannabis genus in one or more respects.

ONEIROGENS
An oneirogen is widely considered to induce, enhance or promote lucid or vivid dreaming. It is sometimes defined as a substance that produces dream-like states of consciousness. These can be profound, and can manifest as realistic or abstract.

EMPATHOGENS
Empathogens and entactogens tend to produce feelings of emotional communion and bonding with others, particularly in terms of empathy and oneness.

This state is most widely reported with respect to MDMA, but is actually created via a substantial number of substances.

EUPHORIANTS
These create a sense of euphoria, elation or bliss, sometimes in association with the empathy produced via an empathogen.

ANXIOLYTICS & SEDATIVES
A sedative can produce a calming or relaxing effect, such that stress, irritability or agitation is reduced. In some cases sedatives can produce hypnotic anticonvulsant and muscle relaxant effects.

Technically, sedatives are depressants, in that they induce depression of the central nervous system (CNS), although many also have antipsychotic properties.

NOOTROPICS
Also referred to as smart drugs, nootropics are substances (chemical or botanical) that improve or enhance cognitive function, including memory and creativity.

DELIRIANTS
This is a class of hallucinogen that induces an *'acute confusional state'*, as opposed to the more lucid state typified by classical psychedelics.

Deliriants generally produce unpleasant experiences, are often toxic, and are prone to expose the user to personal risk, which can be severe.

UNCLASSIFIED
A number of substances produce effects which do not fit comfortably into any of the above. Some, for example, induce a combination of these, providing a very distinct experience. Others create differing effects as the experience unfolds.

Note that there are a variety of other approaches and definitions, and that most, like this one, introduce a degree of subjectivity.

The adjacent diagram presents one view of the relationships between different classifications and some of the most well known chemicals.

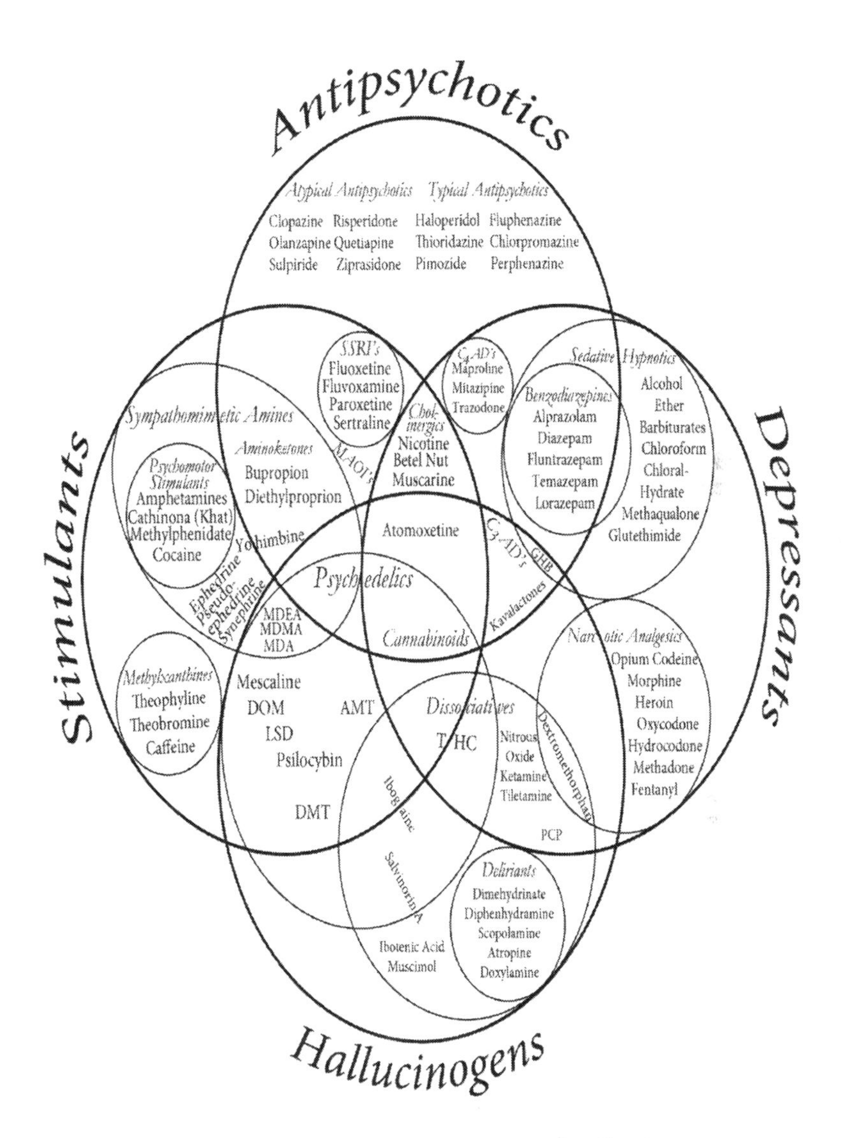

One Representation Of Common Drug Classification
[Public Domain Image: commons.wikimedia.org/wiki/File:Drug_Venn_Diagram.jpg]

1.2.4 Routes of Administration (RoA)

These are the methods by which chemicals or botanicals are introduced to the body, and are thus able to take effect.

ORAL
This is swallowing or drinking. Common methods of the former include bombing, which is wrapping the drug in cigarette paper and consuming by mouth (perhaps with water), or simply eating plant material or swallowing a pill.

QUIDDING
This is chewing the substance (usually a botanical) over a prolonged period and then expelling.

BUCCAL & SUBBUCCAL
This is holding the substance between lip and gum, or in the buccal area (in the cheek), such that it diffuses into the bloodstream through the tissues which line the mouth.

SUBLINGUAL
This is holding the substance under the tongue, again until it diffuses into the bloodstream.

INSUFFLATION
Also known as snorting or railing, insufflating is sniffing the substance hard up the nasal cavity, commonly using a straw or paper tube.

SMOKING
This is inhaling and exhaling the smoke of the combusted substance. Often, the inhaled smoke is held in the lungs for a chosen period of time.

VAPING
This is inhaling and exhaling the vapour produced by heating the substance in a suitable device (usually but not always electronic) or via another pre-determined method.

HOT-KNIFING
This is inhaling the smoke produced when the substance is compressed between the heated ends of two knives, which are pushed through a hole made at the foot of a bottle (usually plastic). There are variations on this, but all involve hot knives and the inhaling of smoke through the mouth of a suitable vessel or container.

TRANSDERMAL
This is absorbing the chemical through the skin, for example, via an adhesive patch.

RECTAL
This is anally inserting the substance such that it is absorbed by the rectum's blood vessels.

INJECTION / INTRAVENOUS (IV)
This is injecting the substance into a blood vein using a needle. It is not recommended, at all.

All the above methods were employed at least once with respect to the sampling of the chemicals and botanicals in the following sections, with the exception of transdermal, rectal and intravenous.

AN IMPORTANT SAFETY NOTE
For most psychoactives, the applicable dose is almost invariably dependent upon the RoA being used. A safe dose via one method can sometimes be deadly via another method. It is imperative, therefore, that when choosing a particular RoA, the safe and appropriate dose for that specific RoA is researched extremely carefully.

This point cannot be over-emphasized, as it is a misstep that the unwary can easily fall foul of, with tragic consequences.

AN UNLIKELY SAFETY NOTE
I don't believe that I have to write this one, but apparently it is necessary. The word *eyeballing* refers to the ill advised practice of measuring a dose based upon its visual appearance. An example would be splitting a gram of powder into ten 100mg doses by separating it into ten equal looking piles.

This is obviously a bad idea, but worse still is sticking the powder into your eye!

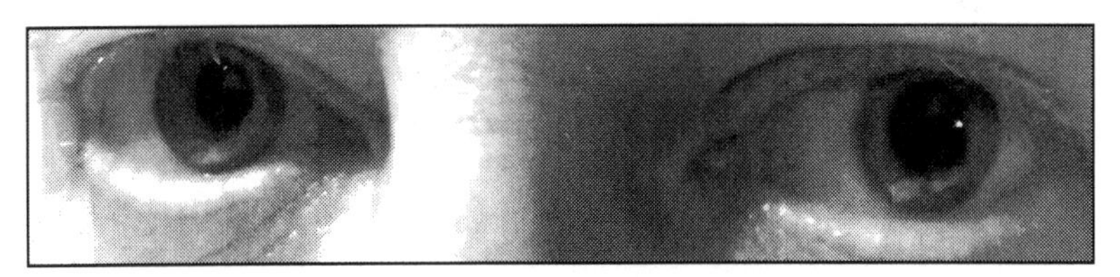

[Eyes are best used for vision]

Incredibly, I once read a forum post in which the author thought that eyeballing was an RoA. In other words, having seen the word frequently in the context of drug use (e.g. "*I eyeballed 10mg*"), he almost blinded himself because he thought it was a method of taking his drug.

Don't do this.

1.2.5 More On Source & Jurisdiction

Most of the chemicals and botanicals sampled for the purposes of this book were directly (and legally) purchased online from UK based websites, using a regular bank card. Regarding safety, this tenuous audit trail to source did at least provide the beginnings of a primitive level of assurance. The specific acquisitions were:

> RESEARCH CHEMICALS
> 1P-ETH-LAD; 1P-LSD; 2C-B-AN; 2C-B-FLY; 5-MeO-DALT; 5-MeO-DIBF; AL-LAD; BK-2C-B; LSZ; 2AI; 3,4 CTMP; 3-FPM; 4-Me-TMP; 4F-EPH; 4F-MPH; IPPH; MPA; NM2AI; PPH; TPA; Ephenidine, Diclazepam; Etizolam; Flubromazolam; Nifoxipam; Pyrazolam; 3-MeO-PCMo; Diphenidine; MXP; MDAI; MEAI; MNA; Mexedrone; Aniracetam; Citicoline; Armodafinil; Modafiendz; Noopept; NSI 189; Phenibut; Picamilon; PRL-8-53; L-Theanine.
>
> BOTANICALS
> Cebil; Chaliponga Leaves; Fly Agaric; HBWS; Iboga; Ololiuqui; Salvia; San Pedro Cactus; Syrian Rue Seeds; Yopo; Ephedra; Ginkgo; Guarana; Guayusa; Kola Nut; Wormwood; Yohimbe; Blue Lotus; Catnip; Damiana; Imphepho; Indian Warrior; Kanna; Lavender; Maconha Brava; Marihuanilla; Morning Glory Seeds; Mulungu; Passion Flower; Skullcap; Valerian Root; White Sage; Wild Dagga; Catuaba; Celastrus Paniculatus; Calea; Mexican Tarragon; Mugwort; Rapé; Ubulawu; Kava Kava; Kratom; Mapacho; Sakae Naa; Sinicuichi; Datura; Entada Rheedii.

The following compounds were legally purchased from UK based head shops (retail outlets), usually located in the North West of England:

> AMT; BK-2C-B; EPH; MXP; MXE; 6-APB; MDAI; 5F-AKB48; AM-2201; AM-694; JWH-018; JWH-073.

All the other substances were tested outside the UK, and where practical, in an authentic setting.

THE INTERNET VENDORS
Whilst the overall number of vendors operating via the Internet during this period was substantial, the vast majority of the above materials were obtained from a relatively small minority:

> RESEARCH CHEMICALS:
> BRC Fine Chemicals, Buckled Bonzi, Chemical Wire, CT High Street, Lizard Labs, Pure Chemicals, Royal Alchemist, Rave Gardener.
>
> BOTANICALS:
> Spirit Garden, Organic Dyes, Element Earth (Mind Foods), PotSeed, Elegant Essence, CoffeeshOp.

These were generally well regarded and provided a timely and professional service.

1.3 GENERAL SAFETY NOTES

1.3.1 If You Are Not An Adult

If you are not an adult, your brain is still growing, and the critical parts involved in decision-making are not fully developed. As a result, the use of recreational drugs can cause disproportionate harm and damage.

Physiologically, they can alter your hard wiring. They can precipitate serious psychological disorders, and can have long term consequences for your mental health. They can change your thinking, your perception and your judgement.

I know how this may sound, and that I may come across as a tedious old straight preaching the same propagandistic lecture you have heard before, but this isn't the case at all (apart from the old bit).

None of this is waffle or exaggeration. A quick flick through the pages of this book will demonstrate where I am coming from. I am providing the truth in simple terms: nothing more.

The stats don't lie and neither does the science, even if the politicians and the media do. If you have any reason to doubt this advice, research directly for yourself. Obtain the facts.

You have a long time ahead of you in which to experience drugs, if this is what you wish to do. There is no rush and no imperative to do it now.

Don't do it now. Now is not the time. This advice equally applies to alcohol.

If other factors are influencing you, for example peer-pressure, try to see the wider context. Try to see these moments in the timeline of your entire life. Take a decision based upon that timescale; because that is the timescale you may be affecting.

If you are confused, or if you have already taken drugs and you fear that you are slipping into addiction or another drug related predicament, seek help urgently. Do not let it continue. I cannot stress this enough.

You simply don't have to take drugs at this pivotal point in your life. It most definitely isn't cool, and I guarantee that in 10 years you will see this, even if you cannot see it now. I also guarantee that if you read these words in 10 years you will absolutely agree with them. Your future self will know what you may not know now.

If this book achieves nothing other than to persuade you to wait, it was worth all the effort to write it.

Don't do it.

1.3.2 Risk Mitigation For IV

As stated earlier, injecting (IV) is a terrible idea from a safety perspective. However, if you are using this RoA regardless, specialist websites commonly offer the following tips to mitigate some of the risks. [Note: Consult these sites directly for greater detail.]

- Only inject in a clean safe environment and make sure that equipment and other items are clean and are readily to hand.
- Prepare in advance for an overdose (e.g. have people around to check on you). If you are using an opioid have some naloxone available, if possible. Also have contact details for the emergency services to hand.
- Always prepare for yourself and always inject yourself.

- Never share needles or equipment, including with your partner.
- Always use a new capped needle.
- Make sure that the injection site on your skin is clean.
- If sharing a drug, split it before use. Failing this, at least ensure that a fresh container is used for each hit (and no re-use or re-dipping of needles).
- Use filters to help remove impurities.
- Remove air bubbles (e.g. point upwards, push gently and flick).
- Use an unshared tourniquet.

- Don't inject into an artery; only a vein.
- If you don't find a vein straight away use a new needle. Take your time.
- Don't inject into your hands (the veins are too small).
- Never inject into an area that's swollen or sore.
- Try to rotate injection sites.

- Insert the needle at a 45 degree angle, injecting towards the heart (in the direction of the blood flow).
- Make sure that the needle's hole is facing upwards.
- Make sure that you are in a vein (you should see blood if you push slightly and then draw-back a little). [Note: only draw-back minimally]
- If the blood is brighter/pink-red, rather than dark/black-red you are injecting into an artery. Abort immediately and stem the bleeding.
- Release the tourniquet and inject slowly, keeping arm straight.
- Remove the needle slowly.
- Apply a light press to the injection site to stem blood flow.
- Secure and recap your syringe ready for return or safe disposal.
- Clean-up everything (e.g. with bleach) and finally clean yourself.
- If you have problems with bleeding or swelling seek medical help urgently.

Remember that this isn't the solution, but these steps may help to reduce risk. The solution is to stop using this RoA. Please do try. Use whatever support services are available and never be afraid to ask for help. I can't stress this enough.

Finally, if you think you may have overdosed, or if you encounter any other sort of medical issue, don't delay: call the emergency services.

1.3.3 Nasal Care

If you insufflate your drugs it is important that you take sensible precautions and that you perform appropriate aftercare. This particularly applies if you use this method regularly. Maintaining a clean environment and sterile equipment is an obvious requirement, but it is surprising how standards can slip whilst under the influence.

Regarding the drug itself, assuming of course that all the steps outlined earlier have been undertaken, it is a good idea to check the constitution of the material. For example, is the powder fine enough? Stating the obvious it is wise to avoid snorting crushed pills, not only on this basis but because they often contain fillers, binding agents and other ingredients, which are not well suited to this RoA.

For nasal irrigation there is a variety of commercial products and tools available. Alternatively, making your own saline solution is a relatively trivial exercise. In either case regular use of this approach is certainly worth considering.

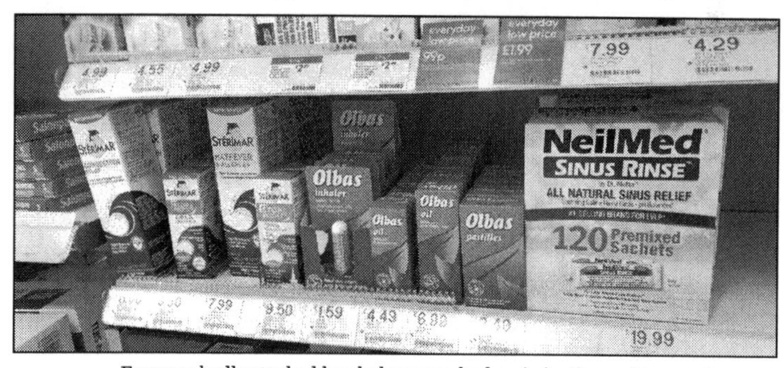

Even my badly stocked local pharmacy had an irrigation option

The operation itself is simple enough, with a common procedure explained on the UKCR forum:

> *"The actual practice of nasal lavage is far simpler and less offensive than it might sound. Placing your head over the sink, tilted to one side, insert the nozzle of the bottle into the uppermost nostril, breathe through your mouth and allow the water to pour into your nostril, whereupon it will flow through your nose and out of the other nostril. Sustain this for 20-30 seconds or as long as is comfortable. Tilt your head to the opposite side, and repeat with the other nostril. Once you've used about half the solution, blow your nose and repeat. This should help to flush out any residual grot and minimise damage to the nasal mucosa."* ~ Magick

Frequency is often a matter of personal preference, but this should not become excessive.

If you habitually insufflate use common sense. Don't disregard the needs of your nose.

1.3.4 Chemsex

Chemsex is generally defined as the consumption of drugs to facilitate or enhance sexual activity, and is a lot more prevalent than most people assume. Whilst this aspect is referred to for individual drugs in the following sections of this book, there are a number of general considerations which are worthy of note at the outset.

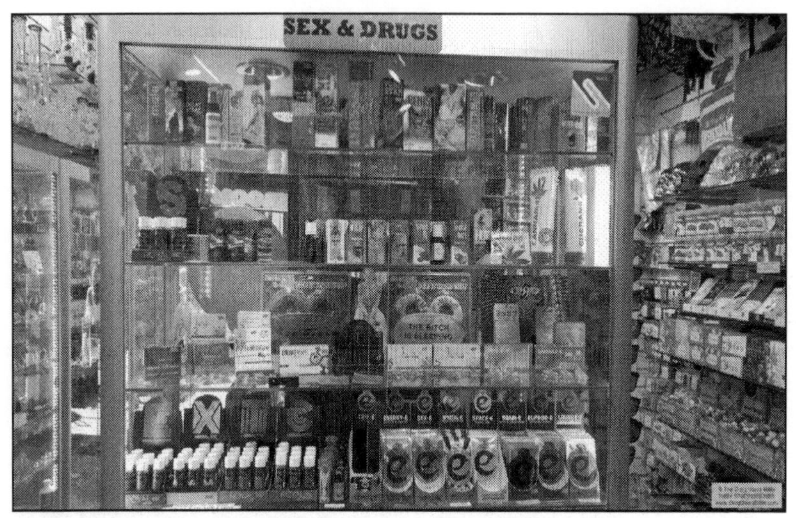

A selection of erotic drugs, Amsterdam

THE CHEMSEX DRUGS
The actual effects and the experience differ significantly from drug class to drug class. I would summarize these as follows:

> Certain stimulants (particularly amphetamines) produce the most primal, prolonged and intensive orgasmic pleasure.
>
> Cannabinoids (cannabis) help you to get lost in the moment and flow with it.
>
> At low doses many psychedelics can take you to a different place, and enhance physical sensitivity.
>
> Empathogens, such as MDMA, tend to take a similar path, with a more muted headspace, but hardly surprisingly enhanced empathy.

I am aware that some people cite alcohol and GHB in this field, but I view these primarily as relaxants, and not as active sexual enhancers. I would not pitch them in the same ballpark as any of the above in this respect.

THE DARK SIDE
If this sounds like an invitation to dive in and to engage, it isn't. As with most joys in life there is a flip side: in this case exposure to significant danger. Drug use carries risk, and drug use for sexual gratification is no different.

Stating the obvious immediately, the usual harm reduction procedures and practices continue to apply. This includes the *10 Commandments of Safer Drug Use* as specified earlier.

I would add to these a number of other considerations which relate specifically to chemsex:

- In some cases, most significantly with stimulants/amphetamines, a high watermark can be reached which is not attainable without the drug. This is a poisoned chalice. It can cause a number of subsequent problems, making normal sexual activity relatively unfulfilling, with obvious and very real implications for relationships.

  Don't trivialise or dismiss this aspect: it is not as uncommon as you might imagine.

- Often related to this is an ongoing craving for the sexual payload of the drug in question. Added to its existing hooks, this potent additional inducement can accelerate the path to addiction.

  Be constantly aware of this and take full account of it.

- It is important to bear in mind that under the influence restraint and judgement are often impaired, and that events can develop quickly and potentially without due deliberation. It is probably not the best idea for a single party to heavily engage whilst the other(s) doesn't.

  Equally, parameters and boundaries should be agreed by all parties beforehand.

- Finally, the compound stress of both sex and drugs on the body should be carefully contemplated, particularly by those with any pre-existing medical conditions.

THE LAST WORD
It is a statement of fact that some drugs can increase sexual appetite and enhance the experience itself. However, my last word on this would be that, if indulging, the real world still exists and so do its risks. Don't suspend logic and always practise harm reduction.

Or alternatively, steer well clear.

1.3.5 What Goes Up Must Come Down

What goes up must come down? In the case of most drugs this is broadly true. Perhaps a better description of this phenomenon is that when you take these drugs, you are borrowing from the future, repayable sometimes with interest; meaning that the comedown and aftermath reverse-compensate for the up and the high.

I would stress that this does not apply to all drugs. Many psychedelics and dissociatives, for example, are immune to this tendency to some extent or another. However, it does apply to most of the common street drugs, such as cocaine, speed, heroin, alcohol and MDMA.

I have given this aspect a great deal of thought over the years, to the point of attempting to create graphs for certain compounds. I gave up on this idea due to the various levels of subjectivity and the difficulty with precision. However, a generic graph might look something like this:

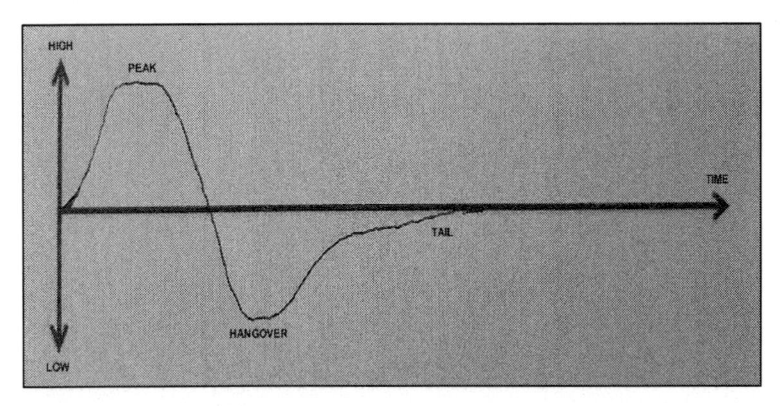

Some drugs may have a gentler dip with a much longer tail (a very slow recovery), whereas others flush relatively quickly but can have a very deep initial hangover. Some can have an extraordinarily high peak, whereas others have a gentle elevation and lengthy period of contentment. There exists, of course, everything in between.

The main point I would make here is that a drug experience covers the whole period, not just the incline and the peak. A typical alcohol binge, for example, will usually deliver a few hours of semi-euphoria, followed by a sedated fuzziness, a hangover in the morning, a day of being under the weather, and perhaps another day (or more) of feeling under par.

When a drug of this type is selected for use, it is important to consider the entire picture, and not be carried away via anticipation of the early part of the ride. You are signing-on for its entirety, come what may: be sure that this is what you actually want.

2

A CHEMICAL JOURNEY

2. A CHEMICAL JOURNEY

2.1 INTRODUCTION

A psychoactive drug is typically defined as a chemical that changes brain function and results in alterations in perception, mood, or consciousness. Whilst the use of such compounds can be traced to prehistory, the modern era has been framed and dominated by the doctrines and brutalities of the *war on drugs*.

In the early years of this century, however, a situation developed in the UK which temporarily created a respite from this unremitting prohibition. This period can reasonably be referred to as the *Legal High Years*.

THE LEGAL HIGH YEARS
Until May 2016, a large and thriving market existed for what were collectively referred to as "*legal highs*", or "*research chemicals*". This was served directly online, and by retail outlets across major towns and cities in the UK.

It had emerged via the pressure of demand, the use of idiomatic terminology, and a stagnant unresponsive legislature.

Wikipedia describes research chemicals in the following terms:

> *"Many pharmacologically active chemicals are sold online under the guise of "research chemicals," when in reality they are untested designer drugs that are being consumed by buyers taking advantage of many of the compounds' transitional or nonexistent legal status."*

And designer drugs as follows:

> *"A designer drug is a structural or functional analogue of a controlled substance that has been designed to mimic the pharmacological effects of the original drug, while avoiding classification as illegal and/or detection in standard drug tests"*

Whilst this is accurate, it is incomplete: the market also offered a number of products which were novel, rather than straight copies (analogues) of traditional and existing drugs.

It is worth noting that the traditional underground drug trade continued as usual, and that historically many of these illegal substances were technically once research chemicals. Some of these are included within this section, with sampling having been undertaken under appropriate foreign jurisdiction.

The transient and dynamic nature of this unique market not only produced an ambiguous legal position, with new legislation unable to keep abreast with the emerging new products, but created a number of bizarre ironies. For instance, chemicals clearly intended for human consumption were routinely labelled NOT FOR HUMAN COMSUMPTION on both front and rear.

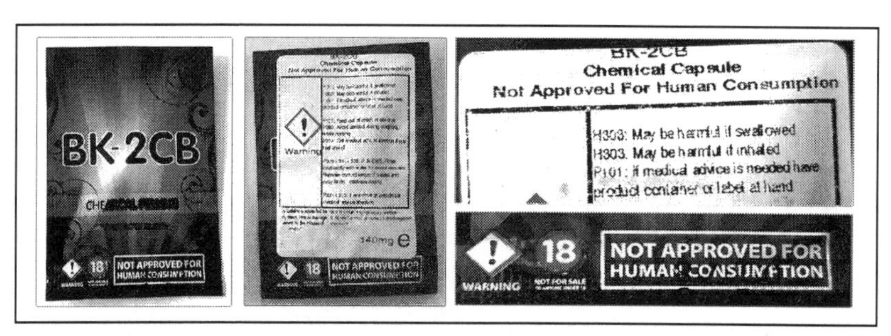

The sophistication of the market developed equally quickly, with internet forums becoming a hive of often detailed discussion. These communities became increasingly important vehicles, and not only through the dissemination of safety information. They were central in framing vendor reputation, which in turn would positively influence the conduct of suppliers.

Such was the open nature of this situation that many vendors engaged in the forums themselves, often exploring entirely new products based upon feedback, commentary and debate.

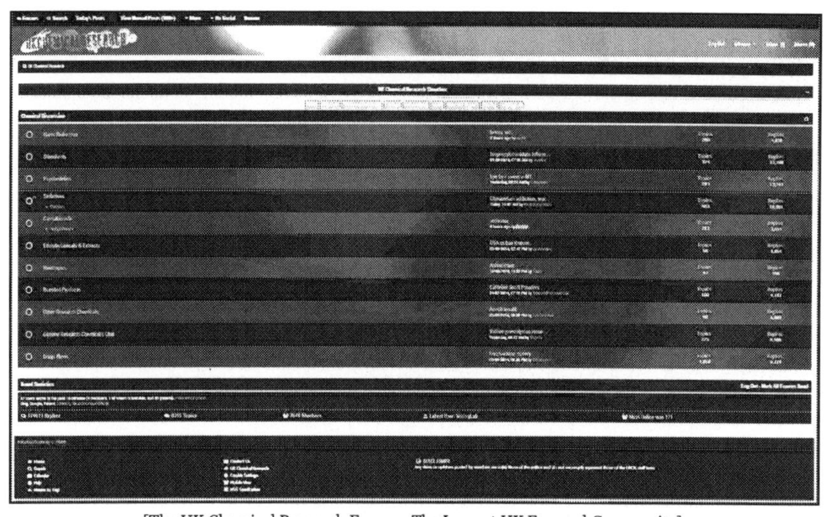

[The UK Chemical Research Forum - The Largest UK Focused Community]

During this period, the UK based user had a huge array of psychoactive chemicals available to choose from, which could be delivered directly within 24 hours. Further, whilst some of these were often new and relatively untested, large groups and communities existed to share information and report early experiences.

The market operated entirely legally, and in most respects, vendors offered their wares in exactly the same manner as any other online supplier of products or services (see Section 1.2.5).

An astonishing scenario of market/public self-regulation flourished, no doubt saving many lives, until the Cameron Government introduced the *Psychoactive Substances Act 2016*, under the blinkered stewardship of Theresa Mary May. This free to access source of developing and life critical information, and of self-sustaining consumer protection, was instantly destroyed, with the inevitable tragic consequences.

A CHEMICAL JOURNEY

This was the background against which most of my chemical research was conducted. As well as becoming academically and intellectually intriguing, it carried a sense of adventure, as I engaged a unique and fertile period of psychoactive exploration and investigation.

At the same time, however, I never lost sight of the dangers inherent to the enterprise. To address these, I identified and developed an entire series of disciplines, procedures and processes to mitigate risk. These are discussed in the introductory section of this book, and referred to throughout.

CHEMICAL CLASSIFICATION

To facilitate reference, the chemicals sampled on the journey have been ordered into the following sub-sections:

2.2 Psychedelics
2.3 Stimulants
2.4 Anxiolytics & Sedatives
2.5 Intoxicating Depressants
2.6 Dissociatives
2.7 Empathogens & Euphoriants
2.8 Cannabinoids
2.9 Nootropics

Where appropriate, indications of chronological order are provided within the text of the individual experience reports.

Reminder: Section 4.8 offers definitions and explanations of many of the acronyms and idioms used throughout this book.

2.2 PSYCHEDELICS

Textbook Definition: *These are substances which alter perception and cognition, creating an experience which is different to ordinary consciousness. The psychedelic state is often related to forms such as meditation, dreaming, yoga, near-death or out-of-body experiences, and access to other realms or dimensions of reality.*

The following chemicals have been sampled and researched for inclusion within this section:

2.2.1 1P-LSD
2.2.2 1P-ETH-LAD
2.2.3 2C-B
2.2.4 2C-B-AN
2.2.5 2C-B-FLY
2.2.6 2C-E
2.2.7 2C-I
2.2.8 4-ACO-DMT
2.2.9 4-HO-MET
2.2.10 5-MeO-DALT
2.2.11 5-MeO-DIBF
2.2.12 AL-LAD
2.2.13 AMT
2.2.14 BK-2C-B
2.2.15 Changa
2.2.16 DMT
2.2.17 LSD
2.2.18 LSZ

Psychedelics produce the most dramatic of experiences, sometimes with life changing influence. They tend to be amongst the safest of chemicals in terms of risk profile, and indeed, are frequently used to treat addiction and other self-destructive behavioural issues.

A huge volume of literature covering their spiritual and therapeutic aspects is also available, and distinctive genres of art and music have been inspired via the psychedelic experience itself.

In terms of a personal journey, psychedelic trips have provided some of the most profound and beneficial experiences of my life. I share the school of thought that sets psychedelics apart from all other psychoactive materials.

The consciousness expanding capability of psychedelics is frequently documented, but rarely in such scientific depth as that presented by Timothy Leary in the 1970's. In his *Eight-Circuit Model of Consciousness* he proposed a framework for consciousness, in which the various levels were articulated in scientifically relevant terms. Robert Anton Wilson later expanded upon this, publishing a number of books.

The eight levels of this model were also presented with reference to ancient philosophies, belief systems and theories, including Hinduism, Buddhism and the chakra system. Perhaps of greater relevance to many readers of this book is that the eight levels have also been associated with psychoactive drugs, in terms of their activation, intensification or enhancement. Thus we have opioids and alcohol, for example, associated with lower levels of consciousness, and psychedelics such as DMT and LSD with higher levels.

The following table represents a broad approximation of mappings as extracted from the literature:

	Timothy Leary	Robert Anton-Wilson	Chakra	Example Drug Stimuli
1	The vegetative-invertebrate circuit	The oral bio-survival circuit	Muladhara	Opioids, Many Sedatives
2	The emotional-locomotion circuit	The anal territorial circuit	Svadhishthana	Alcohol
3	The laryngeal-manual symbolic circuit	The semantic time-binding circuit	Manipura	Stimulants (amphetamine, cocaine, caffeine, etc)
4	The socio-sexual domestication circuit	The socio-sexual circuit	Anahata	Hormones, Entactogens (MDMA, etc)
5	The neurosomatic circuit	The neurosomatic circuit	Vishuddha	Cannabis, MDMA, Low Dose LSD
6	The neuro-electric circuit	The metaprogramming circuit	Ajna	LSD, Mescaline, Psilocybin DMT
7	The neurogenetic circuit	The morphogenetic circuit	Sahasrara	LSD, Psilocybin, DMT (all higher doses)
8	The neuro-atomic metaphysiological	The non-local quantum circuit		DMT, Ketamine

For the lower circuits, mappings have also been created between this model and the work of psychoanalysts like Jung and Freud. For example: Circuit1/Sensation/Oral; Circuit2/Feeling/Anal; Circuit3/Reason/Latency; etc. This is a rich and fascinating field.

Needless to say, this sort of positive scientific research and boundless investigation has always been subject to hostility by the established order. Indeed, Leary himself stated that he had written his book, *Science Faction,* in "*various prisons to which the author had been sentenced for dangerous ideology and violations of Newtonian and religious laws*".

Despite this flagrant and medieval proscription of science, the use of psychedelics for self-exploration has continued. A lengthy list of individuals who have recorded their work via unorthodox methods has emerged, none more prominent or persuasive than Terence McKenna. McKenna used what he referred to as "*heroic doses*", usually of botanicals, and his books, and indeed countless YouTube videos, have documented his experiences and theories in significant depth.

Another aspect suppressed via prohibition is the use of psychedelics in a medical context, to alleviate human suffering and misery. I refer here to ailments such as addiction, depression and mental illness.

As I write these words, after generations of brutal indifference to lost knowledge and remedy, the fruits of another periodic study have slipped through the cracks into the public domain: psilocybin mushrooms can be successfully used to treat depression. This is presented as though the revelation is actually news.

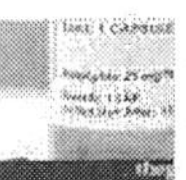

Magic **mushroom** chemical psilocybin could be key to treating depression - studies
The Guardian
A single dose of psilocybin, the active ingredient of magic **mushrooms**, can lift the anxiety and depression experienced by people with advanced cancer for six months or even longer, two new studies show. Researchers involved in the two trials in the ...

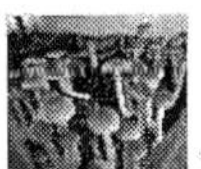

The Life-Changing Magic of **Mushrooms**
The Atlantic
The results of Vincent's **mushroom** trip—and those of 79 other study subjects like her—are now being made public, and they're very encouraging. A pair of randomized, blinded studies published Thursday in The Journal of Psychopharmacology provide the ...

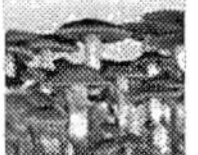

Magic **mushrooms** significantly improves distress and depression in cancer patients
Daily Mail
Magic **mushrooms** significantly improve symptoms of distress and depression in cancer patients, a clinical trial has concluded. The psychedelic drug is a banned substance classed in the same category as heroin and LSD by the DEA. But research at NYU ...

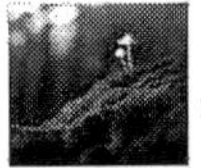

Magic **mushroom** drug helps people with cancer face death
New Scientist
Researchers have shown that a single dose of psilocybin – the active ingredient in magic **mushrooms** – combined with psychotherapy reduces depression and anxiety and increases feelings of wellbeing in people with cancer. What's more, for most, these ...

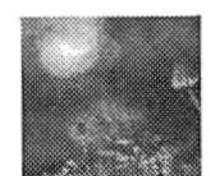

'Magic **Mushrooms**' Compound May Treat Depression in Cancer Patients
Live Science
The hallucinogen found in "magic **mushrooms**" can considerably reduce the depression and anxiety felt by patients who have terminal or advanced cancer, according to new research published in two studies. Both studies showed that just a single dose of ...

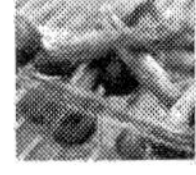

Magic **mushrooms** may ease anxiety and depression in cancer patients, studies find
The Independent
The psychedelic drug in "magic **mushrooms**" can quickly and effectively help treat anxiety and depression in cancer patients, an effect that may last for months, two small studies show. It worked for Dinah Bazer, who endured a terrifying hallucination ...

Despite this flicker of scientific fact reaching the populace, the cruelty of denial continues unabated.

Psychedelics provide unique potential for medicine, for scientific knowledge, and many argue, for the evolution and survival of the human species. It is a tragedy and an outrage that they are damned and misrepresented by those whose motives are anything but altruistic.

However, even against a background of relentless hostility their fundamental value has long been recognised, and not only within the confines of academia and science:

> *"Taking LSD was a profound experience, one of the most important things in my life. LSD shows you that there's another side to the coin, and you can't remember it when it wears off, but you know it. It reinforced my sense of what was important creating great things instead of making money, putting things back into the stream of history and of human consciousness as much as I could."*
> ~ Steve Jobs

> *"It's a very salutary thing to realize that the rather dull universe in which most of us spend most of our time is not the only universe there is. I think it's healthy that people should have this experience."*
> ~ Aldous Huxley

> *"The potential of the psychedelic drugs to provide access to the interior universe, is, I believe, their most valuable property."*
> ~ Alexander Shulgin

> *"They invented LSD to control people and what they did was give us freedom. Sometimes it works in mysterious ways its wonders to perform."*
> ~ John Lennon

> *"Perhaps to some extent we have lost sight of the fact that LSD can be very, very helpful in our society if used properly."*
> ~ Senator Robert Kennedy

> *"With psychedelics, if you're fortunate and break through, you understand what is truly of value in life."*
> ~ Gary Fisher

> *"I think that in human evolution it has never been as necessary to have this substance LSD. It is just a tool to turn us into what we are supposed to be."*
> ~ Albert Hofmann

> *"LSD is simply an exploratory instrument like a microscope or telescope, except this one is inside of you instead of outside of you."*
> ~ Alan Watts

Having stated all this, as with every other psychoactive, it is important to treat these remarkable substances with respect, and always follow the safety protocols documented earlier.

2.2.1 1P-LSD

Common Nomenclature	1-propionyl-lysergic acid diethylamide
Street & Reference Names	1plsd
Reference Dosage	Threshold 20ug+; Light 25ug+; Medium 50ug+ Strong 150ug+ [Drugs-Forum] Light 50ug+; Common 100ug+; Strong 150ug+ [TripSit]
Anticipated: Onset / Duration	1 hour / 10 hours
Maximum Dose Experienced	150ug
Form	Blotter
RoA	Oral
Source / Jurisdiction	Internet / UK
Personal Rating On Shulgin Scale	+++

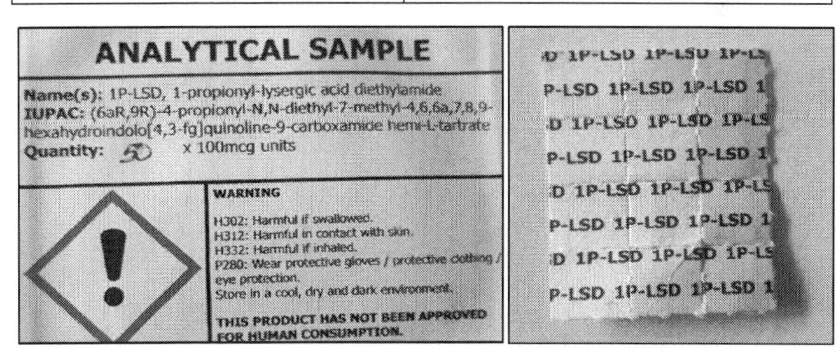

SUBJECTIVE EXPERIENCE

When 1P-LSD appeared on the markets towards the end of 2014 it was immediately recognised that its effects were identical, or near identical, to those of LSD itself.

This was also my experience. Thus, in logging my personal research, it is difficult, perhaps impossible, to add a new perspective to the countless reports and monologues that have been produced over the years. Instead, I will simply map generic features and insights, rather than delve into the content or substance of any single or specific trip.

As with most chemicals of this class, I procured the tabs directly from *Lizard Labs*, which already had a reputation for bringing high quality and novel psychedelics to the online market. IP-LSD was to become its most well known creation, and was widely distributed through other vendors.

As usual with dosage, I started small and built up. In fact I started very small, with a microdose.

Herein lies another dimension to this particular psychedelic: some people microdose on a daily or regular basis. This is commonly claimed to enhance mental or visual acuity or insight, to counter depression, to increase creativity or productivity, and so forth.

That's an aside. My microdose tests were simply intended to dip my toe into the water, to get a feel for the drug, and to gain some assurance regarding its quality and safety.

As I built up the dose the experiences became richer and more influential. Music was dramatically enhanced, as were computer visuals, and vision generally became more interesting. There's something about the vibrancy of colouration on 1P-LSD or LSD which seems to be a universal constant.

The headspace was always extremely pleasant, and a wonderful feeling of oneness with the universe increased with dose. This is an aspect well worthy of focus in its own right, as I found the same as virtually everyone else who has written on this facet: specifically that nature is a truly wonderful place in which to experience it. I frequently gazed around in astonishment, seeing, feeling, indeed witnessing, the interconnectedness, of.... everything.

I recall, on one particular trip, stepping out into the garden during a warm sunny evening. I was at one with nature, as the swarms swirled around plants and bushes, all in perfect harmony. The sky was simply beautiful as clouds drifted effortlessly across. At one point I lay horizontal on the grass and simply watched. Everything evoked a sense of wonder, as I drank in an experience which was all around me.

Goodness knows what sort of spectacle I would have made had anyone been looking through their window and witnessed my astonishment. It was a oneness that only someone who has been there can possibly understand. I didn't just see it or hear it, I was part of it, and actually felt the whole within myself.

This was an entirely different type of ego-shattering drama to the unfoldments of ayahuasca, for example. It was beauty and bliss within its own boundless terms.

Words will always fail, and can never properly describe the quality or depths of the sensations and perceptions which are unlocked. Indeed, I have experienced so many beautiful moments, and I believe learned much, through the use of this remarkable drug.

The onset of a typical 1P-LSD trip usually took about an hour, with indications that changes were afoot beginning well before this. This was a gentle incline, barely perceived during its early stages, with hints slowly manifesting here and there, and steadily strengthening.

The duration was always lengthy, with the often quoted 8-12 hours not being far off the mark. It should be noted that the peak was considerably shorter than this, and fully functional control was always established well before the end.

Mild after effects of lassitude, and a feeling of being drained, sometimes persisted into the next day. However, for me, these minor discomforts were always well worth enduring, given the perceived positives and benefits which came with the overall exercise.

REFLECTION

There's a neat video on YouTube, the chorus of which perfectly sums up the feeling I experience following a 1P-LSD trip: *"I wish I'd gone deeper but I'm not so brave"*.

This is an unspoken desire to learn more, more quickly, by taking increasingly larger doses. It is an intellectual challenge, tempered only by fear of the unknown, and the length of the period of reduced social capacitation.

This innate curiosity and yearning to uncover mystery is what has driven me to slowly push the boundaries, and indeed, to continue to explore this genre.

[*Shulgin Reference for LSD: TiHKAL #26, p490*]

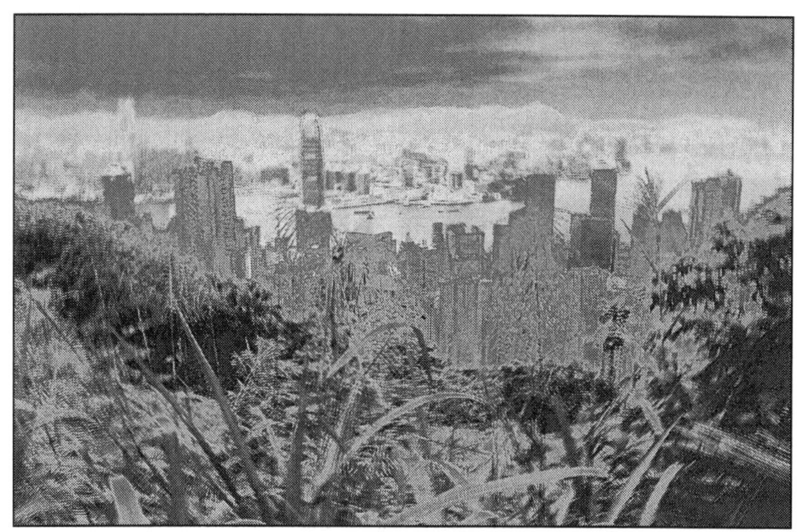

'Picture Yourself'
The obligatory psychedelic image

2.2.2 1P-ETH-LAD

Common Nomenclature	1-propionyl-6-ethyl-6-nor-lysergic acid diethyamide
Street & Reference Names	N/A
Reference Dosage	Light 30ug+; Common 60ug+; Heavy 100ug+ [TripSit]
Anticipated: Onset / Duration	1 hour / 9 hours
Maximum Dose Experienced	75ug+25ug
Form	Blotter
RoA	Oral
Source / Jurisdiction	Internet / UK
Personal Rating On Shulgin Scale	+++

ANALYTICAL SAMPLE

Name(s): 1P-ETH-LAD, 1-propionyl-6-ethyl-6-nor-lysergic acid diethylamide
IUPAC: (8ß)-1-propionyl-N,N-diethyl-6-ethyl-9,10-didehydroergoline-8-carboxamide hemi-L-tartrate
Quantity: 25 x 100mcg units

WARNING

H302: Harmful if swallowed.
H312: Harmful in contact with skin.
H332: Harmful if inhaled.
P280: Wear protective gloves / protective clothing eye protection.
Store in a cool, dry and dark environment.

THIS PRODUCT HAS NOT BEEN APPROVED FOR HUMAN CONSUMPTION.

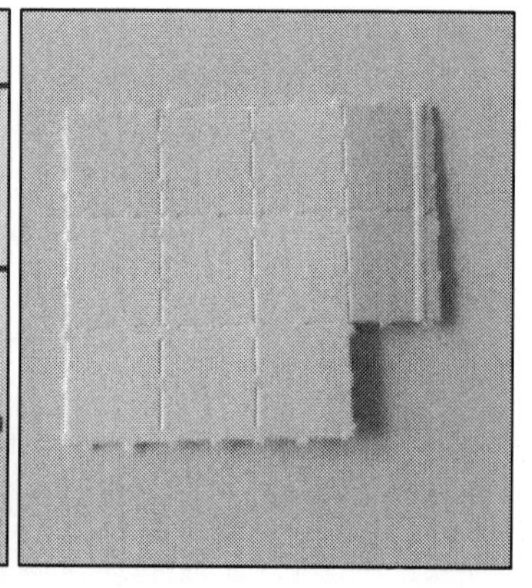

SUBJECTIVE EXPERIENCE

This is a strange trip report to write, not only because this is not the first time I have sampled 1P-ETH-LAD, but because I have used it in combination with AL-LAD and 1P-LSD on several occasions. Although combinations are not something I usually entertain, and certainly don't encourage, I find that lysergamides are not particularly taxing in terms of body load, at least when only mixed together.

The problem I have here is that through mixing these chemicals I have largely forgotten the details of the prior individual 1P-ETH-LAD experience. Given that my memory is flawed, I feel ill equipped to write a detailed report. Hence, this particular log is not reflection of my first experience, but rather, it represents the chronology of a re-visit.

IP-ETH-LAD to ETH-LAD, is what 1P-LSD is to LSD, which are almost universally considered to be indistinguishable. It is probably reasonable to assume, therefore, that 1P-ETH-LAD mirrors ETH-LAD in terms of effect. ETH-LAD itself is a shorter acting analogue of LSD, which was first documented by Alexander Shulgin in his book TiHKAL in 1997.

One issue I have tended to have with lysergamides in general is that I find it hard to tell them apart: meaning that I find the experiences, at least in terms of headspace, to be extremely similar. That said, I have never attempted to log a trip with comparison in mind. I will make the effort this time.

Starting afresh, therefore, what should I dose? Only one of the major online reference sources quotes any figures, and these appear to have been taken directly from the ETH-LAD page. Initially, I therefore looked at the difference between 1P-LSD and LSD, to perhaps enable an ETH-LAD to 1P-ETH-LAD estimate.

Taking the *common* threshold for LSD, both TripSit and Psychonautwiki place this at 75*ug*. The equivalent figures for 1P-LSD are 50*ug* and 100ug respectively, which is a substantial difference. However, the average between them is in fact 75*ug*, which suggests that *1P* does not significantly strengthen or weaken the LSD experience. Against this I note that many subjective opinions across the forums suggest that dose-to-dose 1P is slightly less intense.

Regarding ETH-LAD versus LSD, the *common* threshold for the former is placed at 60ug. This would make it slightly stronger per *ug* than LSD. If the *1P* slightly weakens the experience per *ug* perhaps pitching this dose at 60ug is reasonable, given that I have not consumed a lysergamide for many months. I note also that references on Erowid do not dramatically contradict this figure.

In terms of expectation, forum posts suggest that more visuals are invoked than there are via LSD, with more clarity of mind. Let's see.

> T+0:00 I cut a 100ug tab into pieces, isolating 60ug to the best of my ability. I chew, suck and swallow it. [3pm]
>
> T+0:15 Maybe, just maybe, a bit of headspace is developing. My eyes seem to linger on objects for slightly longer than usual as I move and look around.
>
> T+0:30 There are no further developments to report at this point. Perhaps I feel a little flushed and warm.
>
> T+1:00 I am now unmistakably under the influence of a drug. I feel comfortable but restless, in that I am increasingly distant from normal everyday reality. There may be early indications of morphing and more interesting colouration, but largely a certain headspace is present and is evolving. I am not particularly immersed or uncomfortable, but I am aware of a physical edge.

T+1:15 I am in a sort of mellow and balmy space at this point, with a tingly body sensation. I hear my ambient music occasionally interjecting in the background. It sounds very pleasant, and is definitely enhanced. I feel more comfortable now than earlier.

Walking around, I can feel physically light and, for want of a better word, floaty. In the mirror, my pupils look reasonably normal. There are no serious visuals yet, but the greater appreciation of colour is now unmistakable.

T+1:30 I am now well into ++ Shulgin territory, edging towards +++. It's a heady space, dreamy almost, with tracers hinting in the periphery and a little morphing there too.

T+2:00 At 2 hours I must now be at the peak of the experience. I remain totally functional, but with a meditative and whimsical headspace which I can drift into for lengthy periods. I can also zone in and out of light visual distortion and morphing. The ambient music remains pleasant in the distance, occasionally attracting positive attention and appreciation.

How does this compare to 1P-LSD or LSD? This does seem to support more mental clarity, although I have to accept that this could be auto-suggestion. What 1P-LSD dose does this equate to? I would definitely suggest more than 60ug.

T+2:15 At this point it is a real struggle to engage a conversation without coming across as a tripping zombie. Staying connected and on topic is hard work. I feel strange and smoothly drifting, but in a positive sense, with the feeling that I am not quite *with it*. It is a nice experience, of course, but I feel slightly on the edge, as though something unexpected may happen.

T+2:45 I just drifted away for maybe 30 minutes, awareness of the here and now occasionally coming back into focus. I felt chilly for a few minutes, as I strolled around and wandered, but sat down again and allowed myself to drift back into comfort; into the psychedelic space.

T+3:30 The experience is less intense now, but nonetheless, it remains very pleasant. My pupils are half dilated. I am ready to engage in more complex entertainment, perhaps YouTube videos or similar. My skin feels quite tingly, something similar to the feeling experienced when the hairs stand up on the back of the neck. This sensation has been a feature throughout.

T+4:00 I have just managed to eat a significant meal. The baked potato was hard going, but I got through it. The issue was mainly volumetric, rather than taste or capability related.

I now seem to have emerged into to the down flight of the trip. I am still content and retain the energy to seek some sort of mental stimulation.

T+5:00 I am still under the influence but I am easily functional. In fact, I am functional enough to contemplate walking to the local pool and having a swim. I decide to go for it.

T+5:30 I survived the swim. It felt strangely refreshing in that I was partially numbed to any chill from the water, not that it wasn't reasonably warm. My body was pleased to stretch and exercise.

The walk to the pool brought the familiar feeling that I was indoors; that nature and the exterior were harmoniously interiorised in some way. This wasn't the same feeling of oneness which I have felt with LSD, but was still a comforting inclusiveness of the outside physical world. This could have been a pre-cursor to the oneness experience, which might emerge at a higher dose.

There is less intellectual wonder than I recall with 1P-LSD, and more of a consciously aware feeling of pro-actively witnessing reality and observing it from within. There seems to be more clarity in terms of perceiving and computing the norm.

T+6:00 The duration of a 1P-ETH-LAD experience is usually presented as eight to twelve hours. For me, at this dose, it isn't. I can still feel it, but the ride seems like it is almost over.

I am a little drained, mentally tired, but with a weak after-the-party psychedelic headspace in situ. Does this still count as duration? Given that I am writing in these terms I would suggest not.

This has been a very nice experience. I instinctively know that it was very dependent upon set and setting, and that had I engaged in nature or in a similarly suitable place on a warm sunny day, it would have been absolutely wonderful. This is not to say that it hasn't been extremely enjoyable. It has.

It's now 9pm. I am tired and ready for bed, although I do expect some issues with sleep.

Last but not least, there has been no significant body load at any stage.

In terms of aftermath, I drifted off peacefully and had a surprisingly good night's sleep. In the morning there was no fog or difficulty, and indeed, I felt quite invigorated, which is common with psychedelics.

Whilst a little tired, my subsequent mental status was certainly more positive than the norm, almost as if an internal reset button had been pressed, clearing psychological clutter.

[*Shulgin Reference for ETH-LAD: TiHKAL #12, p442*]

2.2.3 2C-B

Common Nomenclature	2,5-dimethoxy-4-bromophenethylamine
Street & Reference Names	Nexus; Bees; Venus; 2cb
Reference Dosage	Threshold 2mg+; Light 5mg+; Common 15mg+; Strong 25mg+ [Erowid] Threshold 2mg+;Light 10mg+; Common 20mg+; Strong 35mg+; Heavy 55mg+ [Psychonautwiki] Light: 5mg+; Common: 15mg+; Strong: 30mg+; Heavy: 50mg+; [TripSit]
Anticipated: Onset / Duration	1 hours / 6 hours
Maximum Dose Experienced	15mg+3mg
Form	Pill
Form	Oral
Source / Jurisdiction	Dealer / Europe
Personal Rating On Shulgin Scale	++

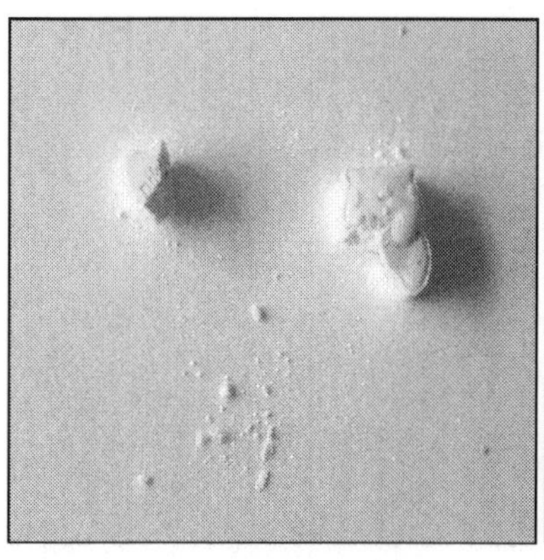

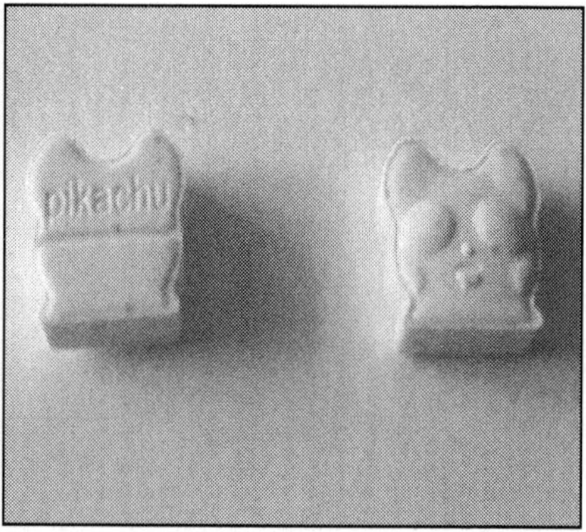

SUBJECTIVE EXPERIENCE
2C-B was first synthesised by Alexander Shulgin in 1974 and became one of his most popular creations. It was initially used in psychiatric therapy, before emerging as a popular recreational drug.

For a period in the late 1980s it was sold as a legal alternative to MDMA, but generally it is now perceived more accurately; as a chemical which induces its own unique experience. At the time of writing it is still widely available, and is sometimes (dubiously) used as a club drug.

It was, in fact, one of Shulgin's personal favourites, particularly in the context of sexual activity:

> *"If there is anything ever found to be an effective aphrodisiac, it will probably be patterned after 2C-B in structure."* ~ Alexander Shulgin

With respect to this, it is interesting to note that it was once sold commercially as an aphrodisiac, under the names *Erox* and *Nexus.*

Research (including with reference to Shulgin's *PiHKAL*) also indicates that this chemical is extremely dose sensitive, with a very steep curve: meaning that only slight changes in dose can result in significantly different experience outcomes.

After due diligence consideration, and with this in mind, I decide to dose at 15mg, which is pitched well above threshold but is reasonably low on the overall scale.

As a backdrop, the particular pill I am sampling was recently the subject of a number of hysterical and misleading UK media reports. It is bright yellow in colour and was allegedly manufactured in the Netherlands.

T+0.00 I crumble the pill (18mg) and put 3mg to one side, swallowing the rest with fizzy water. Note that I am testing on an empty stomach. [3pm]

T+0.40 The headspace is starting to develop. A chilly feeling emerges, and I note that I have cold fingers (indicating vasoconstriction).

I feel a little shivery, apart from my head, which is strangely warm.

T+1.00 The ride seems to have settled. The headspace is now stable and the earlier body sensations linger lightly but gently in the background.

T+1.15 At this point I am still fully functional and can easily suppress the experience, which comprises a mild psychedelic ambiance with no obvious visuals, other than brighter colouration should I focus upon this aspect. Layered on top of this there is a physical awareness which is slowly levelling.

T+1:30 There is no significant change. I am in a solid ++ state, but one which is not unduly exciting.

T+1:45 As this is clearly not going to escalate much further, if at all, I pop the remaining 3mg from the original pill. The total dose is now 18mg.

T+2:00 I test taste, via a bag of plain crisps. There is no particular change or enhancement, and no noticeable loss or increase in appetite.

Now, what about sex and horn, as so frequently referred to?

> There is certainly interest, but it is not overwhelming by any means.
>
> I do feel that sexual human contact would be enhanced as there is a tactile edge to this, but there is no strong or compulsive drive or urge (as per certain stimulants). It is quite subtle in nature, and I suspect that suitable circumstances and intimacy would make all the difference.
>
> T+2:30 I feel content and happy enough, although I am not tripping high or particularly intensively. The shivers and chills have largely dissipated and there is no perceptible discomfort in terms of body load. My skin does feel relatively sensitised, in a strange entactogenic sort of way.
>
> My mind tends to wander and drift, again though it is well under normal functional control if I focus. I feel a little dreamy.
>
> Despite eating so little today, after the crisps and some yoghurt I don't feel at all hungry. Note that I have been drinking plenty of fluid, but for safety reasons rather than thirst.
>
> Regarding visuals, along with slightly enhanced colouration there is a degree of morphing in play, albeit light and transient. This isn't a central feature.
>
> T+3:10 At this point I believe that I am drifting back down towards baseline, which defies most of the published material.
>
> I feel a sense of calmness and serenity: a comfortable and positive mood. There remains a certain sentience which is not quite tingly, but is perhaps a prelude status to this condition.
>
> T+3:30 The effects documented earlier are still present, but are much less pronounced. I am closing in on normality.
>
> T+4:00 To all intents and purposes, I am back to base, with only the usual sort of post-trip afterglow persisting.

Following this pleasant but unspectacular experience, I tired a little earlier than usual and retired to bed early. I slept well and woke up with no hangover at all.

Overall, this was a good ++ experience. I can see how some people confuse it with MDMA, but I found it to be less empathogenic and I was much more body conscious. I found it to be similar to, but less intense than, a 10-12mg dose of 2C-B-FLY (noting that I hadn't tested any of the other 2C compounds at this point).

Given my size and experience 15mg was probably a good introductory dose, but if further testing is possible, I will probably increase this to the 20mg range. Generally, however, as some users do report body load issues, caution is advisable.

[*Shulgin Reference: PiHKAL #20, p503*]

2.2.4 2C-B-AN

Common Nomenclature	2C-B-AN
Street & Reference Names	N/A
Reference Dosage	Light 30mg+; Common 45mg+; Strong 70mg+ Heavy 100mg+ [TripSit]
Anticipated: Onset / Duration	1 hour / 7 hours
Maximum Dose Experienced	55mg+10mg
Form	Powder
RoA	Oral
Source / Jurisdiction	Internet / UK
Personal Rating On Shulgin Scale	++

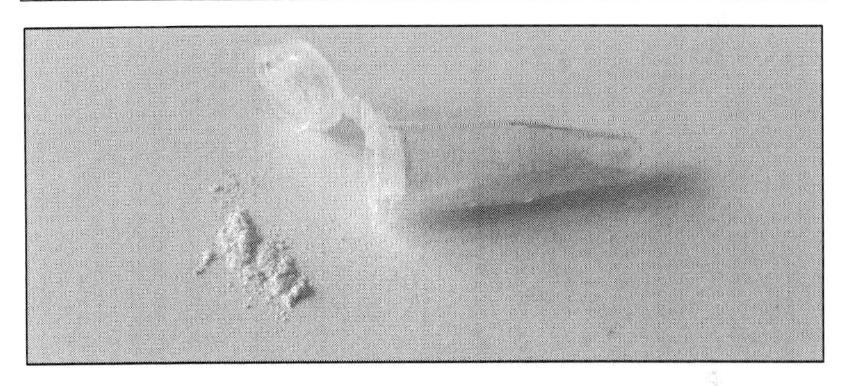

SUBJECTIVE EXPERIENCE
A small supply of this appeared on the market in 2016, shortly before the general UK ban came into effect. I was fortunate to obtain enough for a couple of low-dose trips.

These were pleasant enough: enhanced colouration with minor visuals, a sense of mood lift with mild euphoria, and a tingly body feel as experienced with other 2C-B variants.

The difference between many of these analogues is often subtle and difficult to distinguish, particularly with respect to headspace. It could well be that this one converts to 2C-B itself in vivo, as I have seen suggested.

Overall, this was a very nice foray, with the relatively short duration being a positive in my circumstances at the time. It was certainly trippy in nature, and I was almost back to baseline after about 6 hours.

2.2.5 2C-B-FLY

Common Nomenclature	2C-B-FLY
Street & Reference Names	N/A
Reference Dosage	Light 5mg+; Common 10mg+; Strong 18mg+; Heavy 25mg+ [TripSit] Threshold 2mg+; Light 5mg+; Common 10mg+; Strong 18mg+; Heavy 25mg+ [Psychonautwiki]
Anticipated: Onset / Duration	1 hour / 7 hours
Maximum Dose Experienced	10mg
Form	Pill & Powder
RoA	Oral & Insufflated
Source / Jurisdiction	Internet / UK
Personal Rating On Shulgin Scale	++

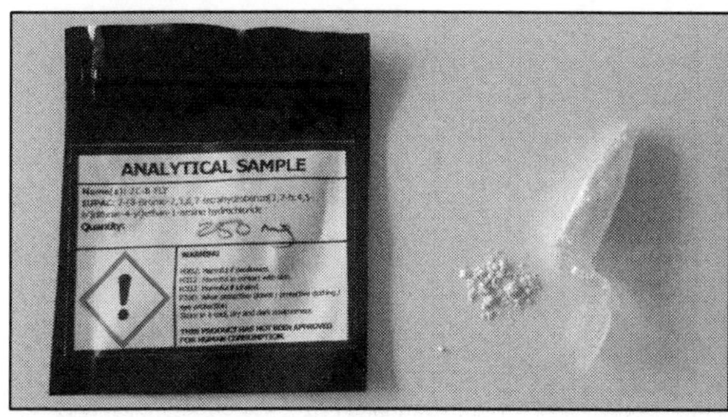

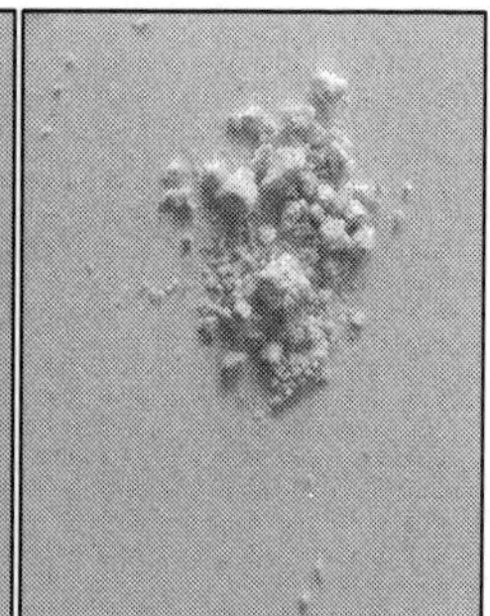

SUBJECTIVE EXPERIENCE

2C-B-FLY was first synthesised in 1996 by Aaron P. Monte, and by 2005 it had become sufficiently popular to merit its own Erowid vault. However, its popularity waned when a couple of deaths were erroneously linked to it, circa 2009. The chemical involved in these incidents was actually *Bromo-DragonFly*, which has a far lower threshold and a much higher toxicity. This had been mislabelled as 2-CB-FLY.

Notwithstanding this confusion, 2-CB-FLY made a comeback at the start of 2016, when it was released online by *Lizard Labs.* It was one of the few working psychedelics readily and legally available on the open market at the time of the generic UK ban in May of that year.

Prior to this date, I sampled this on a number of occasions, usually orally, and largely in the 10mg-15mg range.

Whilst it lacked the depth of 1p-LSD (which was similarly available), it was shorter lasting, and came with entactogenic body tingles and its own feel.

I didn't find the headspace to be as clear or rewarding as that provided by lysergamides: despite a change in perception, it induced less insight, and less of a feeling of oneness and spirituality. This is not to say that these were totally absent.

It was fun in its own right, and was perhaps a twist on 2-CB. Visually, it created a light sheen and enhanced colouration, but there was little in the way of serious OEVs or CEVs. It is possible, or perhaps probable, that these may manifest with higher doses.

Insufflation was agony. I experimented with this RoA on several occasions, and each came with at least 24 hours of subsequent discomfort, which at times seemed to be bordering on the edge of a nasally driven head cold. As would be expected via this route, the onset was much faster and the duration was shorter, but the physical cost was higher and the trip itself was consequently less comfortable. Nasally, I usually dosed at around the 8mg level.

Overall 2C-B-FLY produced a decent ride, providing a more frivolous and physical contrast to my preferred psychedelics. The shorter duration was certainly an attraction, and with expectation set appropriately, it provided for an interesting trip.

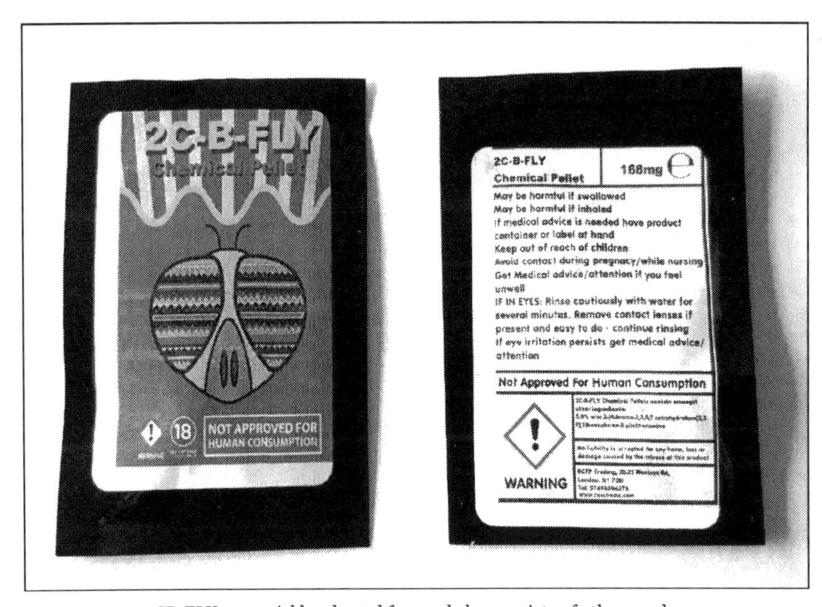

2-CB-FLY was quickly adopted for resale by a variety of other vendors

2.2.6 2C-E

Common Nomenclature	2,5-dimethoxy-4-ethylphenethylamine
Street & Reference Names	2ce; Europa
Reference Dosage	Threshold 2mg+; Light 5mg+; Common 10mg+; Strong 15mg+; Heavy 25mg+ [Erowid] Typical 5mg-15mg [Drugs-Forum]
Anticipated: Onset / Duration	30 Minutes / 8 Hours
Maximum Dose Experienced	9-10mg
Form	Pill
RoA	Oral
Source / Jurisdiction	Dealer / Overseas

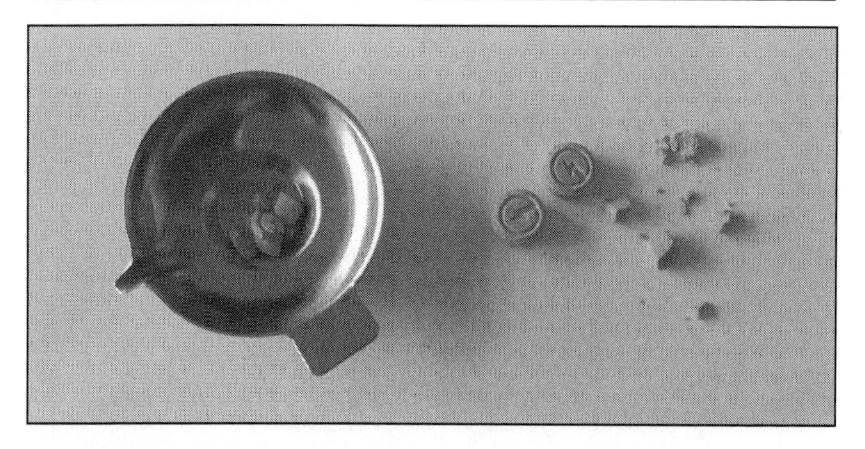

SUBJECTIVE EXPERIENCE
2C-E was first synthesised by Alexander Shulgin, and was documented in PiHKAL in 1991. He rated it as one of the most important phenethylamine compounds, which he referred to as his *magical half-dozen*. For the record, these comprised mescaline, and six of his own inventions: DOM, 2C-B, 2C-E, 2C-T-2 and 2C-T-7.

Recreationally, it became increasingly popular from the early 2000s. However, it was classified in the UK in 2002 and scheduled in the United States in July 2012.

2C-E is often considered to invoke a deeply meaningful experience, with references to this effect present across Internet forums and in a number of books. A good example of the latter is Myron J. Stolaroff's '*Thanatos to Eros: 35 Years of Psychedelic Exploration Ethnomedicien and the Study of Consciousness*', which can be found on the MAPS website.

My 18mg sample was allegedly produced by a Chinese lab, and pressed into pill form in the UK. On the face of it, this seems to be a good dose, but further research leads me to exercise additional caution.

One factor is that for many users 2C-E produces a high body load. Another is that reports across the harm reduction forums repeatedly stress a steep response curve and high intensity low-dose experiences. The following comments, from respected posters on the *BlueLight* forum, are fairly typical:

> *"This one has a VERY steep dose/response curve and I'd imagine every half-milligram can produce a noticeable jump in intensity."* ~ *Morninggloryseed*
>
> *"I tried 12mgs of 2C-E for the first time tonite. Wow! It was really damn intense."* ~ Piper methysticum
>
> *"The 2C-E dose-reponse curve is probably the sharpest I've ever experienced. I have seen a full freakout on 15mg."* ~ Fizzacyst
>
> *" Yes it can knock your socks off at 12mg or be almost irrelevant at 16mg weird that."* ~ B9

In the ideal circumstance I would perhaps plump for 15mg, but today is far from ideal, and a *full freakout* is out of the question. I therefore go for 9mg, but still with a little trepidation.

> T+0:00 I weigh the pill, break it up, and measure half. It is just over, so the dose is somewhere between 9mg and 10mg. I swallow this with a glass of water. [3:20pm]
>
> T+0:20 A mild headspace is developing, with perhaps enhanced visible colouration, but all is minimal. I wonder if I have taken enough.
>
> T+0:35 The headiness has intensified, and a tingly body feeling has emerged, which is particularly evident in my hands. A familiar psychedelic sheen to my vision is also developing. In terms of mood, there may be a little elevation. All these effects are quite mild, but are now very clear.
>
> T+ 1:00 Little has changed. I resist the temptation to swallow the other half of the pill largely on the basis of a couple of outlier trip reports which claimed a two hour onset.
>
> This is in fact reasonably agreeable. The headiness has a drifting quality, as does vision unless I specifically focus. There is definitely an introspective edge here, which flows quite strongly if I take that direction.
>
> T+1:30 The effects I described on the hour mark have strengthened and stabilised. It is a pleasant enough high, with psychedelic edges, and clear scope for introspection. The headiness is of a slightly different nature to the other 2C psychedelics I have experienced. It has a more hypnotic feel to it, with a sense of falling into an internal state of reverie.

The mind play is the predominant feature, with the tingly body sensation playing alongside. The light visual sheen is still present, but there are no real CEVs or OEVs. Clearly, these emerge with higher doses.

T+2:00 There is no significant euphoria or mood lift. There is, however, a great deal of thought and reflection. As my mind casts on to different topics, I find myself immersed in profound consideration and absorbed in pensive contemplation.

This thinking mode can be relatively pleasant depending upon its focus, and I find myself pro-actively changing the topic of my attention to avoid negative subject matter, and thus unpleasantness.

T+3:00 The intensity has now largely subsided, although the deep thought and introspection do continue to roll.

T+5:00 This is slowly fading towards base, but with the drifting headiness still a notable factor.

T+7:00 I am now left with a low level feeling of contentedness and the normal psychedelic lassitude and fatigue. The show is over, but the dying embers ebb and flow in the background. I am tiring and thinking about sleep.

I retired to bed at 11:30pm, some 8 hours after swallowing the crumbled pill. I slept normally, but awoke with a mild headache. This will have been part of the commonly referenced body load, but it passed quickly.

In his book, PiHKAL, Shulgin states "*Several people have said, about 2C-E, 'I don't think I like it, since it isn't that much fun. But I intend to explore it again.' There is something here that will reward the experimenter.*" This is a good summary of my own impression.

This wasn't bouncy or fun but there was a depth there waiting to be explored. I felt as though I was at the door, peeping inside. I was content but not elevated, and I tended to drift into deep thought. The latter manifestation persisted for a large part of the experience.

A higher dose would probably have made for a more interesting ride, albeit with the potential for some bumps. I may return to this chemical should the opportunity arise, but this isn't a priority.

Reminder: 2C-E is extremely dose sensitive, and same-dose effects vary considerably from person to person. Exercise caution.

[*Shulgin Reference: PiHKAL - #24 (Page 515)*]

2.2.7 2C-I

Common Nomenclature	2,5-Dimethoxy-4-iodophenethylamine
Street & Reference Names	2ci; Smiles
Reference Dosage	Threshold 2mg+; Light 5mg+; Common 10mg+; Strong 20mg+ [Erowid] Typical 5mg-20mg [Drugs-Forum]
Anticipated: Onset / Duration	1 Hour / 8 Hours
Maximum Dose Experienced	9mg
Form	Pill
RoA	Oral
Source / Jurisdiction	Dealer / Overseas

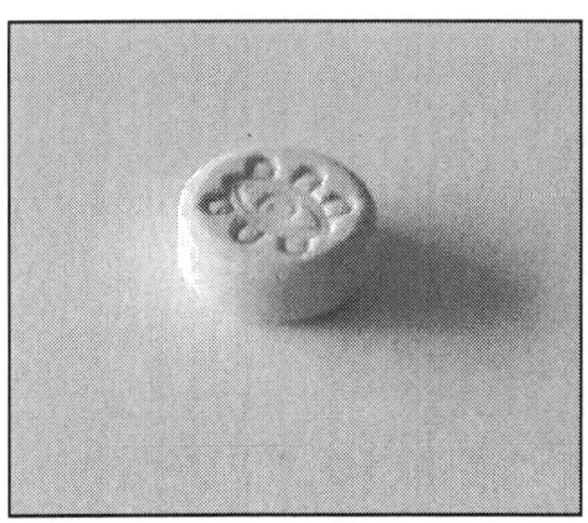

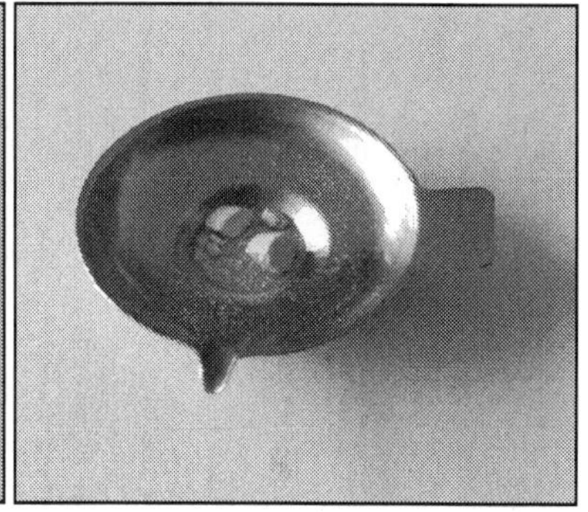

SUBJECTIVE EXPERIENCE
First synthesised by Alexander Shulgin in 1976, 2C-I began to emerge as a popular recreational drug in the late 1990's. Sometimes confused with 2C-I-NBOMe and dubbed with the name *Smiles* by the media, it was no surprise when it was scheduled in the United States in 2012. It had already been classified in the UK in 1998.

My sample came in the form of an 18mg pill, reputedly sourced from China and pressed in the UK. I tested it on a swelteringly hot summer's day; the sort of day on which it is difficult to escape the background heat. This was one of the reasons I went low with the dose: uncomfortable body load could well be multiplied in such conditions.

> T+0:00 I weigh the pill and then break it into pieces, accumulating 9mg on the scales. I swig the crumbled debris down with spring water. The operation isn't particularly clean and I catch the unpleasantness of the taste and constitution of the pill at the back of my throat. [15:20]

T+0:20 Only the mildest of mental stimulation is apparent, but I do feel a little more comfortable with the conditions.

T+0:40 The hazy headspace has only developed a little, but there is now a light sheen to vision.

T+1:00 There is a sweaty touchy feel to this, with the familiar dreamy 2C type of mindset, which is quite smooth, although unexciting. Rationality is fully maintained, although as is often the case with 2C's, concentration upon specific external factors or subject matter can be heightened from time to time.

I hesitate to use the word comfortable again, but that is the general vibe as I walk around. There are no real visuals to report.

T+1:15 This is quite a physical experience: sentient, clammy hands, with horn available. The headspace is now more solid and the sheen on my vision has strengthened, but not into any definable OEVs or CEVs.

It is quite pleasant at this point. I notice that my pupils are semi-dilated.

T+2:00 I have been on a plateau for some time. This will clearly go no further. It is stable with the mild dreamy mood and the tactile body warmth.

T+3:00 I have now started to slide down the gears. The gentle psychedelic headiness remains, as does the warmth and sensuality, but at increasingly lower levels.

T+5:00 I bathe in the afterglow, with the dying embers of enhanced colouration and the soft landing of the head and body high flowing down towards base.

With certain senses enhanced and anxieties chased away a walk into suburbia becomes a genuine pleasure.

I retire to bed at 11:30pm, eight hours after initial ingestion.

T+16:00 I drifted off fairly quickly and the night's sleep was a good one. This morning I feel completely normal.

Overall, on this dose this was a fairly mild and pleasant experience. It didn't have the depth of, for example, 2C-E, or indeed, a great deal of excitement, but for a gentle afternoon sojourn it was positive and enjoyable.

For a fully engaged psychedelic ride I suspect that the consensus, of a dose of perhaps 12-15mg, is probably about right.

[*Shulgin Reference: PiHKAL - #33 (Page 539)*]

2.2.8 4-ACO-DMT

Common Nomenclature	O-Acetylpsilocin
Street & Reference Names	4-Acetoxy-DMT; Psilacetin;
Reference Dosage	Threshold 2.5mg+; Light 3mg+; Common 8mg+; Strong 25mg+ [Erowid] Threshold 5mg+; Light 10mg+; Common 20mg+; Strong 30mg+; Heavy 50mg+ [Psychonautwiki] Light 5mg+; Common 10mg+; Heavy 25mg+ [TripSit]
Anticipated: Onset / Duration	2 Hours / 8 Hours
Maximum Dose Experienced	6mg
Form	Powder
RoA	Oral
Source / Jurisdiction	Dealer / Overseas
Personal Rating On Shulgin Scale	++*

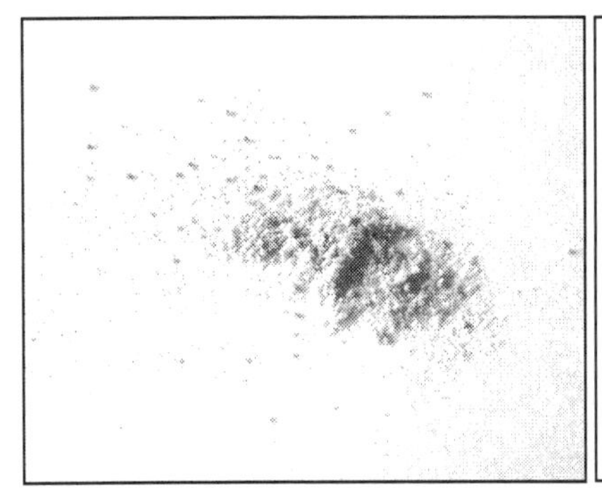

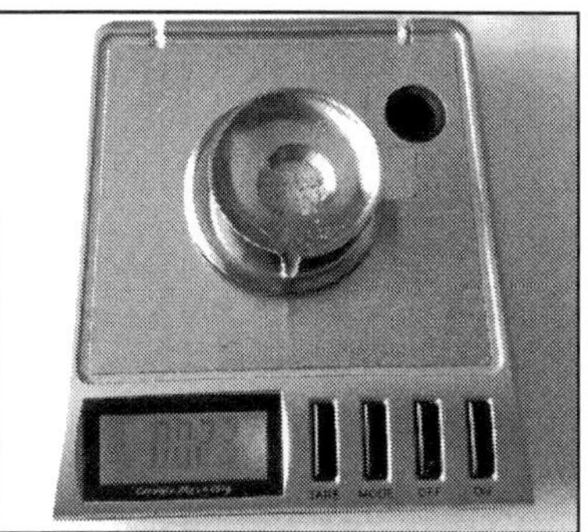

SUBJECTIVE EXPERIENCE

4-ACO-DMT was first synthesised by Albert Hofmann and Franz Troxler in the early 1960's, and was patented by Sandoz Ltd in 1963. It is widely considered to produce an almost identical experience to that of psilocybin containing mushrooms. Indeed, Erowid states that it is "*probably metabolically converted into psilocin in the body*".

At time of writing this report it is increasingly popular, including with researchers seeking to replicate the famed "*McKenna experience*" via doses in excess of 50mg. A word of caution here though: there are a number of reports of ++++ experiences occurring with doses of under 20mg. It is important, therefore, to adhere to standard safety measures even though this chemical is generally considered to be relatively benign.

I do have a large dose experience of 4-ACO-DMT on my future *bucket list*, but today I have to remain broadly functional, as there is potential for social interaction for which I need to be relatively unimpaired. For this reason I will start extremely low, just to get a feel for it.

Note that I am also rather tired this morning, and slightly hung-over. This is clearly not the perfect condition for testing, which is another factor that gravitates towards a small dose experiment.

> T+0:00 I consume approximately 6mg orally: straight down the hatch with water. [11:45am]
>
> T+0:30 I have quickly developed a psychedelic headspace, and already it is a fairly strong one. Colours are brighter and I notice that my focus drifts onto different objects almost of its own accord. In my case, the commonly stated onset period of two hours is clearly not correct.
>
> T+0:45 I feel chilly, so I add an extra layer of clothing. Regarding vision, there is some diffraction and maybe a little morphing in play, with slight tracers and over-currents also appearing.
>
> T+1:00 This would be very pleasant if I wasn't so tired. Checking in the mirror, my pupils are dilated. The headspace is still very apparent.
>
> T+1:30 At this point I succumb to the need for sleep. This is a waste in some respects, but it is needed.
>
> T+3:30 I am well awake now and find that I am close to baseline . I slept deeply for about half an hour and dozed for the rest of the time, basking in the headspace.

There is no doubt that this was the real deal. The feel was close to my experience of magic mushrooms, as expected, and I am surprised that it was so active at such a low dose.

Its short duration was another surprise, even though some of the time projections quoted online suggested that this could occur. This aspect certainly places it into a niche that is under-populated by other psychedelics of this nature.

It was a pleasant ride, despite my poor condition.

I look forward to further experimentation during the coming months, and perhaps a deeper and more spiritually meaningful trip.

[*Shulgin Reference for 4-NO-DMT: TiHKAL #18, p468*]

2.2.9 4-HO-MET

Common Nomenclature	4-hydroxy-N-methyl-N-ethyl tryptamine
Street & Reference Names	Metocin; Methylcybin; Colour
Reference Dosage	Threshold 2mg+; Light 5mg+; Common 8mg+; Strong 10mg+; Heavy 25mg+ [Erowid] Threshold 2mg+; Light 5mg+; Common 8mg+; Strong 15mg+; Heavy 30mg+ [Psychonautwiki] Low 5mg+; Moderate 10mg+; High 16mg+; Very High 25mg+ [Drugs-Forum]
Anticipated: Onset / Duration	30 Minutes / 5 Hours
Maximum Dose Experienced	6mg+5mg
Form	Powder
RoA	Oral
Source / Jurisdiction	Dealer / Overseas

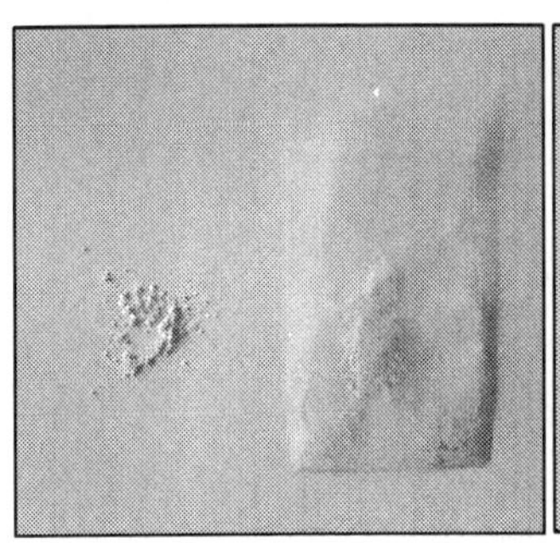

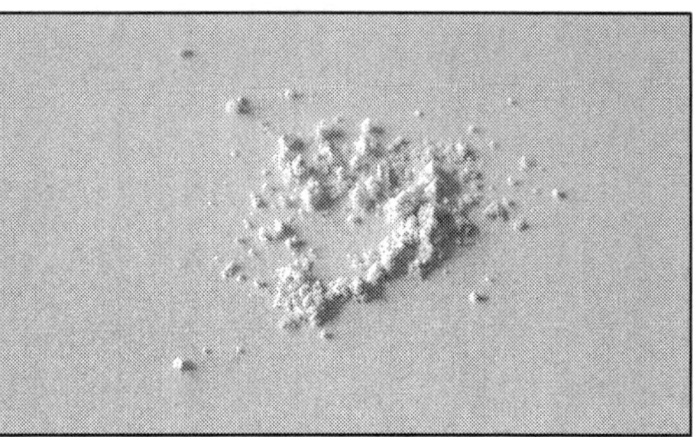

SUBJECTIVE EXPERIENCE
This is described by Wikipedia as *a structural and functional analogue of psilocin*, which in turn is present in most psychedelic mushrooms. Hardly surprisingly, it is generally considered to produce very similar effects. It was first synthesised by Alexander Shulgin, and is documented in his book, *TiHKAL*.

At the time of testing, along with 4-ACO-DMT, 4-HO-MET is increasingly popular, appearing on the *must-do* list of many regular Internet posters. It is often suggested that of the two it offers more head clarity, is less deep, has more visuals, and is therefore more recreational.

Unfortunately, it will be difficult to draw comparisons in this report, having only sampled a low dose of 4-AcO-DMT, but I cannot deny that I have been looking forward to this particular experiment.

My original inclination was to dose at 10-15mg, but social circumstances have again conspired against me, dictating that I retain a reasonable degree of functionality. I therefore dose significantly lower.

T+0:00 6mg is carefully measured from the 11mg that fell out of the small plastic bag as I poured it on to the pan. I retain the other half for potential use later in the trip. [2:40pm]

T+0:30 A headspace is slowly emerging, and I feel clammy, although I am unsure whether I am hot or cold.

T+0:50 A very mild and pleasant headiness has developed, which is verging on serene in nature, suggesting a mood lift. Vision is almost glossy in character, with a mild sheen. Music is not particularly enhanced.

T+1:00 An hour has passed, and given that I consumed on an empty stomach, I suspect that this is as far as it will go. This is fine, but so am I, so I decide to toss and wash the other 5mg.

T+1:40 The gloss I referred to earlier is slightly stronger, I am warm, and the headspace is now very comfortable. It isn't overpowering in any way, and I am easily functional, but there is a rather pleasant ambience to existence.

I am not experiencing any real visuals at this stage, other than the haze referred to above. This is contrary to expectations, and to most general user reports. Perhaps this feature is dose dependent, although it is possible that my sample isn't particularly strong.

No significant pupil dilation is apparent, but there is some tactile sensitivity present. Although I feel that I am definitely playing in low-dose territory, the influence of the drug is well into the Shulgin ++ range.

T+2:00 I am in a reflective state of general psychedelic awareness. The headspace has a gentle character to it, with no perceptible rough edges. Focus on individual tasks is fairly straight forward if required, but the desire to bathe in the overall warmth is stronger.

T+2:40 I am now floating on a plateau, having peaked some time ago. I sense that from here I will experience a slow and gentle come-down, which I expect to last a couple of hours. I remain comfortable however, in a somewhat numbed bubble of contentedness. The body sensation of light tactility is still physically present, but the clamminess is subsiding.

T+3:10 I continue to feel serene but I am now unengaged enough to pro-actively seek some form of extra entertainment, courtesy of YouTube. I purposely avoid the news, as it is generally bad, and I have an eye on set and setting.

At this stage I feel more equipped to draw comparison with the low dose of 4-ACO-DMT which I sampled a couple of weeks ago. This certainly has a milder less intense feel about it, with possibly less scope for introspection. I would have to go deeper with both to offer anything more substantive.

T+4:00 I have just consumed a meal without difficulty. Given that by now I am well into the dying embers of the experience, perhaps it is not surprising that I noticed no particular degradation or enhancement of taste or appetite.

To all intents and purposes the show now appears to be over. I feel largely at base, with a mild psychedelic fatigue and lassitude, as is usual for most members of this class.

In retrospect, I feel that I would have learned far more had I gone with the whole 11mg which fate served from the packet, rather than taking it in two halves. However, this was still a positive low-end experience, with no real negatives or unwanted side effects.

As with 4-ACO-DMT, I hope to return to this in due course.

[*Shulgin Reference: TiHKAL #20, p480*]

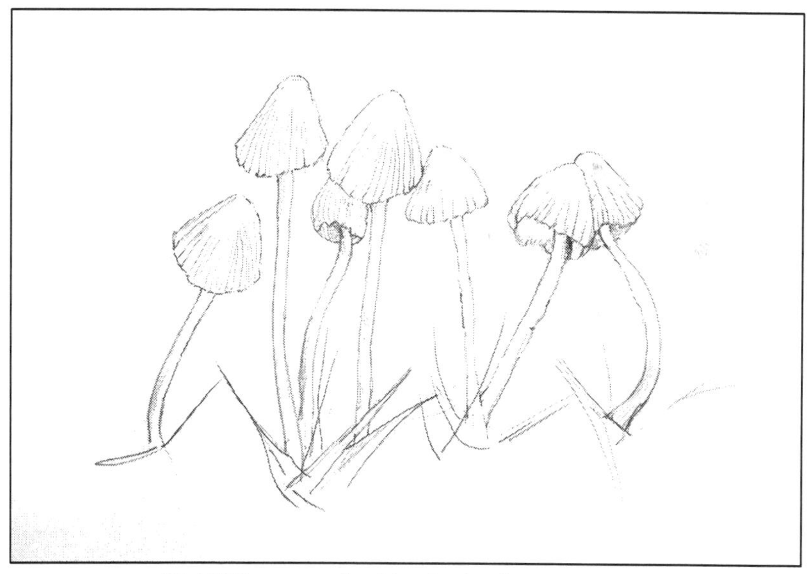

4-HO-MET is a structural and functional analogue of psilocin. Its effects are often compared to those of psilocybin mushrooms.

2.2.10 5-MEO-DALT

Common Nomenclature	N,N-diallyl-5-methoxytryptamine
Street & Reference Names	N/A
Reference Dosage	Threshold 5mg+; Light 4mg+; Common 12mg+; Strong 25mg+; Heavy 35mg+ [Psychonautwiki] Threshold 4mg+; Light 5mg+; Common 12mg+; Strong 20mg+; [TripSit]
Anticipated: Onset / Duration	20 Minutes /5 Hours
Maximum Dose Experienced	100mg
Form	Powder
RoA	Oral
Source / Jurisdiction	Internet / UK
Personal Rating On Shulgin Scale	+

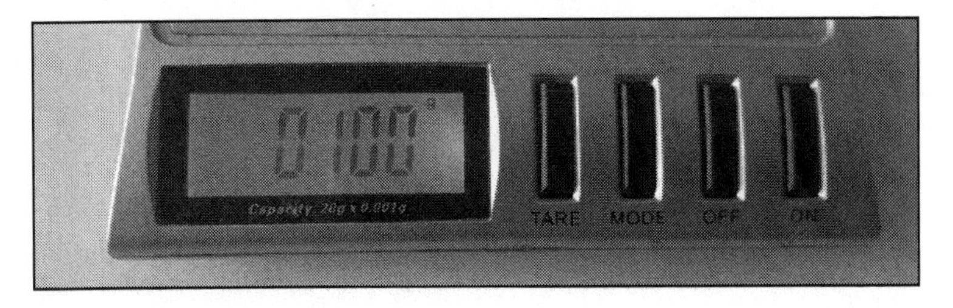

SUBJECTIVE EXPERIENCE
This compound is memorable largely because it represents the most glaring mistake I have ever made with respect to dosing. Given the advice I provide throughout this book regarding this issue, I cannot possibly account for the error. It was a mental aberration, and I was fortunate that it occurred with a relatively benign drug.

The dose I was aiming for was 10mg, hoping for a light and relatively short psychedelic buzz. I went ahead and measured 0.1 on the scales. Yes, this was 100mg; or 10x my intended dose.

Once it was down the hatch I realized what I had done but it was too late. I made efforts to vomit, even drinking salty water, but to no avail. The panic which ensued was far from pleasant, but the onset of the drug itself took the edge away, and I manoeuvred my way through it, consuming copious amounts of water, and eating like a pig.

The trip itself was far from remarkable. It comprised largely a light psychedelic headspace, accompanied by body tingles and perhaps some sedation. There was no significant come-down or hangover; just a lesson never to repeat the same mistake.

2.2.11 5-MEO-DIBF

Common Nomenclature	5-MEO-DIBF
Street & Reference Names	N/A
Reference Dosage	Light 10mg+; Common20mg+; Strong 40mg+ [TripSit Oral] Light 5mg+; Common 10mg+; Strong 15mg+ [TripSit Insufflated]
Anticipated: Onset / Duration	5 Minutes / 6 Hours [Insufflated] 45 Minutes / 9 Hours [Oral]
Maximum Dose Experienced	50mg
Form	Powder / Pill
Form / RoA	Oral
Source / Jurisdiction	Internet / UK
Personal Rating On Shulgin Scale	+

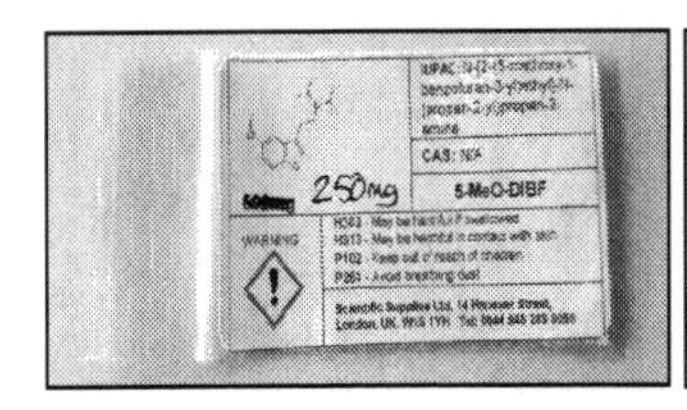

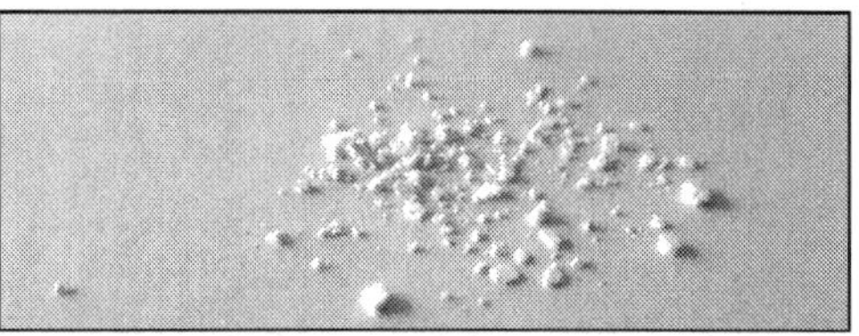

SUBJECTIVE EXPERIENCE
5-MEO-DIBF appeared on the market early in 2015, and was greeted fairly positively, although my own impression was more muted than most. I wrote the following comment on a forum at the time:

> *This delivered a psychedelic headspace, with a mild tactile tingly hornability feel. Urge to redose? It is difficult to say as this was always going to be a short gig, but I felt no real compulsion. I'm not sure where the estimates of a nine hour duration came from, as I seem to be floating down after just four. This was decent enough, and I enjoyed it more than most other recent releases. However, this isn't saying much.*

The last sentence of this probably sums it up quite well. On each occasion it created a general headspace, but other than this, did not appear to be remarkable or particularly interesting. In fairness, this equally applies to the other *5-meo* compounds I have sampled.

Note that there were a few safety warnings in circulation at the time of testing, so caution is advised, certainly with respect to larger doses. Given my less than enthralling experiences and the doubts cast by these, I binned my remaining supply.

2.2.12 AL-LAD

Common Nomenclature	6-Allyl-6-nor-lysergic acid diethylamide
Street & Reference Names	Aladdin
Reference Dosage	Light 40ug+; Common 75ug+; Strong 175ug+; Heavy 250ug+; [TripSit] Threshold 20ug+; Light 50ug+; Common 100ug+; Strong 200ug+; Heavy 350ug+; [Psychonautwiki]
Anticipated: Onset / Duration	1 Hour / 7 Hours
Maximum Dose Experienced	150ug
Form	Blotter
RoA	Oral
Source / Jurisdiction	Internet / UK
Personal Rating On Shulgin Scale	+++

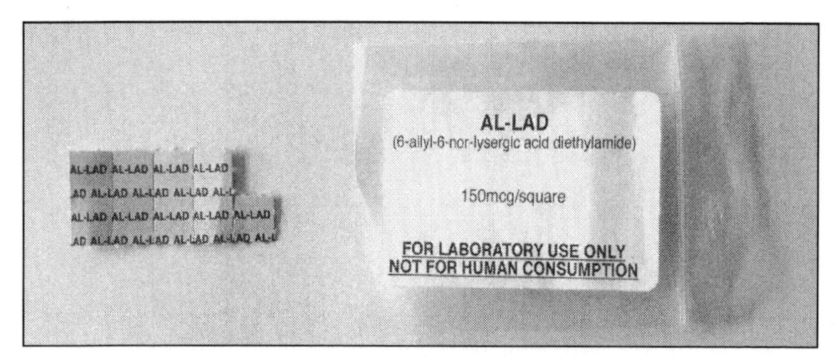

SUBJECTIVE EXPERIENCE
First synthesised in Japan in the 1970s, AL-LAD gained traction as a recreational psychedelic after it was included in Alexander Shulgin's second landmark book, *TiHKAL*. It became particularly popular from 2013, due to its wide scale availability as an Internet research chemical.

I have sampled AL-LAD on a number of previous occasions. I re-test it again today partly to do justice to it in terms of detail, but also because my memory refuses to distinguish it from LSD.

I elect to sample a small dose of 60ug, which is less than half my previous high dose, but nonetheless is within the range suggested online as *common*. I limit myself largely due to personal domestic circumstance: real life intervening again.

I note in reading the literature that Shulgin himself had this sort of cross to bear with this exact same chemical. On testing 50ug of AL-LAD he stated that:

> "*I am aware in twenty minutes, and am into a stoned place, not too LSD like, in another hour. I would very much like to push higher, but that is not in the cards today and I must acknowledge recovery by hour eight.*" ~ TiHKAL

Regarding the nature of trip itself, I don't recall the same degree of LSD-like *oneness* from my previous forays, but rather, more brightness of colours and a shorter ride. I hope that this experiment will clarify.

> T+0:00 I cut a 150ug square into half. I then take one half and also cut it into half. I then repeat this with one of the ¼ pieces, making one half of this a little larger than the other. I therefore have ½, ¼, ⅛- and ⅛+.
>
> I chew and swallow the ¼ and the ⅛+ which should approximate the requisite 60ug. I do realise that this isn't science at its best. [3pm]
>
> T+0:15 I have perhaps the first inkling that something may be occurring: a strange turn of headspace. When I think about it, perhaps colours become slightly more vibrant. We are, however, very much in the margins here. I listen to Alan Watts (philosopher) on YouTube to pass the time.
>
> T+0:40 Something is certainly happening now. The headspace is developing along with a comfort zone. I notice events through the window, such as a bird flying by, which catches my eye, and I actually watch it; which is something, of course, that I don't usually do.
>
> I drift slightly into unconscious thought, with a now dreamy sensibility. Physically the familiar tingly sensation is stirring.
>
> T+1:00 I find myself asking a number of questions: When is a trip a trip? Where exactly is the threshold and how do I define it?
>
> Here, now, I am clearly affected by this drug. The headspace has developed, colours are brighter, and my mind wanders where it would not normally wander. Having stated this, I am more or less completely functional and behaviourally normal if I choose to focus on being so.
>
> I feel like I am in a twilight zone between normality and tripping.
>
> I spot the ⅛- of the tab still on the desk, and given that this is so gentle, I decide to chew and swallow, taking the dose up to 75mg. This is still very much in the shallow end.
>
> T+1:15 I feel warm and content, and to a degree I am wallowing in the headspace.

As I contemplate generally I examine the question of horn. Yes, it is there if desired, but the issue I ponder is that sex is frequently considered to be a significant matter with respect to stimulants, which promote an animalistic lust. It is less debated with respect to psychedelics. Granted, this is possibly due to the more intellectual focus of the latter, and that thoughts can sometimes be too strange or weird to progress, but on the other hand, isn't human sexuality actually played out in the brain, via imagination, anticipation and thought?

I suddenly remember that I am tripping, and thus I am aware that everything I have just typed could be out of court.

T+1:30 I play some music, and it is easy to drift into. I am relaxed, but somehow my mind is hungry for elevation and stimulation. I am drawn to documentaries and information as a source of ideas and knowledge.

There is no adverse body load at all, although at times I feel slightly numb (physically) with ongoing tingles.

I feel the sort of mellow equanimity that I only really fall into via this class of psychedelic. I am usually in a rush, but not so when engaging. It occurs that intellectual stimulation is far easier to achieve if a pro-active decision is taken to stop and explore more slowly.

T+2:15 I am on a plateau and have been for some time, drifting in and out of different areas of interest. I can be functional if I need to be. This is a pleasant level.

T+3:00 A quality I find with most psychedelics is that the come-down is so gracious. You can start to leave the peak, and pass down through the main plateau, yet there is no urge to redose. The contentedness remains, even where the effects begin to dissipate.

This is what I feel now. I am still within the experience, very much so, but the intensity has declined from, for example, an hour ago. I feel fine about that. I am drifting nicely. The headspace is warm, even though signs of fatigue occasionally manifest. I am still in a very nice place.

I should state that this has largely been a cerebral type of expedition. There have been no overwhelming OEVs or CEVS, other than occasional bits and pieces as I stared into the garden. There has been a touch of morphing and some tracers and a little pattern recognition, but not as the central focus of proceedings.

I have an awareness of this aspect, but my mind is largely preoccupied by varying thoughts and inquiries and interests.

T+4:00 I am well on the way back to base, although the warmth and headspace creates the impression that the current state will linger for several hours. I feel a little worn out.

T+5:00 To snap out of the slumber I decide to walk to the local pool and take a swim. I have done this previously under the influence of lysergamides, and have found it to be refreshing and rewarding.

T+6:00 Mission accomplished: I returned from the pool safely, albeit having detoured to savour the outing.

When I do take myself out of the confines of the house, I always have the same feeling: I wish that I had stopped analysing and reflecting and opted for the open-air much earlier. It always takes me by surprise. In a sense it is like seeing the world for the first time; seeing it with new eyes.

I gaze around and I walk in wonder. I feel safe, and can take it all in, as though I am in a personal bubble. The colours, the sounds, the stillness, the entire scene is almost overwhelming in parts. It is beautiful.

The feeling is one of pro-actively observing it as an outsider, but from a vantage point of being within. It is a detachment that isn't really detached: one of being able to actually look, appreciate, and indeed, experience as a consciously separate entity. It is a unique type of awareness. It never fails to fill me with awe.

I promise myself that next time I use this class of chemical I will explore this much earlier in the trip.

I have enjoyed this ride immensely. Even after six hours I still feel positivity and a general vibe of well being.

I retired to bed at 11:30pm (T+8:30) and had a good night's sleep, interestingly, with deeper cycles than usual. There was also some vivid dreaming. I woke in the morning feeling refreshed and on form.

This is a chemical that has consistently delivered insight, fulfilment and positivity, with little or no body load. This occasion was no exception.

Unfortunately, it was formally banned by the UK government in January 2015, following earlier recommendations from its *Advisory Council on the Misuse of Drugs* (ACMD). It is noteworthy and indeed, politically revealing, that this body had failed to identify any harm associated with its use.

[*Shulgin Reference: TiHKAL #1, p391*]

2.2.13 AMT

Common Nomenclature	Alpha-Methyltryptamine
Street & Reference Names	N/A
Reference Dosage	Threshold 5mg+; Light 10mg+; Common 20mg+; Strong 30mg+; Heavy 60mg+ [Erowid] Light 15mg+; Common 25mg+; Strong 40mg+; Heavy 60mg+; [TripSit]
Anticipated: Onset / Duration	1 Hour / 12 Hours
Maximum Dose Experienced	40mg
Form	Pill
RoA	Oral
Source / Jurisdiction	Internet / UK
Personal Rating On Shulgin Scale	++

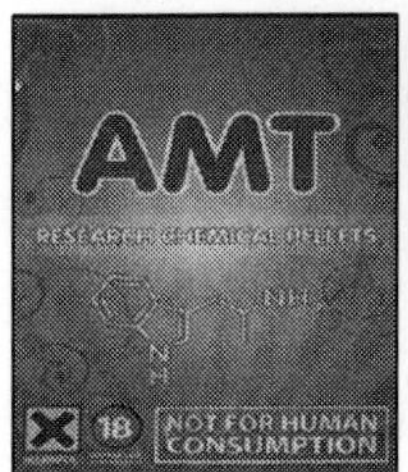

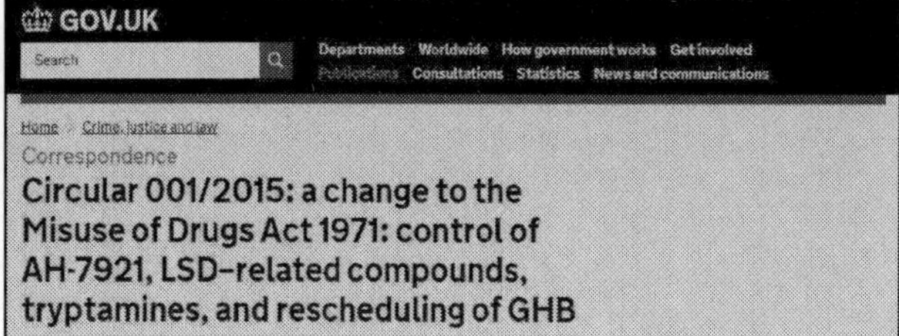

SUBJECTIVE EXPERIENCE

This is one that almost got away. It was a freebie; a single pill in a packet, given to me by a head shop in Manchester after I had purchased a number of other items, and engaged in a chat about the market. It was months later that I decided to try it, albeit with a little trepidation, given multiple online reports of high body load.

I experienced relatively little in terms of nausea or general malaise, but equally, not an all firing or visual psychedelic trip either. Yes, I was psychoactively aware, with a vague psychedelic headspace, but it was not a particularly strong or exciting one.

Unable to have a second spin of the wheel, with AMT no longer available, I could only speculate three reasons: I didn't take enough (despite reference dose sources indicating otherwise), the AMT had degraded by the time I consumed it or the set and setting was wrong for the context of the trip.

If it was still accessible I would probably sample this again, but under significantly different conditions.

[*Shulgin Reference: TiHKAL #48, p654*]

2.2.14 BK-2C-B

Common Nomenclature	beta-keto 2C-B
Street & Reference Names	Beta-keto
Reference Dosage	Threshold 50mg+; Common 80mg+; Strong 100mg+; Heavy 150mg+ [TripSit] Threshold 50mg+; Light 60mg+; Common 80 mg+; Strong 100mg+; Heavy 150mg+ [Psychonautwiki]
Anticipated: Onset / Duration	30 Minutes / 10 Hours
Maximum Dose Experienced	82mg
Form	Pill
RoA	Oral
Source / Jurisdiction	Internet / UK
Personal Rating On Shulgin Scale	++*

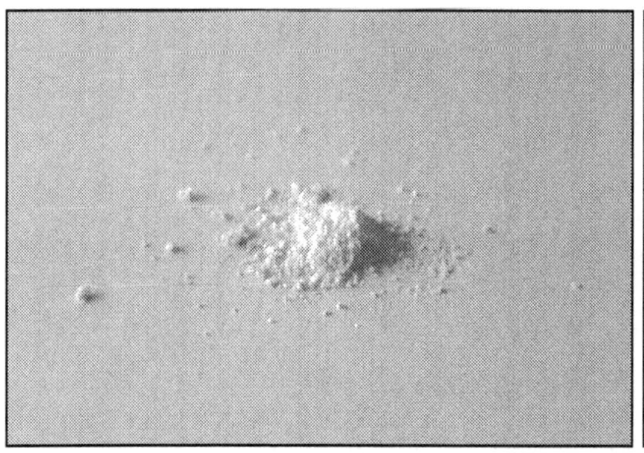
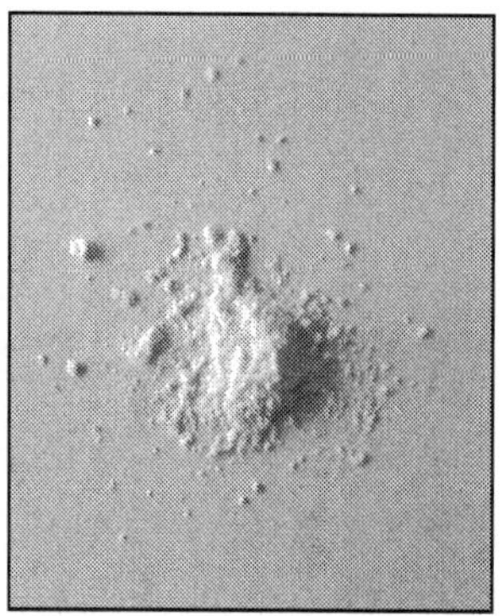

SUBJECTIVE EXPERIENCE
BK-2C-B began to appear on the markets in 2013. Whilst it did not generate any particular fanfare or excitement, it was consistently available, and over the following years was sampled by relatively large numbers.

From my own perspective, its long duration provided something of a deterrent: writing off at least a day to test it wasn't the easiest commitment to make. However, in 2014 I gave it a spin.

The results were disappointing. I experienced a mild psychedelic buzz, with minor body and head stimulation. This was at such a low level that it was difficult to document in much detail.

Subsequently, I discovered that the likely reason for this was that its effects are diluted considerably if it is mixed with water upon ingestion. Further research indicated that the usual *modus operandi* was to bomb it in a gel cap, or in cigarette paper, with an acid based drink.

Regarding dose, online trip reports suggested that the effects were extremely variable. Some people experienced intensity at well under 100mg, whereas others felt very little, replicating my own story.

For this experiment, and after much deliberation, I decided to dose at 80mg. I based this upon my new found knowledge regarding acidity, and on the generic recommendations of the major harm reduction communities.

I had BK-2-CB samples available in both pill and powder form. I chose to proceed with powder, simply because I could weigh this with greater precision.

I embarked upon the exercise with an empty stomach and low expectations.

> T+0:00 I attempt to measure 80mg, but 82mg drops on to the scale. I bomb it in rizla cigarette paper with a glass of orange juice. [3pm]
>
> T+0:40 Earlier than I anticipated something is emerging: a hazy drifty headspace. This is minor but clearly present. I also feel slight physical warmth, and a mild anxiolytic effect is taking hold.
>
> T+1:00 A heady psychedelic feel is now firmly in place. Visually, a blurry sheen has developed, which is emphasised when I change my field of focus. There could be an impression of after-images and diffraction, but there is no significant distortion, and no movement (morphing, breathing, etc). I feel a little distant, but quite relaxed.
>
> I am warm with a general overlay of body tingles. With the latter aspect in play I can understand why some people consider this to be a sex enhancing drug.
>
> T+1:30 All the previous effects are now well established, and this is quite a pleasant journey. I do feel some body strain, but nothing excessive. It is certainly one of the tingliest and most physical psychedelics I have experienced.
>
> Although it lacks the intellectual depth of the lysergamides, the head buzz is quite intense, and the hazy visual sheen is stronger than it was earlier.
>
> I am well into ++ territory on the Shulgin scale, but not quite touching +++. I am functional, but I am at the point at which it is increasingly difficult to hide my tripping status. I certainly have to avoid anything other than brief episodes of communication with third parties.

T+2:00 The onset is definitely complete, and I have stabilised on a plateau. It remains very physical, with almost constant tingles, and the head haze continues unabated.

T+3:00 The experience has calmed, and is drifting towards the lower end of the ++ range. I am comfortable, with the sentient flushes of body awareness interjecting from time to time. The headspace is now sufficiently mild that I could happily socialize in the right company.

T+4:00 I have now moved into a period of lower level psychedelic glow. The headspace is gentle and can be pushed into the background at will, and the physicality is gently tumbling along.

This has been extremely tactile, with body sensitivity greatly enhanced. This facet reminds me of Shulgin's statements with respect to 2C-B and sexuality. Under the right circumstances this aspect would clearly be supercharged.

There is a degree of mental fatigue entering the fray, but given its positivity I seek to make the most of the longevity of the experience.

T+5:00 The show is over to the extent that the main act has left the stage. I am still lapping up the dying embers of what has been an excellent ride. Although there are no more fireworks to be seen; I continue to bask in a lower level psychedelic aura.

It is comfortable and I am relaxed, but all intensity has departed. Even so, I remain in a place from which I am in no hurry to leave. Indeed, I hope that the claims that this lasts for many more hours are accurate.

At this point it seems that *Psychonautwiki* wasn't far off the mark with this comment:

> *"The effects of this compound are described as considerably more stimulating and less psychedelic with a longer duration in comparison to its close structural relative 2C-B"*

Perhaps there is also an empathogenic edge lurking, along with the usual softening of ego.

Although it is rather late in the game I check my pupils in the mirror. They are dilated: the left more than the right. I've no idea what this means, if anything.

T+7:00 The last two hours passed quickly, as I was consumed in a Terence McKenna lecture, courtesy of YouTube.

T+8:00 The headspace still lingers, as does the tranquillity, and I remain quite happy. I notice belatedly that audio seems to be enhanced. I should have explored this earlier.

T+9:00 I take 0.5mg of etizolam as a sleep aid, and retire to bed.

T+10:00 Whilst I lie in bed and close my eyes, mild CEVs are present. This is something else I should have explored earlier!

The night's sleep was undisturbed, but was not long enough. In the morning I was mentally fatigued, and an early nap was already on my mind as I prepared for the day. Unfortunately, I still felt some psychedelic stimulation and edge, so this was not going to be possible.

In terms of duration, this was certainly a long one, and it took its toll. Having said this, my general mood remained elevated and I was relaxed, so the prolonged length was not all negative.

Regarding dose, it transpired that 80mg was plenty, and the fruit juice trick was entirely effective.

For years I looked down on this drug with a snobbish too-familiar attitude: it was so widely available yet there were so few enthusiasts. However, it surprised me. I had an excellent time. Body load was a little too high, but perhaps this was the cost of the thrill and exhilaration of the tactility.

I am glad that I procured enough to engage a few more trips before the counterproductive axe of the *Psychoactive Substances Act* made it impossible to source.

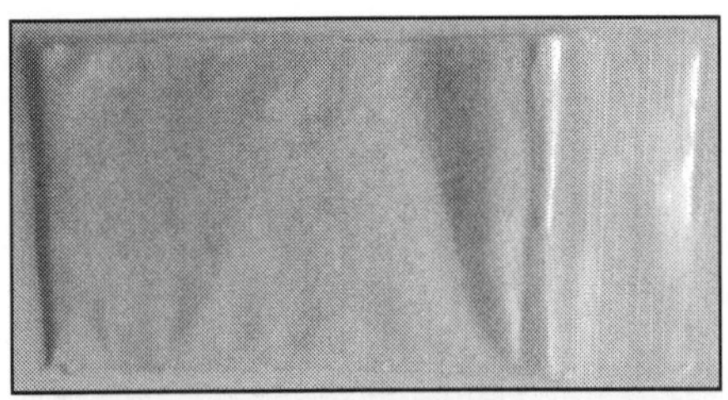

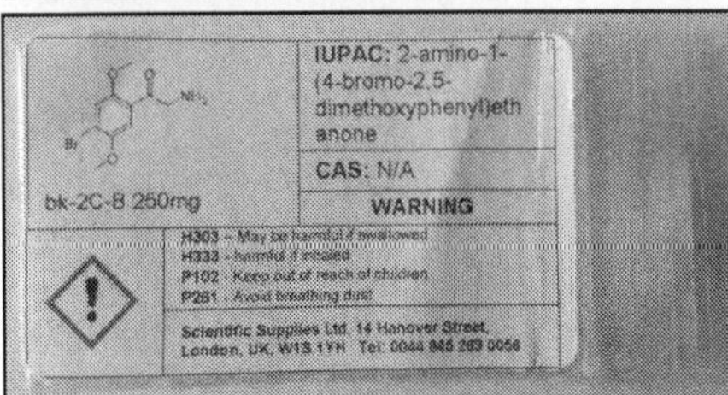

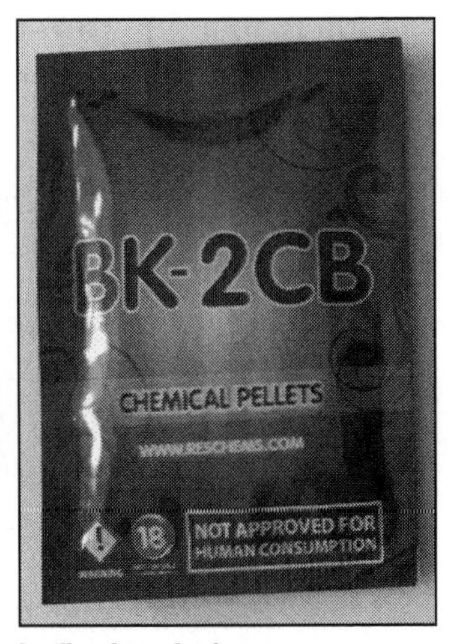

BK-2C-B was commonly available in both pill and powder form.

2.2.15 Changa

Common Nomenclature	Changa
Major Active Compound	DMT (Mimosa Hostilis)
Street & Reference Names	Changa; Aussiewaska
Anticipated: Onset / Duration	30 Seconds / 30 Minutes
Maximum Dose Experienced	Unknown
Form	Plant Material
RoA	Smoked
Source / Jurisdiction	Dealer / Overseas

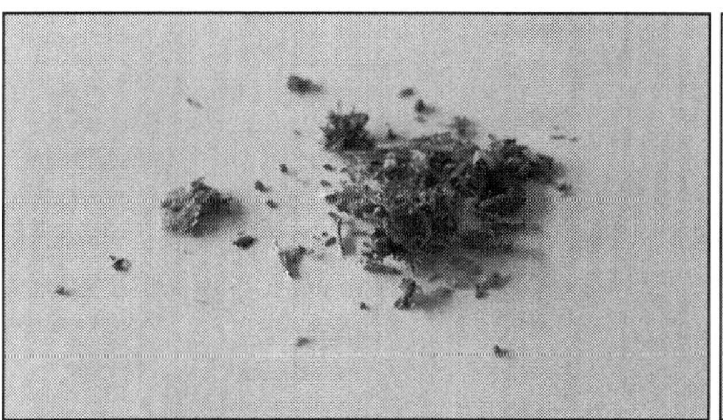

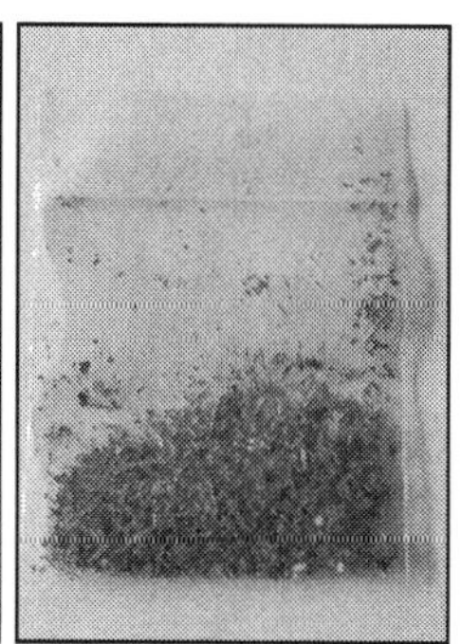

SUBJECTIVE EXPERIENCE

Changa is commonly defined as a DMT-infused smoking blend. More specifically, it is DMT (or a DMT containing plant) combined with a MAOI, the latter being a *monoamine oxidase inhibitor*, which prevents the former from being broken down before it can become psychoactive.

It is believed to have originated in Australia, circa 2001, where enthusiasm for this field of interest can only have increased following a visit by Terence McKenna in 1997. With reference to this, I have also seen changa referred to colloquially as *Aussiewaska* (ref ayahuasca). Note too that locally there are a significant number of DMT bearing plants available, including the national flower, the *Golden Wattle.*

In terms of risk and potential harm, MAOIs must generally be treated with extreme caution. Even cursory research reveals a host of dangers. Wikipedia, for example, is explicit:

> *"MAOIs should not be combined with other psychoactive substances (antidepressants, painkillers, stimulants, both legal and illegal etc.) except under expert care. Certain combinations can cause lethal reactions..."*

The extent of the risk is variable, but this is, absolutely, not an aspect to treat lightly. If you are unable to leave a clear drug-free run before and after using an MAOI, the potential interactions and perils must be investigated thoroughly.

Whilst the most common RoA for DMT is undoubtedly vaporization, the changa smoking method brings its own attributes. For example, it prolongs the duration, and is considered by many to make the experience more coherent in nature.

Regarding my own exploration, my host assured me that the changa was 50% strong. The DMT source, *mimosa hostilis*, was apparently imported from Brazil.

On the issue of execution, YouTube videos suggest that most users smoke from a pipe or a small bong, and usually hold for about 5 seconds or so, albeit with some holding longer. All seem to fall deep into an abyss, but simultaneously retain overall control and an awareness of sober reality, with many able to narrate their experience in real time. It is hard to gauge how much they immerse into the real *McKenna-esque* DMT space, and how much they just skim the surface.

Note that I recorded this trip retrospectively due to incapacity during the journey itself. With an experienced *sitter* in situ I launched the experiment at 7pm.

> Using a small water bong, I filled the bowl, fired up, and inhaled lightly but solidly. It was quite a harsh and not particularly pleasant smoke.

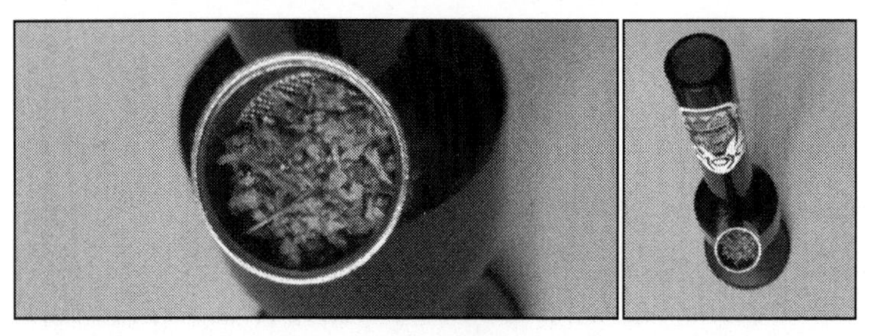

> The general headspace quickly emerged, and was hard to distinguish from that of previous DMT exploits. The visuals, however, were sustained rather than fleeting, enabling a different perspective.
>
> With eyes closed I entered a vibrantly colourful interior chamber, adorned with clearly defined architraved polygonal features, which were drifting gently. This was not threatening, but rather a little unsettling. I was in full possession of my faculties and was able to analyse and contemplate.
>
> When I opened my eyes, the visuals were still there, but only as a semi-transparent sheen. This strengthened and weakened, and hovered between myself and the wall beyond. When I focused upon it, the field solidified and floated towards me, such that the objects seemed to drift into my chest if I followed them downwards to my now horizontal body.

Unlike the strange snake-like intertwining CEVs I had experienced with psilocybe, these comprised a manufactured worldly construct: an actual indoor environment rather than a pattern.

Perhaps 5 minutes into the trip, curiosity got the better of me, and I took another toke. The same phenomena continued but the construct was strengthened and perhaps more stable. My earlier anxiety was dissipating as I came to terms with the alien strangeness.

After another few minutes I re-loaded the bowl and took a third toke, holding for approximately 6-8 seconds.

I was, by now, confident enough to face the exterior world. I walked into what was a typical suburban rear garden, similar to my own back home. I was in for a surprise.

Beneath my feet the lawn presented an incredible sight. I saw it as a mini-forest of individual clusters of grass-plants, which were swaying and moving in unison. They were lush and vibrant and alive as they danced and drifted in harmony before my eyes. The patterns they formed were clearly evident (the technical term for which is appropriately *pattern recognition*).

As I looked towards the wooden lattice on the fence, this too was drifting and swaying, and moving back and forth, with the overlapping wood presenting a rhythmic three dimensional interplay. Again, it was extremely colourful, dollhouse-effect-like in appearance, and seemed almost alive.

Everything in sight was gently ebbing and flowing, with objects shifting seamlessly and elegantly in relation to each other. I felt comfortable, almost in awe, as I watched and gazed.

With the entire visual field in motion, the fabric of reality itself seemed to be coming apart. Indeed, at one point this notion was so plausible that I contemplated what would be behind it should it break any further.

Walking back across the lawn towards the house, I stopped again, as the grass itself was simply astonishing. It really was like a like a miniature woodland in its own right, dancing in the non-existent breeze as I floated over it.

In the house the shag pile rug exhibited a similar moving effect. Although not as rich or marvellous, it was still alive in terms of motion and movement.

I was pro-actively navigating the experience. I could choose to tune into the visuals (OEV or CEV), allowing myself to be semi-immersed, drifting into the headspace and flowing with it. Or I could pull myself out and try, with some difficulty, to manage normal reality and discern the unfolding manifestations from the outside.

I have adopted the word *tuneable* to describe this measure of control, as it does seem to fit the capacity to direct the trip from a higher level of consciousness.

As the effects of the changa slowly diminished I was still able to enter the fading world of colour and pattern when I closed my eyes, and see into the sheen as I opened them, until this too gradually waned.

On a time check I noted that it was 7:25pm: the entire exercise had lasted about 25 minutes. It seemed much longer. I was still experiencing a certain headiness, and a glow, but the visible *other-worldiness* had gone.

An hour after the experience, the headiness was still present, but was less intense. I felt much more relaxed and serene than I had before embarking upon the experiment, and indeed, than I had for some time.

Although not particularly tired, I retired to bed at midnight, about 5 hours after initial inhalation, and fell asleep reasonably swiftly. I awoke a couple of times during the night, with a mild headache, which was wrapped in the heady feel of the trip afterglow. I also experienced a significant degree of lucid dreaming.

During the following morning I felt more tired than usual, with some mental fatigue, and a slight ongoing headache. It may well be relevant that the latter is frequently reported as a side effect of MAOIs.

Overall changa provided an extraordinarily rich and vivid experience. I engaged in a real and distinct journey of colour and wonder. Having stated this, I feel that I skirted the edges of its potential and that I could have gone deeper and immersed more completely. Should future circumstances allow, I will endeavour to do so.

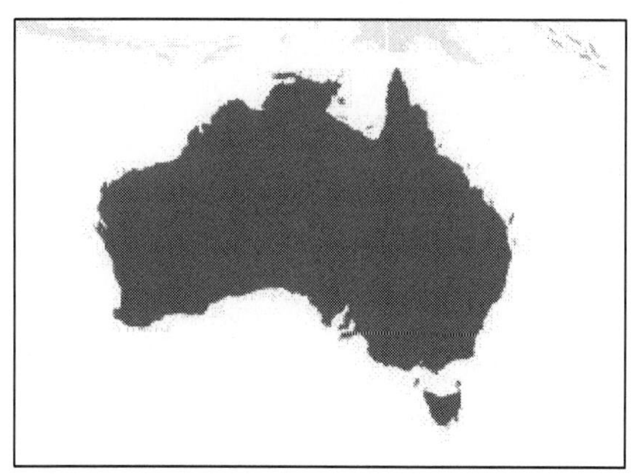

Aussiewaska: an unexpected origin but a predictable name

2.2.16 DMT

Common Nomenclature	N,N-Dimethyltryptamine
Street & Reference Names	N,N-DMT; Dimitri; The Spirit Molecule
Reference Dosage	Threshold 2mg+; Light 10mg+; Medium 20mg+; Strong 40mg+ [Drugs-Forum] Threshold 2mg+; Light 10mg+; Common 20mg+; Strong 40mg+ [Erowid] Threshold 5mg+; Light 10mg+; Common 15mg+; Strong 25mg+; Heavy 35mg+ [TripSit]
Anticipated: Onset / Duration	20 Seconds / 6 Minutes
Maximum Dose Experienced	20mg
Form	Powder
RoA	Vaporised
Source / Jurisdiction	Dealer / Overseas
Personal Rating On Shulgin Scale	+++

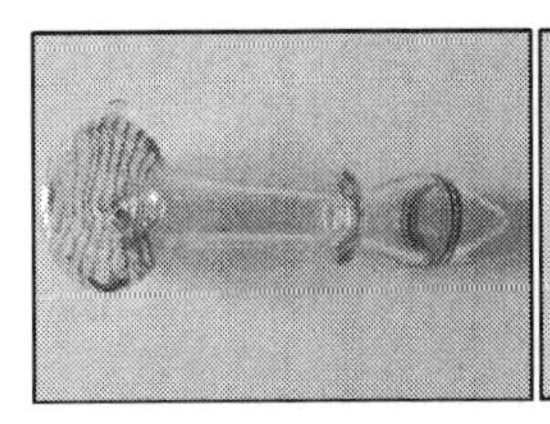

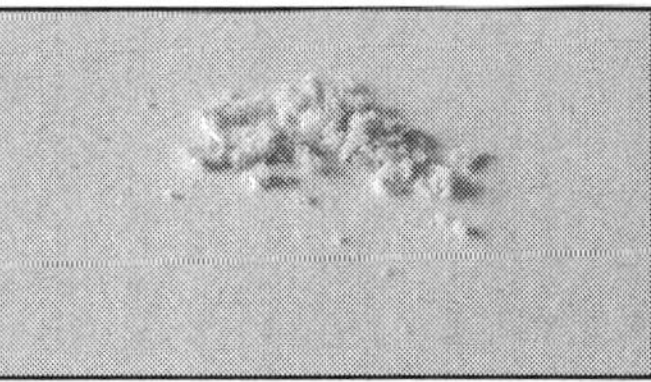

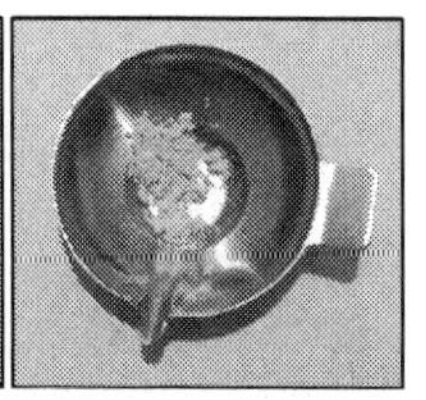

SUBJECTIVE EXPERIENCE
Despite invoking what is possibly the most intense of psychedelic experiences, DMT is found naturally within the human cerebrospinal system and elsewhere. Indeed, it is frequently suggested that it is excreted by the pineal gland (in the centre of the brain). Outside the human organism it is also present in mammals and many species of plants, seemingly permeating nature itself.

Whilst I had previously engaged DMT as an ingredient of ayahuasca, smoking the raw molecule produces a radically different and less gentle type of experience. Unfortunately, smoking an effective *breakthrough* dose to achieve this is frequently reported as being a difficult operation to execute.

The trick is to vaporize the crystals, rather than to burn them, which is apparently easier said than done. Nonetheless, I set about the task with diligence and patience.

BREAKTHROUGH ATTEMPT #1
For this attempt I obtained a glass pipe, courtesy of Amazon, for a grand total of £5.95 (see image above). I began the experiment at 10am.

I placed 20mg of DMT into the pipe, and carefully heated the bottom of the bowl with a lighter. As smoke began to appear, I inhaled, slowly. Nothing happened; so I repeated several times until the crystals had all disappeared.

There were no hallucinations and no trip. There was an extremely mild psychedelic type headspace, which lasted an hour or so. That was it.

My conclusion was that I must have burned the DMT, or even swallowed some of the crystals before they melted. This was an abject failure.

BREAKTHROUGH ATTEMPT #2

Further research led me to buy a *VaporGenie*. This was a much more expensive device, but contributors across multiple forums claimed great success in using it to breakthrough. Regardless, it still sounded like a fiddly exercise to undertake.

The experiment began at 7:30pm. I placed 22mg into the chamber of the VaporGenie on top of a damiana ash bed, and sprinkled some further ashes on top. On heating I inhaled, trying not to suck the flame deep enough into the device to touch the DMT. I held the smoke nervously for 10 seconds and then exhaled. I saw smoke dissipate into the air as I did so.

I knew that I was under some sort of influence almost immediately. I lay down, placed my head on to a cushion and closed my eyes, largely because I was chicken and didn't want to see the world actually disintegrate before me.

The problem was that it didn't. I missed the breakthrough again, and I missed the famed chrysanthemum too (the alleged prelude to entering the main hallucinogenic event).

However, what I did see were some glorious CEVs. There were concave adornments on the walls of wherever I was. They were morphing a little, but were largely stable and were of rich beautiful colours.

As I opened my eyes to check the real world status this vision immediately disappeared. There were no OEVs of any significance, so I closed my eyes again. Unfortunately, I couldn't reach the same clarity or intensity as moments ago. However, what I had seen was *somewhere*; not just patterns, but actual walls with indented window type alcoves (but without transparency). It was like some grand medieval castle-like interior, but bright, perfect and extremely colourful.

I was feeling fine, and not so scared, so I lit up again, inhaled, and held for another ten seconds. This time I didn't notice any smoke or vapour.

I embraced the notion that closing my eyes was a little like tuning into a frequency. I simply chose to go there. It was a strange feeling.

I searched for the other-worldly interior again. There were CEVs but not enough to frame the place. I suspect that the DMT may well have been largely used or burned on the first hit.

I chased it three more times over the next 10 minutes, but all I could find was the headspace and the colours.

I opened the pipe: only ashes remained.

I actually got somewhere with this attempt, but not far enough. However, I was encouraged sufficiently to promise myself that I would try this again soon, using the same technique, but being more careful with the flame, and perhaps holding the smoke for longer.

I would say the duration of the main play was around 6 minutes, as generally advertised.

As an experience it was perfectly fine, with interesting visuals, a nice headspace, a certain contentment, a short duration, no body load, and some afterglow. Without having some knowledge of where DMT can lead when fully charged, I suspect that I would have been extremely happy with this, but I was disappointed not to have broken through. I was determined to be bolder next time.

Note that my subsequent sleep pattern was a little disrupted with several wake-ups and some weird vivid dreams. Retro checking on the Internet, I learned that this is quite a common phenomenon. This continued into a second night, with sleep cycles broken by dreams which were sometimes not very positive.

BREAKTHROUGH ATTEMPT #3

This time I measured 35mg and mixed it with the remaining ashes from *Attempt #2*. I prepared in the same manner and initiated the experiment.

I misfired again, but I instantly understood why. I felt powder enter my mouth as I inhaled. This was DMT and ash; unvaporised. I had inhaled too strongly, and it was apparent that the chemical was not entrenched sufficiently below the ash, which itself was not heavy enough.

The experience itself was much like a re-run of the second attempt, but the visuals were more intense. Was that the initial framing of the famed orange chrysanthemum I saw during the first few seconds? Perhaps, but it dissipated very quickly, just as it started to form.

I felt a strange analgesic numbness of the body as I lay on the ground, and again failed to recapture the same visual intensity once I had opened my eyes. There were OEVs, but the real action was on the back of my eyelids.

Subsequently, Sleep was again disturbed, with strange vivid dreaming.

Retrospectively, I feel that I should try to compare this with salvia divinorum, which was the source of my first alien-reality type of encounter.

My experience of smoking salvia was of being pulled into a bright and lucidly coloured out-of-body domain, which comprised sharp threatening echoed shapes, framed on my original field of vision. I felt that my mind was being dragged outwards into this abyss, as I struggled in absolute terror. This is considered by many to be a form of delirium. However, given that oral consumption produces a different response, I wouldn't classify it as such.

DMT produced similarly wonderful colours, but it presented an actual locale, the timeline was ordered, and there was no fear. Also, at the doses I sampled, I had the capacity to proactively tune in to this construct, rather than being suddenly wrenched into an inferno.

This intelligible character of ordered enfoldment is, in fact, the major difference between DMT and the other psychedelic chemicals I have so far tested. With DMT I wasn't experiencing a variation of where I was at the moment I inhaled, but rather, I found myself in entirely different surroundings, which had appeared from nowhere. I had my faculties intact and my mind was rational, but I was transplanted into an unknown setting, which appeared to comprise some sort of other-reality. This wasn't random patterns or shapes or bright lights, it was an actual place. This, of course, renders it astonishing.

At some point in the future I will be drawn to a 4th attempt.

[*Reference: Rick Strassman DMT: The Spirit Molecule*]
[*Shulgin Reference: TiHKAL #6, p412*]

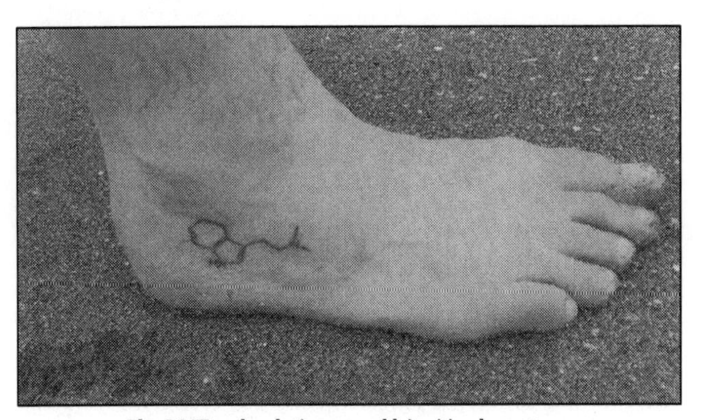

The DMT molecule (on my ankle)... it's a long story.

2.2.17 LSD

Common Nomenclature	D-lysergic Acid Diethylamide
Street & Reference Names	Lucy; Acid;
Reference Dosage	Threshold 20ug+; Light 25ug+; Common 50ug+; Strong 150ug+; Heavy 400ug+ [Erowid] Threshold 25ug+; Light 50ug+; Common 75ug+; Strong 200ug+; Heavy 400ug+ [Psychonautwiki] Light 50ug+; Common 75ug+; Strong 175ug+; Heavy 250ug+ [TripSit]
Anticipated: Onset / Duration	1 Hour / 12 Hours
Maximum Dose Experienced	Not Known [Two Blotters]
Form	Blotter
RoA	Oral
Personal Rating On Shulgin Scale	++

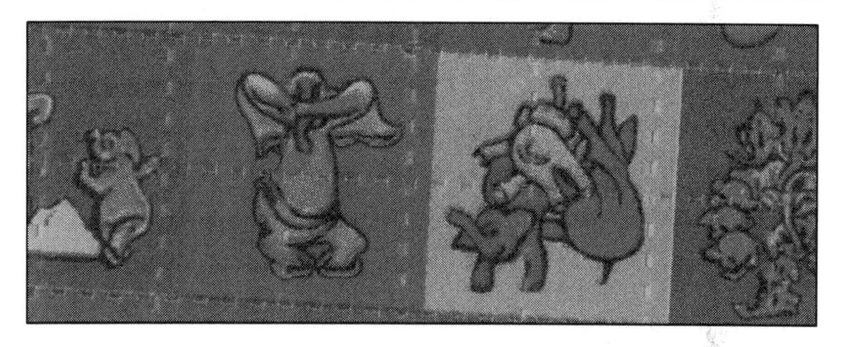

SUBJECTIVE EXPERIENCE
Famously discovered by Albert Hoffman in 1938, the recreational use of LSD exploded in the 1960's. It was central to the counterculture revolution, having a profound influence which spanned far beyond art and music, and eventually touched most facets of society.

Its value in the fields of psychiatry and psychology as an agent to alleviate human misery was quickly established. Countless studies emerged as research flourished, particularly across the United States.

This all came to an abrupt end, courtesy of Richard Milhous Nixon and the *war on drugs*. Indeed, LSD was made an initial and prime target. Research was unceremoniously halted, thousands were imprisoned and psychedelic study and exploration was driven underground.

My own experience with LSD unfolded during the folly of youth. I managed to acquire two blotters, and consumed one of them on a clear warm Sunday afternoon. I remained indoors waiting for something to happen.

After an indeterminate period of time I deemed that the blotter must have been a dud, and I swallowed the second. Within perhaps ten minutes a trip started to materialise. My immediate reaction was to panic: what if this was the first blotter taking effect?

Fortunately, after being informed that I was an idiot, I was reassured by my less than impressed sitter, and I calmed down considerably.

My recollections are somewhat vague, but a fascination with various shapes, patterns and materials was memorable. I also recall that there was some horn present at one point. More radical was my experience when I was eventually taken on an evening walk.

The perspective was something akin to the *dollhouse effect*, in which the exterior appeared to be so tranquil that I perceived it as part of a giant interior. I noticed chimneys, telegraph poles, and items not normally on my conscious visible radar. The sky appeared as a ceiling, almost touchable, and was totally non-threatening.

I felt no nausea or negativity at all. It was a pleasant experience, albeit a gentle one.

This was my first foray into the realms of psychedelia and it would leave a long term impression, although not as a result of any form of trauma or extreme stimulation. It was profound: the temporary shift in perception was to have a permanent and positive influence on my worldview.

> *"I believe it's true to say that everyone who has experienced LSD or another psychedelic would look on that experience, especially the first one, as a major life-changing event."* ~ Ralph Metzner

Now, many years later, I can align elements of this trip with more recent experimentation with 1p-LSD and other lysergamides. That intimate relationship with the outdoors and nature, the wonderment of the visuals, the delicate excitation of the other senses, the aura of the headspace: all ebb and flow to differing degrees between each experience.

As LSD is almost indistinguishable from 1p-LSD, I have attempted to more fully document the trip experience itself within the entry for the latter. Needless to say, I hope to have many more encounters in the future.

[*Shulgin Reference: TiHKAL #26, p490*]

2.2.18 LSZ

Common Nomenclature	Lysergic Acid 2,4-Dimethylazetidide
Street & Reference Names	Diazedine, Lambda
Reference Dosage	Threshold 10ug+; Light 50ug+; Common 100ug+; Strong 200ug+ [Erowid] Threshold 80ug+; Light 100ug+; Common 150ug+; Heavy 300ug+ [TripSit] Threshold 50ug+; Light 100ug+; Common 150ug+; Strong 300ug+; Heavy 400ug+ [Psychonautwiki]
Anticipated: Onset / Duration	45 Minutes / 8 Hours
Maximum Dose Experienced	60ug+15ug
Form	Blotter
RoA	Oral
Source / Jurisdiction	Internet / UK
Personal Rating On Shulgin Scale	++

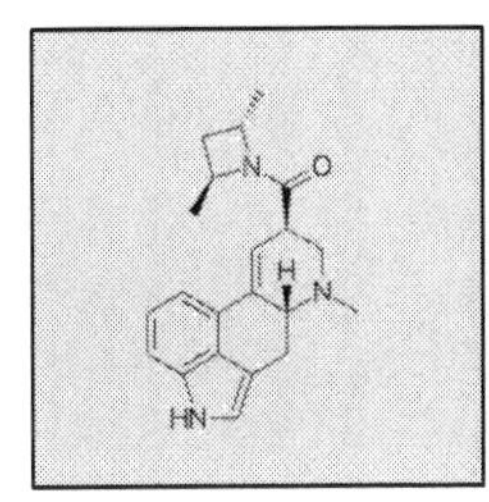

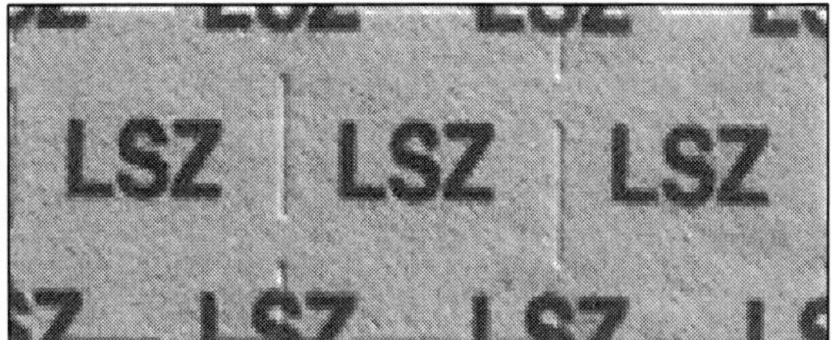

SUBJECTIVE EXPERIENCE
This one is tricky: as in my personal inability to distinguish between the varying effects of the different lysergamides.

I understood that 75ug was a small dose, but I only possessed three blotters in total, and I wanted to test gently. Nonetheless, the familiar headspace soon emerged, as did a nice mood elevation.

It is commonly claimed that LSZ offers more introspection than its more popular sisters, LSD and AL-LAD. I looked for this, but didn't really find it. Regardless, the few low-end trips I experienced were very enjoyable.

In retrospect, I should have gone higher whilst this was still on the market. Having stated this, I have no reason to believe that it would have produced a significantly different experience to that of its close relatives (see previous reports).

2.3. STIMULANTS

Textbook Definition: *Stimulants, or 'stims', enhance or improve mental and/or physical capability or function. Manifestations of this can include alertness, wakefulness, focus, and apparent increased energy. As a consequence, stimulants are sometimes referred to as 'uppers'.*

The following chemicals have been sampled and researched for inclusion within this section:

2.3.1 2AI
2.3.2 3,4 CTMP
2.3.3 3-FPM
2.3.4 4-FA
2.3.5 4-Me-TMP
2.3.6 4F-EPH
2.3.7 4F-MPH
2.3.8 Adderall
2.3.9 Amphetamine
2.3.10 Caffeine
2.3.11 Cocaine
2.3.12 EPH
2.3.13 HDMP-28
2.3.14 Hexen
2.3.15 IPPH
2.3.16 Methamphetamine
2.3.17 Methylphenidate
2.3.18 MPA
2.3.19 NM2AI
2.3.20 PPH
2.3.21 Pipradrol
2.3.22 TPA

There is more to stimulants than meets the eye, or less metaphorically, the nose. In a previous era, if someone had given me something to stimulate, I would simply have expected to be more awake and alert. After all, by definition shouldn't stims always increase energy and improve productivity and functionality?

For some highly functional stims, this is exactly what occurs. They improve focus and drive, and allow tasks to be completed with vigour and efficiency. But many stims have certain *edges*: a hint of euphoria, an empathogenic twist, or an awakened sexual appetite.

Those edges tend to bring joy and pleasure, all experienced on the high octane fuel of the stim itself. They can lead to binges, which can in turn become out of control and run headlong into the danger zone.

The risks associated with misuse of drugs in this class are well documented, with cases of overdose and addiction frequently reported. Increased heart rate and blood pressure can quickly escalate to heart attack, seizure or stroke. Psychosis is also a real threat, and one which should not be underestimated.

Long term use of some of these chemicals comes with a host of potential problems, including respiratory disorders, severe weight loss, gastrointestinal issues, kidney and liver damage, sexual dysfunctionality, tissue breakdown, acute depression, tooth decay, and paranoia.

There are other physical issues to consider too. Loss of appetite can be viewed as positive or negative, but the threat of dehydration is always something to be aware of, and the comedown can be difficult, as can the hangover.

It is always sensible, and strongly recommended, to plan ahead and tread carefully, particularly if larger doses or redosing is being contemplated.

Note also that mixing stims with alcohol is most definitely not a good idea. Research intensively, prior to contemplating any combination.

Be careful.

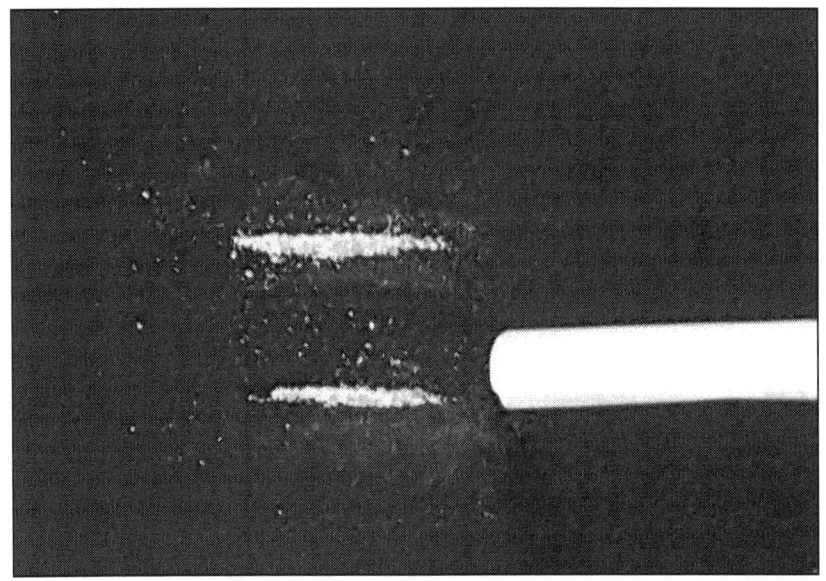

Stimulants are commonly insufflated, but many are ingested.
Attention to dosage for your specific RoA is therefore essential.

THE STIM BINGE
It begins in anticipation of seemingly eternal joy and ends in the curse of guilt and regret. Often, far more often than most non-users imagine, it is co-fuelled by the most carnal of desires and needs, which serve to drive it to even greater heights and subsequent lows.

When interviewed I am sometimes asked why I refer to libido and arousal so brazenly in this book, particularly in this section. The answer is because for so many users it is an intrinsic facet of the experience, for better and for worse. A cursory glance through Internet forums on the subject will confirm the scale, and that it would be wholly remiss to ignore it.

The following Reddit post provides a glimpse into the world of the stim-binge addict:

> *"Just like a romance, a stim binge starts so optimistically, every second is perfect, with so many perfect seconds to come. Then the realization that much time has actually passed, with little notice, or recollection of what exactly filled the time, and all you know is that it was happy time, and dreamily surrender to your most basic desires, the customary shame that accompanies the fulfilment of these desires is absent, you are psychologically shielded from any thoughts that may disturb your impossibly content state of mind, except one nagging thought does occasionally sneak in and remind you that time is passing, and this bliss cannot last forever. You try to prolong your special state, use any pretext you can find to convince yourself that you deserve just a little longer before going back. Your former euphoria is now greatly diminished by the mental (sleep) and physical (food) requirements that you have been ignoring all this time. Your medicine is weaker, and tastes worse, and the thought of the approaching end of the holiday itself ends the holiday. Goodbye lover, until next time. I will remember this feeling, but curiously forget every other specific detail of how 72 hours was spent. "Fuuuuucck 72 hours !? Kill me. Why is my crotch sore?", and other unwelcome observations in succession. The optimism that began the run is vanished completely, replaced with the equally thought dominating consequences of what suddenly seems like a bad trade, a regret, a lesson to not do this again. But in a few days, your desire for another little vacation begins to return at the precise rate that your recollection of the aftermath fades away. The cycle of escapism spins round like a pookie, or some more poetic simile."* ~ Rhinestonecowboyaway, Reddit

And so it goes, binge-to-binge.

Because the above comment is cleverly written it provokes a smile, dark humour. Really though, it isn't funny at all, and it definitely isn't where you want to be. You have a life to live, the pleasure from which shouldn't be driven by a drug which will slowly but surely lead to your physical and mental deterioration.

If you are going to take any of these drugs love 'em and leave 'em. Don't return in the short term, if ever. If you allow them to become routine or your primary source of pleasure in life, you will be in serious peril, and you may not escape it.

2.3.1 2-AI

Common Nomenclature	2-Aminoindane
Street & Reference Names	N/A
Reference Dosage	Threshold 3mg+; Light 5mg+; Common 10mg+; Strong 20mg+ [TripSit] Threshold 3mg+; Light 5mg+; Common 10mg+; Strong 20mg+; Heavy 40mg+ [Psychonautwiki]
Anticipated: Onset / Duration	15 Minutes / 2 Hours
Maximum Dose Experienced	20mg
Form	Powder
RoA	Oral
Source / Jurisdiction	Internet / UK

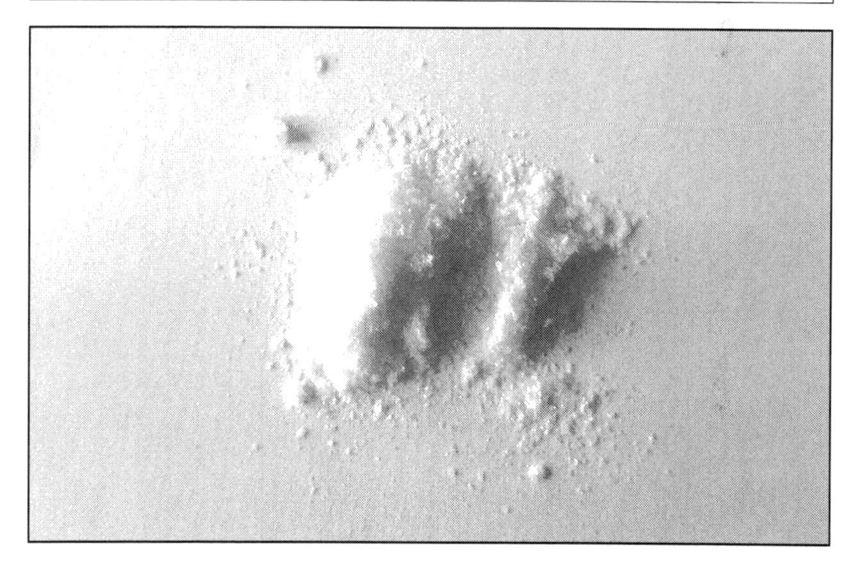

SUBJECTIVE EXPERIENCE
2-AI first emerged in 2003. Although it never became hugely popular in its own right, it remained available throughout the legal high years.

I sampled this chemical on a couple of occasions, circa 2012. Unfortunately, my recollection of these experiments is a little vague, and I didn't record the precise doses. Through the mists of time, a mild, functional, and unremarkable stimulation comes to mind, with a slightly jittery edge.

For the purpose of this book I therefore undertook a final test, in the context of being a little tired and having a less than exciting social event to attend.

The following notes were taken during the experience:

> I dose 20mg orally at 6:15pm. The taste of chemical is always gross, and this is no exception.
>
> After half an hour or so, I begin to feel a mildly stimulated headspace and less fatigue, but I am in no way ramped up. I do feel slightly chilly, suggesting a degree of vasoconstriction, but this soon passes and I become quite warm, a condition which persists for some hours.
>
> The evening is passing rather unspectacularly. I am slightly stimulated, but not in a manner that makes me talkative or active. Certainly, the sleepiness has been chased away, but it has not been replaced by an uplift or mood enhancement.
>
> The stimulation is quite bland; meaning that although I am not drowsy, I am in no way sparking or mentally sharp. I have little interest in proceedings, but this chemical is carrying me through them in a semi-detached and almost disengaged way.
>
> On returning home a few hours later the effects have faded, although some background lag and presence remains.

The following morning I reported that:

> I was able to retire to bed normally, and enjoy a reasonable night's sleep. I feel no ill effects or any type of hangover.

My original assessment appears to have been reasonably accurate, although I didn't feel particularly jittery during the re-run. Perhaps that issue manifested with a higher dose.

In summary, therefore, I found this to be active and functional, but not engaging or exciting. A higher dose might create more stimulation, but I suspect with it a more artificial chemical feel, rather than recreational pleasure.

On the markets, 2-AI tended to be mixed with chemicals such as MDAI and 3FPM, and sold under brand names. Whilst this will certainly have added a more interesting aspect to the experience, it will also have introduced additional variables and issues with respect to safety and risk.

Overall, this chemical did more or less what was expected, but it is not one to which I am ever likely to return.

2.3.2 3,4-CTMP

Common Nomenclature	3,4-Dichloromethylphenidat
Street & Reference Names	34ctmp
Reference Dosage	Threshold 2mg+; Light 5mg+; Medium 10mg+; Strong 20mg+ [Drugs-Forum] Threshold 1mg+; Light: 2mg+; Common 4mg+; Heavy 6mg+ [TripSit]
Anticipated: Onset / Duration	1 Hour / 12 Hours
Maximum Dose Experienced	7mg
Form	Powder
RoA	Oral
Source / Jurisdiction	Internet / UK

VICE
Politics Entertainment Save Yourselves LGBTQ Drugs NSFW Photos Shop
Vice Channels
The VICE Netherlands Designer Drug Awards 2014
A shit ton of new ones came out last year. You're probably wondering what they're about. We asked our friends in Holland to sum them up.

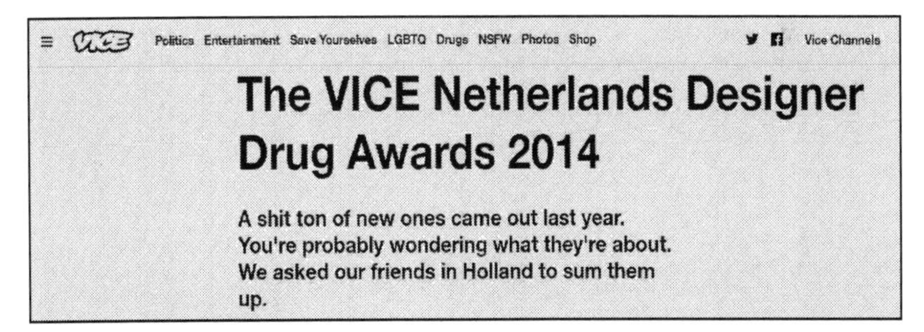

SUBJECTIVE EXPERIENCE

I sampled this in March 2015, shortly before it was banned in the UK via a Temporary Class Drug Order (TCDO). Compared to other stims in its class it was potent, at least mg for mg, but I did not find it to be particularly recreational.

It was certainly functional, in that I was lively and awake under its influence. In line with the durations cited by reference sites, I also recall that I was stimulated for almost the entire day.

Due to the legislation, lack of significant uplift in mood, and occasional warnings of vasoconstriction and associated risks, I only tested it on the one occasion. Despite this, and again demonstrating that experience is subjective, 3,4-CTMP was a winner ('fastest riser') in the *VICE Netherlands Designer Drug Awards* in 2014. It was also the most searched for drug on one of the main Internet forums in 2012, and was sometimes suggested as an alternative to methylphenidate.

By and large, it now appears to have faded into the annals of history.

2.3.3 3-FPM

Common Nomenclature	3-Fluorophenmetrazine
Street & Reference Names	3fp; PAL-593
Reference Dosage	Threshold 5 mg+; Light 10mg+; Common 25mg+; Strong 50mg+; Heavy 70mg+ [Oral, Psychonautwiki]
Anticipated: Onset / Duration	20 Minutes / 6 Hours
Maximum Dose Experienced	200mg (multiple redoses)
Form	Powder
RoA	Oral / Insufflated
Source / Jurisdiction	Internet / UK

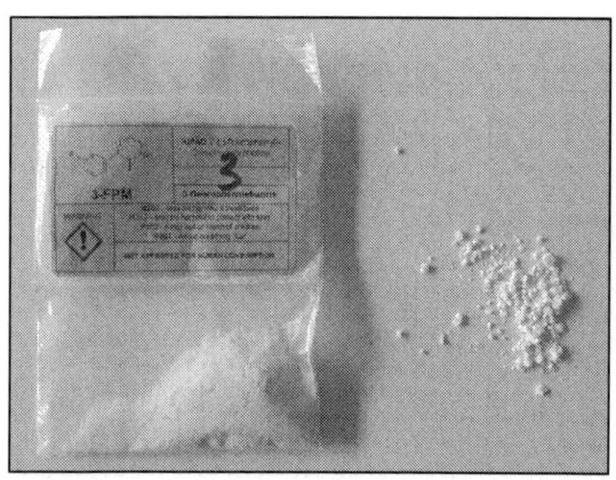

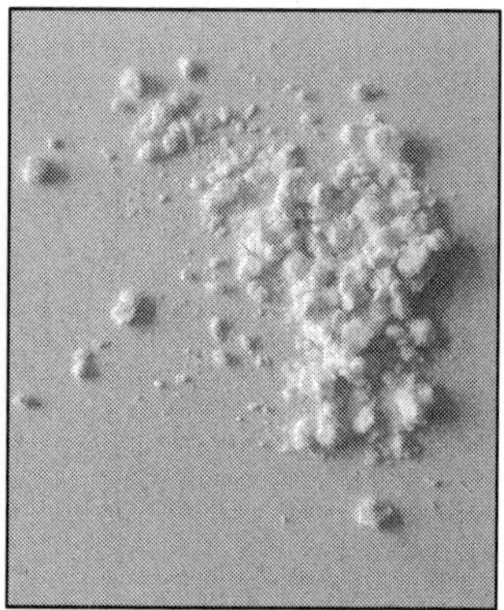

SUBJECTIVE EXPERIENCE
Recreationally, this first emerged in the 1960's. Unsubstantiated claims that The Beatles used it in Hamburg as a functional aid, to enable them to perform for excessively long hours, perhaps illustrate its standing as a street drug at that time. After disappearing for a couple of generations, it re-emerged late in 2014, sold via online vendors and sourced, presumably, from Chinese labs.

I sampled it on a number of occasions, writing on forums over several months. My contributions amounted to the following (edited for continuity):

> Well, that was a nice little experience. I consumed this orally as a series of 50mg doses, to test the water. This produced a mild buzz, confirming other observations what we are probably talking 100mg+ for the full effect, at least via this RoA.

And:

> I insufflated over the course of the evening. The intensity gradually increased to produce an extremely nice ride, although I was still generally functional if I needed to be.
>
> Interestingly, whilst not pleasant, I didn't find insufflation to be so terrible. Certainly, my last snorting exercise, with kanna, was much more problematic. This lack of discomfort could have been mitigated by the fact that I had consumed a small amount orally beforehand, but I was expecting far worse.
>
> Less positive news came with residue stim. I was awake until around 1am, at which point I popped 1mg of Etizolam. This did the trick, and I slept like a baby.

The upshot of what I now consider to be reckless dosing was that this provided a fairly pleasant experience. However, my final post described another side to the coin:

> The thread on this substance is extraordinary. I was one of the early jumpers and was as enthusiastic as anyone. It seemed to be nice and clean, and was certainly the source of an enjoyable buzz. However, it soon became obvious that there was a ceiling, and that I was consuming increasing amounts to get beyond it.
>
> This was a red light for me, so I stopped after a few sessions.
>
> I had cold and flu-like symptoms over Christmas, but although I suspect it was implicated, I can't pin it on this chemical with any certainty. What I definitely experienced was increasing body load, and lower returns in terms of reward. This got to the point where the positive effects were simply not worth the aftermath.
>
> The reports of illness and other reactions are alarming. It really is so easy to fall into the redosing trap with this one, even for experienced researchers who should know better.
>
> Take it easy.

During the following months claims emerged that 3-FPM was the cause of inflammation and that it had detrimental effects upon the immune system. Certainly, it seemed to linger in the body longer than most.

I never returned to this following these early tests. Functionally, there were better options available, and recreationally I felt no inclination to take undue risks.

Notwithstanding the above, at one point this was one of the most popular legal stimulants on the market.

2.3.4 4-FA

Common Nomenclature	4-Fluoroamphetamine
Street & Reference Names	4-FMP; PAL-303; Flux; Flits; R2D2; PFA
Reference Dosage	Threshold 10mg+; Light 25mg+; Common 50mg+; Strong 100mg+; Heavy 150mg+ [Psychonautwiki] Light 50mg+; Common 70mg+; Heavy 115mg+ [TripSit]
Anticipated: Onset / Duration	30 Minutes / 6 Hours
Maximum Dose Experienced	110mg (50mg + 25mg + 25mg + 10mg)
Form	Powder
RoA	Oral
Source / Jurisdiction	Dealer / Overseas

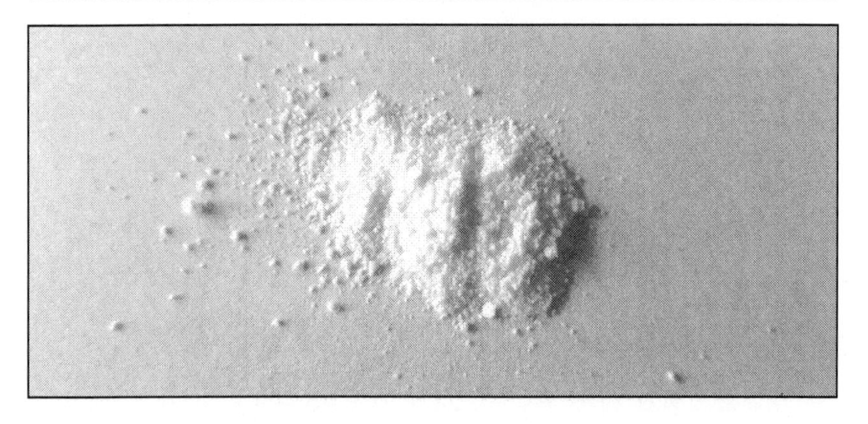

SUBJECTIVE EXPERIENCE
4-FA became commercially available as a research chemical circa 2001. In terms of effect it is often positioned, subjectively, as being somewhere between amphetamine and MDMA. At the time of writing it is increasingly popular, particularly in the Netherlands.

Despite the reference figures above, there are a substantial number of posts across Internet forums citing significantly higher doses, many in the 100mg to 200mg range, and some even higher. In this respect, Azarius.com states:

> *"According to different sources, a dosage between 80-140 mg is considered common; a dose of 50-80 mg produces a mild trip".*

This probably reflects the broad consensus.

I elect to apply a dose limit on the session by measuring 150mg and placing the rest out of immediate reach. Of this, I plan to take 50mg, and possibly redose with another 50mg if the experience is positive enough to merit deeper exploration. The other 50mg is reserved in case the threshold is not reached.

> T+0:00 50mg is bombed orally in rizla paper. I also create two small 25mg packets for the potential redosing, and leave the final 50mg in the scale pan. [2:55pm]
>
> T+0:30 Something may be happening. I am warm, content, clammy and a little sweaty. I feel slightly uplifted and a little light headed.
>
> T+0:45 As there has been no significant change during the last 15 minutes I begin to contemplate the first of those redose packets. I ate a small bowl of muesli about three hours ago, so stomach content shouldn't be having a significant effect.
>
> T+1:00 Although I am not immersed in stimulation or empathy, there does appear to be an upswing in intensity. I therefore hold off the 25mg redose. I walk around occasionally to assess the effects. I do feel quite comfortable and fairly happy.
>
> T+1:15 I decide to redose: 25mg is bombed. I have now dosed 75mg in total.
>
> T+1:30 At 90 minutes the onset of the original 50mg should be largely completed.
>
> I am in a reasonable place, but not firing to the same degree as I was on amphetamine or MDMA, for example. Having stated this, I sampled a far higher dose of those two than I should have.
>
> I will resist the final 25mg for the next 15 minutes to see where this goes.
>
> T+1:45 The final 25mg is bombed. I am now at my planned maximum of 100mg. I will draw a line in the sand here, by taking approximately 10mg of the remaining 50mg, and binning the rest.
>
> T+2:15 The good news is that I don't feel any compulsive urge to redose. This is contrary to my experience with amphetamine and methamphetamine. I feel rather more like I did whilst under the influence of MDMA, in that there is stimulation there, but it is not overwhelming or totally dominant.
>
> I am now fully aware that I am solidly experiencing a drug trip. I am still warm, with the occasional hot flush, and my mind drifts into a mild blissful state. I am generally content. My pupils are dilated, but not fully so. There is no gurning or jaw tension.

Is there any horn?

At this point, not particularly. I didn't experience this aspect with MDMA either, but certainly did with amphetamine. I feel that I could chose to engage on a take it or leave it basis, but at this particular dose I feel none of the wild compulsive sex drive that is sometimes reported for this chemical.

T+3:00 This has now strengthened somewhat. There is slightly more horn and more strength to the overall experience. I am guessing that the final redose is kicking in.

T+3:45 Having become rather more intense the experience has now settled again. I feel that it has reached a plateau, where I expect it to remain for a while.

This is very pleasant, with a sense of positivity and contentedness (including an empathetic edge) without taking me flying.

T+4:15 I remain on the plateau I referred to above. The question is, how long will this last? There are some reports of very lengthy duration and difficulty sleeping, which I hope are false.

I eat a small meal with some fruit juice. Note that I have been sipping water throughout, to avoid any threat of dehydration.

T+6:00 The experience has wound down to a lower level. The effects are still evident, but are of significantly lower intensity than earlier.

T+17:00 The effects continued to fade until I retired to bed at 10:37, which was seven and a half hours after the first dose. I tossed and turned, unable to drop off. As I was wide awake at 1:30 am, I popped 1mg of Etizolam. Thereafter, I slept through until 7:30am.

On rising and heading for coffee, I felt a little groggy, but generally well.

It could be that to fly really high on this I would need to consume a much higher dose, as is suggested by a variety of Internet trip reports. However, at this dose it was nice enough, and I can see the logic of comparisons with MDMA. I experienced quite a mild and gentle journey, with plenty of feel-good factor.

On the flip side, alarmingly, I have recently been reading reports suggesting that 4-FA has occasionally caused cerebral hemorrhaging. In urging caution regarding this, I would particularly stress the need for restraint with respect to dosage.

Finally, note that for a few days following this experiment I experienced a perceptible comedown in terms of flatness. Appropriate planning and aftercare is therefore strongly recommended (see MDMA for further information).

2.3.5 4-Me-TMP

Common Nomenclature	4-Methylmethylphenidate
Street & Reference Names	Threo-4-Methylmethylphenidate
Reference Dosage	Light 25mg+; Common 40mg+; Strong 60mg+; Heavy 90mg+ [TripSit]
Anticipated: Onset / Duration	30 Minutes / 6 Hours
Maximum Dose Experienced	50mg+25mg+50mg
Form	Powder
RoA	Oral
Source / Jurisdiction	Internet / UK

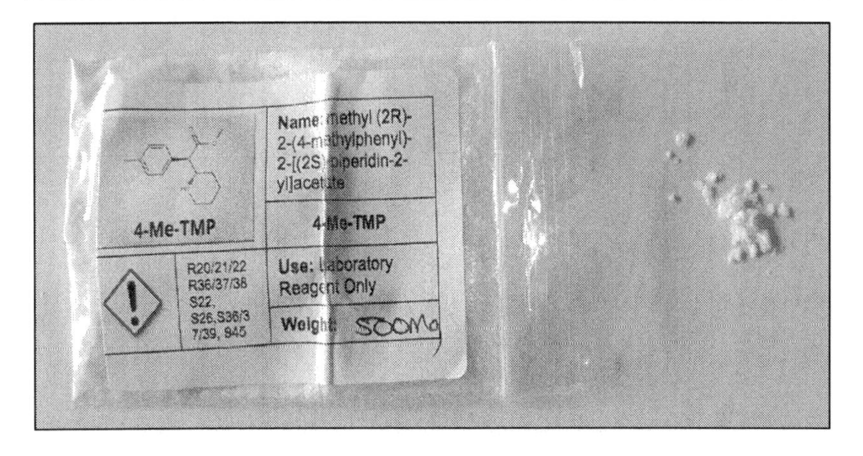

SUBJECTIVE EXPERIENCE
This was on the market for just a few months in the middle of 2015, having been released shortly after the UK ban on EPH and other phenidates. However, I found it to be a little uninspiring and dull, despite a session of fairly hefty redosing.

It provided an EPH-like functional stimulation, with little recreational action. I felt that something was missing, although I am not sure what.

So disappointing was it that I used it on just the one occasion, and left the rest in its baggy for over two years. It was eventually binned.

To be fair, others have reported far more positively than this, with a handful even citing a recreational edge at high doses.

2.3.6 4F-EPH

Common Nomenclature	4-Fluoromethylphenidate
Street & Reference Names	4-FEPH
Reference Dosage	Light 5mg+; Common 10mg+; Strong 30mg+ [Oral, TripSit].
Anticipated: Onset / Duration	5 Minutes / 4 Hours
Maximum Dose Experienced	18mg+10mg+15mg
Form	Powder
RoA	Insufflated
Source / Jurisdiction	Internet / UK

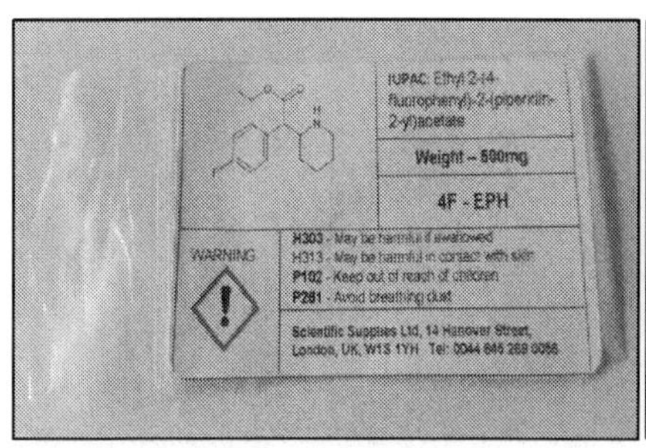

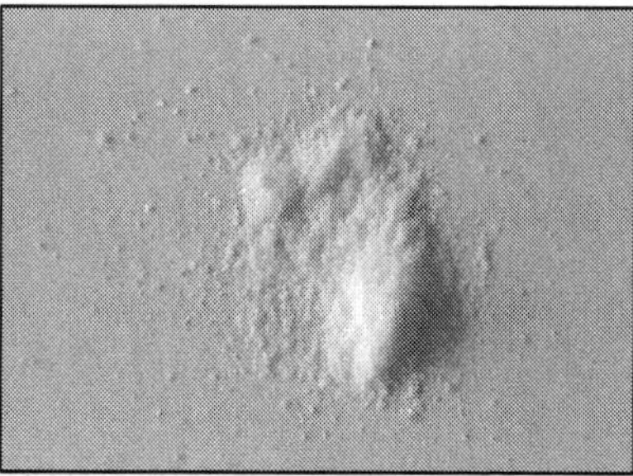

SUBJECTIVE EXPERIENCE
Released at the end of 2015, 4F-EPH was legally available during the same period as 4F-MPH, and for me, it was that chemical's ugly little sister.

Why do I state this?

I do so because, whilst having significant similarities in terms of effect, I found it to provide a less smooth experience, which sometimes had a distinct jittery feel.

I tested it both orally and via insufflation, but both routes led me to reach the same conclusion.

Whilst accepting that this seemed to have many fans who did consider it to be a recreational drug, I largely found it to be functional.

As this is active at relatively low doses, particular caution is advised with respect to this. Note also that as EPH is cited as being caustic to the nasal septum, insufflation is probably best avoided.

2.3.7 4F-MPH

Common Nomenclature	4-Fluoromethylphenidate
Street & Reference Names	4FMPH; 4-FMPH
Reference Dosage	Threshold 1mg+; Light 5mg+; Common 10mg+; Strong 15mg+; Heavy 20mg+ [Oral, TripSit]
Anticipated: Onset / Duration	30 Minutes / 8 Hours
Maximum Dose Experienced	15mg Insufflated; 15mg+20mg Oral
Form	Powder
RoA	Oral
Source / Jurisdiction	Internet / UK

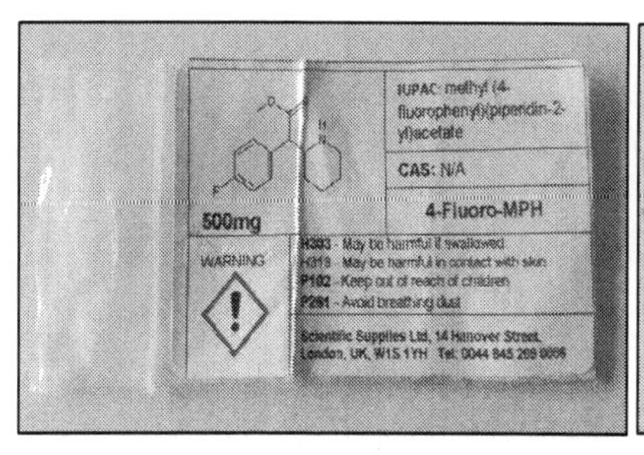

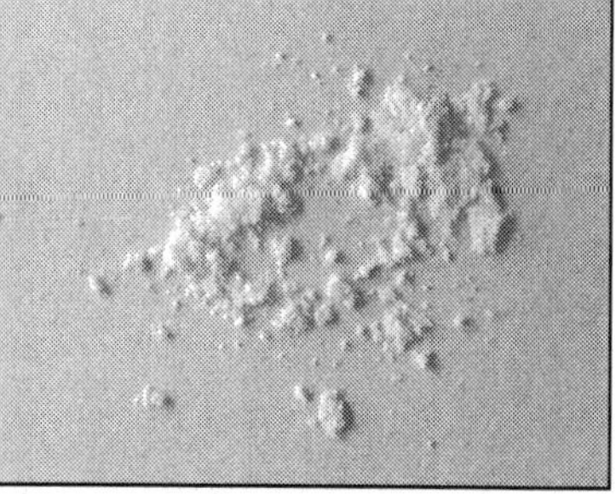

SUBJECTIVE EXPERIENCE
4F-MPH appeared on the markets in 2015, and quickly became popular in its niche. It fits very much into the *functional* category; meaning that it induces little or no euphoria, empathy or mood lift, or indeed, any of those *edges* that make many stims so enjoyable and recreational.

However, there is a significant uplift in terms of energy, alertness and even clarity, and it persists for a very lengthy period. I ought to add here that it is extremely strong at relatively low doses, so caution is the byword.

I used it on a number of occasions, invariably when I had a need to be on my game, yet had been suffering from fatigue or tiredness (mental or physical). For this, it was very much my *go-to* solution, at least for a year or so.

Whilst I found it to be smoother and less jittery than other stimulants in this particular group, such as EPH, it was one which some people abused and eventually became addicted to. Despite its usefulness in certain scenarios, it is not a chemical to make a habit of.

See Section 1.1

2.3.8 Adderall

Common Nomenclature	Adderall
Street & Reference Names	Agent Orange; Blue Lightening
Reference Dosage	Light 5mg+; Common 15mg+; Strong 40mg+; Heavy 75mg+ [Oral, TripSit]
Anticipated: Onset / Duration	30 minutes / 5 Hours
Maximum Dose Experienced	30mg+10mg+10mg+10mg
From	Pills
RoA	Oral
Source / Jurisdiction	Associate / Overseas

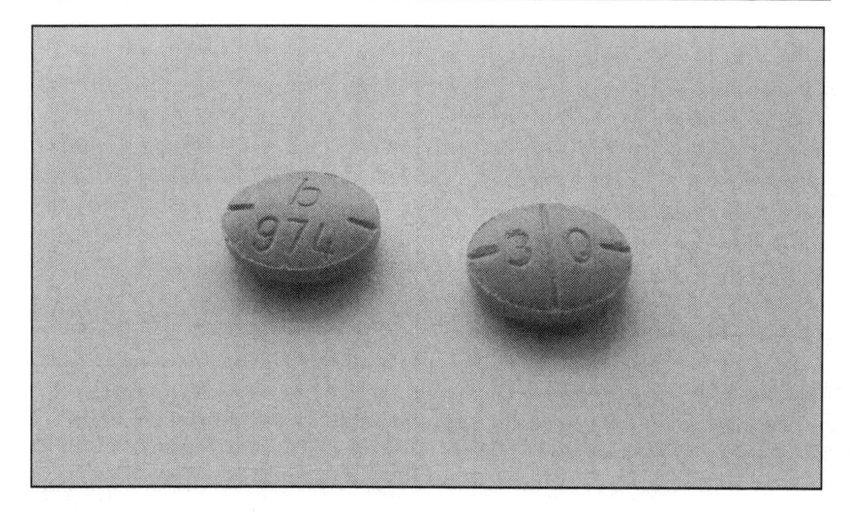

SUBJECTIVE EXPERIENCE
Adderall is a mix of dextroamphetamine and levoamphetamine, in the ratio 75% to 25%, and is prescribed to treat the symptoms of ADHD (attention deficit hyperactivity disorder) and narcolepsy (a sleep disorder). The brand was first introduced in 1996, with a generic version being approved in 2002.

Its recreational use is now well established and unsurprisingly, given its contents, addiction potential and increased tolerance build quickly.

My 60mg supply came in the form of two orange pills. Identity checking their imprints online, drugs.com states that these are: "*b 974 3 0 (Amphetamine and Dextroamphetamine 30 mg)*" and that they were originally supplied by Teva Pharmaceuticals USA.

Coincidentally, Erowid currently uses the exact same type of pill for its illustrative photograph for amphetamine, with adderall listed as a brand name.

Adderall comes in both instant and extended release forms. Here I am covering the IR (instant) version. Also note than some people insufflate, but I am researching this via the oral route. A word in passing on this though: as usual, if you are insufflating, significantly lower doses are required.

With respect to dosage, drugs-forum.com states that:

> *"Adderall is intended to be taken orally, at doses from 5-30mg (measured in instant release). Recreational users do use more, however it is not advisable for inexperienced users to exceed 30mg, if not tolerant to the drug"*

As this is my first experiment with adderall, I obviously wouldn't call myself an experienced user of it, but might do so with respect to stimulants generally, including street amphetamine. Combined with the TripSit and other relevant material I therefore decide to start with 30mg. To help facilitate a faster onset I crush the pills prior to swallowing (a process sometimes referred to as *parachuting*).

In terms of expectation I am anticipating a slightly watered down version of the effects I experienced with amphetamine (of which I took a much higher dose).

T+0:00 I swallow 30mg of my supply with a glass of water [11:50am]

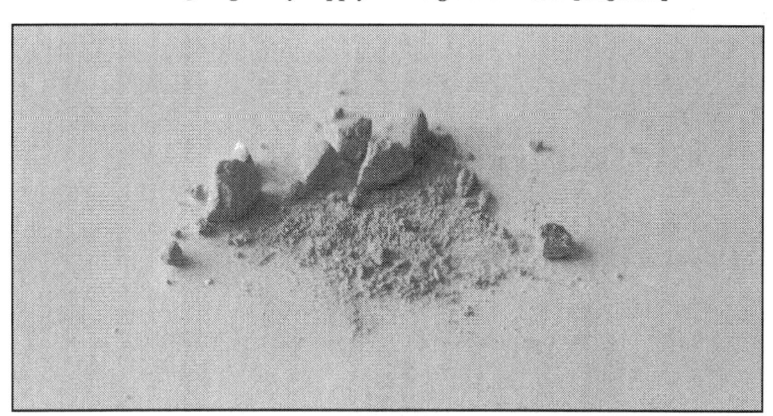

T+0:30 I can feel the usual stim tingles emerging, along with a light head buzz. Already it is quite pleasant, and already I am contemplating another half-pill (maybe 15mg) to top up.

T+1:00 I swill down another 10mg of the crushed orange debris, taking the total to around 40mg. The buzz is currently sustained on a nice level, which I can functionally skate above if necessary.

Unsurprisingly, the major hallmarks of amphetamine are in play now, albeit not very strongly. These include a positive uplift, and indeed horn, if required.

T+2:00 I remain on the same plateau, which is quite nice, but the compulsion to redose is undeniably present. Given that my overall dose is limited to the 60mg I originally acquired I am seeking to control this and spin out the exercise as best I can, which isn't a trivial matter. Despite this intention, I still swallow half the remaining supply, taking the running total to around 50mg.

T+3:00 I now greedily gobble the remainder, hitting the ceiling of my 60mg. Unfortunately this doesn't seem to produce the mild rush of previous re-doses, at least to the same extent, so I hypothesise that I could be hitting some sort of barrier of diminishing returns.

T+4:00 As suspected an hour ago, I have passed the peak, and the buzz and general elevation is slowly fading. I am still in a zone of course, but it is far less intense than it was earlier.

I have little doubt that had I a larger stock available I would continue a little longer, so once again a pre-planned constraint has intervened to save me from myself.

From here I expect a gradual comedown over the next few hours, hopefully a soft and gentle one. I remain warm with a mild head-stim, so this isn't so bad at the present time.

T+5:00 Stim-binge averted, I can now turn some attention to recovery. I am targeting a decent meal in an hour or two, at which point I hope to have at least something of an appetite.

I still feel somewhat fuzzy in a positive sense, if a little unfulfilled. I remain physically warm and generally well.

T+7:00 The ride has basically fizzled out to a flatness. I feel slightly distant and increasingly weary, although not particularly sleepy.

The night's sheep was in fact a decent one, aided and abetted (reluctantly) by 0.5mg of etizolam. The next morning I awoke reasonably fresh, if a little drained.

My expectation was not far off the mark. This was like a weakish re-run with amphetamine; no doubt on account of the dose I was restricted to in comparison. This is not to say that it wasn't decent: it was. It is just that it peaked early, not particularly highly, and then faded slowly over the course of the day, leaving me at a bit of a loose end. In different circumstances I would undoubtedly have enjoyed a better return.

Finally, and it is worth stating the obvious: the warnings I provide for amphetamine also apply to this, so do take care, particularly with dose and frequency of use.

2.3.9 Amphetamine

Common Nomenclature	α-methylphenethylamine
Street & Reference Names	Speed; Speed Paste; Whizz; Amph
Reference Dosage	Light 15mg+; Common 25mg+; Strong 40mg+; Heavy 75mg+ [TripSit]
Anticipated: Onset / Duration	2 Minutes / 6 Hours
Maximum Dose Experienced	150mg
Form	Powder
RoA	Insufflated
Source / Jurisdiction	Dealer / Overseas

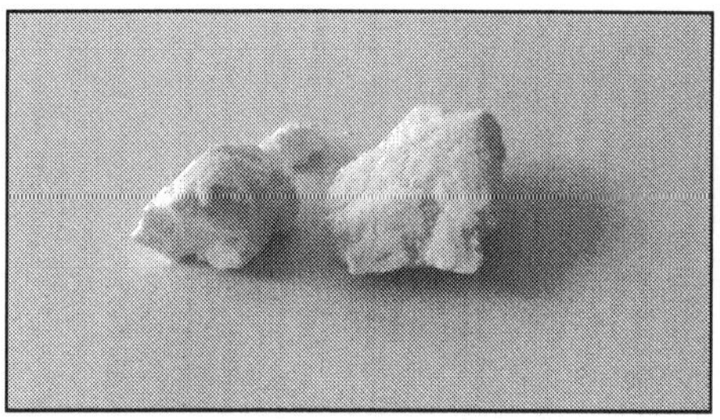

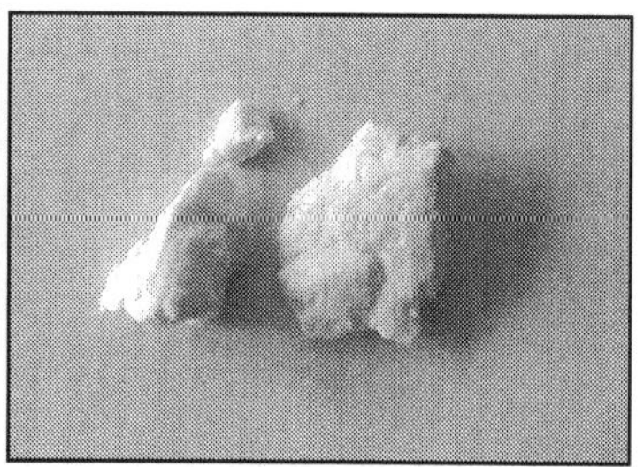

SUBJECTIVE EXPERIENCE
Amphetamine has a colourful history. First synthesised by Lazăr Edeleanu in 1887, it was used medicinally from the 1930's, and was deployed extensively as a performance enhancing stimulant amongst the armed forces during the Second World War. Its recreational use exploded in the 60's, including as a constituent part of the fabled *purple hearts (*drinamyl/barbiturate*).*

Whilst it was one of the first drugs to be scheduled and controlled, it continues to be prescribed for a range of disorders, and remains one of the most popular and widely used street drugs.

My own sample was claimed to be 74% pure, and came in the form of a wet/damp powder, which clumped together, sticking to everything. On opening the sealed plastic I set about drying it over a radiator. Snorting approximately 3mg to test, I quickly noted a heady stimulation. It occurred to me immediately that establishing weight would present an issue, as an unknown amount of fluid would be retained unless it was 100% dry.

On the day of the experiment, I was relatively tired and generally worn out. Another negative was that it was only 8 days since an MDMA test, and my serotonin levels would still have been depleted.

Despite these reservations, the next opportunity to sample this drug might not have presented itself for years, so I proceeded, but with caution.

> T+0:00 I insufflate 15mg. The good news is that this isn't insanely painful on the nose. Note that I haven't eaten for some 4 hours or so. [3pm]
>
> T+0:10 I am now warm, whereas I was quite cold 15 minutes ago. I feel stimulated but not manic.
>
> T+0:25 I snort another line, of perhaps 10mg. I now experience a nice mild headiness with some horn. This is pleasant, but not overly exciting.
>
> T+1:00 The positive feeling has faded onto a minimal plateau. I redose by snorting approximately 20mg, bringing the total to about 45mg.
>
> T+2:00 This is more like it: it is now really quite nice. There is definite stimulation but with an edge which is positive, dreamy and somewhat euphoric. It is rather manic if I want it to be, but I am functional if I proactively concentrate. My pupils are dilated.
>
> T+2:10 I insufflate another line of 15mg or so. This probably now qualifies as a binge, so I'll try to take it easy from here. It is an extremely enjoyable ride.
>
> It reminds me slightly of a combination of MPA and MDAI, which raises the question of how I will sleep and how drained I will be in the morning.
>
> Is there horn? Yes, indeed. This is the stuff of feverish primal sex sessions and never ending porn binges. I have an inclination that there may be some issues with stim-dick, but I could be wrong.
>
> Despite no appetite whatsoever, I eat some food and take a vitamin pill, entirely for health and risk mitigation reasons. I continue to drink a reasonable volume of water, as I always do with this class of drug.
>
> T+3:00 I insufflate another line, and from here I proceed to redose occasionally to remain topped-up over the following hours.

Overall I comfortably consumed more than 100mg before retiring to bed. The next morning, my pupils were still dilated and I felt tired and a little lethargic. However, unlike the aftermath of similar binges on a number of other stimulants, I didn't feel particularly unhealthy. There was no headache and the malaise was minor. Having stated this, the sense that I had been on a drug bender during the previous evening was with me for most of the day.

I can certainly see how some people become addicted to this family of drugs, as I could happily have snorted again and engaged in another session, particularly in the afternoon, had I been foolish enough to do so.

Some days later I did repeat the exercise, with a similar dose. On this occasion, the comedown was more severe and was unpleasant. I woke from spasmodic sleep with a headache and I felt exhausted, dysfunctional, and generally unwell.

This had been a mistake.

The following hangover advice, as researched on the Internet, helped to alleviate some of the discomfort and probably aided my recovery:

- Drink plenty of water. Also drink some fruit juice if available.
- Take some 5-htp supplement pills. This is a precursor to boosting serotonin, which will have been depleted during the binge

  Other supplements and vitamins are sometimes ingested to help rebuild dopamine and restore body nutrients. Pre-investigation can help to identify an appropriate individual stack or multi-supplement.
- Do some light exercise or at least go for a walk, but don't overdo it. It is suggested that this also helps to dissipate anxiety.
- This may be difficult given that speed suppresses appetite, but eat. Eat healthy, to help rebuild calcium for example, and to help dilute what is left of the amphetamine in your system.
- This may seem controversial, but many users smoke cannabis to manage the comedown, calming anxiety and stimulating appetite.
- Sleep, in so far as you are able.

These widely cited recommendations also apply to a number of other chemicals in this class, and are referred to elsewhere in this book.

Subsequently, I encountered the following comment on Reddit:

> *"Amphetamine is amazing but it certainly takes back what it gives. There is no winning with amphetamine - it will come back and bite you in the ass."*

I wouldn't disagree with this at all. With my first experience I may have got away without too much of a comedown, but I certainly didn't with my second.

Tread carefully with this?

You bet!

2.3.10 Caffeine

Common Nomenclature	Caffeine
Street & Reference Names	Tea; Coffee; Yerba Mate; Misc
Reference Dosage	Threshold 10mg+; Common 50mg+; Strong 150mg+; Heavy 400mg+; Lethal 3g+ [Erowid] Threshold: 10mg+; Light 20mg+; Common 75mg+ Strong 250mg+; Heavy 400mg+ [TripSit]
Anticipated: Onset / Duration	5 Minutes / 3 Hours
Maximum Dose Experienced	Unknown
Form	Various
RoA	Oral
Source / Jurisdiction	Retail / UK

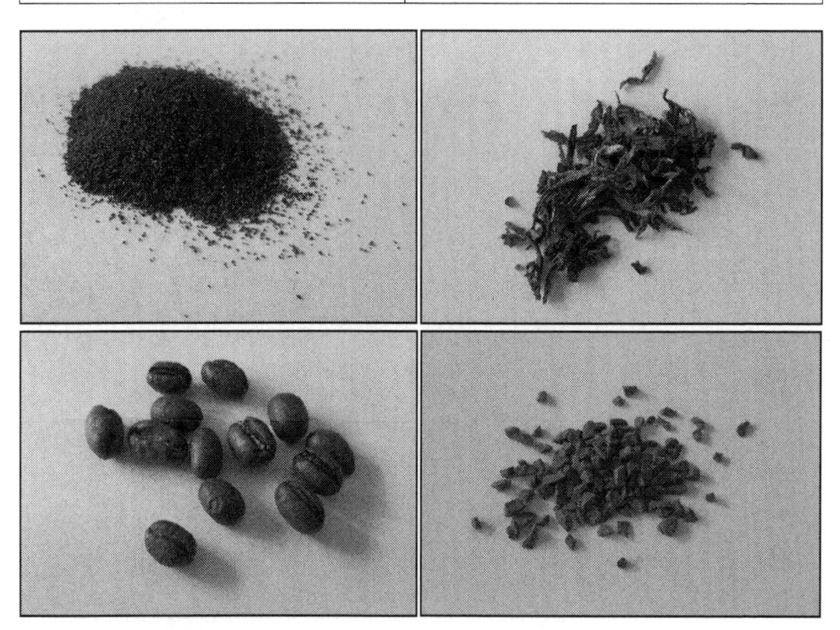

SUBJECTIVE EXPERIENCE
Caffeine is a central nervous system (CNS) stimulant, and is the world's most popular and widely used psychoactive drug. It is available via a vast array of beverages, providing an extremely rich variety of flavours.

Such is the prevalence of the oral form of consumption that there was initial temptation to document each of the major caffeine containing botanicals. However, given the relative subtlety of variation of the caffeine experiences, and that in the modern era it can be purchased in other forms, including powder and tablet, a chemical listing was deemed to be more appropriate.

I find that there are two broad types of caffeine experience. One is a general background stimulation that promotes an alert state of wakefulness. The other provides a jolt: to counter tiredness or weariness in an urgent manner.

The first type, a relatively benign excitation, gives rise to ritual, social bonding, and communication. Connoisseurs of particular beverages have emerged, and sophisticated systems of sub-classification have been honed.

This state of consciousness is also conducive to prolonged individual productive capability, which is consistent with a capitalist based social system.

For millions of people, caffeine consumption is habitual, and for a tiny minority, addictive.

As is generally known, heavy consumption of coffee, or evening consumption, can be an impediment to sleep. However, other potentially more serious issues can also ensue.

High or excessive doses can give rise to jitteriness, or can produce symptoms like dizziness, irritability, headache and sometimes diarrhoea. Should symptoms like vomiting, chest pains, rapid heartbeat, breathing difficulties or convulsions occur immediate medical help should be summoned.

Partially due to familiarity there is little public awareness or consideration of its long term effects, with respect to both health and quality of life. Further, every other stimulant is legislated against, and stigmatised, leaving little scope for rational comparison. None of this, however, is intended to imply that its positive safety profile is not generally merited.

Regarding dosage, as a general guide, a standard cup of brewed coffee is often cited as containing approximately 100mg of caffeine. Erowid lists the caffeine content of a number of other common beverages on the following web page:
https://erowid.org/chemicals/caffeine/caffeine_info1.shtml

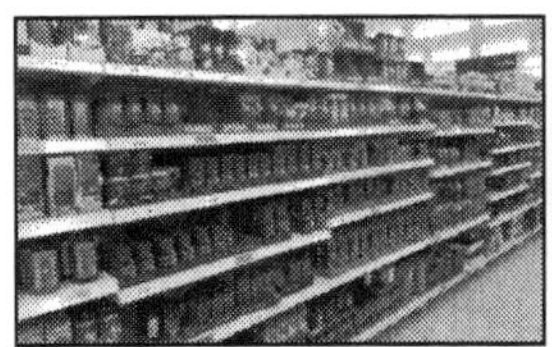
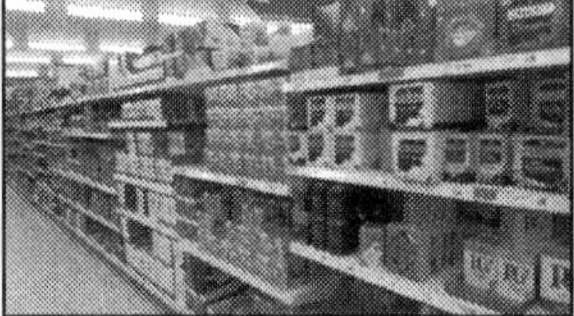
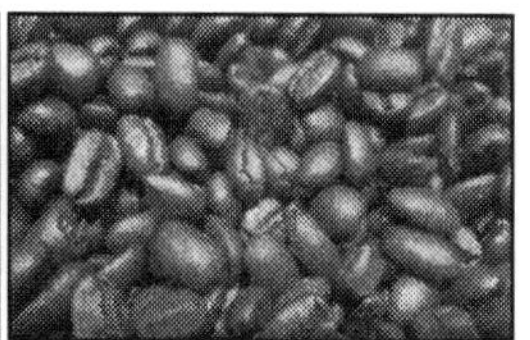

As sourced by your local supermarket (Sainsbury's, Manchester) or coffee shop (Starbucks, Beijing)

2.3.11 Cocaine

Common Nomenclature	Benzoylmethylecgonine
Street & Reference Names	Coke; Crack; Blow; Snow; Nose Candy
Reference Dosage	Light 20mg+; Common 50mg+; Strong 100mg+; Heavy 150mg+ [Insufflated, TripSit]
Anticipated: Onset / Duration	2 Minutes / 90 Minutes
Maximum Dose Experienced	200mg
Form	Powder
RoA	Oral / Smoked / Insufflated
Source / Jurisdiction	Dealer / Overseas

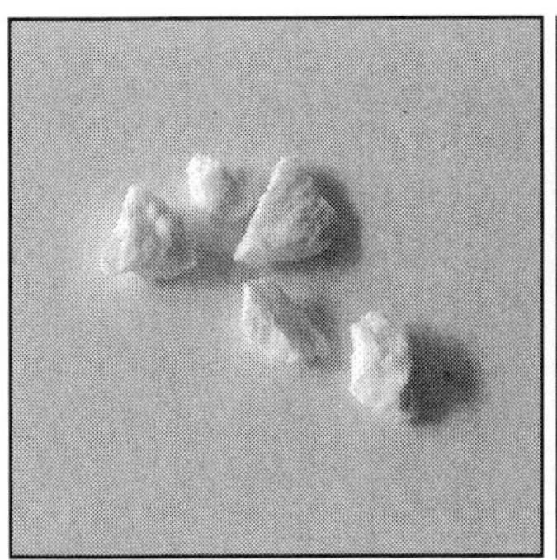

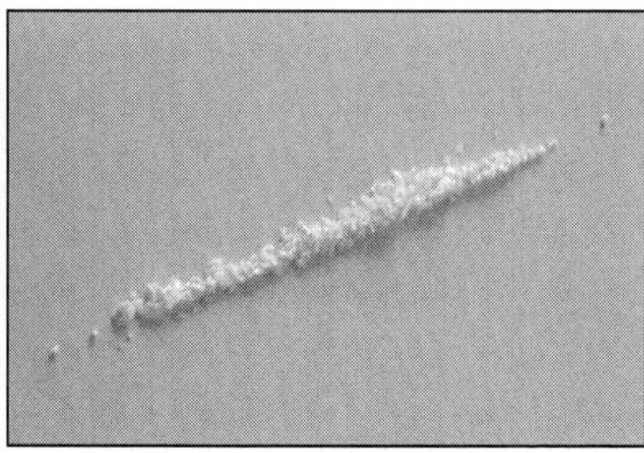

SUBJECTIVE EXPERIENCE
One of the most famed of drugs, cocaine is sourced from the coca plant, and is widely known for its short term high and addiction potential.

In a previous life, in what seems eons ago, I experienced it both orally and by smoking (inhaling its vapours). This was the folly of youth and high risk stupidity, or at least it was on the first occasion.

I found myself in a major North American city where I was offered the substance by a street vendor. It came in the form of a paste/fluid, within a small plastic transparent tube. Having had far too much to drink, I swallowed it. This was naïve, foolish and embarrassing.

The reaction was minimal, certainly during the first few hours. I have since learned that the absorption rate via oral consumption is only about 30%, which may actually have been a positive, given the lack of common sense in such a rash scenario. The alcohol will also have played a part in disguising or suppressing the effect.

The only notable aspect of this mess came the next day, when my head should have been throbbing with an alcohol hangover. It wasn't. Indeed, I felt remarkably functional and healthy.

What I did in mixing was dangerous, but fortunately, I drank plenty of water before sleeping. This may have helped, but was insufficient to explain my luck regarding the missing headache.

Subsequent research did shed some light upon this: cocaine can indeed disguise and mitigate the pain of excessive alcohol consumption. In fact, it is commonly stated on the Internet that *Coca Cola* originally contained cocaine, and was used widely as a hangover cure (orally, obviously). I suspect, therefore, that rather than purchasing a drug induced high, I actually bought my way out of a day's suffering whilst on the tourist trail.

The second cocaine experience occurred in Amsterdam. On one particular evening I found myself in what can best be described as a drug commune, or perhaps in modern lingo a crack house, in an old city centre building. Cocaine and heroin were being shared in tiny white bags (reminiscent of the blue *Salt 'n' Shake* salt packets in a bag of crisps).

The contents of these were placed in a metal bowl, heated and smoked/inhaled. Being careful to take only the cocaine, I engaged. Retrospectively, I now understand that this will have been the free base form of cocaine, commonly known as *crack*.

This experience was a little vague, but by and large, I recall an uplifted feeling and perhaps a short high, albeit not mind blowing in nature. Certainly I wasn't in the realms of wanting more, either then or since.

Zooming forwards to my relatively sane and sensible modern era of risk management and harm mitigation, I finally tested cocaine via its most common RoA: insufflation.

The vendor promised that my 100mg (actually 75mg) was over 83% "*Peruvian Flake*". The substance itself was easy enough to crush into lines, even though its constitution wasn't brittle (it was flaky). I proceeded to sample:

> T+0:00 Two lines of approximately 25mg are snorted. There is no real pain, but mild numbing, so I suspect it is cut with lidocaine or similar. [4:27pm]
>
> T+0:05 Perhaps it is due to exposure to a reasonably high dose of amphetamine three weeks ago, or some other cross tolerance, but the uplift at this point is minimal.
>
> I feel a gentle stimulation, but given no intake of cocaine for over 20 years, I am underwhelmed. Yes, I can feel something coming on, but there is no rush or euphoria. Onset is described as 2-20 minutes, so I will give it a few more minutes before pushing it with the other 25mg.

T+0.10 I snort the last 25mg, so if the purity claimed by the dealer is anywhere near to being accurate, I should be well into the territory of a common dose.

T+0.15 This is more like it. Whilst not feeling mind blown, I do feel elevated. I feel warm, and with a familiar sort of gently elevated headspace, inclusive of a mild visual clarity and a calmness. There is a little horn if I think about it. My pupils appear to be normal when I check in the mirror.

T+0:20 Mentally, I feel that I am in a place from which I could happily socialize, feel comfortable about it, and have a good time. However, staying indoors and doing nothing in particular still provides a mild sense of euphoria and pleasure.

T+0:35 There is no change at this point. I am certainly high, although with a larger dose I would probably be even more exhilarated, with more horn, and so forth. The big question from here is how long will this last?

My experiences with other stimulants have frequently lasted for hours, often too many hours. If this is significantly shorter, as is suggested, I can understand its enormous popularity, subject to the nature of the comedown.

T+0:50 I remain in a very nice place. A heady stim-like buzz pervades, but it is light enough to enable unimpaired functionality.

At the back of my mind is the thought that even though I find it to be rather pleasing, the experience would be even better for anyone new to psychoactives, or even to myself when I was inexperienced and less inured to the world of the drug headspace.

T+1:10 I am coming-down now, fairly gently so far. I am still experiencing an elevated mood, but less so, and the head stim has almost dissipated.

This has been a pleasant experience. It's all about the residuals from here.

The rest of the day passed quite normally and the night's sleep was fine. In the morning I felt no indication of hangover, possibly due to the sensible dose I was restricted to.

On the following day, perhaps because of this lack of negative payload, the thought crossed my mind that I would quite like to snort another line or two. This is not the best sign, as it flashes a big red light.

Note that on a subsequent test, with a dose of 200mg over a number of hours, the aftermath was not as kind. However, it was still significantly gentler than that of many other stimulants. The slippery slope to addiction does appear to be less obvious than for most other drugs in this class. Be careful with respect to this: very careful.

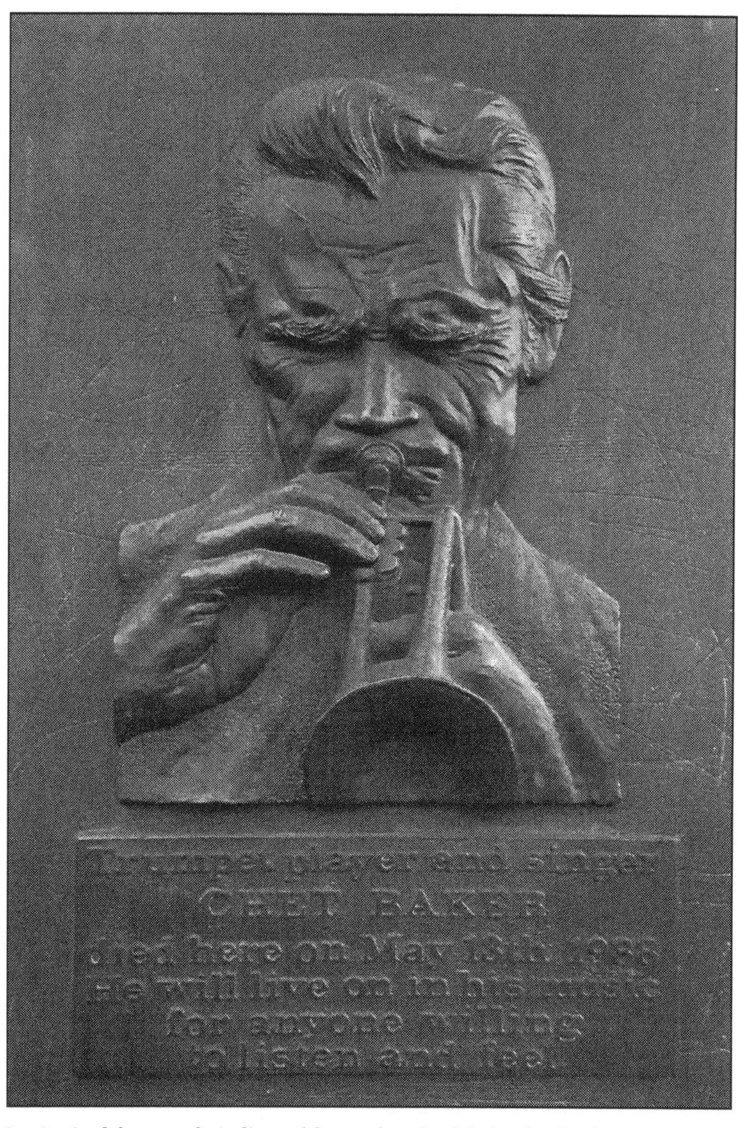

Cocaine is cited frequently in lists of drug related celebrity deaths (see Section 4.3.5). I ran across this plaque outside the Hotel Prins Hendrik in Amsterdam, from which jazz legend Chet Baker accidentally fell to his death with both cocaine and heroin present in his system.

2.3.12 EPH

Common Nomenclature	Ethylphenidate
Street & Reference Names	EP
Reference Dosage	Threshold 10mg+; Light 15mg+; Common 25mg+; Strong 75mg+; Heavy 150mg+ [Erowid] Light: 20mg+; Common 40mg+; Strong 100mg+; Heavy 150mg+ [TripSit]
Anticipated: Onset / Duration	1 Hour / 6 Hours
Maximum Dose Experienced	40mg
Form	Pill
RoA	Oral
Source / Jurisdiction	Head Shop / UK

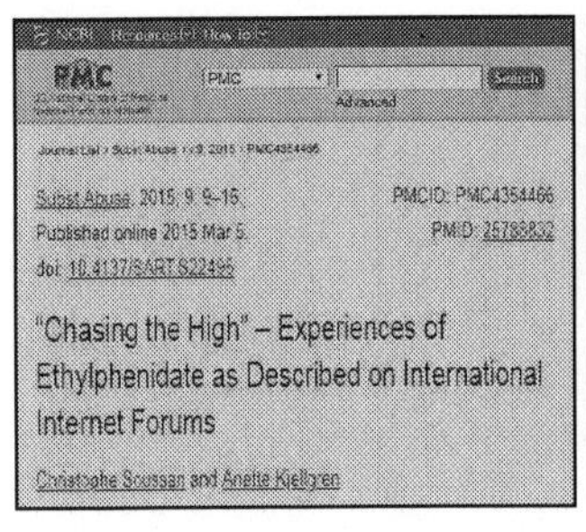

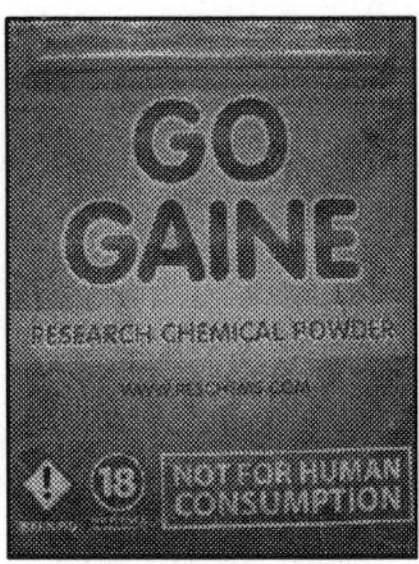

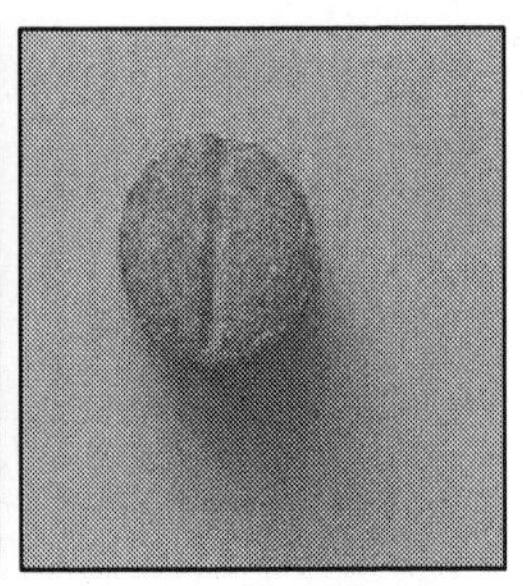

SUBJECTIVE EXPERIENCE
Ethylphenidate emerged on the markets circa 2010/2011, and became increasingly popular over subsequent years. It was banned in the UK via a collective TCDO in April 2015, along with a number of other phenidates.

In 2012, I had been given a complementary pack of four EPH pills in a Manchester head shop, on the back of the purchase of several other items. However, the commentary of the shop assistant on handing them over set an unfortunate tone: "*These are pretty good but they shrink your dick*".

For months I sat on them with that comment swirling in the back of my mind. Did I really want my dick shrinking?

Of course, he was referring to the frequently cited phenomena of *stim dick*: the incapacity to obtain and sustain an erection under the influence of certain compounds in this class. But with far less experience of the *research chemical* scene's lingo at the time, it wasn't an introduction that compelled me to rush home and immediately sample the goodies.

When I eventually did so, I found a sharp jittery unremarkable stimulant.

It was certainly functional, but at this dose (approx 40mg) it lacked even a hint of euphoria or empathogenic edge. Nor did I find much in the way of mood lift. From this perspective I found it to be unrewarding and quite boring.

There were better recreational stimulants around at the time, and much better functional stimulants were soon to emerge, so this wasn't a chemical that I was ever going to test on more than a couple of occasions.

However, there is a *but*.

The *but* is that EPH was an ingredient of a number of the blends commonly sold both in head shops and online. This was the case with one of the iterations of *GoGaine,* which also included MPA, Lidocaine, and Mannitol.

I refer to this particular product because I once had a bad experience with it, which included my unfortunate introduction to the *Shadow People*. See the entry for MPA for further details of this horror story.

EPH, for me, was a stimulant that never really merited the attention it received. It certainly worked in terms of energy and stimulation, but recreationally it offered little else, and always felt somewhat rough around the edges.

I should add that this experience and opinion does run contrary to that of many other users and researchers. My assumption is that they dosed far more heavily than I did, or that they used an EPH containing blend.

ADDITIONAL SAFETY NOTE
This chemical is caustic, and due to the potential for harm to the nasal septum, *TripSit* recommends that it is not insufflated.

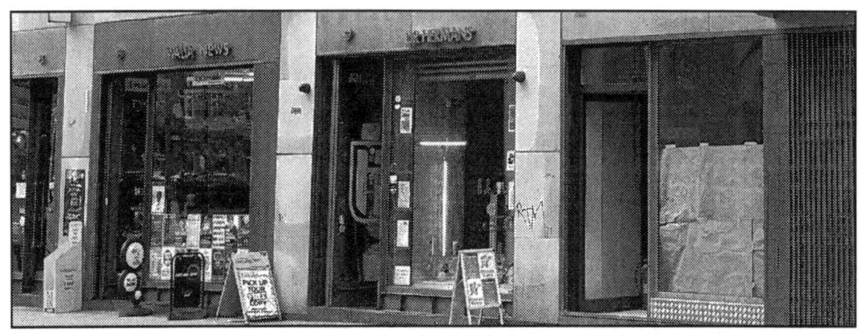

EPH was stocked by head shops in most major cities

2.3.13 HDMP-28

Common Nomenclature	Methylnaphthidate
Street & Reference Names	N/A
Reference Dosage	Threshold 5mg+; Light 10mg+; Medium 20mg+; Strong 40mg+ [Oral, Drugs-Forum] Threshold 8mg+; Light 10mg+; Common 15mg+; Strong 30mg+ [Oral, TripSit]
Anticipated: Onset / Duration	5 Minutes / 3 Hours
Maximum Dose Experienced	10mg+10mg+10mg+10mg+10mg
Form	Powder
RoA	Insufflated
Source / Jurisdiction	Internet / UK

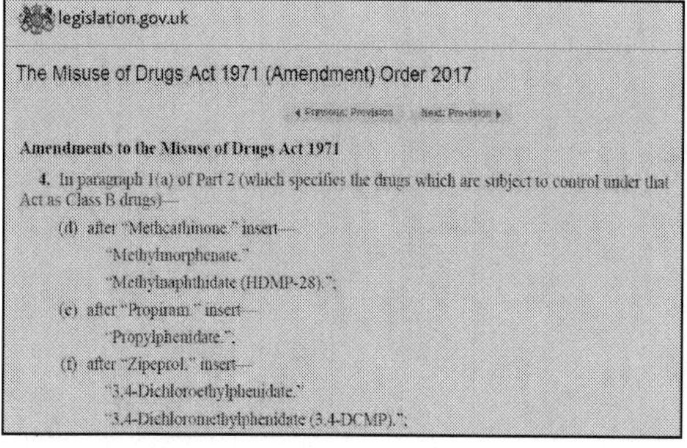

legislation.gov.uk

The Misuse of Drugs Act 1971 (Amendment) Order 2017

◄ Previous: Provision Next: Provision ►

Amendments to the Misuse of Drugs Act 1971

4. In paragraph 1(a) of Part 2 (which specifies the drugs which are subject to control under that Act as Class B drugs)—

(d) after "Methcathinone." insert—

"Methylmorphenate."

"Methylnaphthidate (HDMP-28).";

(e) after "Propiram." insert—

"Propylphenidate.";

(f) after "Zipeprol." insert—

"3,4-Dichloroethylphenidate."

"3,4-Dichloromethylphenidate (3,4-DCMP).";

SUBJECTIVE EXPERIENCE

The supply of HDMP-28 in the UK was strangled almost at birth. It was subjected to a government TCDO shortly after it began to emerge on the markets, during the early months of 2015. The same TCDO schedule also included a number of more established chemicals, specifically 3,4-CTMP, EPH, IPPH, and PPH.

My own sample had been imported from Canada, by a fellow researcher, and was forwarded after his own experiments had disappointed him.

I subsequently reported my experience, in December 2014, in the following terms:

> My usual and preferred RoA is oral, but on this occasion, in an attempt to reduce the anticipated period of residue stim, I decided to insufflate.

I snorted a line of between 5mg and 10mg. I then repeated this exercise approximately every hour for the next few hours. It was a bit of a rough ride.

The experience itself was nice enough, but the body load was high.

The nose-burn was significant. It was much harsher for me than, for example, MPA or 3-FPM. Perhaps I had too much, but later on, a mild headache developed. I experienced the usual stim-dilated pupils, with more than the usual jaw tension.

From reading other reports I was expecting a fairly short residue, but I found it to be lengthy. Ending the tests at approximately 8pm, I was still feeling the influence the following late-afternoon, and I had no sleep at all. This was way too much for my tastes.

Certainly it was a buzz. It was intense, very strong, and long lasting, but I think a lot of work is required to determine the correct dosage, and perhaps the ideal RoA.

I hope this helps other potential researchers, to whom I would advise: be particularly careful with the dose. Start lower than I did, and watch out for compulsive redosing.

Whilst I cannot be absolutely certain that this chemical caused the general malaise which followed this experiment, I have no intention of repeating the exercise to confirm. Take it easy.

I never explored further, and indeed, I binned the remaining powder.

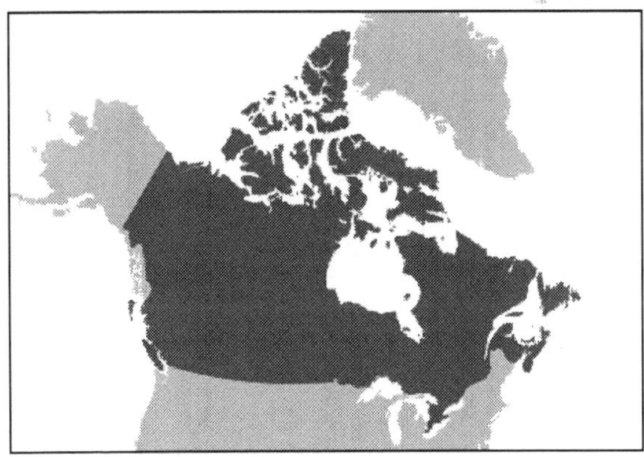

For the committed UK enthusiast Canada was the online source of a number of niche research chemicals

2.3.14 Hexen

Common Nomenclature	Ethyl-Hexedrone
Street & Reference Names	N-Ethyl-Hexedrone; NEH; Hex-en;
Reference Dosage	Threshold 5mg+; Light 15mg+; Common 30mg+; Strong 40mg+ Heavy 50mg+ [Psychonautwiki] Light 10mg+; Common 25mg+ Strong 40mg+ [The Drug Classroom]
Anticipated: Onset / Duration	15 Minutes / 3 Hours
Maximum Dose Experienced	82mg (10+10+10+10+10+8+8+8+8)
Form	Powder
RoA	Insufflated
Source / Jurisdiction	Dealer / Overseas

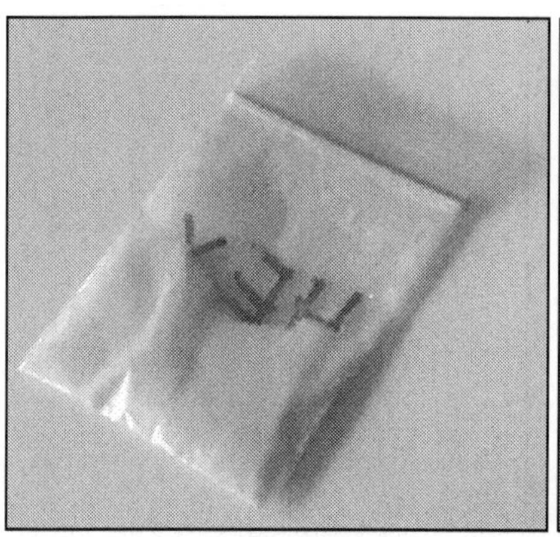

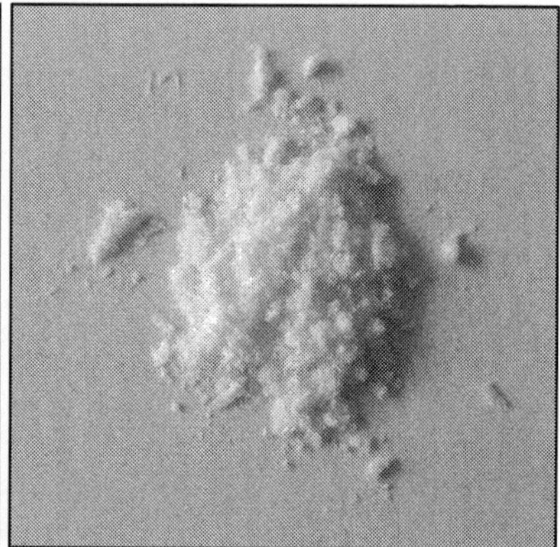

SUBJECTIVE EXPERIENCE
Although it was referenced in the 1960's, hexen wasn't synthesised until 2011. It finally began to appear on the markets towards the end of 2015. Frequently presented as a short acting cathinone with relatively limited residue-stimulation, it rapidly became popular, particularly in the United States

As heavy redosing and compulsive binging is often referred to on Internet forums, I take particular care in this area. As a precautionary barrier, I set aside the maximum I am prepared to sample during this session, and place the rest of the supply well beyond reach.

I divide 50mg into 5 lines of 10mg each. Whether I snort them all depends upon how the afternoon rolls. I place another 32mg in a drawer, in case I decide to extend into the evening.

82mg will therefore be the absolute maximum I can sample today, with a built-in decision point at 50mg.

T+0:00 I insufflate 10mg. [3:15pm]

T+0:15 I feel an ever-so-slight stimulation, and I am noticeably warmer. Noting that I am around threshold at this stage, I decide to insufflate the next 10mg. This should take me into *light* territory, where I should feel something more pronounced.

T+0:45 The previous 30 minutes have flown by. Granted, I was busy installing software, but nonetheless, it whizzed. I feel stimulated and quite happy. As the first 10mg must be fully effective, I insufflate a third line, taking the overall dose to 30mg.

I notice that there is some jaw tension, and that my pupils are slightly dilated.

T+1:00 The experience seems to have settled on to a plateau now. I feel pretty good, with slight euphoria, and I am definitely stimmed, and warm.

I feel the sense of a slight headache in the background, but it isn't sufficient to cause discomfort.

T+1:15 I am quite buzzed and elevated, but not flying. Certainly, I am functional in the sense that I could perform any task required. However, I am well aware that I am wired and I am happy to roll with it.

As it is 30 minutes since the last line, I decide to insufflate the fourth. I am now up to 40mg in total.

Is there any horn? Yes, there is. It is not up to methamphetamine or amphetamine levels, but it is strong, and fully available. Those forum posts on extended porn binges do make sense.

T+1:30 The experience is now slightly more intense than earlier. I am consciously drinking water to keep my fluid intake high, as I am still warm and obviously pumping.

T+1:45 I insufflate the fifth 10mg line. I am now on 50mg, having consumed the whole of the primary batch.

T+2:00 I am well in control of myself and riding on a pleasant plateau. My pupils remain semi dilated.

There is no doubt that I am enjoying the experiment. This has an edge that makes it very recreational, whilst enabling normal functionality to varying levels of capability.

T+2:45 I am still rolling at the same level but I feel a sense of being slightly weary.

As I feel no ill-effects I take the decision to extend. I insufflate 8mg of the optional 32mg batch, splitting the remainder into three equal lines.

T+3:30 As I feel I am tiring again, at least mentally, I insufflate another 8mg, and then another 8mg 30 minutes later.

T+4:15 I insufflate the final 8mg of the secondary batch. The pre-ordained limit of 82mg has now been reached.

I can see how some people binge on this and consume ridiculous amounts. It is very moreish, yet the comparatively painless snorting gives the impression that it is mild, which isn't the case.

It is now 7:30pm. I hope to slowly come-down from here and land towards midnight, and in theory, have a good night's sleep.

T+6:45 It is now 10pm, so as a harm mitigation measure, I eat a bowl of muesli and drink a glass of orange juice.

At 11pm I retire to bed.

The night's sleep was not good, or at least, the first part of it wasn't. I lay tossing and turning for several hours, and could only fall into slumber by taking 1mg of etizolam, which worked well.

In the morning I suffered the usual hangover symptoms. I felt mentally drained and distant, and tired.

I felt nothing like as bad as I did following my forays with some of the infamous hangover stims, or even with MDMA, but regardless, this was a major factor for much of the day. I suspect that had I continued to binge this could have been significantly worse.

I undertook the classic program for recovery, including vitamin pills, 5-HTP, exercise and food.

Hexen is often considered to be relatively forgiving, or even benign. I would suggest emphasis on the word *relatively*. At high doses, it can certainly take its toll, and the urge to redose is definitely strong.

This is not a drug not to take liberties with. The gentle climb and overall placidity can be deceptive. Note also that was one of those occasions upon which I retrospectively believe I dosed too highly.

2.3.15 IPPH

Common Nomenclature	Isopropylphenidate
Street & Reference Names	IPH; IPPD; IPP
Reference Dosage	Threshold 2mg+; Light 5mg+; Common 10mg+; Strong 20mg; Heavy 35mg+ [Insufflated, Psychonautwiki]
Anticipated: Onset / Duration	20 Minutes / 5 Hours
Maximum Dose Experienced	25mg+35mg
Form	Powder
RoA	Oral/Insufflated
Source / Jurisdiction	Internet / UK

O
O
H
N
GOV.UK
Search
Departments Worldwide How government works Get involved
Publications Consultations Statistics
Home > Crime, justice and law
News story
'Legal highs' to be banned under temporary power
Ban on five substances will come into force at 00:01 on Friday 10 April for up to 12 months.

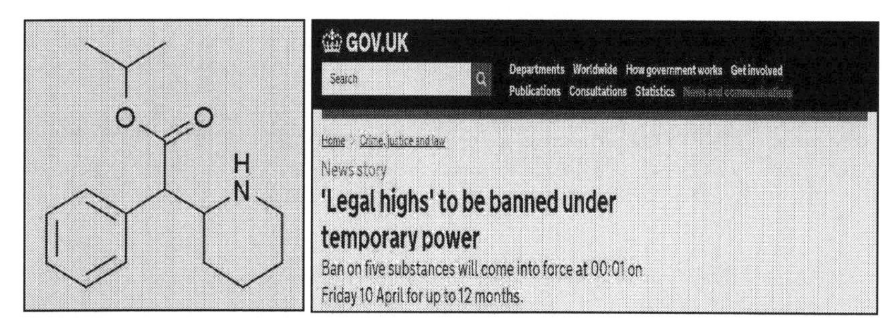

SUBJECTIVE EXPERIENCE
IPPH is a structural analogue of methylphenidate. It appeared on the online markets at the start of 2015, attracting mixed reviews, and was one of five phenidates specifically banned in the UK in April of that year.

I tested it in January 2015, and posted the following report. At the time, most other reports seemed to compare it to EPH, which was one of the most commonly used legal phenidates of that period. I purposely avoided this approach, largely because I subjectively felt that EPH was a little one-dimensional.

> T+0:00 I begin the experiment by taking 25mg orally on a reasonably empty stomach. Given that it is fairly late in the day, I am gambling that suggestions that there is little residue-stim are correct. [5pm]
>
> From the few reports posted so far, this does not seem to be a significant dose. Note also that I have not sampled any chemicals for a week or so, although I did drink a couple of beers last night.
>
> The taste is not the worst, but chems are never really palatable.

T+0:30 Thirty minutes in, there is nothing to note.

T+1:15 Again, there is nothing particularly notable to report. I feel that I could be slightly affected, but equally, this is so weak that it could be a placebo effect.

As others report of full effects within an hour this is somewhat disappointing. I therefore redose with a further 35mg. This takes me to the 60mg maximum I had set aside at the outset.

T+2:15 It suddenly dawns on me: I am indeed under the influence.

It is subtle, mild, and doesn't create the same sort of buzz associated with the currently popular stimulants. I can now see the relevance of third party comments regarding focus and mind-only stimulation with little physical effect.

Perhaps this escaped me on the earlier 25mg dose, as my expectation had been firmly set on a more all embracing and traditional experience.

There is no euphoria, but there is a certain clarity, and gentle delivery.

T+3:00 To finish off I decide to insufflate a couple of lines, to establish if there is a kick via this route. It appears to be kinder on the nose than substances like EPH and 3-FPM.

T+3:30 There wasn't a kick, but perhaps the earlier effects are now a little more pronounced.

I can also confirm that there is no significant dilation of the pupils, and that I am experiencing no jaw tension.

I managed to sleep a few hours later, indicating that as expected residue-stimulation from this chemical isn't excessive. I should also note that there was no horn, but on the other side of the coin, no significant stim-dick either.

All in all this was a fairly pleasant experience with little body load, although I suspect that the mind-set has to be correct to get the most out of it. If you are looking for an all-firing high, or wired excitation, you will be disappointed. It does however seem to be well suited to a situation in which broad functionality is required; perhaps when having to endure a somewhat boring scenario or social event.

Another question is whether it could be used as a potentiator for other substances. It has that sort of feel, but this is probably an area for comment by someone who is more qualified to discuss the chemistry of combinations than I am.

Would I take it again? Yes I would, but in the right setting and with the correct expectation.

2.3.16 Methamphetamine

Common Nomenclature	Methamphetamine
Street & Reference Names	Crystal Meth; Meth; Crystal; Glass; Crank; Tweak; Christine; Ice
Reference Dosage	Threshold 5mg+; Light 5mg+; Common 10mg+; Strong 30mg+; Very Strong 50mg+ [Erowid]
Anticipated: Onset / Duration	10 Minutes / 4 Hours
Maximum Dose Experienced	92mg
Form	Crystal
RoA	Insufflated
Source / Jurisdiction	Dealer / Overseas

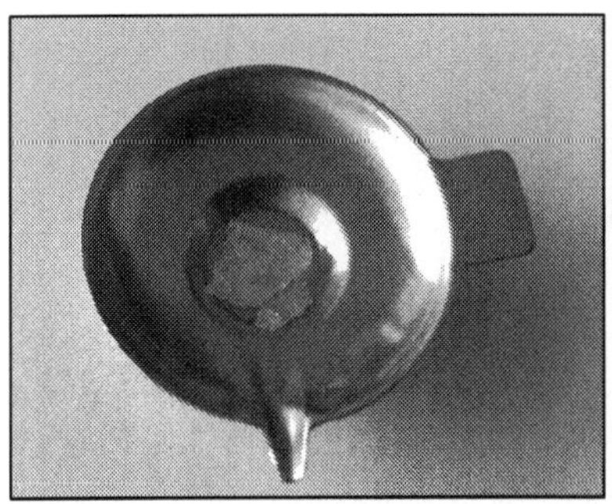

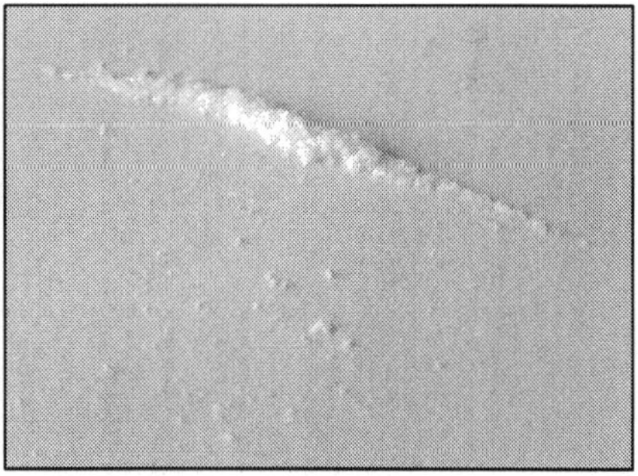

SUBJECTIVE EXPERIENCE
First synthesised in 1893, methamphetamine was, like amphetamine, used during World War II to reduce fatigue and increase alertness amongst combatants. Subsequently, in the 50s and 60s, it was prescribed to treat obesity. Increasing levels of abuse led, inevitably, to various levels of proscription.

In recent years its recreational use has attracted more than its fair share of horror stories and media hysteria. Despite this, and the obvious risk of addiction, it remains extremely popular, particularly as a street drug.

My sample, which was sold as *Crystal Meth Ice Shards*, weighs in at 92mg. I break it in half. I then crush one half and split it into 4 small lines of approximately 10mg each.

> T+0:00 I snort the smallest line, which is probably just under 10mg. [3pm]
>
> T+0:10 Not a lot has happened so far, leading me to believe that I may not have reached threshold. I'll give it another 5 minutes.

T+0:15 There is a low stim-like heady feeling in the background, but not much else. I am also beginning to feel quite warm. Another 10mg is insufflated.

T+0:25 This is very mild, so far. Whilst it is billed as more powerful than amphetamine, I'm finding the opposite. Of course, this could be a weak or adulterated supply, or I just might need more.

T+0:30 I snort the remaining 20mg of the initially crushed crystal. I have now insufflated 40mg in total.

T+0:35 I am starting to sense something stronger. This is headier in nature, I am more charged, and generally I feel a little dreamy. The body warmth is still evident, although it is not uncomfortable.

T+0:50 The increased psychoactivity from those last two lines has not developed any further, and I remain on the same level. Horn? Maybe there is a little, but it isn't compelling.

I now crush the other half of my supply, and snort 20mg (10mg with each nostril). For no apparent reason the left hurts far more than the right.

T+1:00 This is more like it. I am well and truly stimmed, with a bit of a push into the euphoric field, and horn is definitely now available. I can safely say that I have moved up a gear or two.

T+1:25 I'm in a decent place with this. I feel pretty good. There is a nice head buzz, but I still have clarity. It isn't overwhelming or in any way dysfunctional, and I can interact normally if I wish to.

I snort another 10mg, leaving only 10mg of the original 92mg supply.

T+1:45 I snort the last 10mg. This time I experience something of a rush, but it is not harsh. It is worth noting that this is very moreish, with the urge to repeatedly indulge being strong. The policy of only having a fixed amount available is a wise one, as I instinctively know that I would continue to redose and binge if more was available.

The feeling of intense and sustained pleasure is almost overwhelming.

T+2:00 I am still flying nicely, in fact, very nicely indeed. Cloud nine springs to mind. Ecstasy is another good word.

Horn can be extraordinarily intense, to the point that it is completely off the scale. I can certainly see how people engage in mega sex or porn binges with this, as referred to by this comment on TripSit:

> *"Recreationally, methamphetamine is used to increase sexual drive, lift the mood, and increase energy, allowing some users to engage in sexual activity continuously for several days straight"*.

There is a serious danger lurking here though. Given that the heights of such highly charged and enhanced sex cannot be reached without the chemical, the potential for long term disappointment under normal (unintoxicated) circumstances quickly emerges, particularly with repeated use.

I notice that my pupils are dilated. I also haven't eaten since this morning but my appetite has been completely suppressed.

T+2:40 Time has flown and I sense that I have started a slow decline, or at least I am settled on to a plateau. However, I am significantly wired, and I am really enjoying the edge of this, which is a euphoric energised happy buzz.

T+4:00 I am still in the bubble of elation and bliss. I can see why this is so popular.

I was wrong on the earlier comparison with amphetamine. Although different this is actually stronger. My erroneous assumption led to quite a heavy dose. I am somewhat zombified and deep into it, but in a very enjoyable way.

The effects lasted until bed time, and beyond, such that I barely slept. In the morning I felt drained but still slightly under the influence, with a background headache. In other words, I felt rough.

I took the commonly recommended steps to counter this and to speed up recovery, such as taking some 5-HTP, popping a vitamin tablet, eating good food, drinking fruit juice and plenty of water, as well as engaging some exercise and smoking a little cannabis. For more detail on this see the advice offered under the entry for amphetamine.

My head felt drained. It felt strained, like it wasn't at all right and was damaged, but not in a traditional headache sort of way. I also felt de-motivated, and couldn't be bothered to do anything. This was all of concern in itself, but at least I knew that I would recover in time.

Note that the hangover can persist for a lengthy period, and in this case, I was well under par for the best part of a week. Whilst the experience itself was one of great joy and pleasure, the payback during the prolonged aftermath was substantial.

One thing I did right was to make sure that I had only the 92mg available: I could not redose further or take any more. One thing I did wrong was to take 92mg. It was significantly too much: I should have researched harder and assumed that the supply was as strong as it was claimed to be, rather than the opposite.

To be addicted to this must be an absolute living nightmare.

NOTE: If you have just used this drug, and you are looking forward to another hit next weekend, stop. That's the slippery slope straight in front of you.

A FINAL WORD ON ADDICTION
Given the pharmacological complexity of this chemical, I am not certain that the following Reddit user's quote is strictly accurate, but it does broadly capture what can occur with this drug:

> TheJigmeister: "*Also bear in mind that meth floods your brain with serotonin, dopamine, and endorphins. After a while using, your brain burns itself out and your ability to produce those chemicals without drugs drops to near zero. So you quit and you're literally physically incapable of feeling good. It took me over three years to recover to a reasonable level. It does lasting damage to the pleasure you get out of life*"

On a similar theme, from a different thread:

> Wakewalking: "*Your brain does not allow you to reach these peaks again, as it erodes the receptors that allow it to balance the toxic response it gave following your first high. This means your brain now can't feel satisfaction from smaller, normal things in the same way*"

TheFix.Com describes the effect in the following terms:

> "*Using crystal meth is, from a biological perspective, like borrowing from a sadistic loan shark who demands resources faster than you can reasonably replace them—and the interest rate is unimaginably high. When the drug is discontinued, the crash is brutal, the high quickly replaced by a state of bottomless depression and hopelessness.*"

The consequences of this can be appalling. In some cases, they can lead to tragedy, as illustrated by another Reddit user:

> HrIssue: "*My brother was into meth. After three years, when he was at the edge of losing his job he decided to get clean. 4 weeks after getting clean, he hung himself. He kept telling us life was just gray and no color*"

My experience from a single experiment was entirely consistent with this. The high was indescribable; the come-down was horrible. It lasted for days, and even now, in some ways, I still hanker back to it in that I use it as a reference point and comparator for all other drugs in this class.

The picture presented by so many users and addicts is broadly the same: the normal joys of life become less and less special the more you use it. Recovery for heavy users can take years.

This isn't propaganda or media hysteria. Please exercise extreme caution with respect to this drug, particularly regarding regular use.

The aftermath is real, and it can be brutal.

2.3.17 Methylphenidate

Common Nomenclature	Methylphenidate
Street & Reference Names	Ritalin; Concerta; MPH; Medikinet; Metadate; Rubifen; Tranquilyn
Reference Dosage	Therapeutic 5mg+; Moderate 15mg+; Strong 35mg+; Dangerous 60mg+ [Oral, Drugs-Forum] Light 20mg+; Common 40mg+; Strong 60mg+ ; Heavy 80mg+ [Oral, TripSit]
Anticipated: Onset / Duration	1 Hour / 5 Hours
Maximum Dose Experienced	30mg + 10mg + 10mg +10mg
From	Pill
RoA	Oral
Source / Jurisdiction	Associate / UK

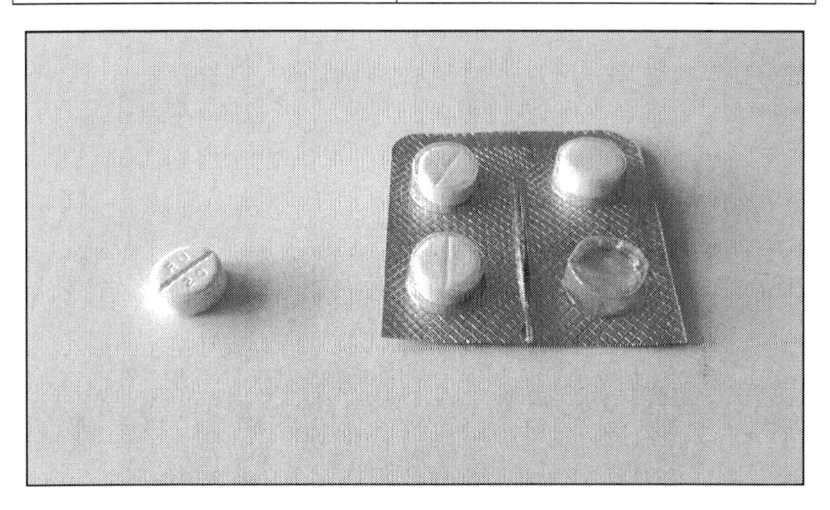

SUBJECTIVE EXPERIENCE

First synthesized in 1944, methylphenidate is a prescription medication which is widely used to treat attention deficit hyperactivity disorder (ADHD) and narcolepsy. During its history it has also been prescribed for a range of other conditions, including chronic fatigue and depression, and at one point was also sold as a pep pill.

As a generic medicine it is available under a large number of trade names, with my own supply branded as *rubifen*. Given that its potential side effects include tachycardia and chest pain in higher doses, I exercised restraint, and placed an absolute lid on my session by obtaining only four 20mg pills.

The question of dosage is a tricky one. Having experience of stimulants like methamphetamine, I am not inclined to go too low, but there are enough hints (not least the Drugs-Forum reference figures) to suggest that jumping in with all four pills would be extremely reckless. I therefore decide to initially start with 30mg.

Note also that these pills are immediate release (IR) and not extended release (XR) versions, so I should feel their effects within a normal time frame (for stimulants)

Regarding my expectations, given that I found that phenidate based research chemicals invariably tended towards the functional end of the spectrum, my enthusiasm is quite muted. I certainly don't anticipate a cocaine or amphetamine like high.

As I begin the experiment I am somewhat tired following what was (for no apparent reason) a poor night's sleep. I also feel a little chilly.

> T+0:00 I break one of the pills in half, and on an empty stomach I pop the 30mg (one and a half pills) into my mouth and swallow with a glass of cold water. [12:20pm]

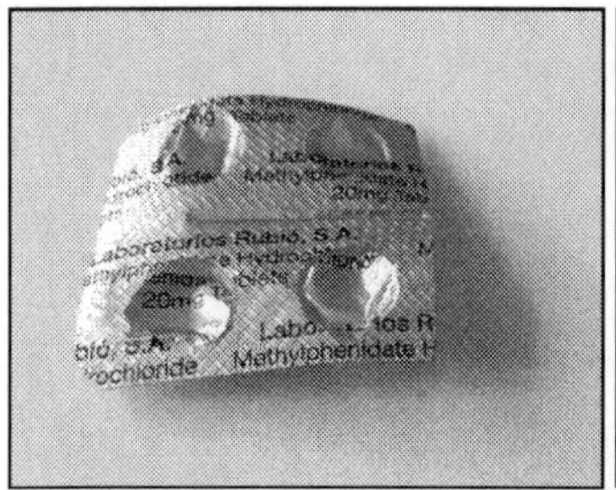

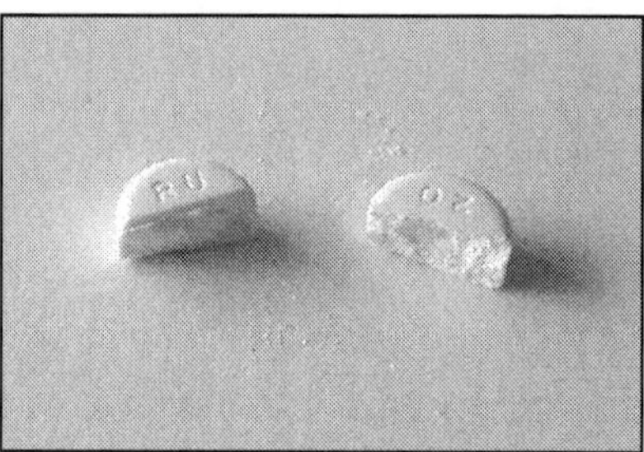

> My plan today is to take the other half-pill in perhaps an hour, and then go from there.
>
> T+1:00 Over the last hour I have gradually warmed-up, and the tiredness has been chased away. I feel much better, sufficient for me to take the next 10mg (bringing the total to 40mg). There is a slight buzz about the head, which at present is relatively gentle.
>
> T+2:00 I remain in a heady-stimulated zone. Within this, I can focus well enough, and I believe that I could easily hide my status in most social scenarios. As expected this is primarily functional rather than recreational, although equally, it is quite pleasant, in that I feel content and energised.
>
> Horn is of only minor interest with no real drive or compulsion. I also notice that the dreaded phenomenon of *stim-dick* is unmistakably present (as per other phenidates)

I now swallow another 10mg, bringing the total to 50mg. Note that I make a point of drinking sufficient water throughout.

T+3:00 I feel like I am on a functional plateau, and that I am not going to find any further recreation or uplift. There is also a hint that I will be exhausted when I come down, perhaps suggesting (rightly or wrongly) that I am on the way down already. I therefore take a final 10mg, bringing the total to 60mg.

I am tempted to flush the rest of the supply, but resist on the basis that the compulsion to take more really doesn't feel that strong.

Physically, my hands are cold, indicating a degree of vasoconstriction. The rest of my body remains quite warm. Perhaps this is psychologically driven, but I occasionally ask myself if my chest feels tight.

T+6:00 The intensity of the stimulation has diminished: it is still clearly evident, but is now milder. I am not in the least bit hungry, but for recovery purposes I force a meal down, with some fruit juice.

T+7:00 I am now closing in on base. I feel generally fatigued but I am still functional on account of the residue effects of the chemical. I am a little heavy headed, as though on the verge of a headache which doesn't quite materialise.

T+9:00 I am pretty much back to baseline now: a bit weary, a slight head presence, but broadly back within normal parameters. I have another bite to eat and then retire to bed.

Contrary to expectation, the night's sleep was better than usual: I dropped off easily, and other than a couple of disturbances I slept through soundly. That the last top-up was much earlier than normal for a stim-outing may have helped, but equally surprising is that I woke feeling refreshed and relaxed, with no hint of hangover or come-down.

The general mood of contentment lasted most of the morning and into the afternoon. Whether this was afterglow from the chemical or just the after effects of a good night's sleep is hard to tell. It could have been a bit of both.

The ride itself was rather bland in comparison to that of the usual standard-bearers of this class, in that it lacked euphoric edge and drive. Instead it seemed to settle onto an energised plateau of contentment. This wasn't bad, but in terms of reward and pleasure, it was somewhat lacking.

Whilst it is unlikely that I will ever revisit this I can see how it does have a place in the medical arena, and why its appeal as a recreational drug is relatively limited.

Finally, again with respect to dosage, this was in fact a little hard going at times: the dose I took was too high. This perhaps serves as a reminder that as with most stimulants overdose is indeed a serious threat. Take it easy if you intend to use this.

2.3.18 MPA

Common Nomenclature	Methiopropamine
Street & Reference Names	N/A
Reference Dosage	Threshold 10mg+; Light 20mg+; Common 40mg+; Strong 50mg+ [Oral, Erowid] Threshold 5mg; Light 5mg+; Common 20mg+; Strong 40mg+ [Insufflated, Erowid]
Anticipated: Onset / Duration	30 Minutes / 6 Hours (Oral)
Maximum Dose Experienced	100mg+
Form	Pill / Powder
RoA	Oral / Insufflated
Source / Jurisdiction	Internet / UK

NH
S
IUPAC: 1--(thiophen-2-yl)-2-methylaminopropane
CAS: N/A
10 x 50mg Pellets
MPA Pellets
WARNING
H303 - May be harmful if swallowed
H313 - May be harmful in contact with skin
P102 - Keep out of reach of children
P261 - Avoid breathing dust
Scientific Supplies Ltd, 14 Hanover Street, London, UK, W1S 1YH Tel: 0044 845 269 0056

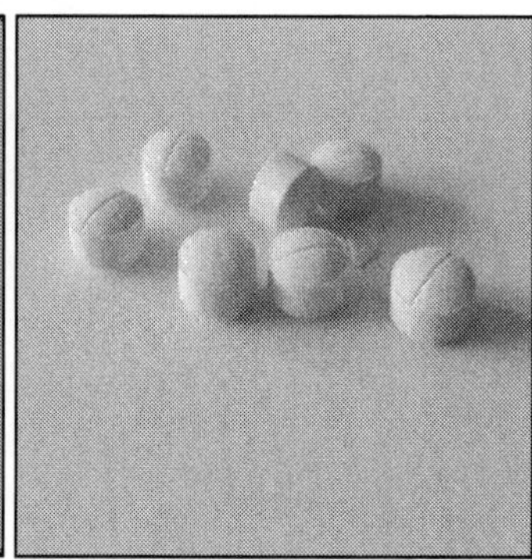

SUBJECTIVE EXPERIENCE
First reported in the 1940s, methiopropamine appeared on the recreational markets at the end of 2010, and was sold in both powder and pill form.

Whilst I engaged periodically over subsequent years, I never found it to be particularly exciting on its own. It was largely a functional stimulant, with only minor edge.

Self evidently, perhaps, I felt stimulated, but also, I felt under the obvious influence of a chemical. On a high dose, there was a bit of euphoric lift, although this did not feel very natural. Subjectively, it wasn't the best or smoothest of rides.

However, when combined with compounds which accentuated or added to its edge, the story changed dramatically.

Over this period, MPA was mixed with a variety of empathogens and similar chemicals. Two that spring to mind, and which I researched extensively, are MDAI and NM2AI.

I sampled a number of such brands, which themselves morphed and changed over time. Amongst these were: *Sparkle-E* (MPA+MDAI, later MPA+5-MeO-DALT), *Pink Panther* (MPA+MDAI+Others), *Green Beans* (MPA+NM2AI), M&M (MPA+NM2AI) and *GoGaine* (MPA+MDAI, later MPA+EPH).

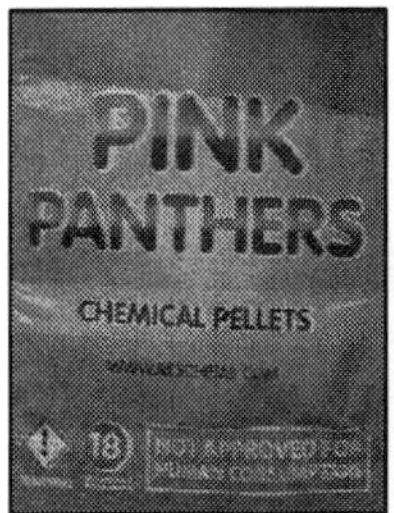

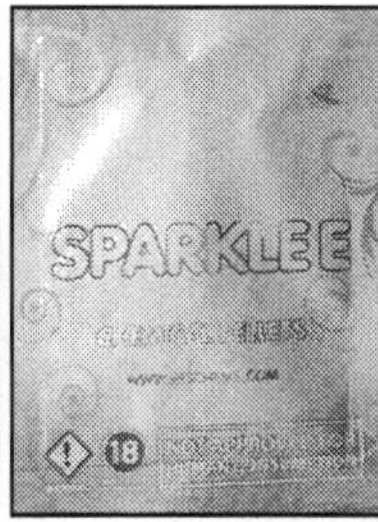
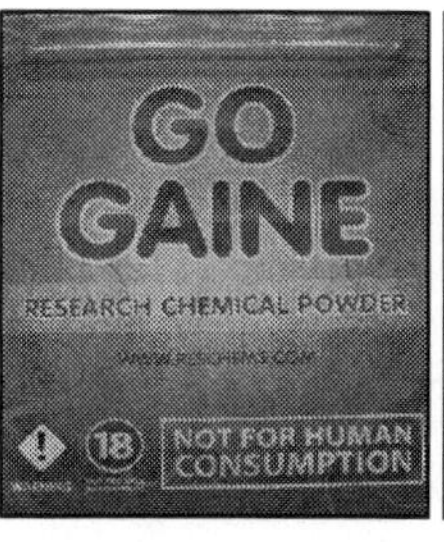

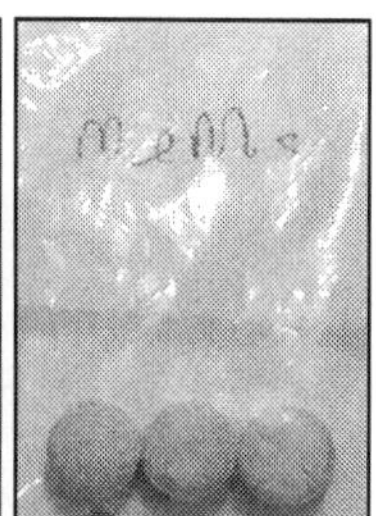

Some of these combinations were extremely effective at inducing experiences inclusive of euphoria, horn, and empathy. At times, their intensity approached that of amphetamine.

In terms of content, an initial wave of change was caused by a shortage of MDAI, which I was told by a head shop vendor was due to the loss of a pre-cursor, resulting from legal issues abroad. Subsequent changes were largely driven by the developing legal landscape in the UK, with MPA itself eventually to become the subject of a Temporary Class Drug Order (TCDO) in November 2015.

Prior to this, there is no doubt that MPA, both stand-alone and combined with other research chemicals, was one of the most widely used substances of the legal high era. I have to admit that I consumed my fair share of this.

THE SHADOW PEOPLE

One last word and it is a word of warning: psychosis is a real disorder, and excessive dosing, usually combined with consequential sleep deprivation, can lead to it.

On one occasion I felt that I was heading there via a foolhardy binge on GoGaine. During this episode I encountered the *shadow people*, a common manifestation, which at the time I had never heard of. The shadow people exist in the corner of your eye, in the semi-dark, and the impression is that they are far from friendly.

Whilst this may sound like an intriguing, humorous or interesting phenomenon, it isn't. It is traumatic and terrifying.

I learned much from that particular episode, and I consider myself to be lucky. Others have not been so lucky. Don't shortcut the safety measures.

2.3.19 NM2AI

Common Nomenclature	N-methyl-2-aminoindane
Street & Reference Names	N-methyl-2-AI
Reference Dosage	Threshold 5mg+; Light 50mg+; Common 100mg+; Strong 150mg+; Heavy 200mg+ [Oral, Psychonautwiki]
Anticipated: Onset / Duration	45 Minutes / 3 Hours
Maximum Dose Experienced	200mg (in combination)
Form	Powder
RoA	Oral / Insufflated
Source / Jurisdiction	Internet / UK

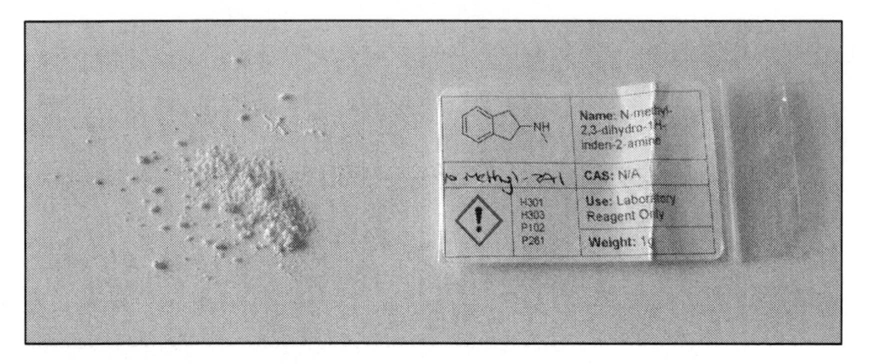

SUBJECTIVE EXPERIENCE
I have sampled this as an ingredient of a number of blends, most notably in combination with MPA. These definitely produced a nice ride, and there is no doubt that NM2AI brought something to the table. The question, therefore, is whether it has any value stand-alone.

A couple of years ago I explored a light dose via the oral route, but got little return. More recently I turned to insufflation. I snorted 40mg, which for this RoA is probably a reasonable first-time dose. The nose burn wasn't as bad as had been suggested online.

There was definite psychoactivity: a slight head buzz, some stimulation, and a minor mood lift. I drifted gently back to baseline after an hour or so. I experienced a very modest but not unpleasant sojourn.

On the question of whether there is a sweet spot for a significant take-off, I join the general consensus in not being sure.

2.3.20 PPH

Common Nomenclature	Propylphenidate
Street & Reference Names	N/A
Reference Dosage	Light 15mg+; Common 25mg+; Strong 60mg+; Heavy 100mg+ [Oral, TripSit]
Anticipated: Onset / Duration	5 Minutes / 2 Hours
Maximum Dose Experienced	36mg (21mg+15mg)
Form	Powder
RoA	Insufflation
Source / Jurisdiction	Internet / UK

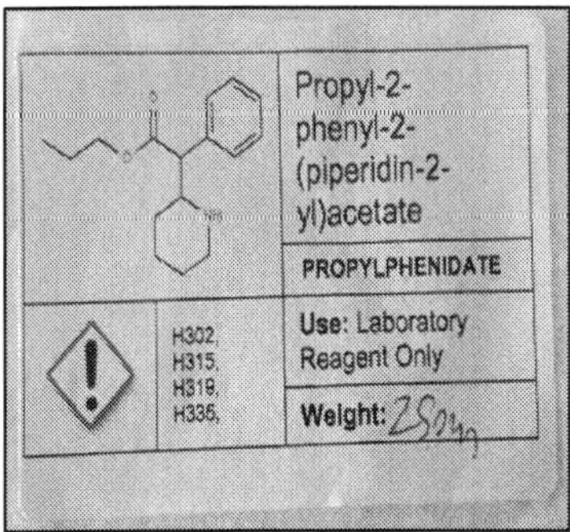

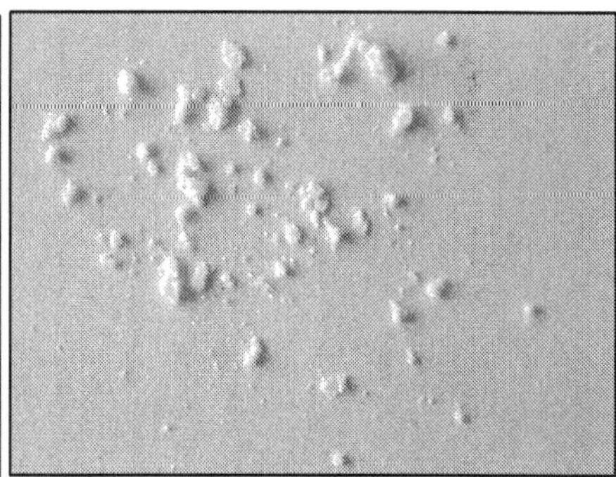

SUBJECTIVE EXPERIENCE

Propylphenidate (PPH) was one of a number of methylphenidate related chemicals banned in the UK via a TCDO in April 2015. As this came shortly after its release, it had a very limited period of open sale. Falling under the same axe were Ethylphenidate, 3,4-Dichloromethylphenidate, Methylnaphthidate and Isopropylphenidate. Fortunately, I had obtained a small sample of 250mg a few weeks earlier, and was able to test it just in time.

Dosage information had yet to become established, particularly for insufflation, so I elected to proceed with particular caution.

> T+0:00 Tipping the packet gently, 21mg pops out of the bag. I line it up and snort. It stings, making my right eye water. I feel the chemical burn as it subsequently rolls down the back of my throat. [4:22pm]
>
> T+0:05 I can already feel something coming-on as the pain dissipates. A mild head warmth emerges, and a general stimulation is suddenly present.

T+0:10 This has settled down now, into a low level background sort of mode. I feel fine, more alive than I did, and perhaps with a slight mood lift.

T+0:15 Thus far this is completely functional, with no horn or other distinguishing features. I still have the foul taste at the back of my throat.

T+0:25 There has been no significant change since the onset. Perhaps my head now feels a strange heaviness, and I am warmer. As this is almost certainly the last time I will sample this compound, I am considering a redose of perhaps 10mg, to move into more commonly referenced territory. Can I face that pain though?

T+0:30 I summon the courage and snort the 15mg that falls out of the bag. I bin the rest as a precaution. This isn't to say that I believe there is much chance of compulsive redosing.

T+0:45 Perhaps I feel more elevated than previously, and I am certainly content. This is nowhere near to the main (illegal) stims, but is fairly pleasing in its own steady way (apart from the now runny nose).

T+0:55 I feel that I have stabilised at this point, as per the last update. I check my blood pressure. It is 152/78: elevated but only slightly. Pulse rate is hovering above 60, which again, isn't far off the mark.

T+1:00 Whilst on this plateau I feel generally comfortable. This isn't bad, but relatively, it isn't a high flying ride. It's just pleasant, at least at this dose. Without the assurance of popular use, I wouldn't really wish to push it any higher.

T+2:00 On the two hour mark I am still under the influence, although perhaps at a reduced level. I feel a somewhat heavy type of head buzz, albeit minor in nature, and a bit of a tingly feel to my face and arms. My hands are a little chilly.

T+3:00 I am slowly coming-down, and hoping that the night's sleep isn't too badly affected. My poor nostril remains uncomfortable. However, I am able to eat normally (so no real appetite suppression), and socialise as usual.

T+16:00 I spent the rest of the evening blowing my nose, and as feared the night's sleep was rather disturbed, at least until the early hours. This morning I feel broadly within normal parameters.

I didn't expect this to light any fires, and it didn't. However, apart from the painful insufflation, it was quite pleasant if a little underwhelming. Had it remained on the market it may have found a niche as part of a combination or blend, but I doubt that it would have ever been a big hitter in terms of popularity. It isn't a chemical I would ever have made a habit of using.

2.3.21 Pipradrol

Common Nomenclature	Pipradrol
Street & Reference Names	Meratran
Reference Dosage	N/A
Anticipated: Onset / Duration	No information available
Maximum Dose Experienced	60mg
Form	Crystal
RoA	Insufflated
Source / Jurisdiction	Gift / Overseas

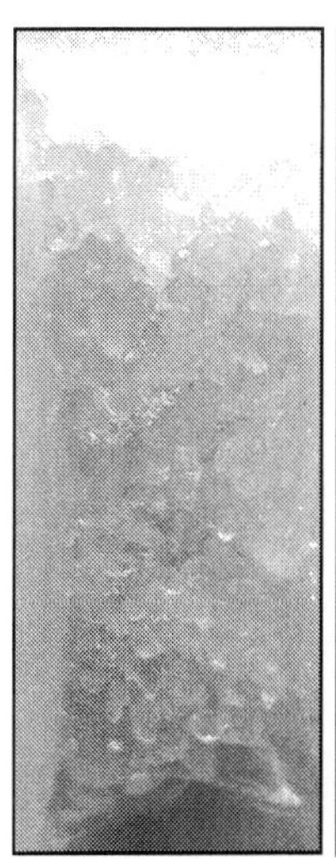

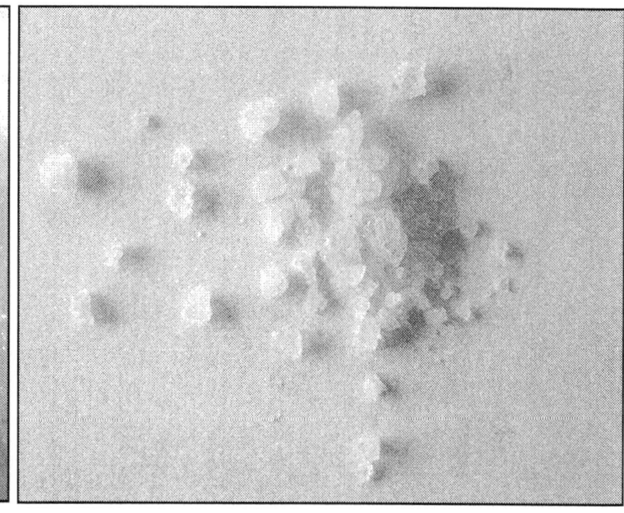

SUBJECTIVE EXPERIENCE
Pipradrol was developed in the 1940's and was used to treat a variety of mental health conditions, including dementia and ADHD. Its abuse potential was such that from the late 70s it was banned across a number of countries, including the United States (schedule IV) and the UK (class C).

A sample fell into my hands more by accident than design. However, despite a lack of reference data and its limited history of recreational use, for the purposes of this book I decided to test it.

> T+0:00 I weigh 60mg of the crystal like structures. They crush easily with a credit card and I arrange them in three lines of approx 20mg each.

I snort a single line. [4:47pm]

T+0:05 I feel nothing other than a slight tingle, which could in fact be a placebo effect. There is a hint of headspace developing: perhaps.

T+0:20 I can now feel a little head stimulation, but nothing intrusive. I insufflate the next 20mg, hoping for more.

This is not painless to snort, but is not a serious problem either.

T+0:40 There has been no change since the 20 minute mark. Given that the first line must now be in full effect, and the second should be developing, I am rather underwhelmed.

T+0:45 The final 20mg is hoovered, taking the total to 60mg.

T+0:50 I'm in that place again, the one which I can only describe as *nice*. It is mildly pleasant, but nothing else. There is no excitement or intensity: just a very minor glow and warmness.

I am hoping that this goes further, but not expecting it to do so.

T+1:00 An hour in and I seem to be at the peak, which is broadly as described on the 50 minute mark.

T+3:00 The glow I referred to earlier continued for a while, and then faded. I am now more or less back to base.

T+16:00 I retired at the usual time and had a normal night. I experienced no problem at all with sleep.

Now, either I am a hard head, which I am not, or there is cross tolerance in play, which I doubt, or this is extremely mild, at least at this sort of dose. It was very disappointing.

Note that in the context of pipradrol as a medicine, Wikipedia states that:

> *"Dosage is between 0.5 and 4 milligrams per day, typically taken as a single dose in the morning as the long duration of effects of pipradrol (up to 12 hours) means insomnia can be a problem especially if it is used at higher doses or taken too late in the day".*

Given this statement, I wouldn't want to push this any higher than I did with this test. I almost certainly went too far.

My verdict, therefore, is that pipradrol offers too little to be of significant recreational interest.

2.3.22 TPA

Common Nomenclature	Thiopropamine
Street & Reference Names	N/A
Reference Dosage	None Available
Anticipated: Onset / Duration	5 Minutes / 8 Hours
Maximum Dose Experienced	120mg
Form	Powder
RoA	Insufflated
Source / Jurisdiction	Internet / UK

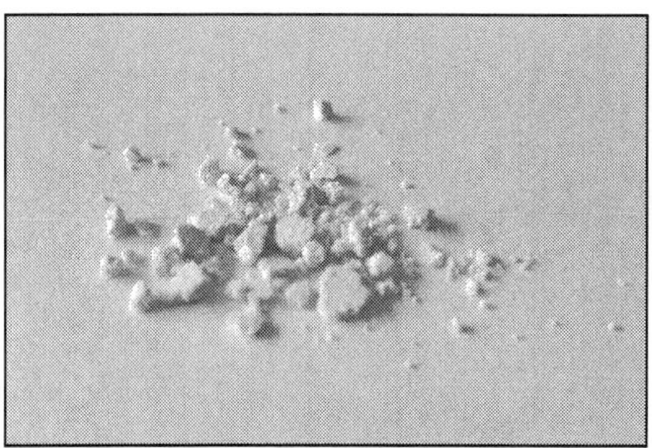
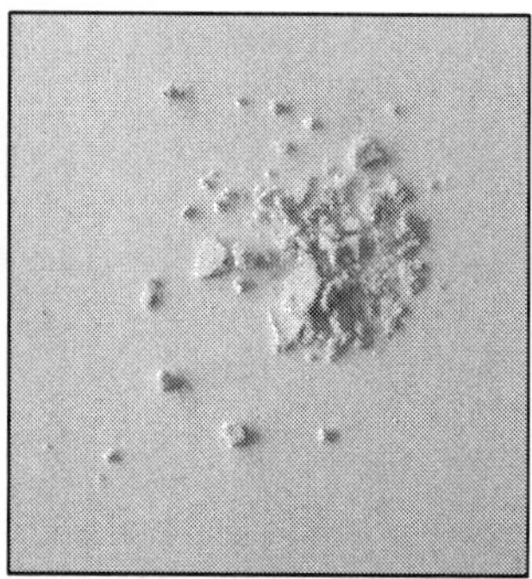

SUBJECTIVE EXPERIENCE
First synthesised in 1942, TPA didn't appear on the markets until early in 2016, shortly after the UK ban on the structurally similar MPA. This came just weeks prior to the implementation of the *Psychoactive Substances Act*, which made its sale and import unlawful (although not its possession).

I only found time to test it after the ban came into force, and wrote the following report the day after my initial experiment:

> I finally tested this one last night. Despite the mixed and sometimes ambiguous reports I dosed at 120mg, via lines of 20, 25, 25, 25 and 25, which were insufflated over several hours.
>
> I started what probably constituted a mini-binge at about 4pm.
>
> The lift on the first 20mg was rapid, and was really quite nice. Nose burn was evident, but I've certainly felt worse.

This was quite functional, but with some euphoria and a slight empathogenic edge, which brought with it a little horn. I must say that, generally, I enjoyed it.

It is quite a long time since I sampled MPA, so this probably has to be taken with a pinch of salt, but it did seem to be a little smoother. A number of amphetamine-like qualities were present, adding to its recreational value.

I was able to consume a light meal in the middle of the ride, which I can't normally face on stimulants, and I had some vitamins earlier in the day, which probably helped what was a reasonably soft comedown.

By 11pm it was fading, and I'd had enough. As I was going to be busy the following day (today) I had a little etizolam and slept like a baby.

On waking this morning I felt pretty good, possibly feeling the tail end of the experience.

Overall, I had an agreeable evening, and indeed, I now regret not stocking more than a single 1g baggy prior to the ban. I should also add that this would have made for a very pleasant sojourn on a much lower dose than I experimented with.

On the basis of my tests, this appeared to be more than just a legal replacement for MPA. It delivered a positive experience in its own right.

Despite arriving on the market late in the fray, I have no idea why it wasn't more popular than it was. It has now, of course, largely passed into the annals of history, as a minor player during the dying embers of the *legal high years*.

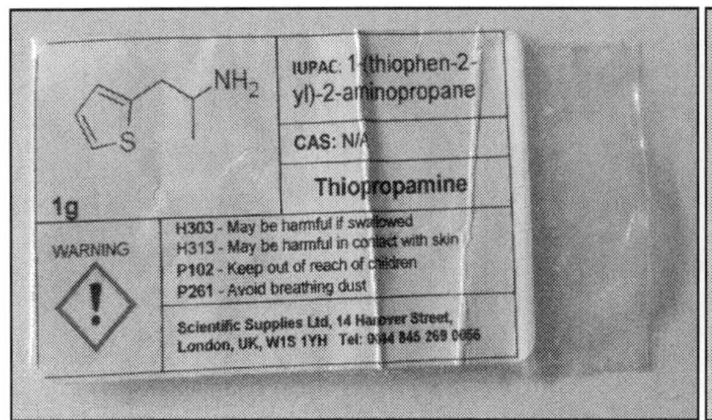

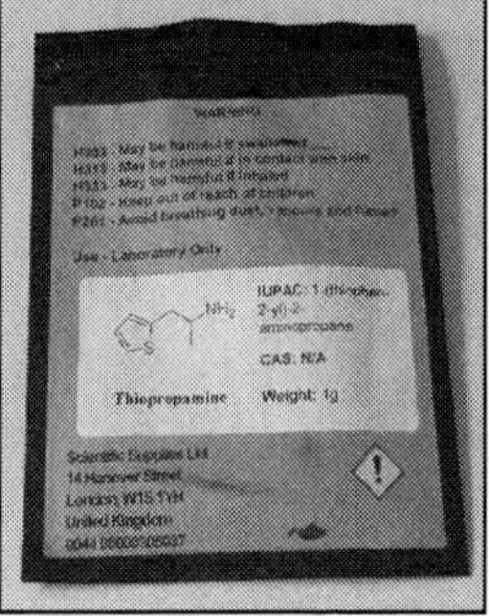

TPA arrived late on the scene, missing the opportunity to become a major force in legal high market

2.4. ANXIOLYTICS & SEDATIVES

Textbook Definition: *A sedative can produce a calming or relaxing effect, such that stress, irritability or agitation is reduced. In some cases sedatives can produce hypnotic anticonvulsant and muscle relaxant effects. Technically, sedatives are depressants, in that they induce depression of the central nervous system (CNS), although many also have antipsychotic properties.*

The following chemicals have been sampled and researched for inclusion within this section:

2.4.1 Alprazolam
2.4.2 Clonazolam
2.4.3 Diazepam
2.4.4 Etizolam
2.4.5 Gabapentin
2.4.6 Pregabalin
2.4.7 Pyrazolam
2.4.8 Others

NOTE: Those CNS depressants which produce contradictory recreational effects to the above, such as opioids and alcohol, have been included in other sections of this book.

During the legal high years benzodiazepines entirely dominated the recreational market for this class of drug. Such was their predominance that I briefly considered using the word in the heading. For consistency, however, I refrained from doing so.

I always associated sedatives, and indeed benzos, with sleep. They are sleeping pills, right? The correct answer to this question is: sometimes.

Sleep is what I originally used them for: etizolam to be specific, to kill a trip to be precise. One day this changed, when a higher than intended dose took me into the realms of the anxiolytic and the hypnotic. I cannot deny that I enjoyed it.

However, by this stage I had already read far too many tragic stories on Internet forums regarding benzo addiction. For this class of drug, I would be particularly careful not to break my personal rules regarding frequency and dose restraint. I therefore skirted the edges and dipped my toes in here and there.

Another area in which to exercise extreme caution relates to combinations, in particular, mixing with alcohol, opioids or other sedatives/anxiolytics. Don't do it.

There is a certain subtlety in this playground. Different drugs do have different effects, but the user sometimes has to be well tuned to recognize and appreciate this. The full catalogue of possibilities is enormous, but in the context referred to above, the risks are all too real.

BENZODIAZEPINES: US FATLALITY FIGURES
The graphs below (courtesy the US Department of Health and Human Services) provide a stark and clear message. The first illustrates the number of deaths in that country involving benzodiazepines. The second has lines overlaid showing the number of deaths involving benzodiazepines and any opioid, benzodiazepines without any opioid, and benzodiazepines and other synthetic narcotics. Benzos are not *soft* drugs. Be careful.

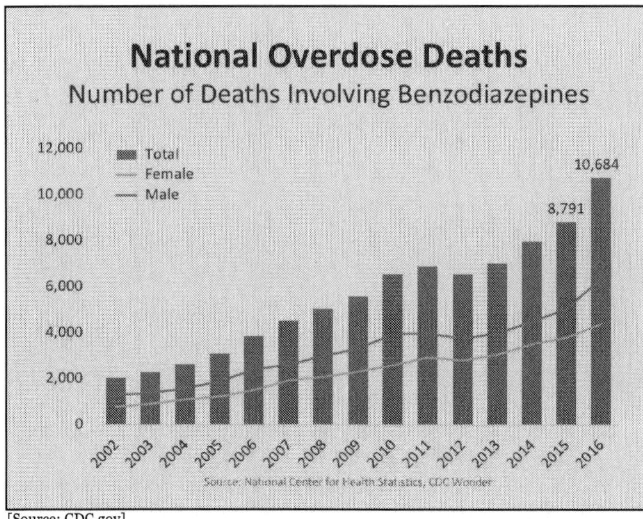

[Source: CDC.gov]

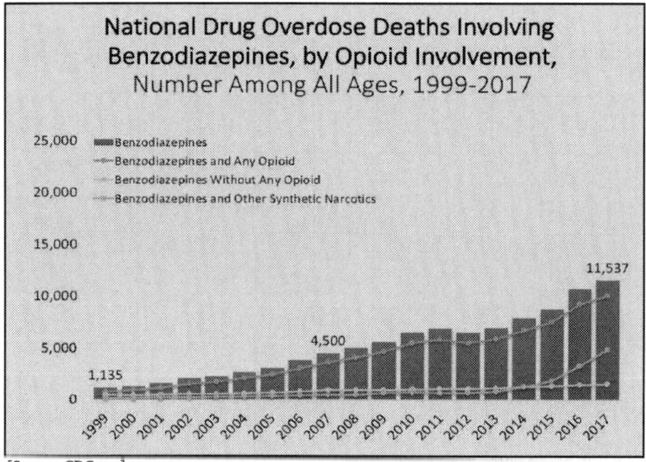

[Source: CDC.gov]

2.4.1 Alprazolam

Common Nomenclature	Alprazolam
Street & Reference Names	Xanax
Reference Dosage	Light: 0.25mg+; Common 0.5mg+; Strong: 1.5mg+ Heavy 2mg+ [TripSit]
Anticipated: Onset / Duration	30 Minutes / 6 Hours
Maximum Dose Experienced	1mg
Form	Pill
RoA	Oral
Source / Jurisdiction	Prescription / Overseas

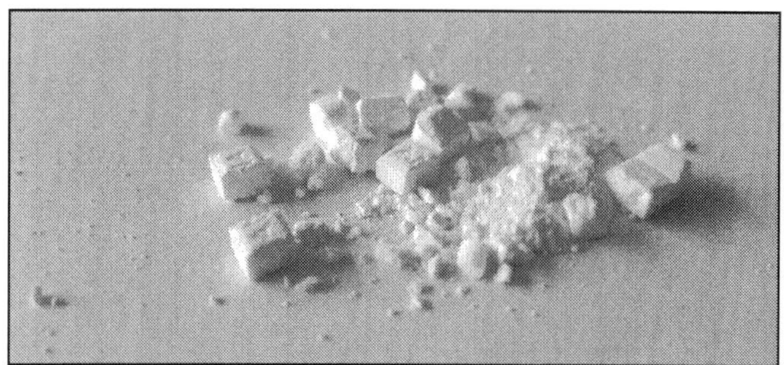

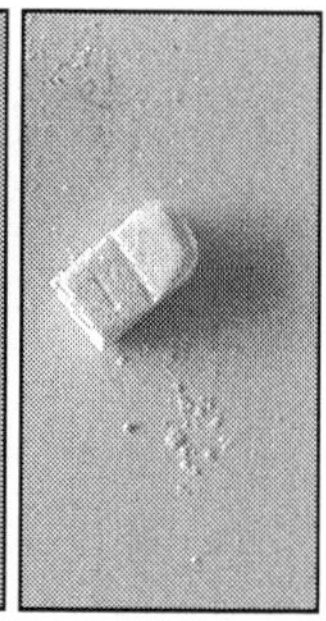

SUBJECTIVE EXPERIENCE
Alprazolam (xanax) is by far the most widely known and popular anxiolytic drug. Indeed, it has long been ranked as the most prescribed psychiatric medication in the United States, with over 40 million prescriptions per year.

Alarmingly, it is also well known for its addiction potential (as are the other drugs in this class). Related to this is the fact that large numbers of people build up a huge tolerance, and dose accordingly.

Another worrying aspect is the number of reports of blackouts and lost hours on higher doses. For a one-off experiment it was this issue which I most concerned myself with during research.

After a great deal of investigation I elect to dose at 1mg. This was not the easiest decision to reach, but I found a disturbing number of forum comments along the following lines:

> *"0.5 - 1 milligrams is optimal for someone with no tolerance. Anything more than that and you'll pass out"* ~ Pasha, BlueLight.org

> *"But from an HR stand point, 2 milligrams is far too potent a dose for someone with no tolerance. That's a fact, not an opinion. In a clinical setting, Alprazolam prescribing regimens begin at 0.250 milligrams. That alone says it all."* ~ Pasha, BlueLight.Org

> *"2mg would put almost anyone with no tolerance on their ass. Swim has been taking Xanax for years and 2mg is still fine"* ~ RaoulDuke32, Drugs-Forum.com

I also noted the following:

> *"Emergency room visits due to the recreational abuse of Xanax more than doubled from 57,419 in 2005 to 124,902 in 2010."* - Addictioncenter.com

Obviously, this is not a drug to treat lightly. I therefore proceed with the utmost caution, clearing my diary and finding a safe space for the rest of the day.

Note that at the time of testing I have no benzo tolerance at all, and my system is entirely clear of all drugs.

> T+0:00 I separate what is probably a little less than 1mg from the crumbled wreckage of my supply, and place the rest well out of reach. I consume this with a glass of cold water, and wait. [3:20pm]
>
> T+0:30 I sense that something coming-on. I feel a mild head driven relaxation and a gentle numbness about my hands, feet and body. It's minor and no threat to functionality, but the change is noticeable.
>
> T+1:00 The head bubble may have evolved slightly, and it is more firmly entrenched in sedation, of the non-fatigued variety. I don't feel any anxiety, but I didn't feel any to begin with.
>
> All sharp edges have in fact disappeared from my worldview as I have moved into a chilled ambience of tranquillity. Vision remains extremely clear and possibly enhanced, which combined with a dreamy headspace makes for a strange feel to the experience.
>
> T+1:20 Time has passed quite quickly, and the above manifestations appear to be fairly stable. This is quite a gentle ride, albeit not a particularly exciting one. The word pleasant probably best describes it, with an overall impression of being a little zoned-out.
>
> I should point out that I don't feel even remotely like keeling over on this dose, or blacking out.
>
> I certainly feel the effects, but not in any negative terms.

T+2:00 I just ate a meal and enjoyed it, so there is no appetite or taste suppression in play. I am content and relaxed, overlaid with a drifting ataractic aura. It's quite a nice background experience.

T+2:45 An unwanted side effect might be that I just spent a large portion of the last hour doing nothing. I couldn't be bothered, so I just lounged around, pinging across YouTube, news sources, forums, and a handful of similar web sites with a smile upon my face. I was totally unproductive.

Now, this could be because I am just bored and at a loose end, or it could be that the xanax has numbed my drive as well as my body. Perhaps I am just chillaxed, which is what I hoped to be, and I could be moaning for the sake of it.

T+3:00 A feeling of drowsiness has started to emerge, and sleep becomes appealing. I will fight this, initially with a cup of tea, and perhaps take a walk in half an hour. I am still partially-immersed but the headiness is morphing into mental fatigue and sleepiness. I make the effort to snap out of it.

T+5:00 I have battled through the drowsiness and now feel like I am approaching baseline. I'm a little worn, and not yet 100% zoned-in again, but broadly I feel like I have had a hard day with general fatigue.

I am most definitely tired and it is certainly a result of the xanax ingestion.

I retired to bed at 10pm, fell asleep very quickly and slept like the proverbial log for a good 10 hours. I awoke feeling a little groggy but a couple of cups of filtered coffee soon addressed this.

Comfortable and cosy are two words I have frequently seen associated with xanax, and I wouldn't argue with them. This was a decent experience, as I floated around the house for a few hours, with no worldly worries on my shoulders. It evolved into tiredness later on, and time began to pass in something of a haze, but there was no hard landing or adverse effects.

Would I take it again, recreationally?

Given that this class of drug isn't really my bag, and the well documented risks commonly presented, I wouldn't. The only circumstance in which I would ever repeat this exercise would be to identify the effects of a larger dose for the purposes of this book. This is unlikely.

I will end by re-emphasizing some of the warnings I made above. It's a nice enough ride in its early stages, but it can be fraught with danger. If you are determined to experiment with it, go easy, and definitely avoid it if you are prone to addiction or struggle to stop when you know you really should. A cursory search on the Internet should persuade you that this isn't one to trifle with.

2.4.2 Clonazolam

Common Nomenclature	Clonazolam
Street & Reference Names	Clam; C-lam
Reference Dosage	Threshold 50ug+; Light 75ug+; Common 200ug+; Heavy 500ug+; [TripSit]
Anticipated: Onset / Duration	20 Minutes / 8 Hours
Maximum Dose Experienced	250ug
Form	Capsules
RoA	Oral
Source / Jurisdiction	Internet / UK

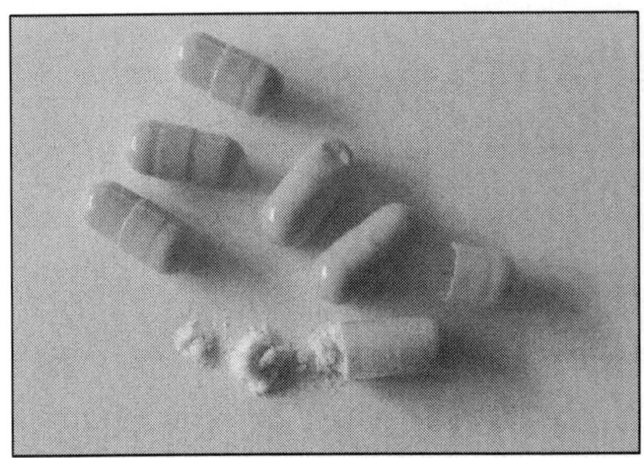

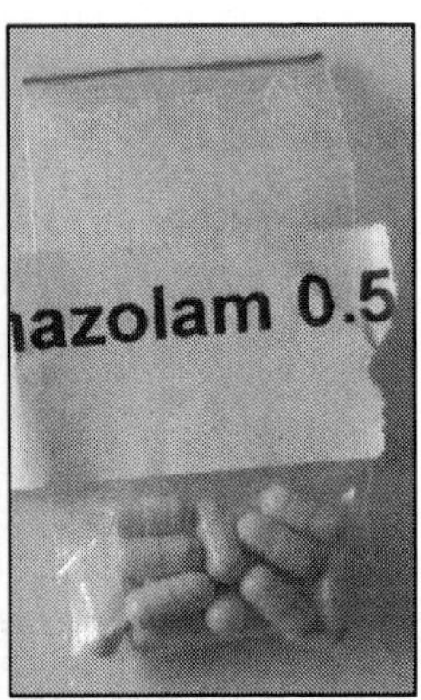

SUBJECTIVE EXPERIENCE
I became aware that this was one of the big hitters courtesy of forum reports. Notably, blackouts were reported here and there, and addiction was cited all too frequently. Accordingly, its fear-factor was set on high, and my foray was always going to be ultra-cautious, and a one-off.

I struggle to report more detail largely because it delivered more or less what I was expecting. This, specifically, was sedation and sleep. The following day wasn't particularly foggy, as I recall.

At time of writing I still have a couple of the little yellow capsules sitting in my drawer of goodies, but as with most benzos, I haven't been particularly motivated to dip into them again.

I suggest that this is one to use only in exceptional circumstances.

2.4.3 Diazepam

Common Nomenclature	Diazepam
Street & Reference Names	Valium; Vs; Diastat; AcuDial; Zetran
Reference Dosage	Light 2.5mg+; Common 5mg+; Heavy 15mg+ [TripSit]
Anticipated: Onset / Duration	1 Hour / 1 Day
Maximum Dose Experienced	15mg
Form	Pill
RoA	Oral
Source / Jurisdiction	Prescription / UK

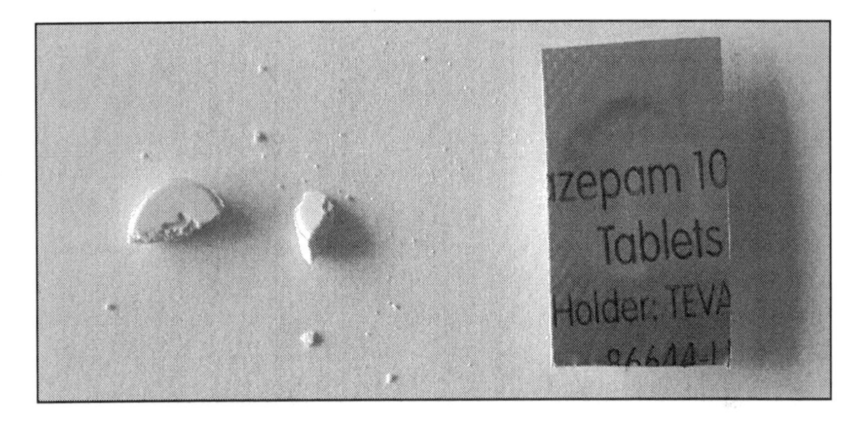

SUBJECTIVE EXPERIENCE
Diazepam was first launched in 1963, and has long been one of the most prescribed medicines in the world. Since its patent expired in 1985, it has been marketed under literally hundreds of brand names.

I was prescribed diazepam in my youth, under the name *valium*, and always found that it created drowsiness, without really alleviating the underlying anxieties, at least in a significant or meaningful way. On the basis of this, my expectations on re-testing it for this book are not high.

As I am entirely clean of benzodiazepines, with no tolerance, I elect to dose at 15mg, a figure which seems to be broadly recommended by a majority of apparently sensible Internet forum posters. This is also within the *common* range according to the online harm reduction communities. Given the fairly lengthy half-life of this drug, this is as far as I really wish to venture.

My physical condition is good, although I am rather anxious today due to domestic events which are outside my control. I am consuming on an empty stomach.

T+0:00 I break one of my two 10mg diazepam pills in half. I swallow one and a half with a glass of water, and bin the remaining half. [5:15pm].

T+0:15. I anticipated an onset of about an hour, yet my mind is already floating with a strange dreamy high, which ebbs and flows in waves. I am clearly under the influence of this drug, and it is a pleasing heady experience, making it difficult to focus or concentrate. The anxiety I was fretting with earlier has now dissipated.

Bodily, there is a mild numbness, which again, isn't unpleasant. I feel a little detached, but in a positive sense. Thus far, this is gentle and kind.

I wonder how far this will go, and hope that it will last, so that I can come to terms with it a little more and perhaps bask in it at my leisure.

Ding dong! Horror of horrors: the doorbell rings. I see through the window that it is a neighbour dropping something off the for the charity shop. I'll be back....

The crisis is over. It was difficult to hide my status but I managed, I think. I doubt that I would have pulled it off had she engaged in a conversation.

I am finding this live report increasingly difficult to write. Walking around is also a bit weird. I feel a drunken type of intoxication, but not with any of the rough or negative aspects. I am just not fully tuned in to my surroundings: I am slightly off kilter, but it is a very mild and gentle offset.

T+0:30 I feel that I am becoming more accustomed to this. My body is comfortable as I meander but I am careful not to sway excessively or walk into a wall, or generally act as a drunk. It's all very gentle but I am aware that at least to some degree I am socially debilitated. Avoiding sustained contact with people whilst in this condition seems to be a good idea.

I put my head down onto the desk and realise that I could drift off to sleep. I fight it and stand up to encounter the strangeness again. I am content and all anxiety remains absent.

T+0:45 I am now adapting to this strange and off-key type of serene inebriation. There are occasional challenges, like negotiating the walk upstairs, but I can float around semi-functionally, enjoying this dreamy sheen on perception. I feel sedated but with some interesting aspects present. I am not significantly tired, but rather, a little dazed with a hypnotic edge.

It is really quite pleasant. The ataractic effects have softened my real life dramas and to some degree they now seem external to my current bubble.

T+1:00 Sadly, I am coming-down from the heady driven weirdness of earlier, and morphing into a traditional type of zoned-out phase, which is relaxed in nature but more akin to normality. I no longer have a problem walking or moving around and physically I am increasingly capable.

There is no urge to work, so drive has been diminished. The anxiety hasn't returned, at least as yet.

T+2:00 In terms of functionality I am back to base. I am composed and chilled, and all stress is absent. This now feels like a regular medicated sedation.

T+4:00 Over the last two hours a real-life domestic drama suddenly bore down upon me from nowhere, through no fault of my own. I managed to navigate it with common sense and relative calm. This broadly sums up where I am with the experience at present: I am sedated and tranquil, but functional. I am tiring a little.

The overall experience was reasonably positive. The first hour was one of strange euphoric type headiness, during which functionality was impaired. Physical movement was tricky but fun and intense social interaction would not have been easy. It was extremely enjoyable.

It then settled into a more classic tranquillised sedation, with calming and anxiolytic properties, but without undue drowsiness. However, after four hours or so I did begin to tire, so much so that I retired to bed an hour later. The night's sleep was, as might be expected, a good one, and I awoke a little subdued but generally fine.

Finally, it would be remiss not to end with a word of caution. Benzodiazepine tolerance is real, as is addiction. Even the most elementary Internet research uncovers stories of struggle and tragedy. From here I will therefore abstain from this class of drug for a considerable period.

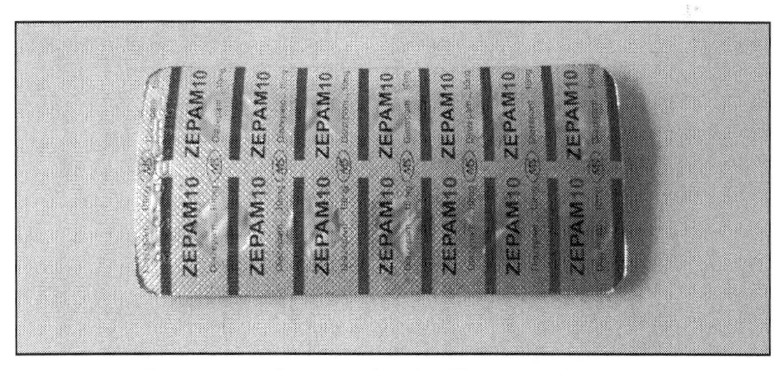

There are currently over 500 brands of diazepam on the market

2.4.4 Etizolam

Common Nomenclature	Etizolam
Street & Reference Names	Etiz; Etilaam; Depas; Etizest; Pasaden; Zoly;
Reference Dosage	Light 0.5mg+; Common 1mg+; Strong 2mg+ [TripSit]
Anticipated: Onset / Duration	30 Minutes / 7 Hours
Maximum Dose Experienced	2mg
Form	Pill
RoA	Oral
Source / Jurisdiction	Internet / UK

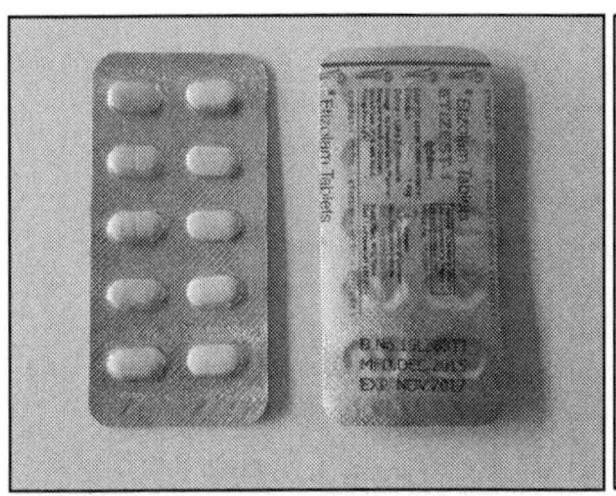

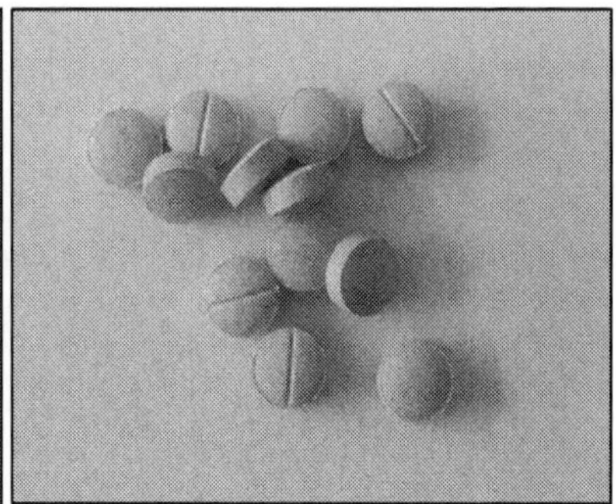

SUBJECTIVE EXPERIENCE
Etizolam is my sleep aid of choice. I use it just occasionally, usually to kill a stim or a trip. It works well, with little or no lag the following day. It comes on quickly, and is effective even at 0.5mg.

However, on one occasion I consumed 2mg, and I learned the meaning of the term *hypnotic*. I slept for 14 hours, and when I awoke, I was zombified. I felt good; floating in a zoned-out headspace. A walk outside was extremely pleasant and the day passed in a splendid haze. Despite this seductive positivity I instinctively knew that, given its addictive tendencies, this was not a habit to get into.

That story perhaps serves as a reminder of the general nature of benzodiazepines: overdose is a very serious hazard and many people struggle with long term addiction, which is extremely difficult to shake off. Be careful.

Note: The general consensus appears to be that 1mg of etizolam equates to about 10mg of diazepam

2.4.5 Gabapentin

Common Nomenclature	Gabapentin
Street & Reference Names	Neurontin; Johnnies; Gabbies
Reference Dosage	Light 300mg+; Common 600mg+; Strong 1200mg+ [TripSit]
Anticipated: Onset / Duration	1 Hour / 8 Hours
Maximum Dose Experienced	300mg + 300mg
From	Capsules
RoA	Oral
Source / Jurisdiction	Associate / UK

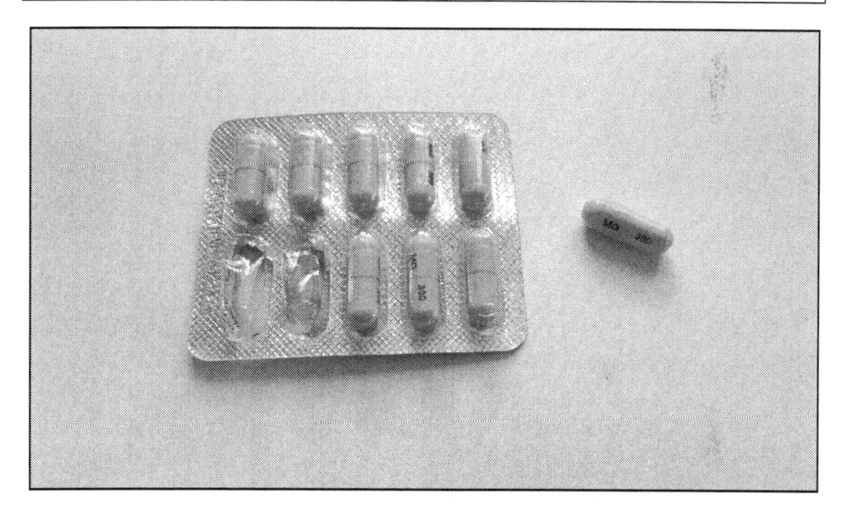

SUBJECTIVE EXPERIENCE
First introduced in the 1970s, and initially approved to treat epilepsy, gabapentin is now prescribed to treat a number of ailments, including seizures, neuropathic pain and restless leg syndrome. However, its anxiolytic and quasi-euphoric effects have also led to its use as a recreational drug. I have seen it described as a *mild benzo*, but with dramatically smaller returns on repeat doses during a session. It is also known for tolerance to build very quickly.

My supply came in the form of 300mg capsules, which is handy given that most online reference sources quote thresholds in multiples of 300. Given that some of these suggest topping the first dose up after perhaps 30 minutes to an hour, I elect to start with 300mg and then perhaps add another 300mg downstream. This should pitch me well into *common* territory, but in two simple stages.

In terms of anticipation, I'm not quite sure what to expect. Further, I am torn with contradiction: I am still tempted to go for a higher dose, yet at the same time I don't really consider this class of drug to be my *thing*. In the end, sense prevails.

> T+0:00 I swallow a 300mg capsule with a glass of water. [1:00pm]
>
> T+0:45 A heady mellow feeling is now emerging. It is minor at present, but certainly noticeable.
>
> T+1:30 I am not euphoric or uplifted, but that head driven aura referred to in the last note is now well established. There are no fireworks, but my headspace has been calmed, and anxieties have disappeared.
>
> T+2:00 I remain in the same warm and softened zone as I decide to take my usual afternoon nap. I have little problem falling into a sleep.
>
> T+3:00 I am now awake again, and mentally I am back into a similar place. There is a hint of physical analgesia with this, and the gentle ambience of the sedation persists nicely. I eat and enjoy a decent meal.
>
> T+4:00 The intensity has now reduced significantly, and despite having left it much later than intended I am left wondering whether to redose. After some consideration I open a capsule and take another 300mg.

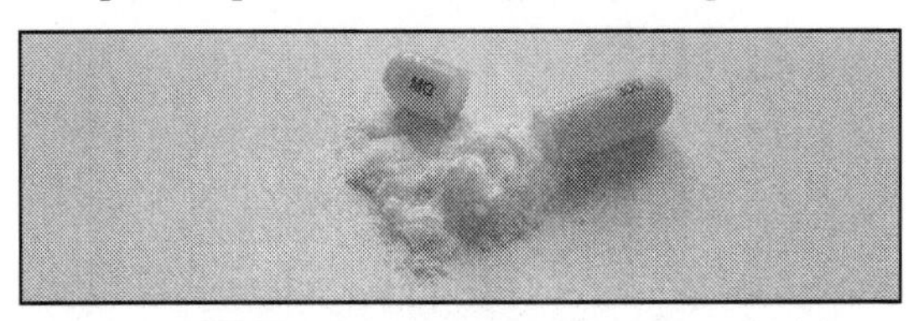

> T+5:30 I am experiencing a sort of cerebral numbness, but without a real high. I feel tranquillised without being tired or weary. There's been no obvious kick from the second dose, but perhaps it has intensified the plateau.
>
> T+8:00 Given the slightly unworldly sense that pervades vision, there is a minor hypnotic feel in play. My hands remain a little numb too. The intensity is now lower, but I remain in a gentle bubble of neutrality.

I retired to bed at about 11pm, 10 hours after the initial intake. The night's sleep wasn't bad, and the headache that I thought I had in the middle of it wasn't really there in the morning, although I felt a bit flat. This flatness lingered all day.

I found this to be strongish at times, in a hypnotic rather than a euphoric sense. It delivered both a mood and a physical numbness, which produced contentment rather than enjoyment. This isn't to say that it wasn't a reasonably pleasant ride though, and I should note that the second dose was totally unwarranted.

With respect to a comparison with benzodiazepines, it subjectively carried less lift, although this could have been partly due to my prevailing mood and circumstance.

2.4.6 Pregabalin

Common Nomenclature	Pregabalin
Street & Reference Names	Lyrica
Reference Dosage	Threshold 75mg+; Light 150mg+; Common 450mg+; Strong 750mg+; Heavy 1400mg [Drugs-Forum] Light 150mg+; Common 300mg+; Strong 600mg-900mg [TripSit]
Anticipated: Onset / Duration	1 Hour / 10 Hours
Maximum Dose Experienced	300mg+300mg
From	Capsules
RoA	Oral
Source / Jurisdiction	Associate / Overseas

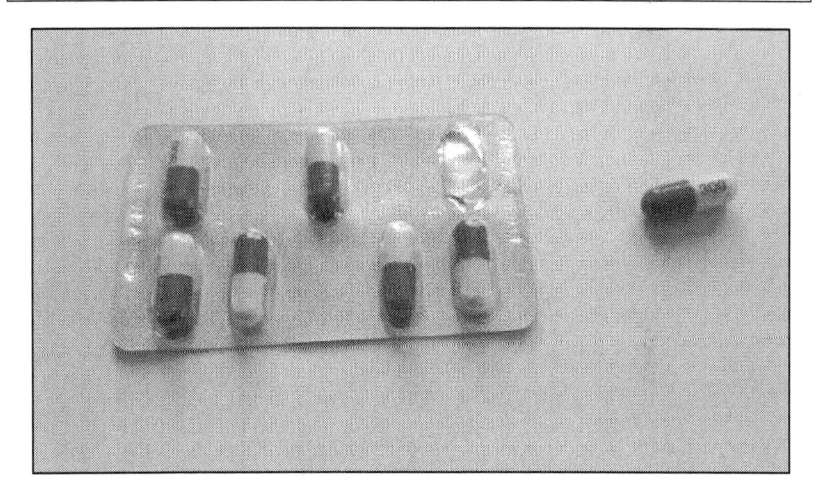

SUBJECTIVE EXPERIENCE
First synthesized in 1990, pregabalin appeared on the market as a prescription drug under the brand name *lyrica* in 2005. It is used to treat a variety of ailments, including anxiety and pain.

Descriptions of its psychoactive effects vary somewhat. Whilst it is commonly classified as an anxiolytic, a sedative and a relaxant, I have sometimes seen references to hypnotic properties, and occasionally I have encountered suggestions that it can induce euphoria. Despite the US government currently regarding it as having a low potential for abuse (Schedule V), it is clear that this is a serious recreational drug.

Regarding dosage, my initial inclination was to go for 450mg, but I subsequently found too many forum posts stating that sub-300mg doses were more than sufficient. [e.g. "*150mg gives me a nice little high while 300mg gets me crazy high*" ~Silenced, Bluelight.org]. I found these hard to ignore.

Given that pregabalin was developed as a successor to gabapentin my expectations today are not great. I tested the latter a few weeks ago, and found it to be generally relaxing and calming but without anything in the way of uplift. I am also feeling a little washed-out and tired, which won't help matters.

T+0:00 I swallow a single 300mg capsule with a glass of water [2.00pm]

T+1:00 Anxiolytic effects have emerged in the form of a comfort bubble, and a heady sense of well being. As I am not "*crazy high*" I pop another 300mg, to hopefully intensify proceedings.

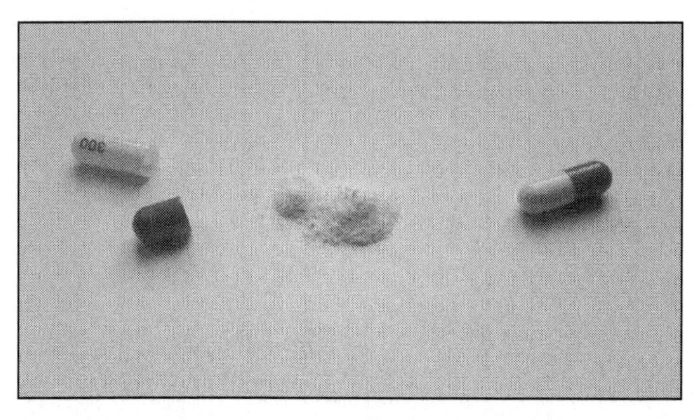

T+1:30 This is undeniably a nice benzo-like vibe, with a touch of inebriation. I feel warm and contented, with the headspace flowing here and there under a gentle dreamy sedation.

T+2:00 At this point I am heavily inebriated and groggy. The dreamy headspace now carries a hint of nausea and some dizziness, to the extent that I lie on my bed for 15 minutes. This is rapidly becoming very uncomfortable and is definitely not pleasant. I soon hit the bed for a second time.

T+ 4:30 The second recovery nap turned into a deep two hour sleep. I awoke feeling horrible: dizzy, groggy, and unable to function properly. I staggered to the bathroom, and then downstairs, trying to avoid contact with anyone.

I place my head on my arms, lean forward and rest on the desk. I occasionally manage to lift myself up and struggle to type some words. Incredibly I am barely able to function. This is an awful experience and I wonder how much longer it will last. My fingers are trembling and I feel dreadful.

To be in a public place in this state would be a nightmare. I would have to slump somewhere, appearing as a severely intoxicated drunk.

I totally underestimated this drug. I am basically zombified and largely mistuned to what is going on around me, which appears to be distant. My hands are numb and I am, essentially, stupefied, with head spinning.

My efforts to browse the Internet for more information on pregabalin fail miserably: I am simply not capable. The excessive inebriation is way past the point of serious discomfort. Yes, I desperately want this to stop.

T+5:30 Somehow I have just about managed to eat a pizza, which I ate almost mechanically to avoid making too much of a mess. This was a real challenge, but I got through it courtesy of the motivating thought that a bit of food might bring the unwanted-high down faster.

There is no doubt that any effort to hide my intoxicated state in a social scenario would still fail badly.

T+6:00 I finally feel slightly less out of it, and I can just about type these notes without recovery breaks. It is far from easy, but I am able to sit up in my chair again without hunching forwards. Gradually I am integrating back into the normality around me.

T+7:00 I am very much coming down; thank goodness. The dizzy inebriation can now be forced into the background with relative ease. I am quite stable again as I walk around, although I still feel generally woozy and not fully tuned back in to my surroundings, which have an unreal edge to them.

T+7:30 I note that time seems to have passed rather quickly. This has been an extremely long ride in terms of the continued psychoactivity of this drug, but it doesn't seem like it. It has now evolved into a mild queasiness about the head and some disorientation, both physical and mental.

Throughout this, anxieties and worries have been generally absent. I might add though that there was a degree of anxiety at the peak in terms of the experience itself: this was worry about when I would recover and if I was actually okay. Yes, it was that intense.

The inebriated headiness is now mild but is constantly present, and at times it can still be sickly and nauseous. I believe that I could now pass as sober again in a complex social situation, but I would have to concentrate to do so.

T+8:00 The intensity continues to wind down, albeit very slowly. I am astonished that it hit so hard and I feel a significant degree of relief.

T+8:30 At 10:30pm I am closing in on my usual bedtime. I expect a difficult night's sleep, not on the basis of the current effects of the drug, but because I slept for over two hours from 4pm.

Despite several wake-ups with a dry mouth, the night's sleep wasn't too bad. The next morning, however, I was still not fully with it and although I wasn't ill, I was not particularly well. I felt like I had a hangover but without the headache, and I was occasionally slightly dizzy and a tad nauseous. A sea-sickness-like feeling lingered for most of the day.

This one was a shock. I clearly took far too much and paid a price in terms of a strong intoxication which at times was extremely uncomfortable. I found myself struggling for some hours, hoping that the ride would wind down and end. Clearly a dose of 300mg or less would have been more than adequate.

Although this was a bad experience, it was an instructive one, from which the lessons are self-evident. If you use this drug be very careful with the dose, and of course don't make a habit of it. It can bite, and not in a pleasant way.

PREGABALIN ADDENDUM
Subsequent to this experience I took the trouble to further investigate the track record of this drug. What I found was alarming. Despite having only appeared relatively recently, the rate of fatality associated with its use was on a steep upward trajectory.

The following graph illustrates the number of cases in which pregabalin was mentioned on death certificates in England & Wales for the period to the end of 2017:

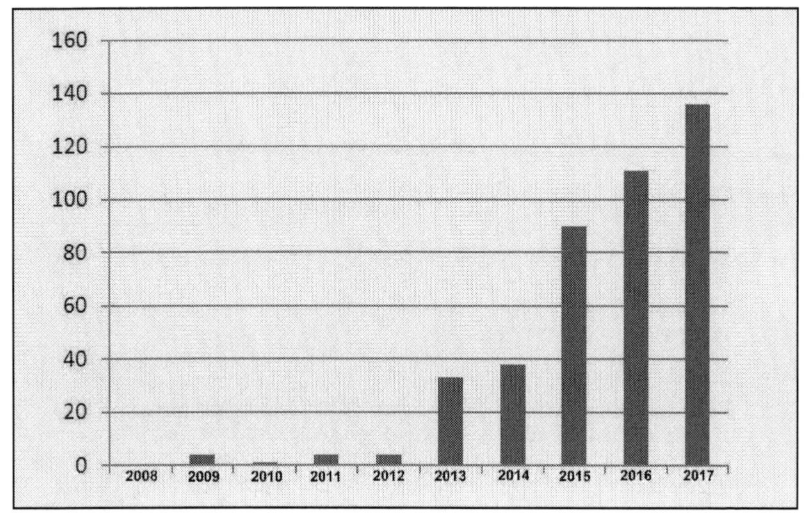

[Source: Office for National Statistics (ONS), UK]

The message could hardly be more obvious, and it re-enforces my words above. This is a serious drug and should not be underestimated.

2.4.7 Pyrazolam

Common Nomenclature	Pyrazolam
Street & Reference Names	N/A
Reference Dosage	Light 1mg+; Common 2mg+; Strong 3mg+ [TripSit]
Anticipated: Onset / Duration	15 Minutes / 6 Hours
Maximum Dose Experienced	1mg
Form	Pill
RoA	Oral
Source / Jurisdiction	Internet / UK

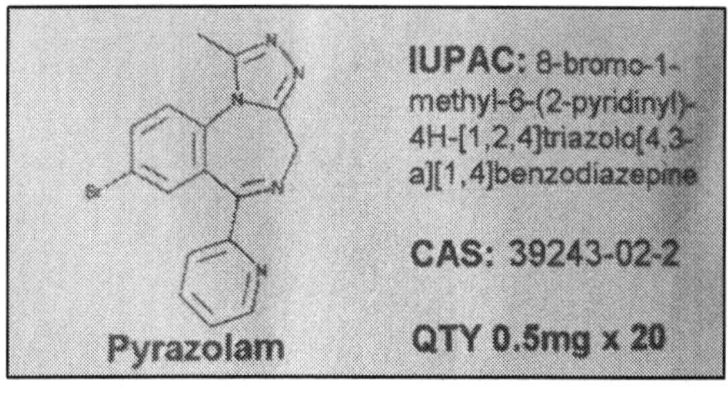

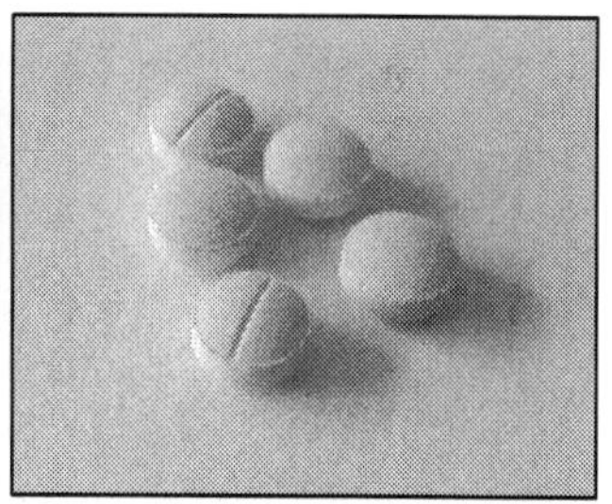

SUBJECTIVE EXPERIENCE

Pyrazolam was developed during the 1970s at Hoffman-La Roche, and became widely available via the online markets circa 2012.

I originally purchased it as a potential sleep aid, but research, prior to consumption, revealed its true niche. It counters anxiety, and is active even at relatively small doses. I don't suffer from undue social anxiety but I have tested it in a number of stressful situations. I have always been impressed.

Its strength for me is that whilst acting as an anxiolytic, it doesn't cause drowsiness. It is functional, or at least has been every time I have sampled it.

It is one of only two benzodiazepines I have used on more than a couple of occasions (the other being etizolam).

In December 2016, despite the prior implementation of the *Psychoactive Substances Act*, pyrazolam and a number of other specifically named benzodiazepines were the subjects of a UK TCDO banning order, which made personal possession, and not just import and supply, illegal.

2.4.8 Others

From a personal perspective, this class of drug doesn't provide significant scope for recreational differentiation. Sedatives sedate, and anxiolytics counter anxiety, with little granularization within the respective functionalities. Attributes such as duration and half-life take a more central role on the stage.

I do accept that some of this commentary may constitute heresy to aficionados, but those members of this class which I have sampled and which are not individually documented on previous pages have merged in terms of effect: my memory has categorised them into a fuzzy and fairly uninteresting *much of a muchness*. I cannot, therefore, wax lyrical about them or expand beyond listing those that I have tested with, at best, a one-liner.

Chlordiazepoxide
7-chloro-2-(methylamino)-5-phenyl-3H-1,4-benzodiazepine- 4-oxide
[Brands: Librium]
I was prescribed this instead of valium in my youth, and found it to be similar, but with less drowsiness.

Doxylamine Succinate
(RS)-N,N-dimethyl-2- (1-phenyl-1-pyridin-2-yl-ethoxy)- ethanamine
[Brands: Unisom]
I slept, although not as deeply as I had hoped.

Diphenhydramine (DPH)
2-(diphenylmethoxy)-N,N-dimethylethanamine
[Brands: Benadryl, Nytol]
This does its job in terms of sleep, although perhaps not as effectively as etizolam.

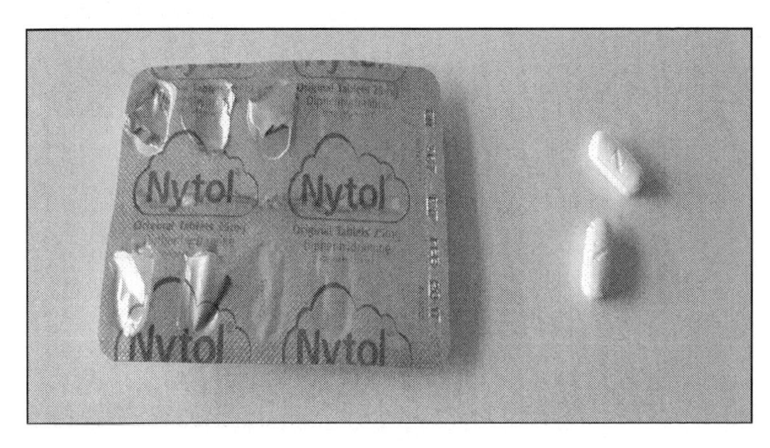

Diclazepam
7-Chloro-5-(2-chlorophenyl)-1-methyl-1,3-dihydro-2H-1,4-benzodiazepin-2-one
I barely recall this one, which probably means that it did a job, but with few if any interesting features.

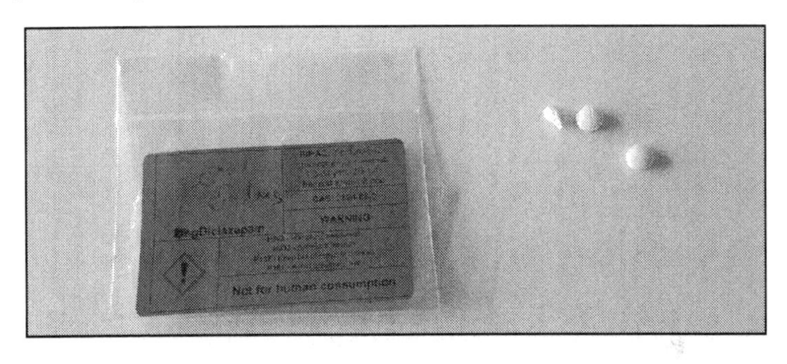

Flubromazolam
8-bromo-6-(2-fluorophenyl)-1-methyl-4H-[1,2,4]triazolo[4,3-a][1,4]benzodiazepine
As diclazepam.

Nifoxipam
5-(2-fluorophenyl)-3-hydroxy-7-nitro-1,3-dihydro-2H-1,4-benzodiazepin-2-one
As diclazepam.

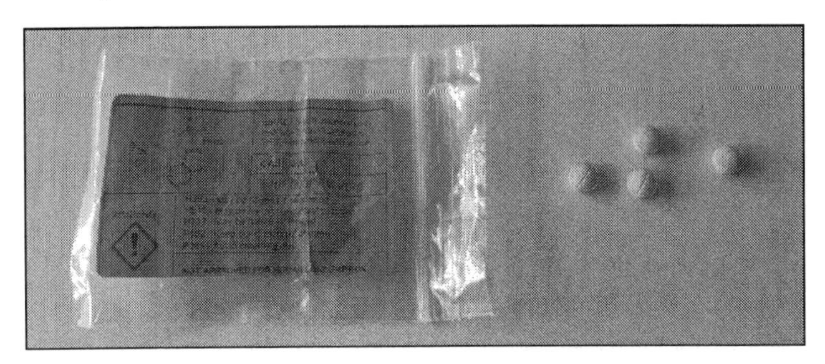

Finally, at one stage, solely for the purpose of this book, I purchased a sample of a benzo called *Flubromazepam*. However, I subsequently encountered numerous Internet reports which stated that this stays in the system for an extraordinarily long period of time. Given my ongoing research, I therefore elected, on safety grounds, to dump it prior to use.

2.5. INTOXICATING DEPRESSANTS

Textbook Definitions: *Depressants induce depression of the central nervous system (CNS), which reduces arousal or stimulation. This slows down the activity of the brain and nervous system, with the physical and psychoactive effects often dependent upon dose. Intoxicants excite or stupefy to the point where physical and mental control is diminished. Intoxicating depressants tend to combine these experiences, with their effects transforming and morphing towards the former, as the timescale unfolds.*

The following chemicals have been sampled and researched for inclusion within this section:

CNS depressants are often referred to as "*downers*", which for most drugs thus classified aligns entirely with the nature of their effects. I refer here to anxiolytics and sedatives, for example. For others, however, the early stages of the experience can appear to be entirely contradictory to this. Alcohol provides a good example, in that initially it tends to create a euphoric or energised feeling of intoxication.

This section embraces this latter category, with sedatives and chemicals with antipsychotic effects being covered earlier in the book.

Included are opioids, although I should point out that I purposely did not sample carfentanil, fentanyl or u-47700. This decision was taken purely on a risk and return basis. During the period from 2015 the number of deaths associated with these particular analogues increased to alarming proportions, which is hardly surprising given their dose sensitivity. As I am not much of a fan of opioids generally, skipping them was a no-brainer.

I would also add that the need to exercise caution with this entire class of psychoactive is further emphasized by the data produced via a range of studies, as illustrated in *Section 4.2* of this book. That these drugs constitute a high proportion of media headlines in terms of addiction and death is not a coincidence. Be extremely careful, particularly with respect to dose and frequency of use.

Finally, I would stress that I do include alcohol, in its many forms, in making these statements.

US FATALITY FIGURES

The U.S. Department of Health & Human Services produces a range of statistics relating to death rates for most members of this class of drug. The following graphics provide something of an overview. Bear in mind that these refer to real people.

For alcohol, *chronic causes* include liver disease, strokes and so forth, whereas *acute causes* include accidents, suicide, poisoning, etc. Interestingly, I found that the alcohol figures were less current and were far more difficult to locate on the CDC website than those for opioids, despite the numbers being significantly higher.

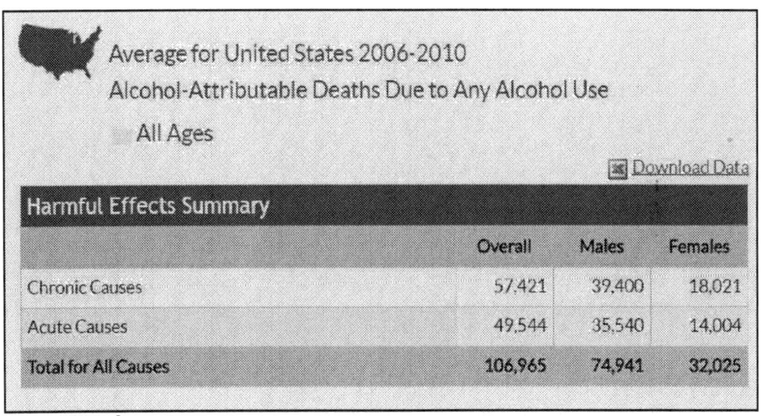

Average for United States 2006-2010

Alcohol-Attributable Deaths Due to Any Alcohol Use

All Ages

Download Data

Harmful Effects Summary

	Overall	Males	Females
Chronic Causes	57,421	39,400	18,021
Acute Causes	49,544	35,540	14,004
Total for All Causes	**106,965**	**74,941**	**32,025**

[Source: CDC.gov]

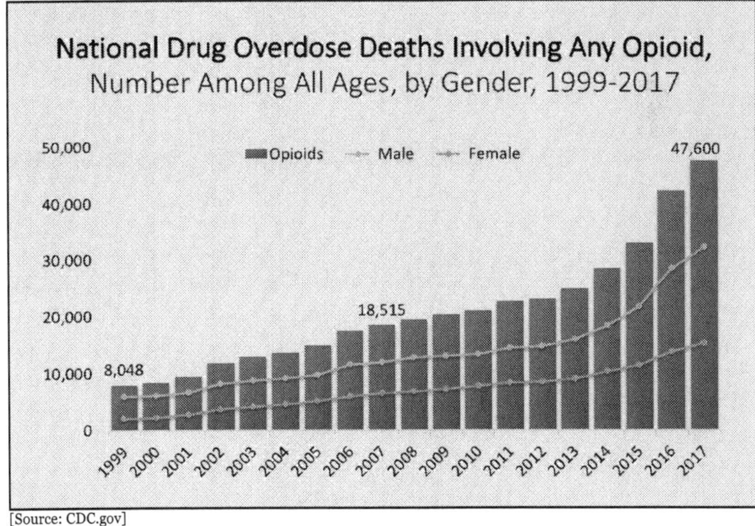

[Source: CDC.gov]

2.5.1 Alcohol

Common Nomenclature	Ethanol
Street & Reference Names	Ethyl Alcohol, Alcohol
Reference Dosage	See the table below
Anticipated: Onset / Duration	Dose Dependent
Maximum Dose Experienced	20+ Units
Form	Fluid
RoA	Oral
Source / Jurisdiction	Dealer / UK & Overseas

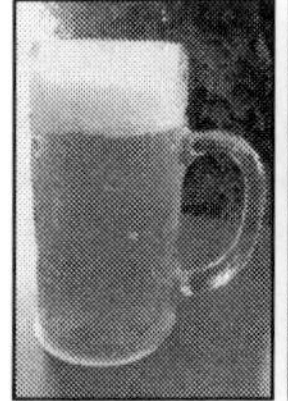
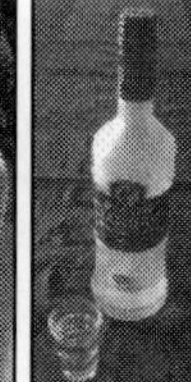
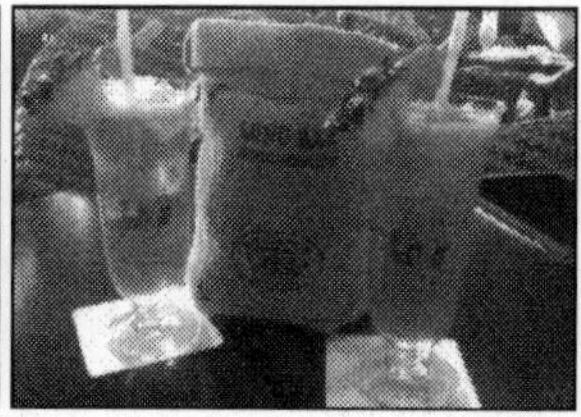
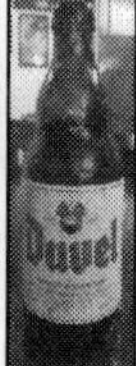

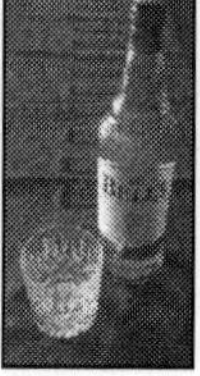
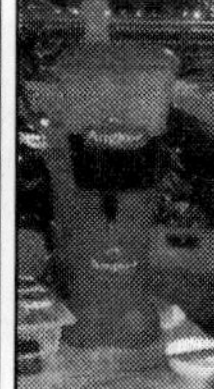

SUBJECTIVE EXPERIENCE
Where should I start with this monster? Perhaps with Terence McKenna:

> "*It lowers sensitivity to social cueing, at the same time as it gives an empowered sense of ego. In other words, it makes you into a jerk. It gives you the courage to say and do what, if you are a decent person, you would otherwise never say and never do.*"

Unfortunately, as everyone who is reading this is already well aware, this is just the start. Alcohol is a hard drug, whatever criterion is used to define this. Its ratio of effective to fatal dose is low, it is highly addictive, and it causes serious physical and psychological harm when used frequently or long term in high doses.

This is what the NHS website tells us:

UNITS	SHORT TERM EFFECTS
1-2	Your heart rate speeds up and your blood vessels expand, giving you the warm, sociable and talkative feeling associated with moderate drinking.
4-6	You become more reckless and uninhibited. Your reaction time and co-ordination are adversely affected.
8-9	Your reaction times will be much slower, your speech will begin to slur and your vision will begin to lose focus. Your liver will be unable to remove all of the alcohol overnight, so it's likely you'll wake with a hangover.

10-12	Your co-ordination will be highly impaired, placing you at serious risk of having an accident. The high level of alcohol has a depressant effect on both your mind and body, which makes you drowsy. This amount of alcohol will begin to reach toxic (poisonous) levels. You will feel badly dehydrated in the morning, which may cause a severe headache. You may also experience symptoms of nausea, vomiting, diarrhoea and indigestion.
>12	You're at considerable risk of developing alcohol poisoning, particularly if you're drinking many units over a short period of time. Alcohol poisoning can cause a person to fall into a coma and could lead to their death.

What is a unit of alcohol? *Drinkaware* defines this as follows:

> *"One alcohol unit is measured as 10ml or 8g of pure alcohol. This equals one 25ml single measure of whisky (ABV 40%), or a third of a pint of beer (ABV 5-6%) or half a standard (175ml) glass of red wine (ABV 12%)"*

Alcohol and tobacco are by far the most deadly drugs in the UK, with a citizen's life lost to alcohol approximately every hour. For example, in 2014, 8,697 alcohol related deaths were registered. This is similarly reflected across the world.

DOSE & EFFECTS

What is my personal experience? It is probably much the same as the majority. I used to drink too much, too often. I regularly engaged in binge drinking. I suspect, to some degree, I fell into the regular trap: familiarity breeds complacency.

It usually begins innocently enough. Assuming a normal rate of consumption, there is a gentle alleviation of stress and tension, increased self-confidence and a mild uplift of disposition. This is sufficiently pleasant to tempt redosing, prolongation, and pursuit of intensification. The session, all too often, is on.

Continued redosing leads to an increasing sense of euphoria and well-being, with certitude and self-esteem growing rapidly. Worries seem to evaporate and inhibitions are released. This high can be extremely pleasurable, but it cannot be sustained.

If sense prevails and redosing stops at an early stage, a period of sedation kicks in. A background drowsiness emerges, perhaps a hint of tiredness, and a relative loss of focus. A night's sleep is a natural adjunct, albeit with reduced restorative quality. The aftermath will range from barely noticeable to tolerable.

If redosing doesn't stop, the experience careers into an array of difficulties. That confidence boost, along with ego, is increasingly inflated. Simultaneously, cognitive performance and sharpness diminishes, sensory inputs are dulled, and behavioural changes become ever more obvious to third parties. Increased disorientation and confusion begin to manifest within a general haze.

Here, we are at the point at which I am likely to embarrass myself, and create regret after the event. Some people are liable to become loud, aggressive or even violent.

Continued redosing exacerbates these tendencies, and the effects materialize into ever more visible and obvious representations, including difficulty in keeping balance and slurring of words. Mentally and consciously, at this point you are lost, largely along with your rationality. The experience is no longer a pleasant one.

At these and higher levels of intoxication some people vomit during the session itself, some fall unconscious or into a stupor, others manage to stagger to bed. The possibility of personal harm, and potentially death, is significantly increased.

The subsequent comedown and hangover is severe, and following a very high dose, is absolutely brutal. I am sure that many readers of this book will recall the indignity of waking in a dysfunctional nightmare, retching and vomiting into a toilet, and generally feeling like death. The headache can be horrific and sustained, and a drained feeling of illness and lethargy can last the entire day, and to a lesser degree, beyond. A background listlessness and relative depression can in fact linger for some days.

I have suffered this drama too many times. Far too many. In our society it is just so easy to fall into the binge-drinking pattern referred to earlier, or alternatively, integrate this drug into a daily lifestyle. Both these paths are fraught with danger, and represent a disaster waiting to happen.

If you are looking forward to your next binge, or need a drink every day to unwind, you might not want to hear this, but you have a problem. It is better to confront this now than to let it roll. For further information on the excessive use of alcohol, and on alcoholism, see *Section 4.3.3*.

One of the outcomes of researching for and writing this book has been that I learned to treat alcohol as every other drug, meaning that I began to assess the relative value and pleasure of its experience, and understand its risk profile. Accordingly, I now rarely use it.

Finally, at higher doses alcohol bears certain similarities to heroin, both in experience and aftermath, with a similar profile of addiction and overdose. Despite this it is available and advertised at every social turn.

On this theme, I will end as I started, with McKenna:

> *"How can we explain the legal toleration for alcohol, the most destructive of all intoxicants, and the almost frenzied efforts to repress nearly all other drugs?"*

I should point out that whilst I may appear to be *anti-alcohol*, I am not: I am *anti-ignorance*. Ignorance of the real nature of alcohol destroys countless lives, and kills so many people each year. Don't be one of them.

WHAT'S YOUR POISON?
Beer, wine, spirits, and even food: alcohol is offered in forms to tempt every palate.

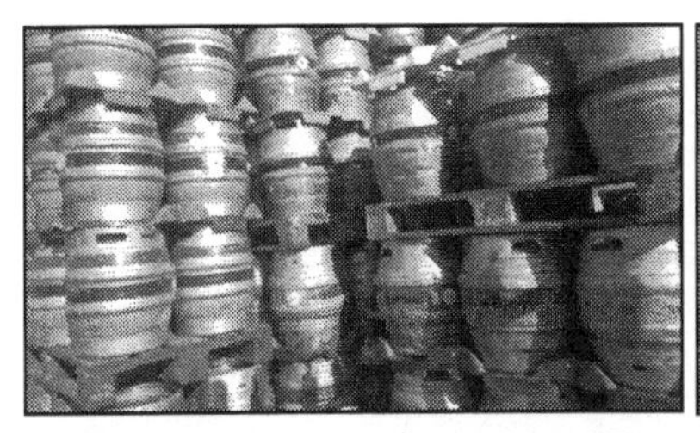
The Titanic Brewery, Stoke-on-Trent, UK

Czech Beer Museum, Prague

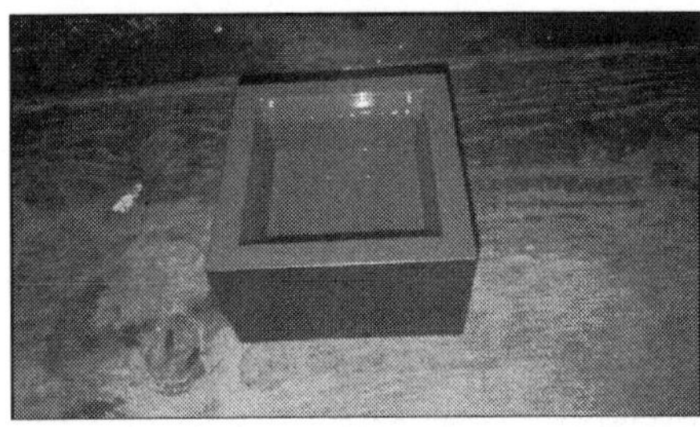
Sake, Tokyo, Japan

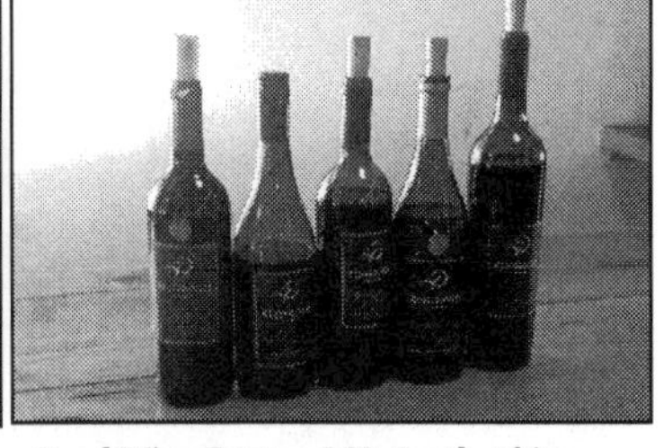
Paarl Wine Estates, WC, South Africa

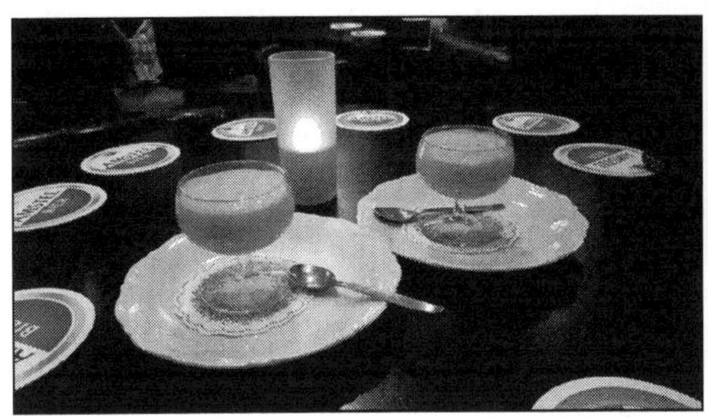

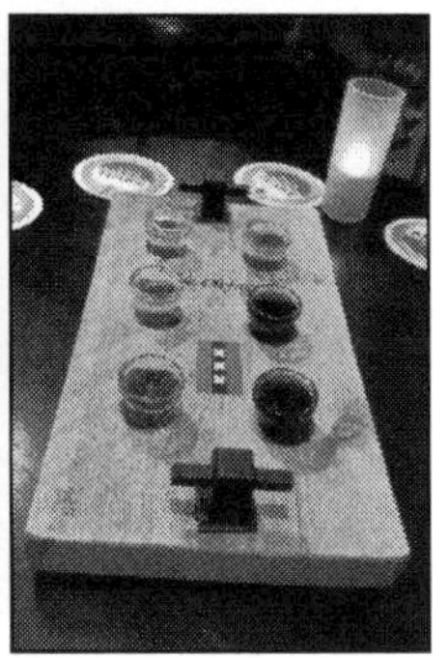
Advocaat and a gin board, as served at *In de Olofspoort*, Amsterdam

Enjoy your preferred presentation of ethanol, but never fool yourself into believing that you are not using a hard addictive drug.

The introductory images at the start of this entry comprise the following: German beer stein, Russian vodka, Singapore sling, Belgium beer, Scotch whisky, Cambodian beer dispenser.

2.5.2 Codeine

Common Nomenclature	3-Methylmorphine
Street & Reference Names	Codate; Codephos; Codamol
Reference Dosage	Light 50mg+; Common 100mg+; Strong 150mg+ [Oral, TripSit]
Anticipated: Onset / Duration	30 Minutes/ 4-6 Hours
Maximum Dose Experienced	100mg
From	Pills
RoA	Oral
Source / Jurisdiction	UK

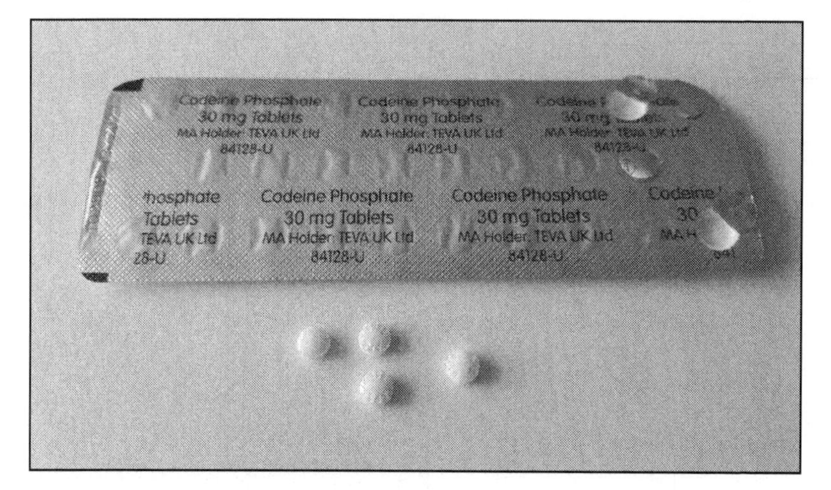

SUBJECTIVE EXPERIENCE

Discovered in 1832 by Pierre Jean Robiquet, codeine is one of the most commonly used members of the opiate family, and is on the World Health Organization's *List of Essential Medicines*. It is generally used to treat pain.

Possible side effects include drowsiness and constipation, whilst less frequently, conditions such as itching, nausea, dry mouth and urinary retention can arise.

As with other opioids, addiction is a serious threat, as is the risk of overdose. A further risk is sometimes presented with codeine in that it is often supplied in combination with paracetamol, ibuprofen, or similar. At high doses these in themselves can cause serious health issues and even death. Please do not brush these warnings aside.

Regarding dosage I elect to target the low end of what is regarded as (recreationally) common, with a figure which is frequently recommended across social media forums: 100mg. This is apparently equivalent to about 15mg of morphine.

As luck would have it, either bad luck or good luck depending upon perspective, I have a fairly bad cold at the moment, with a dry cough. Usually, this would flash a big red light for any sort of drug expedition, but given that codeine is sold openly as a cold remedy, usually as part of a cough syrup, this presents something of an opportunity to kill two birds with one stone. Or alternatively I am using flawed logic to sell the idea to myself, given that for purely medicinal purposes the dose I propose is ludicrous.

From prior research, my expectation is of a period of relaxation, a feeling of well-being, and possibly some euphoria. Later, this may morph into sedation, a sense of heaviness and some sleepiness. Hopefully, along the way this will also mitigate the discomfort of my current ailments.

> T+0:00 I swallow three 30mg pills plus 1/3 of a fourth (weighed not eyeballed). All are swilled down with a glass of water [2:30pm].
>
> Note that I ate an average sized meal about 90 minutes ago.
>
> T+1:00 It is far more difficult to analyse the effects of a drug whilst not in full health, particularly shallow end subtleties. What I can state at this point, however, is that I feel warmer, and some of the pain is being masked. The usual heady opioid comfort bubble is in play, but weariness is suppressing much of the uplift.
>
> T+2:00 I feel sedated, relaxed, and content, with a hint of heaviness and analgesia thrown in. I remain warm, and I am generally apathetic.
>
> T+4:00 Although a less intense version of the above remains, the wretchedness of the cold has now re-established itself. I am tired, shivering, and a bit dizzy, with a headache in situ courtesy, I believe, of excessive coughing. This has certainly taken a turn for the worse.
>
> T+5:30 At 8pm, five and a half hours into the ride, I go to bed. I am still experiencing the residue effects of the drug, but I am now too poorly to sit at my desk and suffer.

I had a terrible night: a headache, a fever and coughing fits. I was basically ill. Ditto the next morning: it felt hangover-like in parts. The question I ask myself is how much of this was created by or exacerbated by the codeine? Was 100mg too much? I cannot believe that this was all down to the cold/flu, although it is possible.

This has been a real mess. It was a reminder that opioids are not my bag. It was also a lesson not to use a recreational drug outing to treat a medical condition, unless certain of the outcome.

2.5.3 GHB

Common Nomenclature	GHB; Gamma Hydroxybutyrate
Street & Reference Names	G, Grievous Bodily Harm, Liquid Ecstasy, Harm
Reference Dosage	Light 0.5g+; Common 1g+; Strong 2g+; Heavy 3g+; Overdose 5g+; Poisoning 10g+ [Erowid] Light 0.5g+; Common 1g+; Strong 2g+; Heavy/Death 5g+; [Psychonautwiki] Light 0.5g+; Common 1g+; Strong 2g+; Heavy 3.5g+; Dangerous 7g+ [TripSit]
Anticipated: Onset / Duration	15 Minutes / 2 Hours
Maximum Dose Experienced	.75g + .75g + 1.2g
Form	Paste
RoA	Oral
Source / Jurisdiction	Dealer / Overseas
Personal Rating On Shulgin Scale	+***

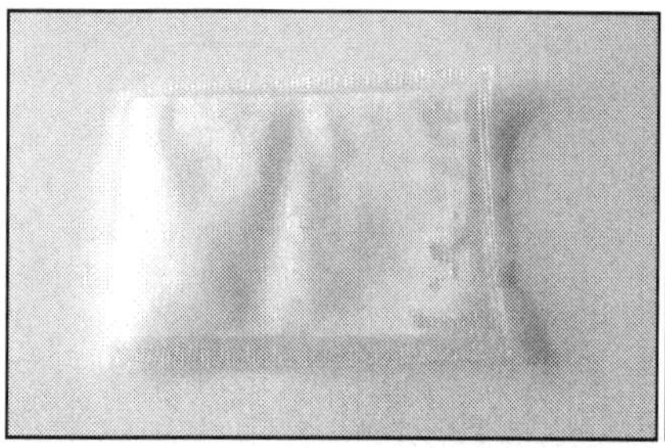

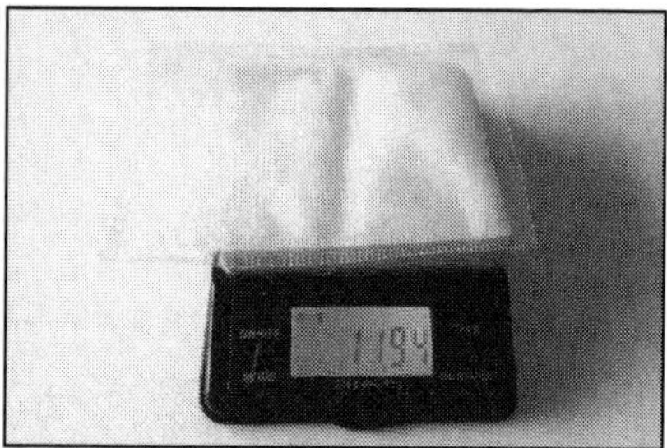

SUBJECTIVE EXPERIENCE
GHB has a colourful history. It was first synthesised in the 1920s, was used as an anaesthetic in the 60s, and was sold as a weight loss and muscle development aid in the 80s. Eventually it was to emerge as a recreational drug at the end of the 90s. It was scheduled in the United States in 2000, and in the UK in 2003.

Whilst commonly used as a club drug, it gained notoriety with the public as a *date rape* drug, following a sustained period of media reporting. Its use has declined considerably over recent years.

Researching the safety of GHB via the Internet immediately rang alarm bells. On the fundamental issue of dosing, *Erowid* bluntly states that: *"If you take 3 - 4 times the normal dose, you may find yourself unconscious and vomiting. If you take more than 3-4 times your normal dose, there is risk of death."*

With this in mind, it is also important to note that the threshold figures given above are for GHB powder, and not for liquid. For GHB in liquid form, it is essential to establish the concentration and work from there.

Another stark warning is not to mix this with alcohol or other depressants. This is an absolute *must-not-do*. It has resulted in tragic consequences all too often.

On purchasing my sample, the dealer was gushing regarding its effects, promising untold joys and delights. His recommended dose was equally forthright, suggesting 2-3g mixed with warm water, and then 1-2g every 20 minutes until *"absolute bliss"* was encountered. In my case, this recklessness was obviously not going to happen.

My 10g supply came in a watertight plastic sachet. It was a soggy wet powder, rather like the constitution of the amphetamine paste I had tested some months earlier. Perhaps it was a little gooier.

Placing this on the scales produced a reading of 11.94g, which indicated that the purchase weight was more or less correct. However, the fact that it wasn't powder, and was damp, raised issues and uncertainty. Erring on the side of caution I therefore weighed wet and dosed low.

T+0:00 I carefully measure 0.75g, which is cited as light-common by the harm reduction websites, and mix it into warm water. It dissolves almost immediately as I stir. There is a slightly salty taste as I swig it down. [3:35pm]

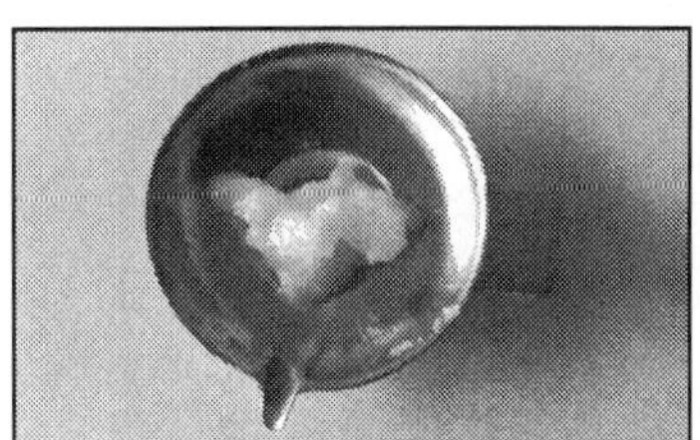

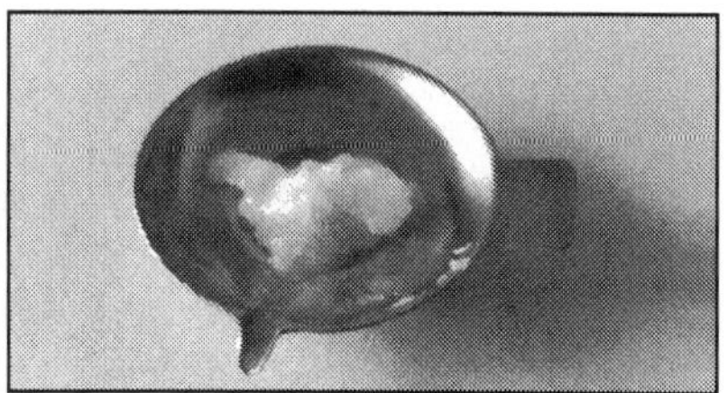

T+0:15 A mild and heady inebriation has already emerged. I hesitate to compare it to alcohol, because there isn't the fuzzy headed accompaniment or loss of clarity. I feel warmer than I did, and the anxious edge I was feeling earlier has been extinguished.

T+0:30 It has not developed significantly, but rather, has established itself on a plateau: the mild intoxication, the anxiolytic calmness, and the slight body warmth are all stable. It is pleasing in nature.

On the issue of sexual stimulation, this can be apparent if I allow my mind to drift into that area. An issue I tend to have here is that it is difficult not to compare drugs alleged to have aphrodisiacal properties with amphetamine or methamphetamine. Against these they are always liable to reflect poorly.

> Whilst this is also the case with GHB on this dose, there is certainly potential in this area.
>
> T+1:00 The experience is positive and basically, quite nice. There is temptation to redose and head into more intensive territory, but this already has warmth and pleasantness to it at its current level.
>
> T+1:30 Whilst the sedation is now more evident, the mildly inebriated feel has diminished. Seeking to re-establish this I dissolve and drink another 0.75g of the sticky white paste. The total dose is now 1.5g
>
> T+2:15 The tranquil feeling with an overtone of lucid intoxication has solidified again. Although I wouldn't describe it as euphoria, my mood is good and there is no anxiety in play. This is quite a nice feeling.
>
> T+3:00 I mix and drink a final clump of 1.2g, making the total 2.7g.
>
> T+3:15 I am now at a similar level to an hour ago, but perhaps a little more zoned-out with less clarity. The headiness is probably more intense. There is no enormous sexual urge, but again, the inclination is there if I take it in that direction, and there is no stim-dick. As I haven't eaten since lunch time I eat a large bowl of muesli.
>
> T+3:45 Unexpectedly, given that I dosed over a gram just 45 minutes ago, I feel that I am on the way down. Perhaps the food contributed to this.
>
> T+6:00 Over the last hour or two the effects have worn down almost to base, leaving some tiredness. I am ready for bed a little earlier than usual.

The night's sleep was reasonably good and I experienced no significant comedown. This was far milder and gentler than I anticipated, and there was no hangover whatsoever.

Following the initial surge, I generally felt a heady sedation, and a degree of mellow inebriation, but with far more clarity to it than alcohol. A term that occurred to me during the experience was *sober intoxication*, as I was far more in control of myself. Regarding the general ataractic effect, this was an underlying factor throughout.

I can fully understand how some people chase this, to try and get more out of it, by redosing repeatedly and heavily. It feels painless and safe, with little hint of the dangers that are there. I sense that this trap would be particularly easy to fall into in a social situation. The same applies to mixing with alcohol. It feels so benign that it misleads. Be careful.

A REMINDER
My personal dosage figures reflect GHB paste and not powder. Powder equivalent doses will be significantly lower.

2.5.4 Heroin

Common Nomenclature	Diacetylmorphine; Diamorphine
Street & Reference Names	Junk; Smack; H
Reference Dosage	Common 5mg+; Heavy 20mg+ Redosing 5mg-10mg [Erowid] Light 7.5mg+; Common 20mg+; Strong 35mg+; Heavy 50mg+ [TripSit]
Anticipated: Onset / Duration	10 Minutes / 6 Hours
Maximum Dose Experienced	50mg
Form	Powder
RoA	Insufflated
Source / Jurisdiction	Dealer / Overseas
Personal Rating On Shulgin Scale	++

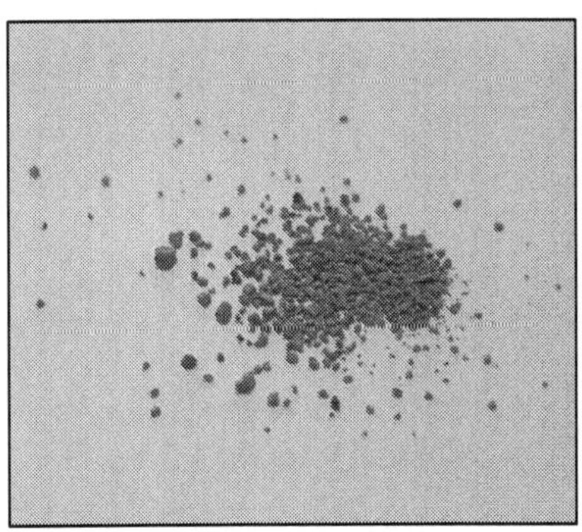

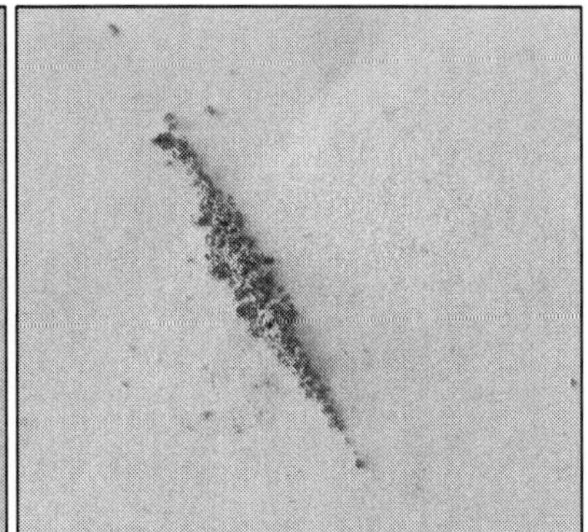

SUBJECTIVE EXPERIENCE
Heroin is probably the most infamous drug in the world. It is refined from morphine, which itself is extracted from the opium poppy, and it was first synthesised in 1874. Erowid describes it as a *euphoric depressant* and an *analgesic*, and there is no doubt that the consequences of abuse can be grave.

For most of my life I never saw the slightest possibility that I would ever use this drug. It never entered my head. The media had done a fine job in frightening my sub-conscious, and simultaneously ensuring that I didn't have a clue what the risks actually were, or how to manage them.

The word *heroin* had become synonymous with addiction and death.

As I increasingly grasped that mainstream drug reporting comprised largely of outright propaganda, a more objective outlook emerged. This solidified as I noted that personally experienced substances, which I knew to be benign, were routinely presented using the same toxic terminology. It was impossible to differentiate any grain of truth from the endless catalogue of misinformation.

With this in mind, I eventually approached heroin in the same rational and cautious manner as I had with every other chemical and botanical. Safety was paramount.

Armed with 100mg of what was purported to be *87% pure uncut #4 heroin*, I embarked on the pre-requisite research, which was from a start point of almost no knowledge at all.

Whilst online literature suggested that most #4 originates in Burma or Colombia, I was totally unaware of the geographic origins of my supply.

Further, what on earth did #4 mean? I quickly learned that #3 was the rawer freebase form, which would not dissolve in water, but that #4 was heroin salt, which would. This distinction is important because the salt form renders the drug suitable for insufflation and IV.

A note in passing: smoking, which is the usual RoA for #3, attracted mixed reports, including many that suggested it was particularly bad for the lungs.

For dose, 5mg-10mg was commonly suggested, and it aligned with the *light* threshold on the harm reduction websites. I therefore decided that 10mg was probably a sensible starting point, with the potential to redose. I noted that additional 5mg-10mg lines were referred to by Erowid:

> "*Heroin users describe chopping out "pin"-thin lines of heroin and then redosing every 30-60 minutes: getting high, coming down a little, snorting another line to get high, coming down a little. This is done over the course of an evening or a day and may feel like chasing the peak high that is achieved*".

Regarding expectation, I anticipated euphoria and a sense of well being, over a period of about 3-5 hours.

> T+0:00 I prepare a 10mg line and insufflate [3:43pm]
>
> T+0:02 I may feel the slightest of something, although this isn't really significant. The thought occurs that this substance may actually be #3.
>
> T+0:05 Perhaps I under-dosed. Given that there is no obvious adverse effect, I snort a little more (10mg). This produces a mild effect: a rather sedated headspace, but no euphoria or high.
>
> T+0:20 I insufflate another 15mg, with no excessive nasal discomfort. I snort deep with my right nostril, and I continue to wait, impatiently.

T+0:30 There is now a clear effect. I feel sedated and a little distant, but not sleepy. This isn't a massive high, but it is a nice light buzz. I am fully functional, in control of myself, and comfortable with the experience.

I perform a few checks. Pupils? They are constricted. Horn? There is nothing abnormal and no real interest. Appetite? No change, in that I am not really hungry. My head is definitely in a lightly inebriated state and I am relaxed.

T+0:40 As I am at ease with this, I decide to snort a final 15mg. Based upon Erowid and the other safety oriented websites, this will take me to a fairly large but not excessive dose, circa 50mg in total. It is probably wise to stop at this point. Again, there is no discomfort in the railing operation itself.

T+0:50 I'm into this more deeply than previously, but the overall character of the ride appears to be set. I am relaxed; my headspace is drifty and unengaged. Physically, I feel a little numbed (analgesic). I am not euphoric but I am tranquil and content.

T+1:10 I am in an ataractic-like comfort zone, in which problems are dissolved and all is good. At this stage, it's a nice drug in terms of effect, but not exciting or compelling in any particular way.

T+1:50 One of the effects mentioned in reference sources was a dry mouth. I can confirm this to be the case: I had to chat to someone for a few minutes, and this came on quickly. Beyond this, there are no significant changes from earlier, although I now feel a little woozy with a hint of fatigue.

T+2:30 The general characteristic hasn't changed, but the fatigue has increased, as has the grogginess. I feel a little like I am suffering from motion sickness. It is not horribly uncomfortable, but it is there in the background, nonetheless. Overlaying this I am still chilled and relaxed.

T+2:35 A meal has arrived. This could be a challenge.

T+3:10 I got through it, meaning that I ate it, but with little enjoyment. There may be a degree of appetite suppression in play here, and certainly, taste isn't accentuated.

I am now fading somewhat. The feeling of queasiness remains, and I am increasingly tired. Indeed, I feel I could fall asleep easily if I lie down. I am still functional but clearly zoned-out, and I am now sweating a little. This isn't particularly pleasant, and I am relieved not to have snorted any further lines.

T+3:15 This has now taken a further turn for the worse. The dizziness continues to increase, as does the sleepiness, so I head to bed. I lie in the dark, drifting and feeling quite unwell. I attempt to rise a couple of times over the next half hour, but I fail, as the spinning head and general malaise is too intense.

T+3:50. I force myself up and head downstairs. I suddenly feel heaviness in my gut, and I vomit: not repeatedly, but I expel the most recent contents of my stomach. I lie down again for 10 minutes before rising once more. This is not good, at all.

T+4:00 I begin to feel slightly better. I am still dizzy, but less intensely, and I am less somnolent, although I could easily have continued to sleep had I wished.

These aspects have taken me by surprise. I Google *heroin* and *vomiting*. This is common; so common that I can't believe that I was unaware of it. For example, *'Talk To Frank'*, which is always quick off the mark with negatives, points out: "*The first dose of heroin can bring about dizziness and vomiting*."

It appears that nausea and vomiting are common features for many, and not only for the first dose. *HowToKickHeroin.Com* describes it like this:

> "*Strangely enough, getting nauseous and throwing up is part of the heroin addict lifestyle. Actually, many addicts glean pleasure from throwing up because they perceive it to mean "strong heroin"*," and "*In hospitals, nausea is expected to occur in 25 – 30 percent of patients treated with opioid drugs. However, since heroin involves greater average dosing and subsequent amplified effects it results in higher than average nauseating events.*"

Well... now I know.

T+5:20 I still feel ill. I suffer a further bout of vomiting. The motion-like sickness persists. It is awful.

I am thinking with clarity and can function, but I am poorly. One decision is taken already however: the rest of the 100mg is binned. Perhaps I took too much of it. Regardless, this body load is far too high to justify any further testing or experimentation.

T+6:00 Slowly, too slowly, I am heading back to baseline. This has not been a good experience. The onset and peak were nice but not particularly wonderful, and the aftermath has been horrible.

Overnight, sleep was sparse and in the morning I woke with a headache. A low level hangover persisted through the early part of the day.

Why on earth do people put themselves through this, and how do they repeat it frequently enough to become addicted? Never again!

WARNING: At the time of writing this page, reports of heroin having been cut with fentanyl and similar chemicals are all too common. Given that fentnyl is typically 30-50 times more potent than heroin, the consequences are inevitable. Test, measure and allergy check your gear carefully before even thinking about using it.

FATAL DOSE COMPARISON
If this picture doesn't paint a thousand words you are not paying attention. In part it explains the wave of opioid related deaths which is currently sweeping the United States. It also surely emphasises why the safety information in this book should be common knowledge, rather than tucked away in the shadows.

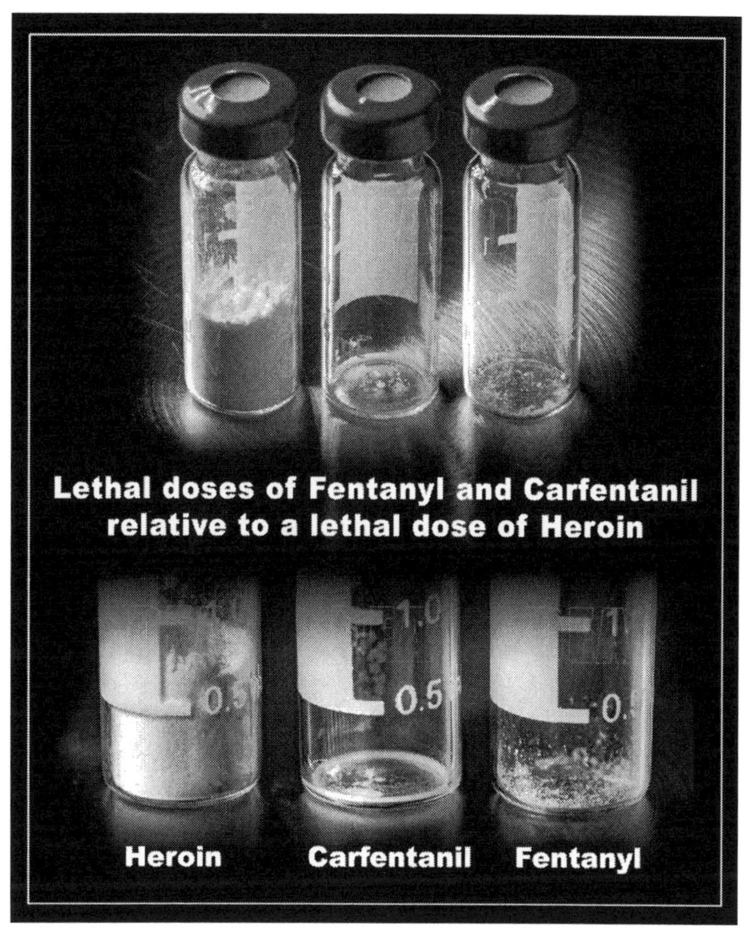

Note that the photograph itself comes courtesy of the DEA (Drug Enforcement Agency). On contacting them regarding its use, I asked if they would place it into the public domain rather than simply grant permission to reproduce, as this would be more likely to have a positive impact upon public health. Their response was affirmative. Credit where it's due.

2.5.5 Lean

Common Nomenclature	Lean
Street & Reference Names	Lean; Sizzurp; Purple Drank; Texas Tea; Dirty Sprite
Active Ingredients	Codeine; Promethazine
Reference Dosage	LEAN: Start With 50mg codeine, 30mg promethazine. No more than 2 doses. [DrugsLab] PROMETHAZINE: Common 25mg-75mg [TripSit] CODEINE: Light 50mg+; Common 100mg+; Strong 150mg+ [TripSit]
Anticipated: Onset / Duration	30 Minutes / 6 Hours
Maximum Dose Experienced	100mg Codeine; 62.5mg Promethazine
From	Fluid
RoA	Oral
Source / Jurisdiction	Associate / UK

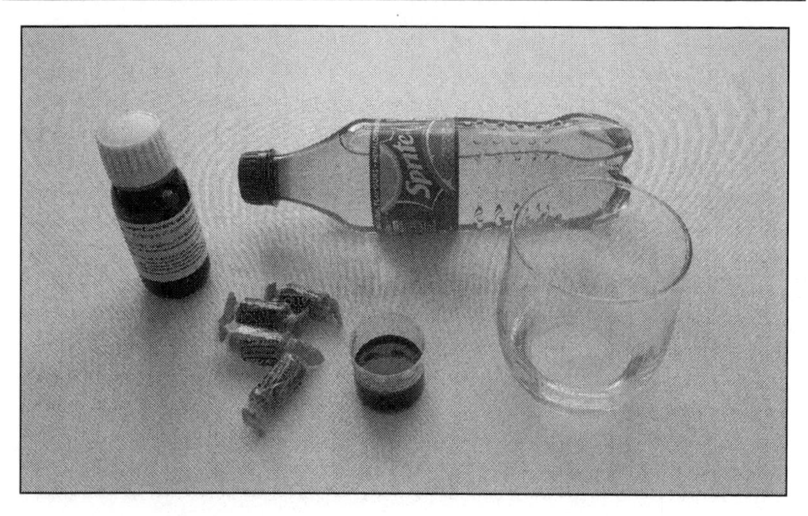

SUBJECTIVE EXPERIENCE
Originating in Texas, lean is codeine and promethazine (in the form of cough syrup) added to soda (typically sprite) and then mixed with fruit-flavoured sweeties (typically *jolly ranchers*). With its active ingredients being widely available, it gained substantial popularity in the 1990s as a cultural accessory, particularly via association with rap and hip hop music.

It is prone to both overdose and addiction, and has claimed a number of high profile casualties. I should also stress that, in particular, it should not be mixed with other CNS depressants (e.g. alcohol), or indeed stimulants or dissociatives.

During research for this experiment I decided to make the exercise as authentic as possible in terms of content. I managed to source some genuine codeine & promethazine cough syrup (as used in the Southern States), some sprite, and even some jolly ranchers. All I am missing is the all-American styrofoam cup to drink from, which is a luxury I will have to forgo.

I admit that I am not really looking forward to this one. I anticipate a sort of sickly sweet sedation which goes nowhere. If I am calling it incorrectly it won't be the first time.

Regarding dose, I found very little available in terms of guidance. I therefore decide to base my calculations upon the data for codeine and promethazine as individual drugs. For the common range, which is what I will punt for, these are broadly cited as 100-150mg for codeine and 25-75mg for promethazine.

My syrup contains 10mg of codeine and 6.25mg of promethazine per 5ml. The full 50ml bottle therefore contains 100mg of codeine and 62.5mg of promethazine. Is this too much? As the vendor himself suggested that as a first time user I should start with half-a bottle (25ml), perhaps it is. I will therefore dose initially with about 30ml (60mg of codeine and 38mg of promethazine) and take the rest a little later if all goes well.

> T+0:00 I measure the mix and pour it into a glass, topping up with sprite. I pop in a couple of jolly ranchers and stir it around for a few minutes, before starting to sip. [2:05pm]
>
> 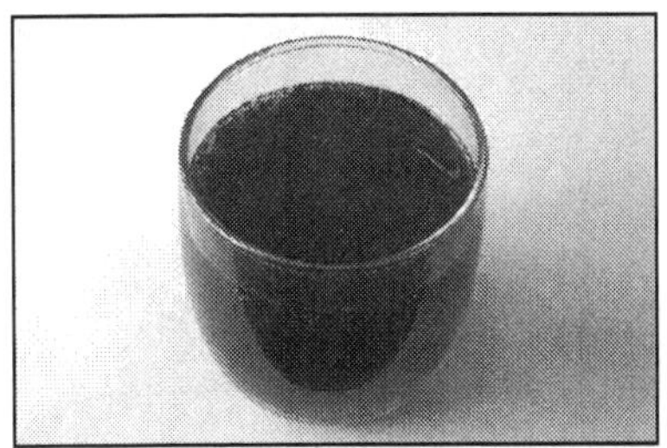 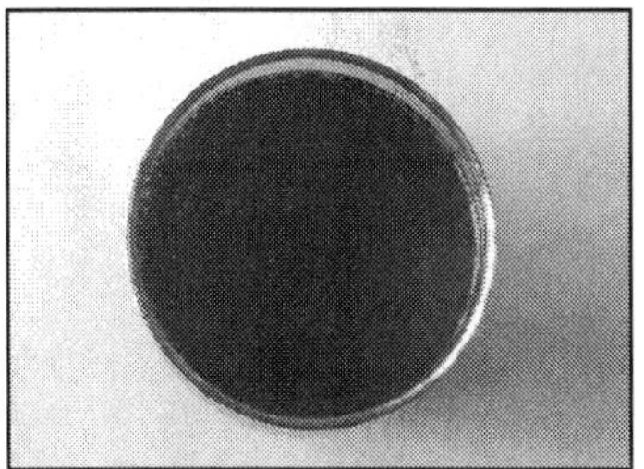
>
> It tastes a little sweet but becomes more palatable as I dilute further with sprite. It is relatively easy to drink.
>
> T+0:15 I am not sure how long users are supposed to take to savour this delight, but I have drunk it all in under 15 minutes. I feel a minor head inebriation emerging, with may be accompanied by a little sedation, but nothing beyond this so far.

T+0:35 I feel relaxed, a bit heady, and basically okay, in a mildly drifting sort of way. This is not unpleasant and it is not overbearing, which leads my thoughts to the remaining 20ml of syrup. Before jumping into this though, I will wait another 15 minutes to see if there are any further developments.

T+1:00 As there's been no significant change I pour the final 20ml of syrup and top it up again with sprite. Rather like I was drinking a fine ale, I swig this down during the next 5 minutes or so.

T+1:30 I am calm and relaxed, if a little distant, and there are no ill effects so far. Subjectively at least, I feel physically and mentally unimpaired.

I wouldn't really describe this as a high as such: there is a sense of comfort, anxieties have dissolved, and the mellow headiness is gentle and pleasing, rather than euphoric.

My face feels a little flushed and hands slightly cold, and maybe there is the tiniest hint of numbness.

T+2:00 The second dose seems to have increased the intensity. I am very aware that I am under the influence now, but that influence is akin to a mildly detached sort of sedation, or a benign form of serenity with a slight sense of uplift. No lethargy or tiredness has emerged, at least at this point.

T+2:30 The heady inebriation is not slacking. It is perhaps now dreamier in nature, creating a numbed distance from the world around me: a cloak of well-being. My face remains flushed and hands chilly. I have the impression that this would lend itself well to certain types of social setting.

T+ 3:30 The intensity has now passed, and I am left with residue in the form of a calm relaxed background aura. There is nothing negative about this, but as I close in on baseline I am becoming increasingly sleepy.

T+8:00 The tiredness became a more dominant feature as the evening progressed, and the dying embers have gradually faded to almost nothing as I retire to bed (10pm).

Without being mind-blown in any way, this was a nice enough ride. It lifted my mood, removed anxieties and provided a decent comfort bubble for a few hours. Whilst it was better than expected, a bonus was that it didn't really carry any noticeable negative payload. Rather than an enormous high, it delivered more of a sustained elevation. As stated earlier, perhaps a different setting would provide for more return from it, or alternatively a higher (more dangerous) dose might add a degree of euphoria.

Finally, whilst touching this aspect, I would again stress that this is addictive and prone to overdose. Don't let the relatively smooth ride that I experienced fool you. Be careful.

2.5.6 Morphine

Common Nomenclature	Morphine
Street & Reference Names	M; Dreamer; Miss Emma; Mr Blue, Morpho; God's Drug; Monkey; Aunti; Unkie; M.S; Emsel
Reference Dosage	IV: No reference figures available from usual sources. Dependent upon the strength of the solution and the attributes of the individual. ORAL: Light 5mg+; Common 15mg+; Strong 30mg+ [TripSit]
Anticipated: Onset / Duration	30 Seconds / 4 Hours
Maximum Dose Experienced	Not Known
Form	Liquid Solution
RoA	Injection
Source / Jurisdiction	Hospital / UK
Personal Rating On Shulgin Scale	++

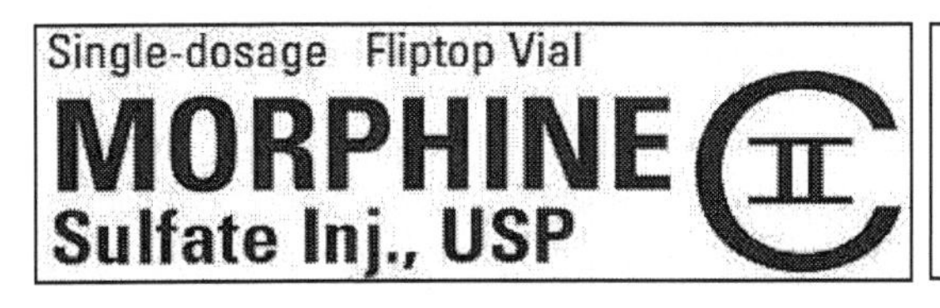

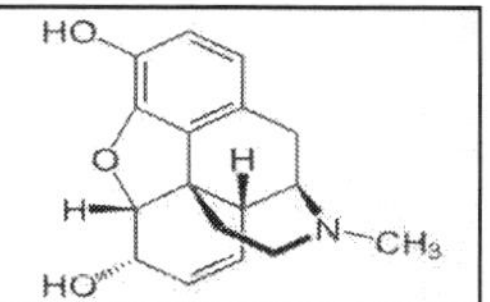

SUBJECTIVE EXPERIENCE
Extracted from the opium poppy, morphine has a long history of medicinal use, and indeed, recreational abuse. By including it in this book, however, I cannot deny that I feel somewhat fraudulent. Yes, I have experienced it, but not recreationally: it was administered courtesy of the NHS, in the Royal Liverpool University Hospital.

I was 21, had recently had my tonsils removed, when I was rushed back to the infirmary due to re-bleeding. On being injected with an unknown dose, presumably to calm my distress and agitation, a semi-euphoric mood lift immediately engulfed me.

It did its job medically, and was extremely pleasant: so much so that I harbour the embarrassing recollection that I may have asked for more.

Notwithstanding this, and despite its wide scale use in this context, this isn't a drug to approach with anything other than extreme caution. Heed the warnings provided in the entries for the other opioids and more generally. It is highly addictive and ultimately destructive.

2.5.7 Oxycodone

Common Nomenclature	Oxycodone
Street & Reference Names	Oxy; Oxynorm; Oxycotten; Ocycontin; Hillbilly; Hillbilly Heroin
Reference Dosage	Light 2.5mg+; Common 5mg+; Strong 10mg+ [Oral, Erowid, Assumes No Tolerance] Light 2.5mg+; Common 10mg+; Strong 25mg+ [Oral, TripSit]
Anticipated: Onset / Duration	30 Minutes / 6 Hours
Maximum Dose Experienced	10mg
From	Pill
RoA	Oral
Source / Jurisdiction	Associate / Overseas

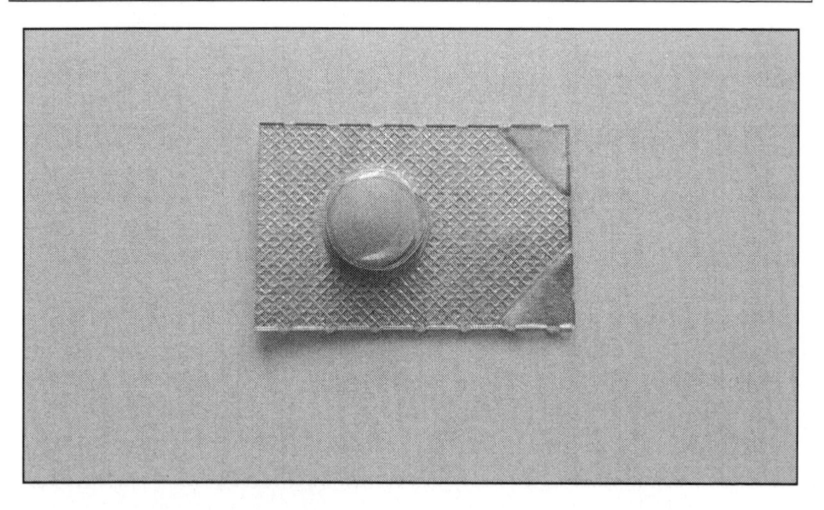

SUBJECTIVE EXPERIENCE
Oxycodone is an opioid medication which is prescribed to treat moderate to severe pain, and is available in both instant and extended release forms. It was first synthesized in Germany in 1916, and was first used clinically in 1917.

As would be expected, it comes with a variety of potential side effects, and clear risks with respect to overdose and addiction. Indeed, according to the CDC (the US Government's *Centers for Disease Control and Prevention*), among drug overdose deaths that mentioned at least one specific drug it ranked #1 in 2011. The message here is extremely clear.

This is certainly one which I will be treading carefully with. Also note that it is not a drug to mix with alcohol, or in fact, other medicines. In addition, grapefruit is commonly cited as a potentiator, and should be avoided.

As a street drug it is sometimes referred to as *hillbilly heroin*, due to its abuse in the Appalachian region of the US and its cultural reputation as a poor man's heroin.

My supply comprises a single 40mg pill, which is actually quite alarming, as even a cursory check reveals this to be a dangerous dose for non-tolerant users. I note also that it is marked "*prolonged release*" and is thus of the extended release variety.

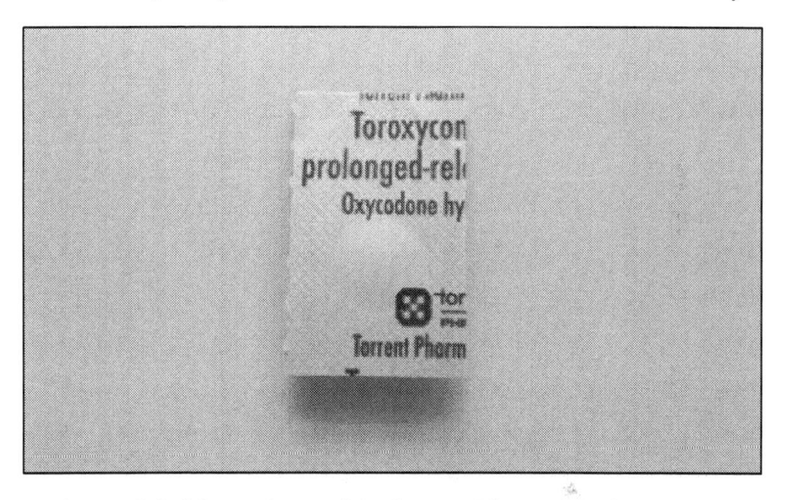

The vendor was helpful enough to explain that I could snort this if I wanted to. All I had to do was remove the wax coating and crush the contents. Given the significantly increased dose sensitivity of this drug when insufflated this isn't a route I will be taking.

So what should I take? Looking at the generic threshold figures, and taking into account my own physiology, my non-tolerant status, and my lack of enthusiasm for opioids generally, I decide to pitch in at no more than 10mg.

For more precision, rather than simply cutting the 40mg pill into four approximate quarters, I use my scales. I weigh the entire pill (148mg) and then cut it into four. I then weigh each quarter and select one which is just under the requisite weight (36mg). Note that, as much as I can, I also make sure that the wax coating is distributed evenly across the four quarters. Overall I am confident that my dose, if anything, is a tad under the 10mg maximum.

The left-over debris is a combination of white crusty powder and yellow coating. It may seem a shame, but I bin it as an obvious safety precaution.

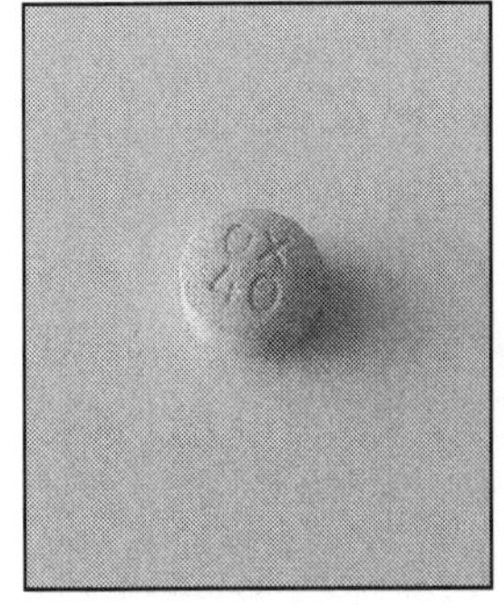

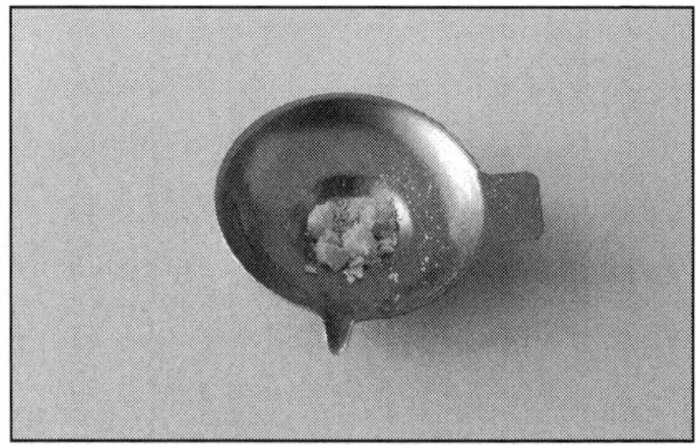

One thought that occurs before starting is that this operation may have neutralized the extended release mechanism of the pill. Regardless, I am now ready to go.

T+0:00 I spoon approx 10mg of oxycodone (the 36mg quarter) into my mouth and swill it down with a glass of water [2:10pm]

T+0:30 A mellow-headedness is starting to emerge and I am warmer. I feel less anxious and slightly more relaxed than I was.

T+1:00 This hasn't evolved very far. It remains a gentle bubble of warm tranquillity, which is pleasant but not euphoric. I'm not complaining: it's a nice enough vibe with an undeniable uplift and it isn't too strong. It also carries a gentle touch of numbness.

T+2:00 I am still floating along quite nicely with no flip side so far.

T+3:30 The intensity is now lower than it was earlier, although I remain in a very comfortable zone. Even though I feel that having more would tip me over into nausea and illness, I do have a worrying sense that I would redose had I not binned the remainder of my supply.

T+6:00 As with some of the other opioids I have experienced, as I tire I still feel slightly dizzy and a little queasy. This is not particularly heavy on this occasion, but it comes and goes, and is noticeable.

I retired to bed at 10pm (T+8:00), exhausted and feeling down about everything in sight, which was no doubt part of the come-down. The night's sleep, however, wasn't so bad, despite a couple of wake-ups in need of water.

I believe that I just about got away with this one. I have made some bad decisions with opioids, usually overdoing it, but here I found a dose which delivered a good few hours of pleasantness with a payback which was apparent but manageable.

Finally, the warnings with respect to oxycodone are particularly stark and I was wise to heed them. If you do intend to use this, I would urge you to do the same. The statistics I referred to earlier tell their own tale.

2.5.8 Poppers

Common Nomenclature	Alkyl Nitrites
Street & Reference Names	TNT; Liquid Gold; Amyl; Rush
Reference Dosage	Not Available
Anticipated: Onset / Duration	10 Seconds / 2 Minutes
Maximum Dose Experienced	Not Known
Form / RoA	Liquid (Vapour) / Inhaled
Source / Jurisdiction	Retail / UK

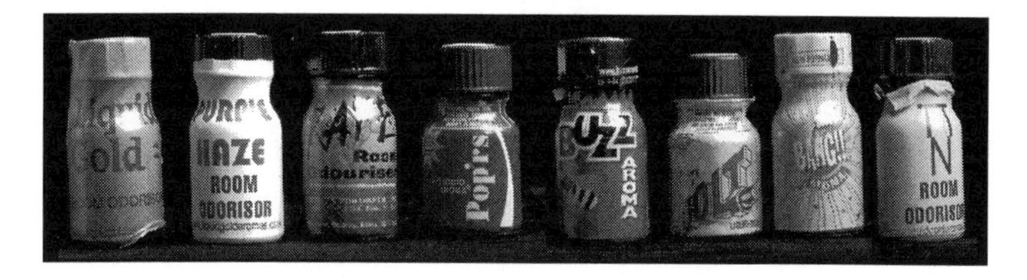

SUBJECTIVE EXPERIENCE
I can't help feeling that I am scraping the barrel by including these. Are they even psychoactive?

Certainly, on inhaling I felt a rush: but it didn't go anywhere. I also felt flushed, and warm, but not in a healthy sort of way. Then it passed, quickly. I was left wondering whether I had done something wrong.

I hadn't.

Alkyl nitrites do not have a direct action upon the brain: they simply increase blood flow. Indeed, this is considered to be so "*peripheral*" by the UK government that poppers were specifically exempted from its psychoactive blanket ban.

Poppers tend to be used during sex, as they relax muscles in the vagina and anal sphincter. Some people also subjectively claim that the head rush can intensify or prolong orgasm, although this was the last thing on my mind during my experiment.

Finally, it is reported that the use of poppers can cause headaches and nausea, and that they should be avoided by anyone with pre-existing cardiac or circulatory problems. Also bear in mind that the fluid itself is can burn the skin, and is highly flammable.

This is not an experiment I am ever likely to repeat.

2.5.9 Tramadol

Common Nomenclature	Tramadol
Street & Reference Names	Ultram; Zytram; Tram; Ralivia
Reference Dosage	Light 50mg+; Common 100mg+; Heavy 250mg-400mg [Oral, TripSit] Threshold 25mg+;Light 50mg+; Common 75mg+; Strong 250mg+ [Oral, Erowid]
Anticipated: Onset / Duration	1 Hour / 6 Hours
Maximum Dose Experienced	100mg
From	Capsules
RoA	Oral
Source / Jurisdiction	Associate / UK

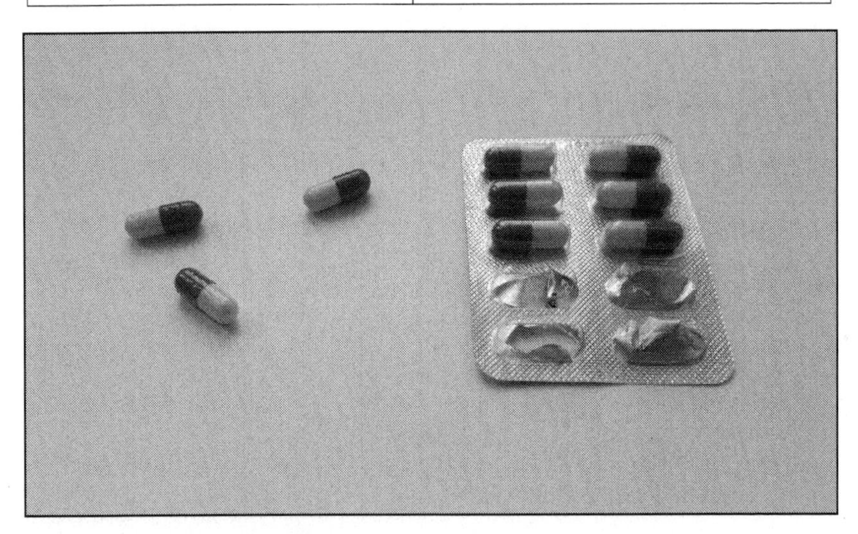

SUBJECTIVE EXPERIENCE
Launched under the brand name *tramal* in 1977, tramadol is a synthetic opioid analgesic which also acts as a serotonin reuptake inhibitor. It is currently marketed as a generic medication under a variety of brand names and is a common prescription drug.

My supply came via an accident: someone else's accident. As per standard practice, it was prescribed as a painkiller, and I was offered a blister pack to photograph for another project. Rather than discarding this after the event, I chose to put some of its contents to a constructive use.

Straight off the bat it is important to stress that this must be treated with a great deal of caution, particularly regarding dosage. TripSit categorically states that there is a "*Risk of seizure at doses over 300mg*". This is echoed by Erowid thus: "*Doses over 300 mg can be physically dangerous in non-tolerated or smaller users.*" Don't ignore this paragraph.

Wikipedia's contribution on this is as follows:

> "*Common side effects include constipation, itchiness, and nausea. Serious side effects may include seizures, increased risk of serotonin syndrome, decreased alertness, and drug addiction*".

With words like these ringing in my ears, and with less than pleasant experiences in the bank with respect to other opioids, I decide to tread carefully, and head to the lower end of the *common* threshold, with a dose of 100mg.

> T+0:00 I take two of the 50mg capsules from the pack and swill them down the hatch with a glass of cold water. [15:50]
>
> T+1:00 Gradually, over the last hour, the effects have emerged: a sort of heady relaxed feeling, with anxieties dissipated. I am able to function completely normally as far as I can tell. This is not unpleasant at all.
>
> I am warm, with mouth becoming slightly dry from time to time. Looking in the mirror I may be flushed and a little glassy eyed.
>
> T+2:00 I have now settled into a slightly dazed comfort zone, with a little uplift. As I find with opioids generally a want for more intensity is present if I think about it. It is hard to measure, but I have an impression that my speed of thought has slowed down.
>
> T+3:00 I am not as hungry as usual for this time of day, but I manage to eat a small meal (vegetarian of course). The comfort zone may be of a slightly lower order now, but I am still warm and contented.
>
> T+7:00 Slowly but surely the effects have wound down over the last few hours, although I still experience a calm dreamy and restive afterglow. I retire to bed at about 10:30pm.

The night's sleep was a good one, and I awoke with no hangover, other than a little fogginess. This was largely chased away by the morning coffee, although some tiredness did persist for a few hours.

Overall this was quite a pleasant ride. There was some sea-sickness-like dizziness at times, suggesting that I may have been borderline on the dose with respect to negative payload, but on the 100mg I just about got away with it.

Finally, a reminder on both the dosage and the addiction potential: be cautious and of course, never make a habit of it.

2.6. DISSOCIATIVES

Textbook Definition: *A dissociative produces a sense of detachment from normal sights, sounds and experiences of self. This dissociation from environment is often classified as an hallucinogenic experience.*

The following chemicals have been sampled and researched for inclusion within this section:

There was something about *the idea* of dissociatives which just didn't appeal. I couldn't understand what could possibly justify the enthusiasm of their users. The fact that the headline member of this class (ketamine) was allegedly a horse tranquilizer hardly helped to add positivity to my subjective negative perspective.

Then there were the disturbing reports of the mind being detached from physical sensory input, and the user effectively falling into a mental void (the so-called *k-hole*). That sounded like the opposite of LSD: instead of a wonderful oneness and connectedness, all is disconnected and an inglorious isolation ensues.

None of this was compelling, so it was through duty rather than desire that I metaphorically jumped into the hole (although no, I didn't *hole*). Needless to say, I was taken entirely by surprise.

Generally it was fun, and even more surprisingly, it was sometimes profound. I found that my mind was not closed down, but rather, was freed to contemplate and explore. I simply never saw this coming.

I was well aware of the dangers presented by this class, including in terms of mixing with alcohol and other drugs. I had read the stories illustrating what can happen if the brain is no longer fully conscious of the active body, which is fuelled by some other chemical. I therefore elected to play in the shallow end, where I enjoyed many rewarding experiences.

A slightly eccentric aspect of my journey was that it was *back-to-front*: ketamine was one of my final dissociative experiments rather than my first. The reason for this was access, in that it was illegal in the UK. I thus had to travel. Whether the order influenced my comparative report on K itself is open to question.

2.6.1 3-MeO-PCMo

Common Nomenclature	3-MeO-PCMo
Street & Reference Names	N/A
Reference Dosage	Threshold 50mg+; Light 100mg+; Common 200mg+; Strong 300mg+; Heavy 400mg+ [Psychonautwiki] Light: 50mg+; Common: 80mg+; Strong 125mg+ [TripSit]
Anticipated: Onset / Duration	30 Minutes / 4 Hours
Maximum Dose Experienced	100mg
Form	Crystal
RoA	Oral
Source / Jurisdiction	Internet / UK
Personal Rating On Shulgin Scale	++

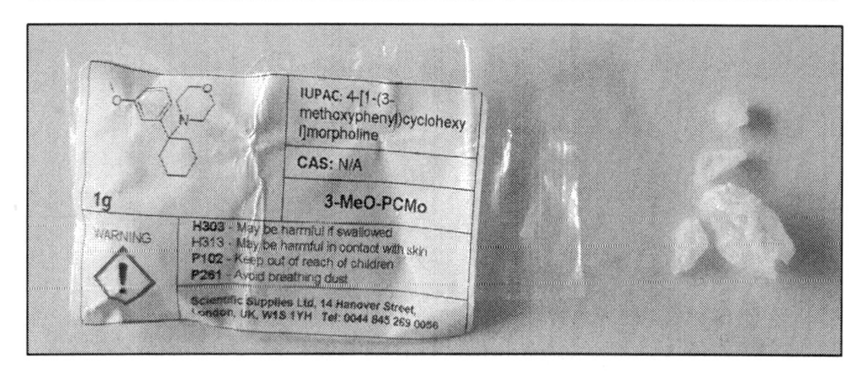

SUBJECTIVE EXPERIENCE
This is an analogue of the more widely known 3-MeO-PCP, and is generally described as a *dissociative anaesthetic*. Given that there are warnings on harm reduction websites stating that heavy doses of 3-MeO-PCP may result in psychosis and mania, and that the doses generally suggested for that chemical are considerably lower than those mooted for 3-MeO-PCMo, the need for caution is well sign-posted.

I sampled this about a year ago, snorting 45mg, but with only minor effects. I have no idea why I chose that RoA, particularly as this was a new compound and it was crystal, but I will take the more familiar oral route this time around.

Forum posts seem to be mixed, with many, but not all, suggesting no or little activity (via any route).

On the basis of this my first inclination was to dose at 200mg. However, even though I purchased from a relatively trusted vendor (BRC) the red flags referred to above persuade me to go low.

Having consulted with a colleague (online), I dose at 100mg.

> T+0:00 I crush the crystals into smaller shards, and then bomb them down the hatch. [4:30pm]
>
> T+0:15 Is a tingling in the head developing? It does seem to be: a sort of benign heady anaesthesia. It is barely noticeable, but it is there nonetheless.
>
> T+0:30 My head feels comfortably warm, which may or may not be a prelude to something more significant. There may be a tiny anxiolytic effect, or perhaps not.
>
> This is all very shallow at present.
>
> T+1:00 That heady anaesthesia has intensified and a gentle dissociation is now in play. The familiar numbing of my hands has emerged, albeit mildly at this stage.
>
> It is beyond question now that I have passed the threshold dose for this substance. I am comfortable with it, so I hope it will go further, although I don't expect it to.
>
> T+1:30 I sense that this has definitely hit a plateau. I am slightly off kilter, but in a pleasant way, and there is numbness to the experience, both physically and mentally.
>
> T+2:00 By most accounts I should be peaking about now, although I feel that I did so an hour ago. Indeed, this now has a coming-down feeling about it, and appears to be tapering towards normality, although I remain calm and somewhat dreamy in a slightly insentient bubble.
>
> T+3:00 The mild physical detachment and pleasant headiness are lingering, albeit at the lower level. Mentally, I feel in a better place than I did before I sampled this, so long may it continue.
>
> T+4:00 I now feel that I am more or less back to base.
>
> T+16:00 I retired to bed, tired, at around 11pm, and had a reasonable night's sleep. This morning, if anything, I feel more relaxed and refreshed than usual.

There was nothing unpleasant about this, in that at this dose the ride was quite nice throughout, if a little unspectacular. I suspect that it would be better still on perhaps 150-200mg, but those red flags and the existence of more market tested alternatives will probably dissuade me from experimenting further.

2.6.2 Diphenidine

Common Nomenclature	Diphenidine
Street & Reference Names	1,2-DEP, DPD, DND
Reference Dosage	Threshold 50mg+; Light 70mg+; Common 85mg+; Heavy 110mg+; [TripSit]
Anticipated: Onset / Duration	60 Minutes / 5 Hours
Maximum Dose Experienced	25mg+15mg
Form	Powder
Form	Oral
Source / Jurisdiction	Internet / UK
Personal Rating On Shulgin Scale	++

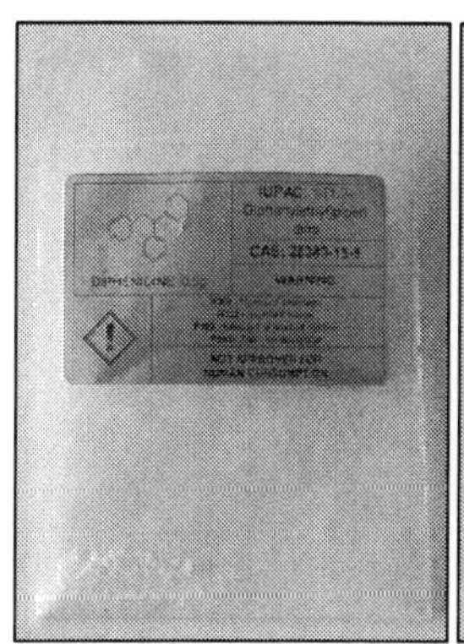

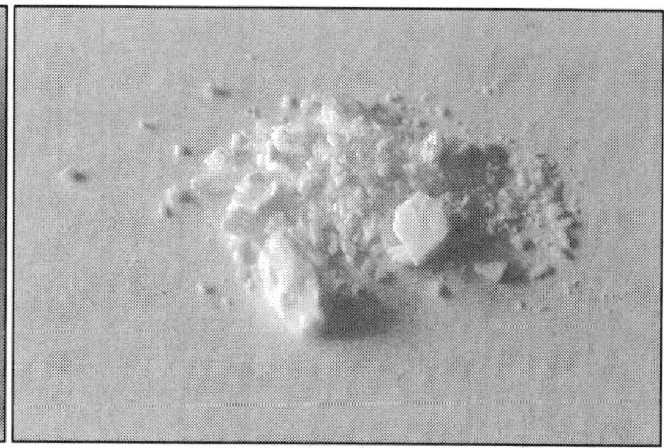

SUBJECTIVE EXPERIENCE

Diphenidine began to appear on the markets in 2013, shortly after the UK ban on ketamine came into effect. However, as it is much longer lasting and is usually taken orally, it is not generally considered to be a direct replacement. The headspace created is also reported to be notably different.

This chemical gave me my first experience of a dissociative, and this was certainly not what I was anticipating. My expectation had been framed by the fact that the aforementioned ketamine, which was the most well known dissociative, had been widely reported by the media to be a horse tranquilliser. On the basis of this I naively assumed that I would fall into a deep relaxing sedation, with significant drowsiness, and perhaps, eventually, sleep.

I wasn't even close.

The psychoactive effects took a significant time to materialise. Indeed, much longer than almost any other compound I had experienced at the time. However, when they emerged they were both immersive and distinctive.

My notes from the time were as follows:

> When I am sat down, focusing upon something cerebral, I can lose myself within the topic for lengthy periods, which is usually a very rewarding and positive experience.
>
> When I stand and walk around I am immediately aware of the disjointed weirdness of the world which I now perceive. This initially invoked some fear, but familiarity has tended to soften it.
>
> Now that this adjustment has occurred, and I have reminded myself that this is just a trip, and thus is a temporary phenomenon, it has become interesting and intriguing. The feeling of general numbness adds to this aspect, in that movement, the simple act of walking, feels more like a seamless floating enterprise.
>
> Overlaid on this, a feeling of general contentment has also taken hold and anxieties have dissipated.
>
> I can now see why dissociatives are such popular recreational drugs.

The overall experiment was both intriguing and enjoyable. I found diphenidine to be multifaceted, in that on the dose I opted for I could solicit different aspects of the experience almost at will.

On the flip side, it should be noted that there have been some reports of tragedy with respect to the use of this drug, which were always in the back of my mind. It also felt less smooth than its cousin, ephenidine, which I have subsequently sampled and explored more frequently.

Diphenidine provided a very strange ride indeed, but with edges which caused sufficient concern to prevent me from going too deep. Whilst I was under the influence, those edges, perhaps jittery in nature, were very mild. Indeed, they could, at least to some degree, have been invoked by familiarity with those reports, and by the negative PR which this class of drug tended to attract from the media at the time. I suspect that had ephenidine not emerged, I would have overcome them and used it for more comprehensive exploration.

Playing exclusively in the shallow end, this was a good introduction to the world of dissociatives. It was one from which I certainly derived a degree of insight and pleasure. Research, however, indicates that it should always be approached with care, and never binged.

2.6.3 DXM

Common Nomenclature	Dextromethorphan
Street & Reference Names	DM; Robo
Reference Dosage	Light 100mg+; Common 200mg+; Strong 300mg+ Heavy 600mg+ Risk of Death 2500mg+ [Erowid] First Plateau 1.5-2.5 mg/kg; Second Plateau 2.5-7.5 mg/kg; Third Plateau 7.5-15 mg/kg; Fourth Plateau 15 mg/kg+ [TripSit]
Anticipated: Onset / Duration	1 Hour / 8 Hours
Maximum Dose Experienced	225mg
From	Fluid
RoA	Oral
Source / Jurisdiction	Retail / UK
Personal Rating On Shulgin Scale	++*

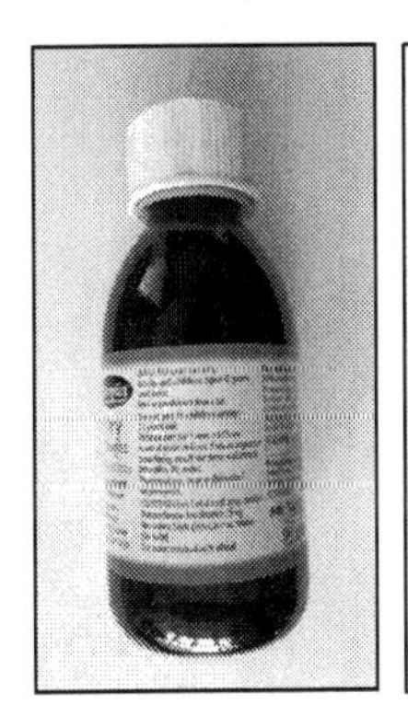

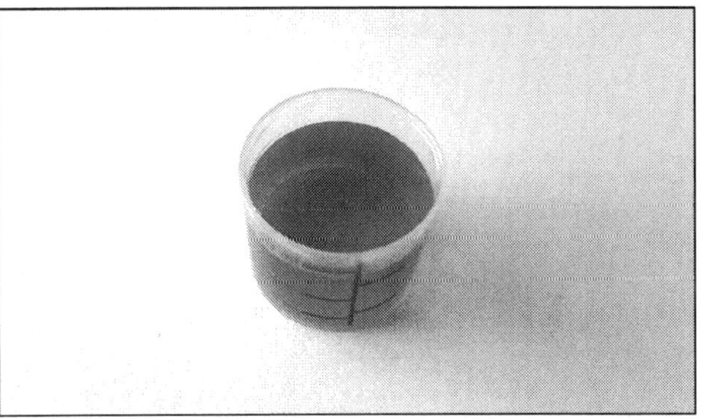

SUBJECTIVE EXPERIENCE
I never really fancied DXM; meaning that having experienced dissociatives like ketamine and ephenidine it didn't really seem to have anything interesting to offer. Further, in some quarters at least it had a reputation for being a *dirty drug* and a poor unclean cousin of other members of this class.

However, after the first edition of the book was published I decided to put this prejudice behind me and to take the plunge. A driving factor in this decision was that I could see some pretty conspicuous safety issues even prior to researching.

As a street drug, DXM is usually taken as part of a medicinal syrup, as purchased from a pharmacy. A number of brands are available, but herein arises the first challenge: to identify a product which doesn't also include other active ingredients, or at least, any problematic ones. This is an aspect not to treat lightly, as some additives can present significant dangers when taken in large (DXM trip) doses.

I eventually found a brand which contained liquid glucose and sucrose, but with only DXM and ethanol as its active ingredients. This explicitly stated that "*Each 5ml of cough syrup contains: Dextromethorphan hydrobromide 7.5mg.*"

From this I deduced that the 150ml bottle contained 225mg of DXM, which moves us on to the question of dosage. For DXM this issue is particularly interesting, as its effects have been commonly divided into four *plateaus* or *stages*.

Descriptions of these vary somewhat between sources, but they are broadly presented as:

> First Plateau: A sense of euphoria, with perhaps some distortion and enhanced music appreciation, and a feeling of heaviness.
>
> Second Plateau: Stronger manifestation of the first plateau effects, possibly with some disorientation, disconnection and mild hallucinations.
>
> Third Plateau: Stronger manifestation of the second plateau effects, but now in terms of a more dissociative experience. There is a possibility of anxiety, delusions, nausea, and memory suppression.
>
> Fourth Plateau: This is an encounter with full dissociation, and the symptoms related to it. This is sometimes referred to as a deep meditative state, often with associated hallucinations
>
> Fifth Plateau: A range of negative effects are encountered, possibly including blackout, delirium, dysphoria, psychosis and even death.

The second plateau is often cited as the place to be, and accordingly I decide to target this range.

So what is the dose? For an 80kg person TripSit presents a range of 200-600mg (with risk of death in excess of 2.2g). Given that at 76kg my 225mg bottle would fit nicely into my target band, I decide to glug the lot.
[Note: TripSit also provides a handy tool for calculating doses on the following URL: http://dxm.tripsit.me]

With all this worked out, I am now good to go.

> T+0.00 I open the bottle and drink its entire contents. It doesn't actually taste so bad; rather like a sweet chocolate liqueur. [1:35pm]
>
> T+0:15 The mixture felt a little heavy when it first landed on my stomach, but a fuzzy warmth is slowly starting to emerge.

T+1:00 A warm inebriation has taken hold, at least in terms of headspace. There is a visual clarity to this when I focus, with maybe a hint of disconnection and even derealization. The mild intoxication comes with some numbness, particularly of the hands as I write these notes. Anxieties also seem to have dissipated.

There appears to be no loss of control (functional or mental), and with concentration I believe (perhaps subjectively) that I could pass as sober in most social situations. My pupils are slightly dilated and face is a little flushed.

T+2:00 As DXM is reputed to enhance appreciation of music I play something in the background. Rather than being an annoyance, which I sometimes find, it is in fact pleasant, and catches my attention positively from time to time.

The earlier effects are still in play, with the heady disorientation and accompanying numbness firmly established. I am more lethargic than anticipated with little motivation to explore or engage, although this could be influenced by a degree of pre-existing tiredness.

T+2:30 All the effects documented thus far continue to strengthen, with some dissociation now evident. This is unlike that of the other dissociatives I have tested in that it has a rather distant feel to it, as though the weirdness is experienced through a haze, rather than immediately around my persona.

With the music playing gently in the background, and a drifty aura surrounding me, this is strangely pleasant. I am no longer convinced that I could manage a difficult or prolonged social scenario without my condition becoming evident.

T+3:00 I remain somewhat distanced from the exterior world, but still connected. I flow with the sensory inputs which tend to hit me as waves of sound and vision. I am not *off my head* as such or high in a euphoric sense, but I am riding with it, with reasonable comfort.

T+4:00 At this point I am past the peak: the intensity is gradually fading.

T+7:00 The effects have slowly wound down, with only residue lingering in the background. It is also worth noting that I ate a lighter meal than usual in the evening, so there was possibly some appetite suppression involved.

The night's sleep was a good one, and the next morning I awoke quite refreshed, with a mild afterglow present, which made for a pleasant morning.

Overall, DXM provided a more immersive ride than I was expecting. This was rather dizzy in places, but generally it was an interesting experience of inebriation and quasi-dissociation. Whilst I doubt that I would repeat the exercise, my initial negativity was a little misplaced. That said, the need for dose restraint and care is obvious. Also note that I was a little down for some days following the experiment, which may have been connected.

2.6.4 Ephenidine

Common Nomenclature	Ephenidine
Street & Reference Names	EPE
Reference Dosage	Light 50mg+; Common 75mg+; Strong 110mg+; Heavy 150mg+ [TripSit] Threshold 50mg+; Light 60mg+ Common 110mg+; Strong 150mg+; Heavy 200mg+ [Psychonautwiki]
Anticipated: Onset / Duration	2 Hours / 6 Hours
Maximum Dose Experienced	75mg+15mg
Form	Powder
RoA	Oral
Source / Jurisdiction	Internet / UK
Personal Rating On Shulgin Scale	+++

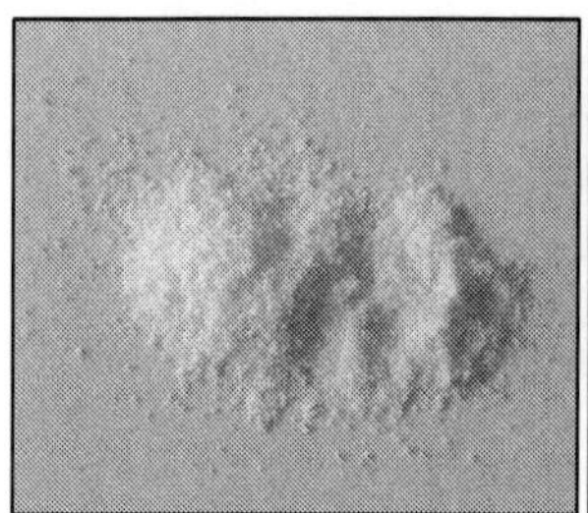

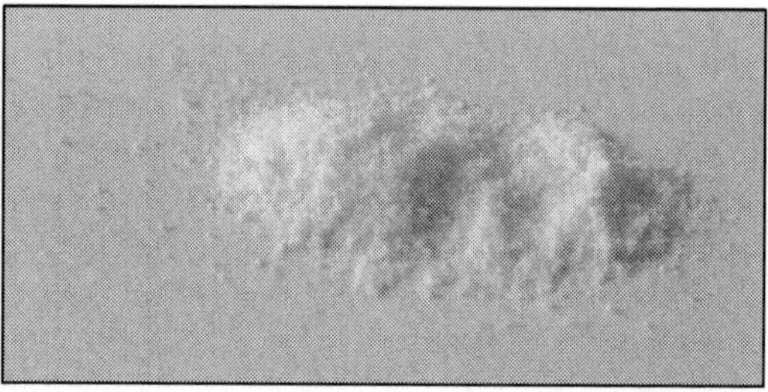

SUBJECTIVE EXPERIENCE
Ephenidine appeared on the markets at the start of 2015, and was purported to produce a state of *dissociative anaesthesia*. It was widely reported to be a smoother dissociative alternative to the other compounds legally available at the time, specifically MXP and Diphenidine.

My own experiences have aligned with this suggestion. I have invariably found that it produces a very pleasant and interesting few hours.

The onset is slow. I find that it doesn't kick in for about 2 hours, contrary to suggestions published in a number of contemporary reports. Its peak lasts perhaps 2-4 hours, and the come-down is slow and soft.

Consuming (orally) at about 4pm, I can find it difficult to sleep at midnight without an aid. I also tend to find the following night to be slightly disturbed, inclusive of vivid dreams. However, the afterglow, which is positive, lasts for several days.

The experience itself, at the level I dose (typically 80mg), is of a slightly euphoric dissociation, at which I am just about able to hold myself together (in a functional sense). A factor here is numbness and a slight impairment of motor functions.

At these doses I feel somewhat *misaligned* with the real world, but I am able to enter various states of focus, introspection and concentration. The accompanying analgesia and mood-lift makes this a very nice ride.

Visually, reality has an edge of distortion, but not in terms of any deterioration or loss of clarity. The world appears to be rather alien and off-key, which, due to the anxiolytic properties of the chemical, is not threatening. The bodily insentience adds to this impression, as normal walking, for example, becomes a smooth, floating and comfortable exercise.

I sense that higher doses would significantly increase the weirdness of the dissociation, and obviously its intensity too, but the ataraxic comfort and curious edges at this level have been sufficient for me not to go deeper, so far.

Finally, whilst this is probably my favourite member of this class, its status as a relatively unknown research chemical, rather than a tried and tested recreational drug, has deterred anything other than (very) occasional use.

Note that at high doses this drug is capable of producing internal hallucinations, so due care and attention is warranted with respect to this. In common with other dissociatives, certain combinations can also be problematic, hence the need for appropriate research and caution.

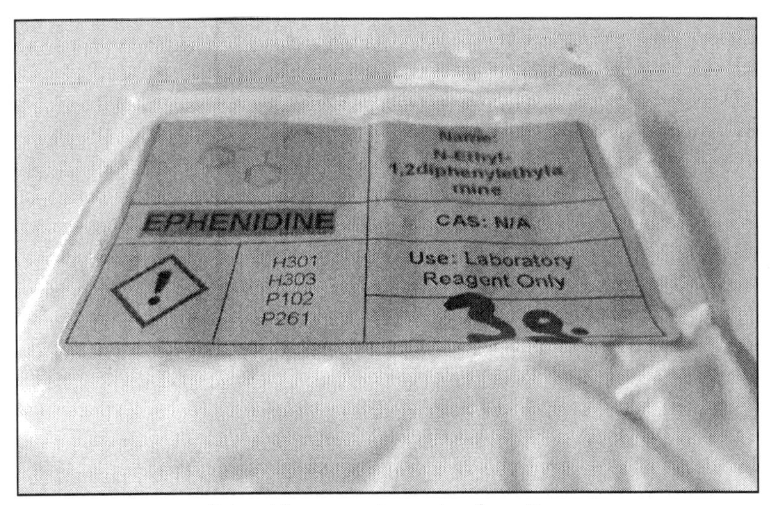

Internet forum reports were largely positive

2.6.5 Ketamine

Common Nomenclature	Ketamine
Street & Reference Names	K; Ket; Special K; Ketalar
Reference Dosage	Threshold 10mg+; Light 15mg+; Common 30mg+; Strong 60mg+; Heavy 100mg+; [Erowid] Threshold 5mg+; Light 20mg+; Common 50mg+; Strong 125mg+; Heavy 175mg+; [TripSit]
Anticipated: Onset / Duration	10 minutes / 2 Hours
Maximum Dose Experienced	50mg
Form	Powder
RoA	Insufflated
Source / Jurisdiction	Dealer / Overseas
Personal Rating On Shulgin Scale	+++

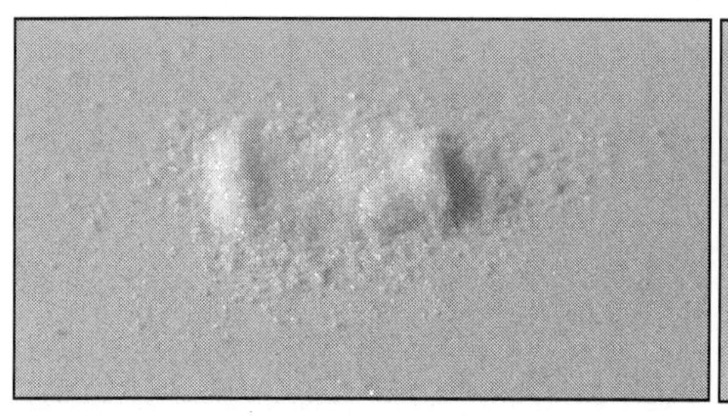

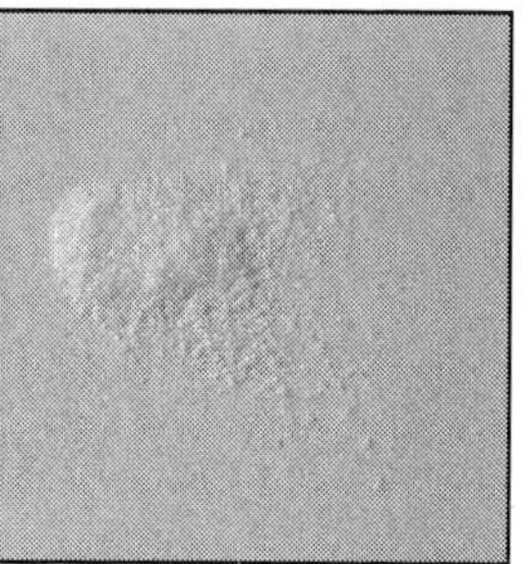

SUBJECTIVE EXPERIENCE
Ketamine emerged as a recreational drug in the 1990's, having been first synthesised in 1962. It was scheduled in the United States in 1999 and classified under the UK's *Misuse of Drugs Act* in 2006. It remains the most famed and popular dissociative.

Its effects are reported to vary according to dose. The most intense state, on a large dose, is known as a k-hole. This is an extremely subjective state of mental dissociation from the body, which has been compared to *near-death* and *out-of-body* experiences. The world becomes increasingly distorted and distant, time is suspended, and hallucination or indescribable perceptions may ensue, along with a sense of disorientation and derealization.

Every k-hole experience will be individual, with factors such as personal psychology, brain chemistry, physiology, set and setting, and personality, all being pertinent. It is not an exploit that should be contemplated lightly, or without significant research and investigation, and is certainly not one for the inexperienced.

It should be stressed here that the k-hole is not the normal or usual recreational ketamine pursuit. This is achieved at much lower doses, which invoke a variety of interesting experiences.

In this respect, it is important to take care not to overdose and enter the k-hole unintentionally, particularly in a public or insecure location. This can result in serious consequences.

If you are intent on using ketamine, my advice is to play in the shallow end, dose with caution, and avoid use with other drugs. Larger doses should only be considered on the basis of planning and preparation, and with a specific and clear objective.

Regarding my experiment, the dealer described his supply as *83% Pure S-Ketamine*, and was predictably positive regarding its quality, claiming that it was "*about twice as potent as racemic ketamine*" (racemic being the other type of ketamine).

With respect to the thresholds suggested across the Internet and given my experience with other dissociatives, 50mg seemed to be a reasonable first time dose. I measure this in preparation.

> T+0:00 I snort the 50mg line. [4:42pm]
>
> T+0:05 I am starting to sense some minor changes in perception.
>
> T+0:10 The show is definitely on the road now. I am feeling a rather disjointed headspace, as visually everything seems to be a little weird and slightly off-key, but in a comfortable way.
>
> Any concerns I had about taking ketamine have already dissipated under its influence.
>
> T+0:15 I am still entirely functional, even though I am not fully *with it*. For no particular reason I check my eyes in the mirror: the pupils are normal.
>
> My body feels a little numb, perhaps a little detached: it is fully operational but the numbness is obvious. For example, hitting the keyboard to type these words seems awkward, with my fingers feeling strange and too large. Walking around the room produces a smooth floating impression.
>
> T+0:20 The headspace bears definite resemblance to the other dissociatives I have sampled. I am inside a zone, but looking through it into the external world. None of this is disagreeable however. I am generally relaxed.
>
> T+0:25 This is quite strong now. I can still, functionally, talk and type, using auto-pilot, but the headspace is intense in a way that is hard to describe. The thought occurs that I can almost feel my brain as an individual organ, which is obviously bizarre.

At the same time, the degree of numbness of the rest of my body has further increased.

T+0:30 I sense that I have found a plateau, in that the experience has stopped intensifying, and I have come to terms with its effects. The physical aspect, largely the insentience, is similar to other chemicals in this class, but it seems to be more apparent. Predictably, the experience has also developed much more quickly than the others, which were all ingested orally.

T+0:40 I play some music to test audio. Pink Floyd is a standard test, and in a bizarre manifestation of synchronicity, *Comfortably Numb* appears on YouTube as a suggestion. The listening experience is not particularly enhanced, so I elect to return to silence and self reflection.

T+0:45 I take a short walk. I feel lumbering and I am aware of my gait. My movement is probably outside my normal walking parameters, but my condition isn't absolutely obvious to others, as far as I can tell.

Talking is fine, but I know I would struggle with anything requiring responsive intensive thought or perceptive social cueing or etiquette.

I am possibly just touching +++ on the Shulgin scale at this point.

Underlying is a property which is also familiar to other dissociatives: it is the distinctive quality of the weird distortion of normal reality. The strangeness in how everything is just offset could be frightening if I didn't know I was under the temporary influence of a drug. Because I do, I can easily suppress any anxiety and ride it, but it is there, nonetheless.

T+0:55 Time has flown. It is already closing in on an hour since I snorted the line. It doesn't feel like that at all.

T+1:05 The hour mark passes and I have passed the peak. I am still rolling, but the headspace is now fully manageable and in the lower ++ area. The numbness has diminished. It is still there, but has changed in character, and is less intrusive.

T+1:15 I am rapidly coming-down the hill towards baseline, and I am chilled and calm. It feels like it may take a while to get fully home, but I have certainly got all my faculties back in place and could easily deal with issues as though I was sober and normal.

It's been an enjoyable ride, and I feel rather like I have been on a highly compressed ephenidine trip.

The comedown doesn't seem to be too drastic thus far.

> T+1:30 I am almost back to base, with those after-trip feelings of glow, tingles, calmness and well being. I wonder what I will recall from this last hour? That's a question to self, because a known feature of ketamine is that it is hard or sometimes impossible to remember the contents of the experience (which I believe is known as *state bounded*).

I have used ketamine on a handful of occasions since this first experiment, and it is a drug that I have increasingly come to terms with regarding expectation. The earlier ephenidine experiences created a mindset of longevity to my dissociative endeavours, which of course ketamine could not meet. However, after the first couple of experiments the two hour duration became less of a disappointment and more a feature. It became increasingly acceptable and positive.

I have never chased ketamine (via redosing), but instead, I identified a niche use for it, in which it was capable of providing both insight and pleasure. Having stated this, my ranking of ephenidine as my favourite dissociative has not changed.

Whilst I enjoy this chemical, there is a *but*. This is that there are definite side effects to prolonged or frequent use. For example, regular ketamine use is reported to cause kidney and/or bladder damage. These are extremely serious issues, and they are what prevent me from pushing this chemical too far, or dipping into it too often.

Tread carefully.

CLINICAL USE: DEPRESSION

Notwithstanding the risks noted above, at time of writing evidence is emerging that, when taken medicinally, ketamine can be used to treat acute depression.

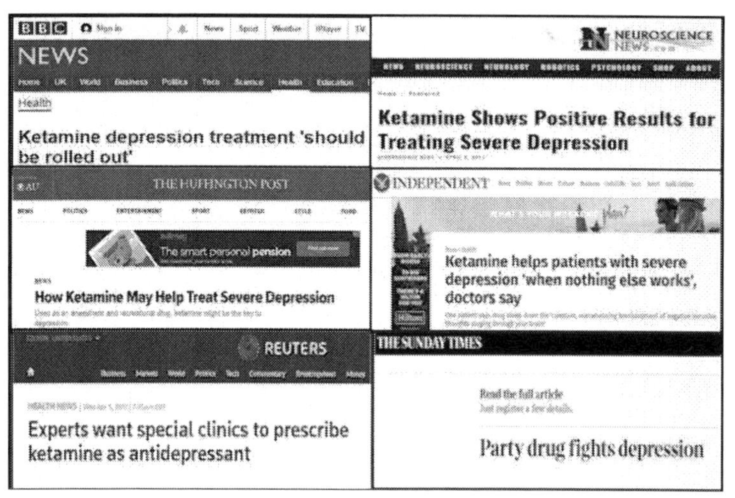

BBC NEWS

Health

Ketamine depression treatment 'should be rolled out'

NEUROSCIENCE NEWS

Ketamine Shows Positive Results for Treating Severe Depression

THE HUFFINGTON POST

How Ketamine May Help Treat Severe Depression

INDEPENDENT

Ketamine helps patients with severe depression 'when nothing else works', doctors say

REUTERS

Experts want special clinics to prescribe ketamine as antidepressant

THE SUNDAY TIMES

Party drug fights depression

2.6.6 MXE

Common Nomenclature	Methoxetamine
Street & Reference Names	Mexxy; Roflcopter; 3'-MeO-2-Oxo-PCE
Reference Dosage	Light 10mg+; Medium 20mg+; Strong 40mg+ [Drugs-Forum] Threshold 8mg+; Light 10mg+; Common 40mg+; Strong 50mg+ [Erowid] Threshold 10mg+; Light 15mg+; Common 25mg+; Strong 40mg+; Hole 75mg+ [TripSit]
Anticipated: Onset / Duration	30 Minutes / 4 Hours
Maximum Dose Experienced	50mg
Form	Pill
RoA	Oral
Source / Jurisdiction	Head Shop / UK
Personal Rating On Shulgin Scale	++

GOV.UK
Search
Departments Worldwide How government works Get involved
Publications Consultations Statistics
Home > Health and social care > Public health > Health improvement > Drug misuse and dependency
News story
Government bans methoxetamine or 'mexxy'
The government has used a temporary class drug order for the first time to ban the 'legal high' methoxetamine, also called 'mexxy' or MXE. From...

MXE
18
NOT FOR HUMAN CONSUMPTION

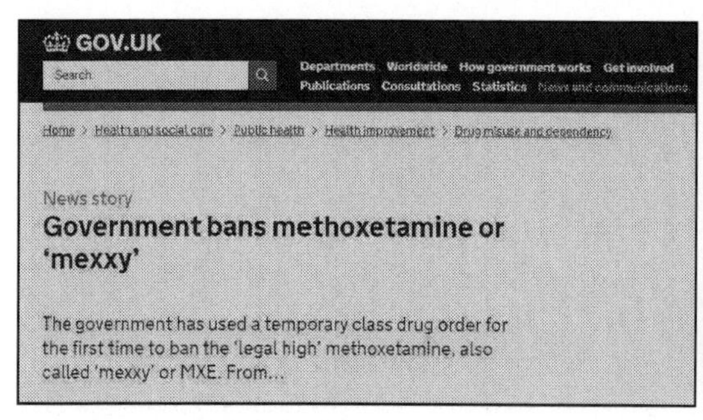

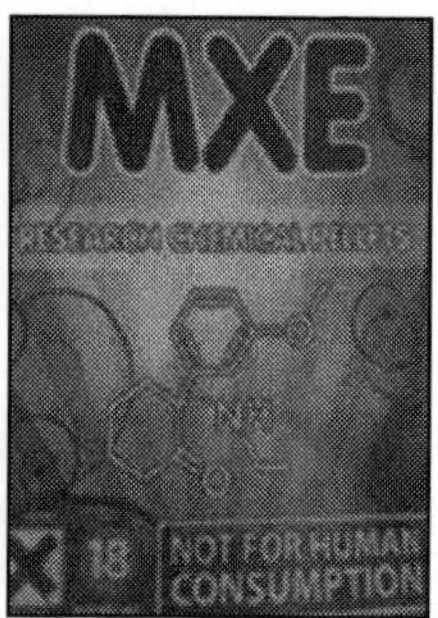

SUBJECTIVE EXPERIENCE

MXE began to appear on the markets at the end of 2010, and was to become popular in a relatively short space of time. It has recently acquired something of a cult status; due in part to production being banned at source (China), causing it to became increasingly difficult to obtain.

At time of writing, its legal status in the United States is unclear, noting that it could be considered to be an analogue of PCE or ketamine. In the UK it was the subject of a TCDO in April 2012, and was classified in February of the following year. I was fortunate to have obtained a sample just a few days prior to this ban.

This was one of my first dissociative adventures, and given its sudden disappearance from the market, my only one with this chemical.

My regret in this context is that I was not able to explore it more deeply, as it was a very positive experience.

Dissociation was not something I approached lightly, and I had read a number of horror stories of people mixing dissociatives with alcohol. I was therefore a little nervous in shovelling perhaps half of my 50mg supply down the hatch.

The action took just a short while to commence: considerably less than an hour. However, as one of the first manifestations was to alleviate my anxiety, the rest of the pill was rapidly consumed. For a period though, there was still a slightly scary edge to proceedings, as everything around me was becoming rather strange.

What followed was a positively charged dissociation, under a mindset of the world around me not being normal, and my perspective not being quite *with it* in this realm. *Weird* is such a lame word to use, but it does capture the essence of the ride. At the same time, I was absolutely comfortable with this.

I felt strangely high but not tuned in. I was able to fall into a period of introspection, but also able to focus upon, for example, academic related pursuits on the Internet. This was indeed significantly different to other forms of intoxication.

There was an *Alice in Wonderland* edge to life: I was fully conscious and aware whilst everything around me had warped slightly, giving it an alien feel. I had retained all my marbles, my clarity and my rationality, but I was witnessing reality as though I wasn't fully in it. Certainly, I enjoyed it.

Another positive came in the aftermath: I suffered no hangover or noticeable come-down, with a mild afterglow lasting a day or two. I was sorry not to have sampled it earlier.

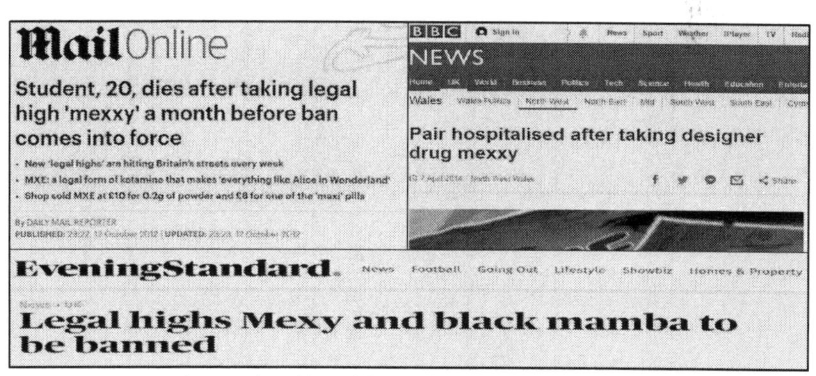

Mail Online

Student, 20, dies after taking legal high 'mexxy' a month before ban comes into force

- New 'legal highs' are hitting Britain's streets every week
- MXE: a legal form of ketamine that makes 'everything like Alice in Wonderland'
- Shop sold MXE at £10 for 0.2g of powder and £8 for one of the 'maxi' pills

BBC NEWS

Wales

Pair hospitalised after taking designer drug mexxy

Evening Standard

News Football Going Out Lifestyle Showbiz Homes & Property

Legal highs Mexy and black mamba to be banned

MXE became the subject of the usual sort of adverse media reporting

2.6.7 MXP

Common Nomenclature	Methoxphenidine
Street & Reference Names	2-MeO-Diphenidine
Reference Dosage	Threshold 15mg+; Light 40mg+; Common 75mg+; Strong 120mg+; Heavy 200mg+ [Erowid] Threshold 30mg+; Light 50mg+; Common 75mg+; Strong 120mg+; [TripSit]
Anticipated: Onset / Duration	30 Minutes / 7 Hours
Maximum Dose Experienced	50mg
Form	Pill
RoA	Oral
Source / Jurisdiction	Internet / UK
Personal Rating On Shulgin Scale	++*

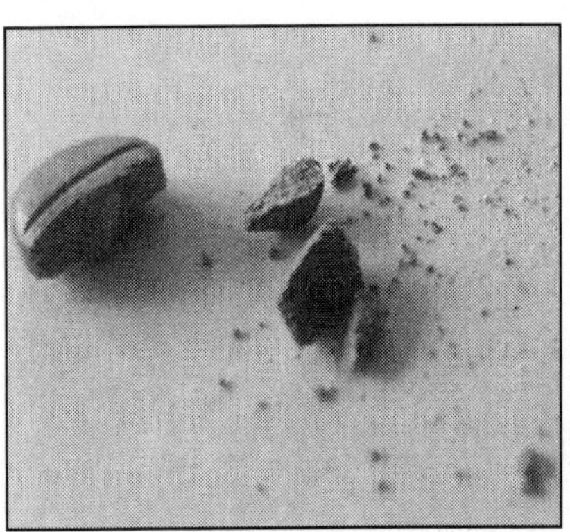

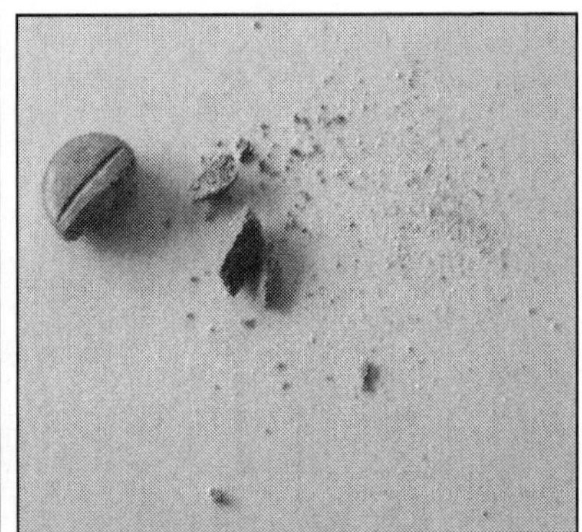

SUBJECTIVE EXPERIENCE
First referenced in a 1989 patent, MXP appeared on the recreational markets at the end of 2013, and became widely available during the following year.

My first experience with this chemical, a couple of years ago, was an early expedition into this field. I was well immersed, I enjoyed it, and I recorded it as a solid ++ on the Shulgin scale. However, other than its dissociative weirdness, and that I felt no ill effects, I recall very little about it.

Fortunately, I still have one old MXP pill of 75mg left in a desk-drawer. A decision is therefore required: what dose should I choose to re-sample with, given the threshold data above?

After the allergy test, there is perhaps 70mg remaining. As I recall Internet reports referring to seizures on high doses, there is an obvious need to proceed with more caution than usual. Further, the *BlueLight* forum warns of unpredictability and inconsistency, and suggests a starting dose of 50mg. I decide to heed this advice.

T+0:00 I break the pill into pieces, separate approximately 50mg, and bomb it down the hatch with water. [2:45pm]

I dispose of the rest to prevent redosing under the influence.

T+0:30 Already I am feeling a sedated headspace, and I dreamily drift off focus now and again. Whilst onset is commonly suggested to be 30-60 minutes, the odd report refers to two hours, which would put it on a par with my experiments with ephenidine. However, this has started to take effect much more quickly than anticipated.

T+0:45 I have now definitely entered the zone. Reality is a little weird, and a degree of anaesthesia is present. I am warm and comfortable, feeling a mellow headiness and physical insentience.

T+1:00 The headiness is pretty solid now, and quite pleasant. The physical feeling is interesting in that there are occasional tactile sensations amidst the overall numbing effect. Time is passing rather quickly. I am already enjoying it.

T+1:15 As weirdness would have it a David Bowie track rolls in the background with: *"Please trip them gently, they don't like to fall, Oh by jingo"*. I certainly feel that I am tripping gently at this stage, and floating.

T+1:30 The disconnection is now increasingly strong. I check my blood pressure: 163/91. It's quite high but not alarming. My pulse is a normal 53bpm. I am not happy about the former, but in the interest of not increasing it further via stress, I choose to navigate my mind away from it rather than dwell upon it.

I take the experience into a more relaxing realm by playing some YouTube videos and reading.

T+1:45 Shock horror: a phone call! This takes me by surprise and I make the mistake of picking up the handset. The real world interjects and I desperately attempt to act like a normal human being. I engage a conversation to the best of my ability with the lady on the other end, but with difficulty. I believe that I am rational and lucid, but I am far from certain. I think the acronym I am looking for here is *OMG*.

With this trauma over, I try to put it behind me and settle back down into the experience.

> T+2:00 I now feel that I have reached a plateau. The two hours have flown by. Although I am still a little haunted by thoughts of the mess I made of that phone call, I am in a fairly happy place.
>
> I am a little chilly and my hands are cold, so there appears to be some vasoconstriction in play.
>
> T+2:30 I feel a little more grounded, and have probably peaked, but I am still flying. There is a sense of wonder to everything as I float from one focus of concentration to another.
>
> T+2:45 I am coming-down. Physically I still have cold and clammy hands, but mentally I am totally functional if I choose to be.
>
> I can still ride the trip if I want to but step off it if I need to.
>
> T+3:30 Time is still passing quickly. There is still some numbness and headiness but I am in a much gentler state of dissociation.
>
> I find that I can choose a subject or topic, focus, and then fall into it for a period, before emerging back into self awareness.
>
> I am now very much in control.
>
> T+4:00 I seem to be winding down in the usual manner for a dissociative, but even at this level, the headspace, body analgesia, and tingles, continue to make this a gentle floating pleasure.

For the rest of the evening I drifted slowly but pleasantly down. Despite the bumps on the road I felt physically well and was able to navigate my mind into positive directions at will. The 50mg dose was clearly sufficient.

The night can best be described as comprising two deep sleeps of 3-4 hours each. The first began with chilliness and the need for an extra cover, and ended with a vivid nightmare. Theorising on the latter, I would speculate that, with the MXP still active at a low level, the intensification of focus upon subject matter took me deeper into the story of my dream than usual. This resulted in an extension of the dream beyond the point at which I would have normally woken, with greater immersion within it. I suspect that this phenomenon may also manifest across other dissociatives.

Notwithstanding the fact that generally I had a very good experience, research demonstrates that this is a chemical which clearly carries risks. Erowid, for example, reports that there have been several deaths associated with its use.

Dose moderation and appropriate caution is strongly advised.

2.6.8 N2O

Common Nomenclature	Nitrous Oxide
Street & Reference Names	Hippy Crack; Nitro; NOS; Laughing Gas; Nangs
Reference Dosage	N/A
Anticipated: Onset / Duration	30 Seconds / 3 Minutes
Maximum Dose Experienced	2 Canisters
Form	Gas
RoA	Inhaled
Source / Jurisdiction	Internet / UK
Personal Rating On Shulgin Scale	++

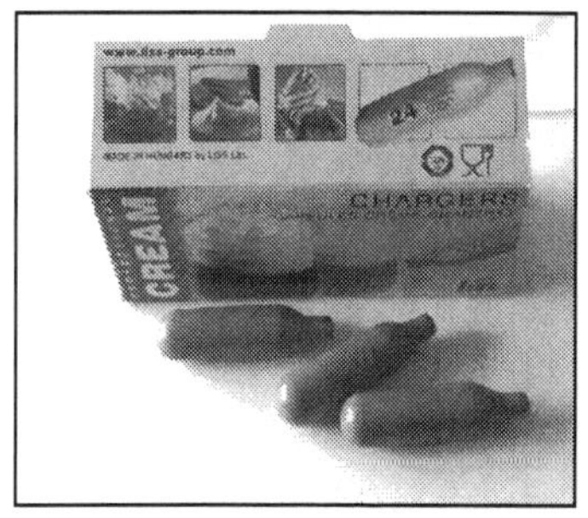

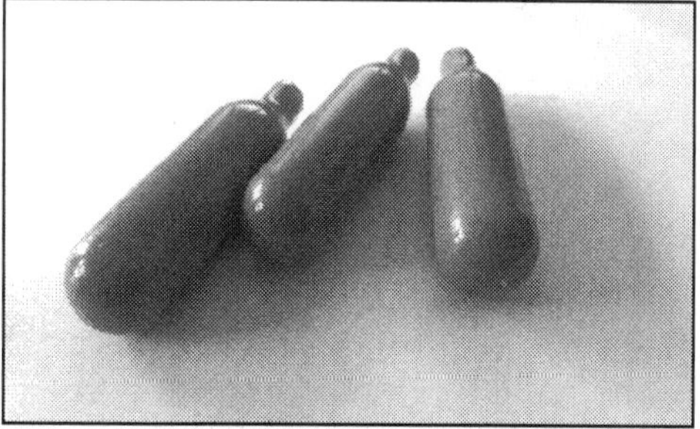

SUBJECTIVE EXPERIENCE
At time of writing (2017) this is extremely popular, particularly on the club scene.

For my own experiment, I elected to use the *balloon method*, which is commonly considered to provide one of the safer forms of inhalation. Using a device known as an *N2O Cracker*, two canisters were blown into a balloon. The content of this was then inhaled and held. This had an immediate effect, in that my headspace dissipated and appeared to distance from my physical being, but it was quick; too quick. It was a *wham bam* type of hit, with little fulfilment or pleasure.

During the aftermath I felt strangely calm and was almost sedated for a period, at least to a small degree. Perhaps this is part of the attraction, but for me, it wasn't a particularly rewarding experience.

I have an inkling that starting from a different state of mind might provide a more positive outcome, and in some cases, act as a reset button in terms of mood. I should add, however, that this is largely speculation.

2.7. EMPATHOGENS & EUPHORIANTS

Textbook Definition: *Empathogens and entactogens tend to produce feelings of emotional communion and bonding with others, particularly in terms of empathy and oneness. This state is most widely reported with respect to MDMA, but is actually created via a substantial number of substances. Euphoriants create a sense of euphoria, elation or bliss, sometimes in association with the empathy produced via an empathogen.*

The following chemicals have been sampled and researched for inclusion within this section:

2.7.1 6-APB
2.7.2 MDA
2.7.3 MDAI
2.7.4 MDMA
2.7.5 MEAI
2.7.6 Mephedrone
2.7.7 Methylone
2.7.8 MNA
2.7.9 Mexedrone

The first research chemical I ever sampled was an empathogen, even though I didn't understand this at the time. The experience was one of warmth, touchiness, attraction, well-being, pleasantness, love, and the *n-word*; niceness. This was MDAI, and I liked it.

The n-word is often very appropriate to describe members of this class. There are no DMT-like hallucinations, no k-holes to fall into, and few super-functional binges to engage. There is euphoria, emotional communion, and empathy, sometimes with a touch of an effect from other classes, such as a slight stim here, or a bit of psychedelic headspace there.

This resonance with other classes also leads some users into the realms of combinations; meaning mixing with other drugs. Some of these are themselves widely used and extremely well known. Examples include candy-flip (MDMA and LSD), sugar-flip (MDMA and cocaine) and hippie-flip (MDMA and shrooms). It should go without saying that these should only be approached with extreme caution.

Despite the deceptively benign nature of some of the chemicals in this class, others can bite, so the general harm reduction rules should not be relaxed under any circumstances. Indeed, a number of specific safety regimes have been established, which should be followed (see the references within the MDMA entry, for example).

These are not drugs to take liberties with. Do not underestimate them.

2.7.1 6-APB

Common Nomenclature	(6-(2-aminopropyl)benzofuran
Street & Reference Names	Benzo Fury; 6APB
Reference Dosage	Threshold 30mg+; Light 40mg+; Normal 50mg+; Strong 80mg+ Heavy 100mg+ [Drugs-Forum] Threshold 15mg+; Light 40mg+; Common 80mg+; Heavy 100mg+ [Erowid] Light: 50mg+; Common 75mg+; Heavy 125mg+ [TripSit]
Anticipated: Onset / Duration	1 Hour / 12 Hours
Maximum Dose Experienced	50mg
Form	Pill / Powder
RoA	Oral
Source / Jurisdiction	Internet / UK
Personal Rating On Shulgin Scale	++

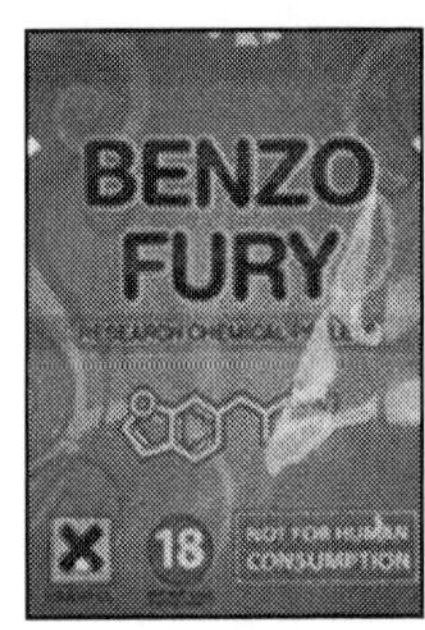

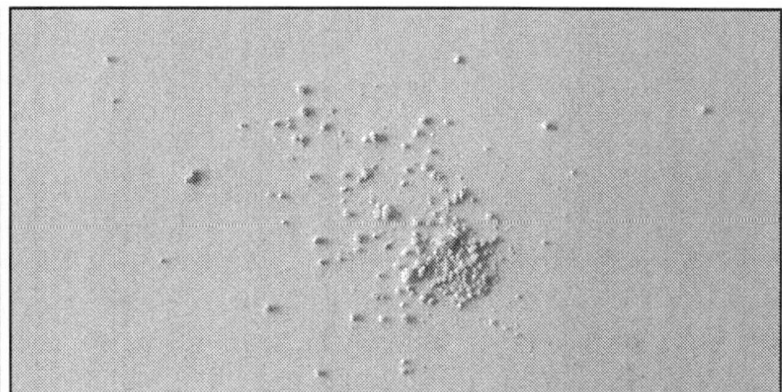

SUBJECTIVE EXPERIENCE

Someone, somewhere, had the dubious idea of calling this chemical *Benzo Fury*, presumably for marketing purposes. It was subsequently promoted in bright orange packets, which became instantly recognizable. Indeed, the combination was so garish and catchy that it was bound to attract the attention of a hostile media. During its heyday, it was to become one of the most cited research chemicals of the media's unremitting campaign against the spurious evils of legal highs, and was subsequently banned in the UK via a TCDO in 2013.

I originally sampled this as a pill circa 2010. It was one of my earliest forays into the research chemical market and as such the experience was under-documented. I recall a really pleasant high: a definite mood-lift and a perspective that all was well with the world.

Some years later I obtained the chemical in powder form, and was able to document it in more detail, albeit at a lower dose.

> T+0:00 Given reports that this may be cardio-toxic, at least with heavy or regular use, I elect to dose at a moderate 50mg. Another consideration here is the anticipated duration, which in my current circumstances is on the long side. I measure the beige coloured powder and bomb it in cigarette paper. [2:35pm]
>
> T+0:25 A body warmth and a dreamy type of ataractic bliss seem to be emerging. I sip on a glass of water to ensure appropriate hydration.
>
> T+1:00 I am warm and slightly sweaty, and the passive heady feeling is now established. It brings with it a general mood lift and a positive empathogenic edge. It isn't strong, and I am entirely functional, fully able to concentrate on tasks as I choose.
>
> T+1:30 This isn't very intense, but on the other side of the coin I had a rare alcohol session last night and was feeling fairly wretched: I now feel much better. My impression is that this isn't as strong as the 6apb I sampled back in 2010.
>
> T+2:00 Whilst this is a very light experience, I can see clear similarities to MDMA, which hardly comes as a surprise. As with MDMA, there is no stim-dick or related issues, and horn is available.
>
> I have often seen claims that 6-APB creates a sense of well being, and I would agree with these. At this point, the body warmth has dissipated a little, but the headiness continues unabated.
>
> T+3:00 The positive contentment flows at a nice and gentle level. I am beginning to feel the odd hunger pang, so there doesn't appear to be any appetite suppression in play.
>
> T+4:00 Whilst I feel that I am still on a plateau of comfort, it is at a lower level than it was earlier.

I slowly descended towards base during the rest of the evening, and retired at about 11pm. After a variable night's sleep I awoke with no ill effects or significant hangover.

At this dose it turned what would have been quite a miserable and slightly hung over day into a pleasant one, and didn't seem to hinder my functionality or my general level of competence. A negative is that for several days subsequently I felt rather down and irritable.

A higher dose would undoubtedly have delivered the extremely pleasing high I recall from my first experiment. However, with TripSit advising an intake of no more than 200mg per night, this isn't something I will push. I should also stress that it is not a chemical to make a habit of.

2.7.2 MDA

Common Nomenclature	3,4-methylenedioxyamphetamine
Street & Reference Names	Sally; Sassafras; Sass; Tenamfetamine
Reference Dosage	Threshold 30mg+; Common (Most People) 100mg+; Required By Few 145mg+ [Erowid] Threshold 20mg+; Light 40mg+; Common 60mg+; Strong 100mg+; Heavy 145mg+ [Psychonautwiki] Light 30mg+; Common 40mg+; Strong 80mg+; Heavy 120mg+ [TripSit]
Anticipated: Onset / Duration	30 minutes / 5 Hours
Maximum Dose Experienced	80mg
Form	Crystal
RoA	Oral
Source / Jurisdiction	Dealer / Overseas

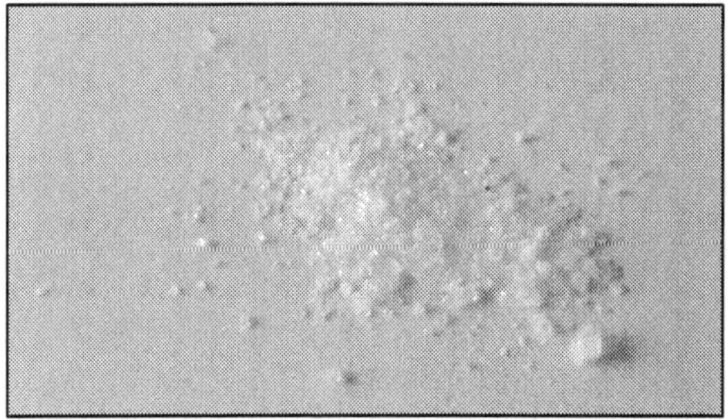

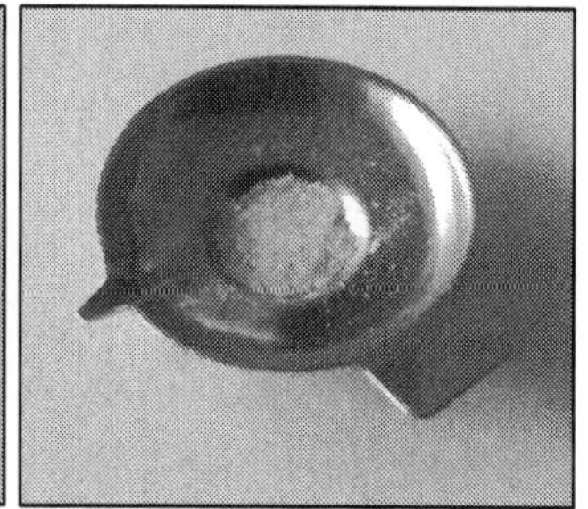

SUBJECTIVE EXPERIENCE
Whilst MDA was first synthesized in 1910, and was subsequently tested and used for various medicinal purposes, it didn't emerge as a recreational drug until the 1960's. Its effects are often compared to those of MDMA, although there appears to be a number of significant differences, not least its apparent variability, a greater stimulation and a stronger psychedelic edge.

It is currently a Schedule 1 controlled drug in the US and a Class A drug in the UK.

Regarding dose, MDA is often cited as requiring about half as much as MDMA to approximate the same level of effect. Listed in PiHKAL (#100), Shulgin referred to a dosage of 80-160mg, whilst across Internet forums a decent dose is sometimes claimed to be 1mg per kg (about 75mg for the average man). This is broadly what I will be pitching at.

Note that at time of testing I have become particularly cautious with drugs in this class due to hangovers following a couple of recent experiments. Internet references to neurotoxicity, with some citing MDA specifically, have further tempered my enthusiasm for a more substantial foray.

T+0:00 I measure 80mg and bomb it in folded rizla paper. [4.00pm]

T+0:30 A mild headiness is developing along with a slight tingling of the skin, which is enveloped within an increasing general comfort. This is coming on quickly.

My pupils are already partly dilated.

T+0:40 I am now high. There is a very strong cognitively immersed euphoric feel to this, and a strong empathogenic drive. Horn is also clearly available.

I am heating up quickly, so I am keeping well topped up with water, even at this early stage.

I already know that 80mg was a plentiful dose and wonder with a little trepidation how much further this will go.

T+1:10 This is a heady, sweaty, serene-like experience, with a sex drive and a trippy edge. I am probably in the upper ++ Shulgin range at the moment, hovering towards +++.

I can just about interact sensibly, but would fail with any complex or serious social challenge, at least in terms of hiding my condition.

It is a pleasant enough roll, but with a little anxiety surfacing now and again on the basis that it could go higher and beyond my ability to manage it.

T+1:20 For the first time I feel that I may be getting on top of this: possibly.

I am rather hot and clammy, my mind is high with a strong drifty aura, and I feel very empathetic. There is a touch of psychedelia lurking there too, which impacts upon clarity.

T+1:40 I am now in more control of the experience, which remains strong. Whilst the general warmth is a heavy physical feature, there are occasional shivers. I know in these cold snaps that it would be a mistake to add clothing as my temperature is clearly elevated.

The empathetic quality of the high is still a dominant factor, with a strong urge for intimacy. It is glaringly obvious why its sister, MDMA, is sometimes referred to as the love drug. I should stress though that in most respects MDA does seem to be more cognitively embracing than MDMA.

I am in the middle of ++ territory, as it ebbs and flows.

T+2:00 Although I am still in command of my mindset, I am warmer than ever: I am actually sweating. I don't feel uncomfortable with this, with the buzzing high carrying me along. However, I can absolutely understand how people become dehydrated, and indeed over-hydrated, as measuring the appropriate intake of fluid is not a trivial task. I sip sensibly rather than gulping heavily.

T+2:45 I am very much rolling, and perhaps still in the midst of a ++. The headspace remains in situ as a nice rounded high, and I am still hot and still drinking fluid. Drinking alcohol with this would clearly be reckless and dangerous.

I do feel jaw tension and the urge to gurn, but I am able to resist.

T+3:10 I manage to eat a full meal without too much difficulty. It was very slow going but there were no issues, and taste was fine.

T+4:00 I have moved down a gear or so, but I am still drifting along.

T+6:00 I am now floating down towards base. However, a sudden unexpected visit from a neighbour demonstrates that I am still, in fact, quite heavily influenced.

During the next few hours I edge towards normality but still sustain a drifting headspace as I retire to bed at midnight (T+ 8 hours).

The night's sleep wasn't too bad, with only a couple of disturbances, largely caused by the volume of water I drank.

In the morning my head was slightly heavy, and I was still a little warm. My pupils were also partly dilated, particularly the left. Presumably this all indicates that the MDA hangs around in the system for quite a while. The accompanying tiredness and mental fatigue eased during the day.

Perhaps also noteworthy is that a couple of nights later I had an extremely vivid dream, the nature of which indicated that this intake of MDA may have been related, particularly with respect to the stimulation of those receptors associated with hallucinogenic effects.

Make no mistake about it, this was a strong roll. 80mg came on fast and whisked me away with a head and body high that took me to the edge. Had I taken what is purported to be a strong dose I have little doubt that I would have careered off the path.

Caution should be exercised both with dose and frequency of use.

2.7.3 MDAI

Common Nomenclature	5,6-methylenedioxy-2-aminoindane
Street & Reference Names	N/A
Reference Dosage	Threshold 20mg+; Light 60+; Common 100mg+; Strong 175mg+ [Erowid] Threshold 20mg+; Light 40mg+; Common 100mg+; Heavy 150mg+ [TripSit]
Anticipated: Onset / Duration	45 Minutes / 5 Hours
Maximum Dose Experienced	100mg+
Form	Powder
RoA	Oral
Source / Jurisdiction	Internet / UK
Personal Rating On Shulgin Scale	++

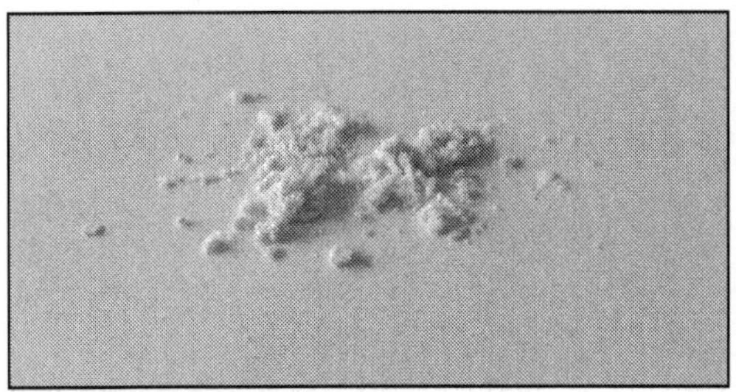

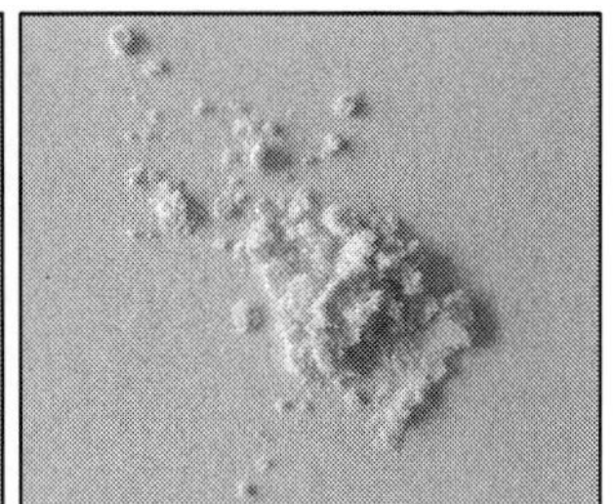

SUBJECTIVE EXPERIENCE

As MDAI was my first ever research chemical, it will forever hold a special place in my heart. Purchased from a well known head shop, it came as 100mg of powder, tucked away within a gelatine capsule.

These were naive and reckless days, and at the time I had little grasp of what to expect, other than some sort of pleasant experience. Fortunately, in terms of relative risk, MDAI is not particularly problematic, so I had chosen to dip my toe into fairly benign waters.

I dosed small: perhaps half a capsule. It was mild and it was indeed pleasant, albeit in a non-intrusive and generally weak way. I had, of course, barely reached threshold. However, I gained confidence from the exercise: I had taken an RC, survived, and actually enjoyed it, albeit superficially.

Life continued, but I still had another 100mg capsule burning a proverbial hole in my drawer. I had binned the rest of the first capsule.

The day came upon which I finally decided to try the *full monty*. Down the hatch it went, and I waited in some trepidation.

This was a significantly stronger experience. After an hour or so I felt a very nice uplift, with yes, an empathogenic edge. I felt good.

Shortly thereafter, I recall walking to a takeaway for some food. Sitting across from me, as I waited, was a woman: a stunning woman, possibly the most beautiful woman I had ever seen. I was well aware that this must be a bi-product of the MDAI, as I tried not to stare.

This took me by surprise. Can drugs really do this? Indeed they can, and I liked the feeling.

Over the following months I bought and consumed a couple more capsules, but then, suddenly, the head shop had no more: apparently there was a problem with manufacture in India. Instead, I was offered a branded product called *Sparkle-E*, which included MDAI, and was claimed by the vendor to be a good substitute.

The other ingredient was in fact Methiopropamine (MPA), which consequently became my first research chemical stimulant.

As the MDAI shortage took hold, *Sparkle-E* soon became MPA + 5-MEO-DALT; as was the world of branded legal highs. This, of course, is another story.

Downstream, circa 2015, MDAI re-emerged via a new lab, allegedly in China. As is frequently the way with such chemicals, in terms of effect it never again seemed to reach the wonderful high of those first few experiments. Somehow, whether perceptually or in reality, the body appears to adjust and move on, beyond what one could attribute to tolerance.

The magic dissipated, but the memory remained.

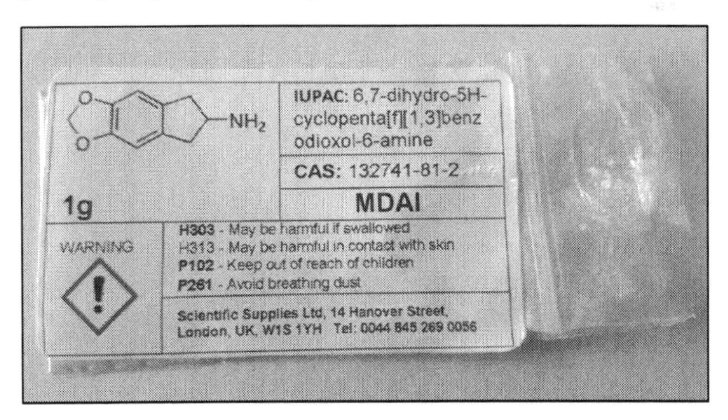

2.7.4 MDMA

Common Nomenclature	3,4-Methylenedioxymethamphetamine
Street & Reference Names	Molly, Ecstasy, XTC, Mandy, E, Pingas
Reference Dosage	Threshold 30mg+; Light 40mg+; Common (average sized people) 75mg+; Strong 150mg+; Heavy 200mg+ [Erowid] Light: 40mg+; Common 75mg+; Strong 125mg+; Heavy 175mg+ [TripSit]
Anticipated: Onset / Duration	45 Minutes / 5 Hours
Maximum Dose Experienced	80mg+30mg+55mg+55mg
Form	Pill
RoA	Oral
Source / Jurisdiction	Internet / UK
Personal Rating On Shulgin Scale	++*

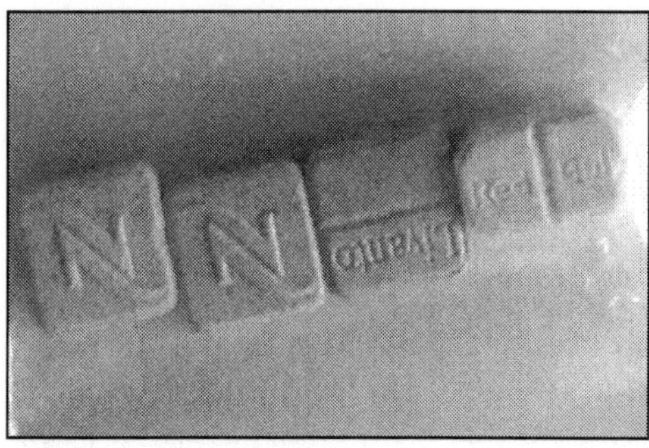

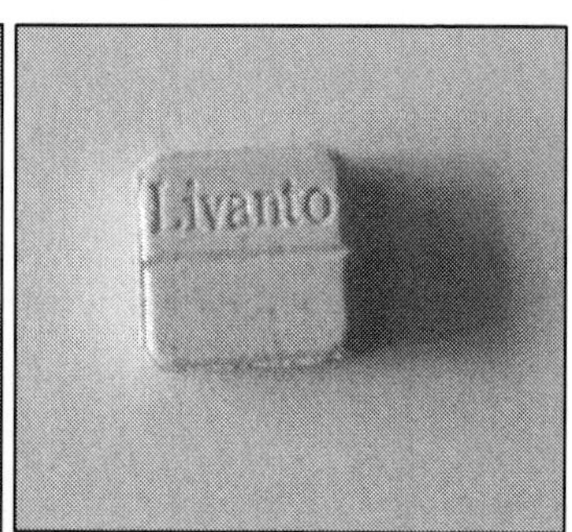

SUBJECTIVE EXPERIENCE
Whilst it was first synthesised in 1912, and famously re-synthesised by Alexander Shulgin in 1965, MDMA only emerged as a street drug in the late 1970s. It became known by a variety of terms, including ecstasy and E, and was eventually to become one of the most popular recreational drugs in the world.

I planned my own foray reasonably well, and consumed with fruit juice, as recommended across a number of forums. I also ensured that I had water readily available to reduce the frequently referenced risk of dehydration. I drank about half a litre every hour or so, noting that over-hydration is also a serious matter.

Even though I was not in a hot environment, such as a club, I also kept an eye on temperature to avoid overheating. I had earlier prepared for the adventure by consuming some vitamin pills (including magnesium).

The pill itself weighed in at a hefty 220mg, so I broke this up, with the intention of redosing into the experience at a gentle rate, assuming all was well.

T+00 I swallow 80mg with fruit juice

T+30 I am coming-up: a definite headspace is emerging.

T+40 The commonly stated 40 minute uptime is correct. It's coming on strong, with an obvious mood lift.

T+60 One hour in and I am significantly elevated, with my head in a positive place. I am somewhat sweaty, but I am drinking a little water to compensate. I am still able to respond sensibly to social cues if necessary. I pop another 30mg from the original pill.

T+1:30 I am experiencing a happy pleasant buzz. This really is nice. I feel confident and I am certainly rolling. I swallow another 55mg, bringing the running total to 165mg.

T+1:50 I am semi-euphoric; glowing with a dreamy high and a sensual edge. Is there horn? There is, but certainly not on the scale of a stim binge. Capability appears to be intact, but there is no compulsive interest, although I sense that human interaction could well change this. This isn't commonly referred to as a party drug for no reason, and I can understand how most forms of intimacy would be vastly enhanced in this state of mind.

Common advice on redosing is not to do it, but if compelled to, to do it as quickly after T+00 as possible. I therefore consume the final 55mg of the now fully crushed pill.

T+2:05 A meal unexpectedly arrives. This isn't what I expected, but being aware that food is sometimes recommended for safety reasons I eat it. It seems fairly normal, so MDMA doesn't appear to enhance taste. Nor does it completely suppress appetite, as many stimulants do.

T+2:14 I'm flying: hot, sweaty, euphoric and struggling to stay functional. My eyelids flicker of their own accord, and I strain to focus and stay with it. The redosing was not a sensible move, particularly on a first-time experiment.

At this point, which I believe and hope is the peak my debilitated state would be obvious to any third party. The experience is now very intense. It is extremely pleasurable but I feel that it is a little too close to the edge. This unease is perhaps exacerbated by thinking in this way. If I was distracted by my immediate environment I suspect that I might just be as high as a kite, without the same degree of anxiety and self-awareness.

T+2:56 My jaw clenching (bruxism) is now unmissable. I am just about functional but badly impaired. I still bathe in a very nice and comfortable headspace, I am still sweaty, and I am still drinking water.

> T+4:00 I am slowly on the way down. This remains pleasant, with a warm glow, and I continue to sweat and drink water (in moderation).
>
> T+5:45 I am now riding on a lower plateau. I am still under the influence, but I can now push this into the background if I absolutely need to. The waves of euphoric well-being have dissipated.
>
> T+7:30 It is getting late, so I head to bed. I feel comfortable and fall into sleep quite easily.

Whilst I slept reasonably soundly, a headache emerged during the night, which persisted into much of the morning. It had disappeared by lunch time, and I was left with a slow and gradual comedown. This wasn't particularly hard, but included a strange offset feeling, and a general heady malaise. It wasn't very pleasant.

The background depression and lack of general positivity lasted for several days, which aligned with the general consensus amongst the user population.

Backtracking on the overall experience, I broke several of my own rules, the main one being the size of the dose. 220mg was excessively large, particularly for a first experience. This was extremely foolish. The primary cause of this was the redosing: I failed to remove the residue from immediate accessibility. This no doubt contributed to the overwhelming nature of parts of the trip, and to the subsequent headache and discomfort.

The lesson here is a general one. Take it easy on the dose, especially if you are not a seasoned user.

MDMA is not a drug to trifle with, and requires sensible consideration, including with respect to aftercare. Entire websites are dedicated to safety, including *rollsafe.org* and *rollingpro.com*. The advice given is usually sensible, and includes the use of supplements, such as 5-HTP, to help restore serotonin levels. I followed most of these measures fastidiously.

A decidedly sage piece of advice is to leave a significant gap between MDMA experiences. Three months is commonly suggested, with six weeks stated as an absolute minimum. It is hard to overstate the importance of this.

Finally, MDMA has attracted more than its fair share of dishonest and false media reporting. This has tended to hide two of the most serious risks associated with its use: relatively toxic chemicals (such as PMA/PMMA) being sold as MDMA, and MDMA adulteration. Testing and appropriate pill research* is therefore of vital importance, as are the other measures listed in the safety section of this book.

* Pill research references: *ecstasydata.org* and *pillreports.net*

[*Shulgin Reference: PiHKAL #109, p733*]

AN ANECDOTAL TALE (THE UNWANTED SWEETIE)
During the dark and seemingly endless years of the *war on drugs* era, some places have earned a reputation for even greater brutality than the norm. One example is Bangkok, in Thailand.

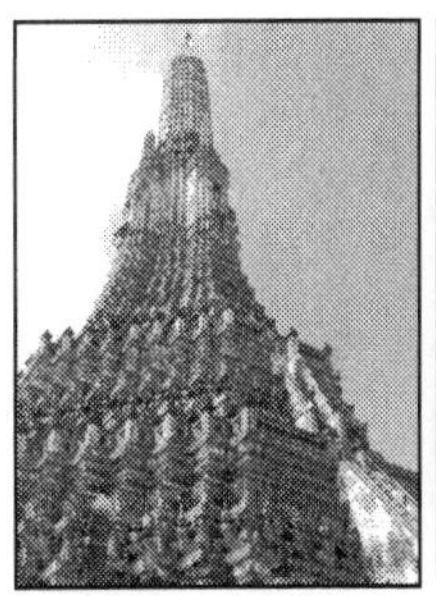

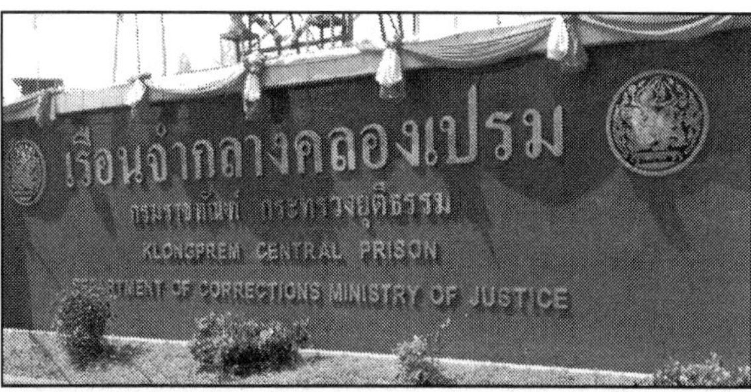

I have found myself stranded at Suvarnabhumi Airport a number of times, either passing through, or having taken a short stopover as a tourist. On one of the latter occasions, I hooked up with an Australian woman and her daughter. We eventually made our way to customs, to proceed to our respective flights.

As we queued in line, we had almost reached the customs desk for our passport checks, when I noticed the unmistakable sight of an ecstasy pill on the ground, just inches from my foot. Someone had obviously found it in their possession as they waited, and discreetly bailed it.

I did exactly what everyone in front of me had done. I pretended that I hadn't noticed it. To my shock and absolute horror, however, the elder of my female companions made to pick it up, presumably to offer it around, and to find who might have dropped it.

The scene raced in my mind. This was almost directly in front of a customs officer, security cameras were clearly rolling, and the woman with me was about to take possession of ecstasy, in Bangkok!

"*Stop!*" I squealed.

"*Mum!*" the daughter gasped. "*Don't even think about it!*"

Fortunately, she did indeed stop in her tracks, and I was able to explain the folly of trying to be helpful in this particular situation. I believe that it went along the lines of "*Aargh! Do you want to spend the next 20 years here, it's a ****** drug!*"

I suspect that one of my nine-lives was being traded, right there. The moral of the story is never to pick up a brightly coloured sweetie in an airport.

2.7.5 MEAI

Common Nomenclature	5-Methoxy-2-indanamine
Street & Reference Names	Chaperon
Reference Dosage	N/A
Anticipated: Onset / Duration	2 hours / 4 Hours
Maximum Dose Experienced	25mg+15mg+15mg
Form	Powder
RoA	Oral
Source / Jurisdiction	Internet / UK
Personal Rating On Shulgin Scale	+

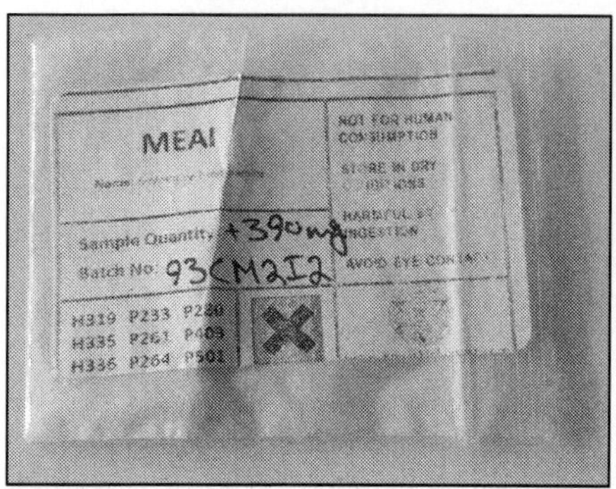

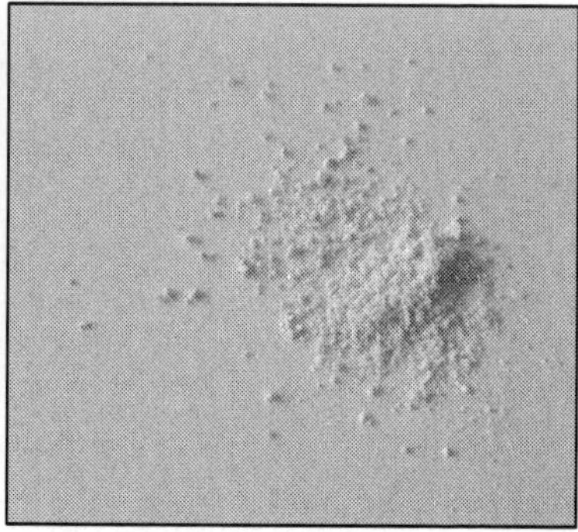

SUBJECTIVE EXPERIENCE
The development of MEAI was greeted by the unprecedented: positive reports by the mainstream media. Even the most insidious of propagandists, the Daily Mail, refrained from its usual hysteria, with a report under the banner headline "*Could a legal high that mimics ecstasy stop people from boozing? Party drug is patented for use as "binge mitigation agent*". The more credible New Scientist led with "*Could a legal high that mimics ecstasy stop people from boozing? Party drug is patented for use as "binge mitigation agent*".

MEAI was reputedly designed by the inventor of mephedrone, Dr Zee, and donated to Professor David Nutt's charitable research group *DrugScience*. However, the chemical itself didn't find its way to the clearnet for over a year. Strangely, when it did, despite this free publicity, the uptake was muted.

Trip reports were also extremely thin on the ground. Other than the initial dose-unspecified sorties covered in the above media articles, I could only find a couple of direct first-hand accounts, both of which were posted on the same forum.

The first post specified a dose of 13mg, with an additional 10mg added later. The second report cited 15mg. The threshold dose stated on the vendor's website was 5-8mg.

For my own experiment, I weighed 20mg on my scales, which was possibly 2-3mg more, given my clumsiness. Whilst this was the highest single dose I had ever seen posted, this did appear to be reasonable, given the overall context. Note that I had performed a small allergy test a month or so earlier.

> T+0.00 Bombing it on an empty stomach with water, the taste is a little like MDAI, but not quite as foul. I sit around, tinkering on my PC, and wait. I occasionally stroll around the house. [6pm].
>
> T+0.30 I feel nothing at all, which is expected, given the anticipated 2 hour onset. I put the kettle on and sip on a cup of chamomile tea.
>
> T+1.00 A slight buzz-like haze has developed, but with clarity if I focus. I also feel a degree of contentedness. It is very mild, but it is there.
>
> T+1.30 There is no significant change at this point, other than an increase in intensity. It has a mild drifty feel, but with the ability to sharpen at will. There is also some sort of mellow intoxication emerging. I am content, but hoping for more to happen.
>
> I deliberately think about alcohol. Would I like a beer? Not really, but I didn't want one beforehand, so perhaps this doesn't add much. Could I actually drink a beer? Yes, I believe so.
>
> Is there horn? Is there any particular enhancement or additional libido or drive? There could be something minimal, but it's not manic by any means. However, unlike with alcohol use, I would be functional.
>
> T+2.00 The effects appear to have become more established. I note that I have dilated pupils, although not full saucers. Simultaneously, I feel like I am on a plateau and that this will go no further.
>
> I feel a little intoxicated, and as the online reports mentioned, if I thought of this from a certain perspective I could describe it as being slightly drunk, but without being groggy. In other words, a mild inebriation, with clarity, and no urge to act like an ego-inflated jerk. There is not really any euphoria, but there is a head buzz and a little sedation.
>
> Would this stop me drinking if I had a nice pint of beer in front of me, as suggested by the media? Not at this point.
>
> Would I drink a pint of fluid instead of beer, if it contained MEAI and tasted pleasant? Yes, I probably would.

I am hungry, which has nothing to do with the MEAI: I haven't eaten since lunch time. However, this chemical clearly doesn't suppress appetite, as many stimulants do. The food itself tastes normal.

This is not unpleasant, but it is not particularly thrilling either. Quite nice is probably a good way of putting it. There's psychoactivity there, via a hazy high and other mild symptoms, but there is no significant oomph. I feel content and what could probably be termed *slightly merry* in an alcohol context (but with less fuzz and more clarity).

I'm quite capable of holding a conversation in an unimpaired manner. I am also capable of precise and rational thought, and performing non-trivial tasks, but at the same time I feel that I am under the influence. In a social setting this could provide the basis for positive interaction and relaxation.

T+3.00 The show now seems to be over, in that I am settling back to base. There is nothing negative to report. I still feel well and relatively positive, but the buzz is dissipating.

This was a decent sojourn, with some parallels to alcohol, but with the worst elements missing. This makes it fairly mild and gentle, but not particularly exciting, at least at this dose. However, I do like its short acting nature, which presumably could be extended by redosing.

It could be argued that these effects lie somewhere between MDAI and alcohol.

A social setting may well provide its niche, as apparently targeted. Bear in mind that for my experiment I was sat at a PC and moving around a house, which wasn't going to light any fires. It would be interesting to learn what it is like when used outdoors, or in company (either with soberistas or alcohol drinkers).

Would I use it again? Yes. I might well explore in the latter scenario, or increase the dose (although this remains tricky to gauge, as no-one else seems to be using it).

A FEW MONTHS LATER: EXPERIMENT #2
A dose of 55mg over several hours was not noticeably different to the above. Indeed, possibly due to other factors, the effects were less pronounced, and a minor feeling of malaise was felt. These could easily have been coincidental.

Whilst I dropped off fairly easily, the night's sleep was a little disturbed, which again, could have nothing at all to do with the substance. I awoke feeling absolutely normal.

On the basis of the above experiences, I suspect that had this been released by one of the bigger vendors, and a year or so before the generic UK ban took effect, it may well have flown. Equally, like MDAI, it may have become an ingredient of a head shop or online blend.

2.7.6 Mephedrone

Common Nomenclature	4-MMC; 4-Methyl methcathinone
Street & Reference Names	Mcat; Mkat; Meow Meow; Drone; Bubbles
Reference Dosage	ORAL Threshold 15mg+; Light 50mg+; Common 100mg+; Strong 150mg+ [Erowid] Light 50mg+; Common 100mg+; Strong 150mg+; Heavy 300mg+ [TripSit] FirstTime 100mg+; Average 150mg+; Strong 250mg [Drugs-Forum] INSUFFLATED Threshold 5mg+; Light 15mg+; Common 20mg+; Strong 75mg+ [Erowid] Light 15mg+; Common 20mg+; Strong 75mg+; Heavy 125mg+ [TripSit]
Anticipated: Onset / Duration	30 Minutes / 4 Hours
Maximum Dose Experienced	250mg
Form	Crystal Powder
RoA	Oral, Insufflated
Source / Jurisdiction	Dealer / Overseas

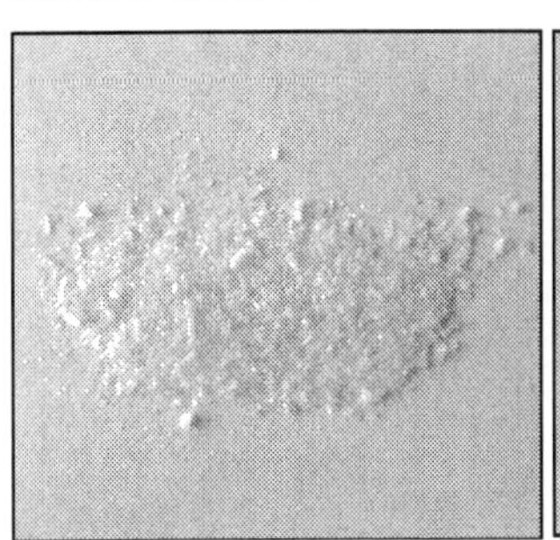

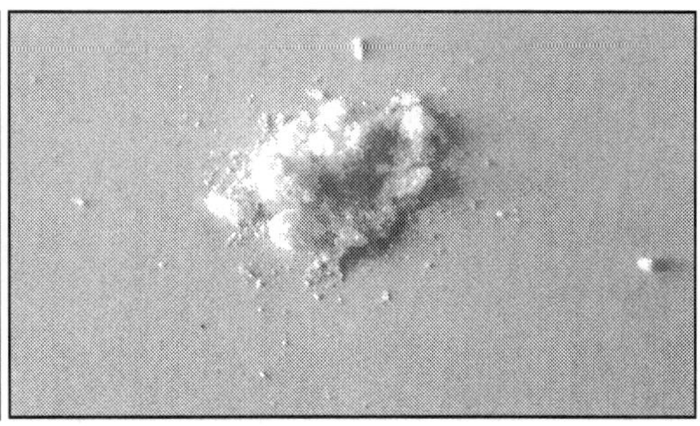

SUBJECTIVE EXPERIENCE
First synthesised in 1929, mephedrone was rediscovered in 2003 (credited to Dr Zee). It became extremely popular from 2008, and indeed, at one point surveys suggested that it ranked alongside MDMA in terms of number of UK users.

This situation was greeted by a lengthy period of media hysteria, inclusive of flagrant exaggeration and outright propaganda, which even extended to deaths being falsely attributed to it. Inevitably it was soon classified in the UK (2010) and scheduled in the United States (2012).

Online, Erowid describes it as "*a stimulant with empathogenic qualities*", whilst TripSit refers to it as "*a short lived euphoric stimulant*". Drugs-forum.com offers this sensible suggestion

> "*Insufflating mephedrone can dramatically increase the urge to redose, therefore it is important users set out a maximum amount for the night and stick to it*".

This is advice which I will certainly heed.

I measure approx 150mg (156mg on the scale) and divide this into doses of 75mg, 25mg, 25mg and 25mg. I measure another 100mg for the scenario in which I wish to explore further. My absolute upper limit is therefore 250mg. I throw the rest away.

Insufflation is the most popular RoA. However, I elect to experiment initially via the oral route, and then subsequently snort a few lines. This approach does appear to be fairly common, particularly for lengthy sessions.

> T+0:00 I wrap the 75mg in cigarette paper and bomb it with water. [2:50pm]
>
> T+0:15 Other than the occasional shiver there has been no response to this point.
>
> T+0:30 I perceive an increase in body temperature, and perhaps there is a minor heady feeling. These early signs, which indicate a slow-burning onset, are enough for me to hold off with the insufflation plan.
>
> T+0:45 I now feel somewhat elevated and relaxed. There is a nice mild buzz to this: a certain high and uplift of mood. There are no rough edges or body load apparent so far, and this is certainly manageable. My pupils are half dilated and I am comfortably warm, apart from my hands, which are cool and clammy.
>
> This is a nice level, although a little higher might be even better. I'll see where this goes during the next 15 minutes and then take a further decision regarding the redosing.
>
> T+0:55 I check my blood pressure for no reason other than curiosity. It is 175/89 with a BPM of 65. Whilst I brush this aside under the influence, I do realise that it is of concern.
>
> T+1:00 An hour into the experience, I believe that the onset is complete. This is quite a happy level, and it isn't too intense. I am feeling stimulation, euphoria and some empathogenic edge, which are all very pleasant.
>
> Horn is available in terms of interest, but there is no amphetamine type hunger or compulsion. There does appear to be some drive enhancement, so I fully understand those users who articulate this aspect, although stim-dick seems to be a factor too (but not to the point of total dysfunctionality).

I am looking forward to the insufflation, as an increase in intensity would surely be enjoyable, but at the same time, online warnings that the snort is painful are fresh in my mind.

T+1:10 I bite the bullet and rail 25mg. This takes me to 100mg, 75mg of which was ingested orally. The snort wasn't at all bad, and certainly nothing like as painful as some users suggested.

T+1:25 Surprisingly, there was no instant rush. Perhaps there has been a minor increase in intensity, but this seems to have crept up slowly rather than appearing suddenly.

I am as high as I have been, probably a little higher, but it has been a gentle incline throughout.

T+1:50 I am subjectively in a similar place to an hour ago, but with a greater sense of depth. My blood pressure is now 162/98 and my BPM is 69.

T+1:55 I snort the next 25mg. As this is proving to be extremely smooth and enjoyable, I also prepare the 100mg which I had put aside for a potential extension.

T+2:00 I insufflate the final 25mg of the primary batch. My total consumption is now 75mg oral and 75mg insufflated, which is well into *common* territory according to the harm reduction websites.

Within a couple of minutes this latest hit has elevated the high and noticeably increased its intensity. This is undoubtedly what is referred to as the rush. It has the same feel as earlier but is significantly headier in nature.

I am now flying high. It would appear that 150mg, at least of this particular sample, is my take-off threshold. This is consistent with a significant number of forum reports.

I would suggest that this is closer to MDMA than amphetamine. It is smoother and less physical than the latter, but not really as empathogenic as the former.

T+2:20 I am still at the new high, very warm (physically), and in a very contented and comfortable bubble.

It occurs to me that this would beat alcohol hands down if I was socialising. It has the feel of a drug to share with friends, although I am quite happy regardless.

T+2:30 I can understand how the desire to stay at this level leads to compulsive redosing, particularly as the duration is presented as short. Coming-down will be a drag. This is a danger of course, but it doesn't feel like it whilst actually engaging.

T+2:40 There is some jaw tension now along with the urge to grind (resisted).

Although I am higher my pupils seem to be less dilated than earlier, which I find to be curious.

T+2:50 I insufflate the first 25mg of the 100mg reserve.

I feel that I now have a better understanding of this drug. There is indeed a rush, like an influx of euphoria, which is extremely rewarding. There is real temptation to chase it, again and again, as per the various reports and warnings.

It is very easy to see how users got through multiple grams of this over a weekend binge session when it was at the height of its popularity.

T+3:10 The second line of the 100mg reserve is fiendishly insufflated. The grand total has reached 200mg.

I am as high as the proverbial kite.

I check my pupils again: they are now more dilated than at any point previously.

T+4:20 The third line of the 100mg reserve is gleefully snorted, and 15 minutes later the final 25mg is hoovered.

T+5:20 I am still rolling, but not as intensely. This is slowly winding down.

T+5:40 I am gently returning to base. I feel no hangover or ill effects so far, and the urge to redose has dissipated. This is certainly one of the shortest acting chemicals of this class, which of course can be a positive attribute for some social occasions.

T+7:00 The show is almost completely over. There are some residue effects in play, including a little stimulation, but simultaneously I am becoming weary. My pupils are back to their normal size.

Following this adventure, I slept reasonably well, and there was no hangover in the morning. This was an entirely different aftermath to those I had endured with amphetamine and MDMA.

This was a very enjoyable experience, and one which confirmed the reputation of mephedrone for short term effect and the temptation to sustain the euphoric high via compulsive redosing. I suspect that this would be harder to resist in a more recreational environment, which in turn may have led to a less gentle landing. I would therefore re-emphasize the need to set a maximum dose in advance. It is probably also wise to stress the need for caution in terms of mixing this with other drugs, and of course, don't skip the usual safety measures (Section 1.1).

2.7.7 Methylone

Common Nomenclature	3,4-methylenedioxy-N-methylcathinone
Street & Reference Names	MDMC; βk-MDMA; M1; Ease; Explosion
Reference Dosage	Threshold 60mg+; Light 100mg+; Common 100mg+; Strong 160mg+; Very Strong 250mg+ [Drugs-Forum] Light 100mg+; Common 150mg+; Strong 200mg+; Heavy 300mg+ [TripSit]
Anticipated: Onset / Duration	30 Minutes / 3 Hours
Maximum Dose Experienced	130mg+45mg
Form	Powder
RoA	Oral
Source / Jurisdiction	Dealer / Overseas

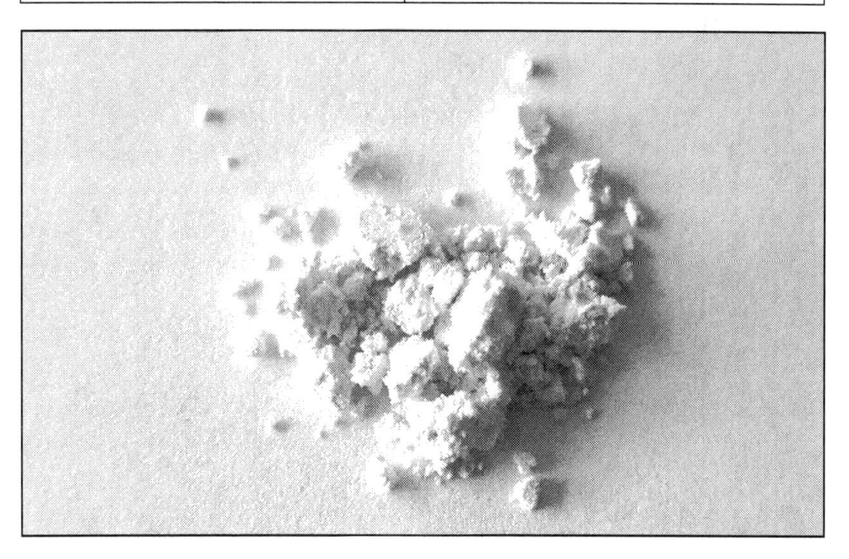

SUBJECTIVE EXPERIENCE
Methylone was first synthesised in the mid 1990's by Peyton Jacob III and Alexander Shulgin. Under the name *explosion* and various others it was to emerge as a popular recreational drug a decade later.

Whilst it was legally available, methylone was often mis-sold as MDMA, although it is widely suggested to be less empathogenic and more stimulating. Certainly, it produces a shorter experience.

It was classified in the UK in 2010 and scheduled in the US in 2011.

As Erowid cited reports of "*worrying heart rate and blood pressure increases*" as well as chest pains at higher doses, I elected to go low. This decision was re-enforced by the relative scarcity of dosage information, and in some cases, its ambiguity.

Note that I had allergy tested with approximately 5mg some weeks earlier.

> T+0:00 175mg of the clumpy white powder is carefully measured. 130mg is bombed in cigarette paper with a glass of water. [16:50]
>
> The remaining 45mg is held back for a potential redose, to be taken should events proceed along a steady and enjoyable path.
>
> T+0:15 There are familiar signs that something is afoot, with my hands feeling slightly cold and clammy.
>
> T+0:20 A headspace is starting to emerge. There is a general drifting feeling, which is fairly neutral but not unpleasant.
>
> T+0:30 I am now unmistakably under the influence. My head has a nice buzz about it, and I feel slightly uplifted, albeit not enormously so. My hands are still a little clammy but I feel increasingly content.
>
> T+0:40 I feel quite ramped up, and indeed high, although I am fully functional and lucid if I need to be.
>
> The vibe is quite pleasing and I feel a general warmth, and certainly, the mood lift is very evident.
>
> I do feel slight chest trembles but nothing alarming at this stage.
>
> T+0:50 The experience seems to have settled on to a plateau of general well being with a dreamy stimulation in play. The word to describe it is probably *nice*, given that it is not overly exhilarating or exciting.
>
> T+1:00 I can see why there are comparisons with MDMA, as it does have a mild empathogenic feel, and it would probably come into its own in a social situation, particularly amongst other users.
>
> I consume the remaining 45mg, taking the total dose to the pre-determined 175mg.This is well into the *common* range according to the harm reduction websites, edging towards strong.
>
> Given the health warnings referred to earlier, this will be sufficient. I have no intention of diverting from my original plan.

T+1:20 There has been no significant change for the last half hour, and I remain in a place of relative contentment. I still feel warm, and of a generally positive disposition, with the semi-euphoric buzz remaining steady.

The minor chest discomfort, which I experienced earlier, has now faded.

T+1:45 There is now slightly more intensity to the headspace, which is presumably due to the extra 45mg kicking in.

All other aspects remain at the same or similar levels.

There is no compulsive horn, but no stim-dick either.

I check my pupils and they remain relatively normal. My blood pressure and pulse are elevated at a worrying 183/94 and 69 respectively.

T+2:15 I believe that the experience is now at a lower level of intensity than it was earlier. I am still enjoying the serenity of the high, which is pleasant and fairly gentle in nature.

T+3:00 I am now drifting back to baseline. The headspace is dissipating slowly but surely, and the body warmth is fading.

T+3:15 I drink some fruit juice, have something to eat, and I am more or less back to base.

In line with expectations, this was a fairly gentle ride. Whilst the comparisons with MDMA are hard to escape, it was much shorter acting, and as suggested in advance, there was more stimulation and a clearer uplift.

It hinted at going further, but given the dose restraint, it remained within sensible parameters. It was positive and pleasing throughout.

The following morning I had a slight headache, and for a couple of days I was aware that I was still experiencing the aftermath. To some degree sleep was also interrupted, with a not too pleasant headiness evident when I awoke. These symptoms occurred despite the usual self-practiced aftercare, such as exercise, vitamin pills, plenty of healthy food, and so forth.

Having stated all this, these ailments were not on the scale of a heavy MDMA come-down, but they did linger.

Although this was a good experience, one or two worrying signs were clearly evident. The body load and the potential risks should not be dismissed lightly.

Tread carefully if you intend to use this.

2.7.8 MNA

Common Nomenclature	Methamnetamine
Street & Reference Names	PAL-1046; MNT
Reference Dosage	Light 60mg+; Common 80mg+; Strong 120mg+; Heavy 150mg+ [TripSit]
Anticipated: Onset / Duration	45 Minutes / 5 Hours
Maximum Dose Experienced	120mg
Form	Powder
RoA	Oral
Source / Jurisdiction	Internet / UK
Personal Rating On Shulgin Scale	+

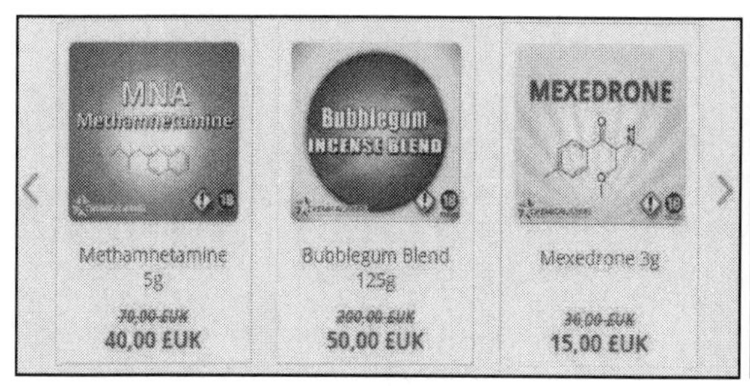

SUBJECTIVE EXPERIENCE
Methamnetamine first appeared at the start of 2015, being offered by a couple of online vendors. Whilst it never gained significant popularity, it remained available in the UK until the passing the *Psychoactive Substances Act* in May 2016.

The following forum post, which comprises both a live element and a subsequent review, was written shortly after its launch:

> I ate a light breakfast mid-morning, got some jobs out of the way, cleared my desk, and began the adventure.
>
> I set an absolute maximum dose of 120mg, separating it from my 500mg bag. This should be more than sufficient to hit the mark, or at least pass threshold, judging from earlier reports.
>
>> T+0:00 Starting cautiously, I orally consume 50mg. It has the usual sort of chemical taste: absolutely horrible, but just about tolerable. [11:50am]

T+00:30 There is no effect to report so far. Waiting impatiently, I sip on a cup of herbal tea.

T+00:40 Still nothing.

I wonder about dose. From reviewing the earlier field reports it does sound like 80mg may be a common threshold point, so I swallow another 30mg.

Somehow the taste is even worse than it was the first time.

T+01:00 I may be registering the slightest of effects at this point, but this is possibly placebo driven. Are colours more distinct, or is that because I want them to be? Is my head and mood nicely at ease?

It all appears to be marginal, so I continue to wait for a solid journey to begin.

I toy with the idea of taking the last 40mg of the 120mg I set aside. I resist, deciding to wait another 15 minutes or so.

T+01:15 I do feel quite content, but it is a very mild form of contentment. I consume the final 40mg.

T+02:45 I feel comfortable, dreamy and chilled. Indeed, the last hour seems to have disappeared without being noticed. It drifted past.

At this point I perform some basic checks.

Is there horn? It is available but there is no real drive. On the other side of the coin, there is no stim-dick.

Is appetite suppressed? No.

T+03:10 I head for bed to take my afternoon nap, wondering if the stim property of this chemical will thwart this plan.

T+04:10 I slept quite well. There appears, therefore, to be little or no stimulation in play.

Interestingly, and unexpectedly, I noticed some extremely mild CEVs whilst lying on the bed. They were nothing to write home about, but they were there

I think that much of this experience was influenced by expectation. This is perhaps very mildly psychedelic, but it isn't a psychedelic. Neither is it a stimulant. I didn't feel any great empathy at this level either.

So what is it?

If it is approached with the expectation of stimulation, it will produce disappointment. Ditto if a psychedelic ride is anticipated.

Sedating? Relaxing? Euphoric? For me, perhaps a tiny bit of all of these, at least on this dose. I felt well enough: mildly happy, with a dreamy headspace in the background and the tiniest hint of psychedelia.

For someone with little or no experience in this field, I suspect that it could induce a significant and enjoyable response.

I certainly couldn't claim that I didn't like it, as it was pleasant, and it could have a place for functional or semi-functional chilling and relaxation.

I can also see why some people have suggested combining it with a little MPA or similar chemical, and it would be interesting to read any reports for higher doses.

One final aspect relates to the potential sedation. I note the following comments on the UKRC forum:

> *"150mg bombed around 2:30pm. Immediately felt surprisingly tired, but a little ethylphenidate sorted that out."*
>
> *"Feeling tired all of a sudden."*

I also note that those members who did not comment on this aspect tended to experiment during the early evening, shortly prior to normal sleep. I, of course, had a nap half-way through.

Statistically, this is obviously insufficient to prove anything. However, at this early stage it is worth bearing in mind.

I certainly felt more than the usual fatigue after my experience and a little flat the following day. Either or both could be unconnected, but I look forward to more contributions to the data pool.

Overall, this seemed to be a fairly mild and pleasant MDAI-type chemical, with some interesting edges, but which never really took off. These were clearly discernable at times, however.

I would have explored this further, but with the all embracing PSA coming into force the following year, further opportunities to sample it didn't materialize.

[Note: The image above (left) is a partial screenshot as taken from the website of popular vendor Chemical Wire, circa 2016.]

2.7.9 Mexedrone

Common Nomenclature	Mexedrone
Street & Reference Names	N/A
Reference Dosage	Light 50mg+; Common 80mg+; Strong 120mg+ [Insufflated, TripSit] Threshold 50mg+ Light 100mg+; Common 150mg+; Strong 250mg+ [Oral, Psychonautwiki]
Anticipated: Onset / Duration	5 Minutes / 3 Hours
Maximum Dose Experienced	50mg+ 100mg+ 100mg+ 100mg
Form	Powder
RoA	Insufflated
Source / Jurisdiction	Internet / UK
Personal Rating On Shulgin Scale	+

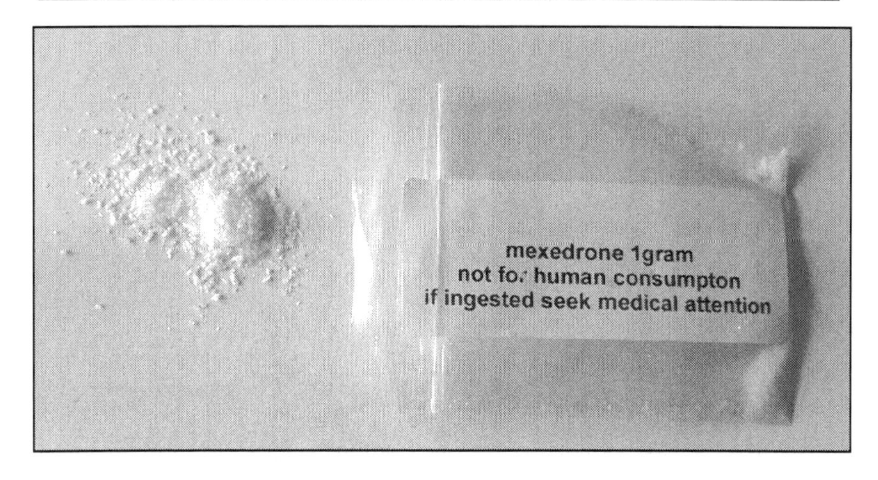

SUBJECTIVE EXPERIENCE
Mexedrone's release in 2015 was accompanied by a sustained period of Internet generated hype. This included the suggestion of close association with mephedrone, with domain names even being registered along these lines (e.g. mcat2.com). Market expectation was therefore extremely high.

However, it was to prove to be disappointing, with only mild effects, and for many, none whatsoever.

The following is a compressed version of my own trip report from that time, as posted on a popular forum:

A joy of a short acting RC is that it can be experienced during a smaller window of opportunity. Courtesy of a sample generously provided by a well known vendor, I was able to perform such a test yesterday afternoon.

My chosen RoA was not my usual preference, which is oral. I insufflated simply because I had eaten a heavy lunch, which I felt might dilute the effect of the drug.

> T+0.00 I crush the crystals and insufflate 50mg to establish the broad headspace and the feel of the experience.
>
> T+0.05 I sense my mood being gently elevated. There is no stimulation at this point, just a barely perceptible shift towards positivity.
>
> T+0.30. As the same sort of mild background feeling has persisted for the best part of half an hour, I insufflate a further 100mg.
>
> T+1.00 The warm positive feel has returned but it is a little stronger. It is quite nice, which is perhaps the best description I can find. There is a minor mood enhancement and a warm pleasant feeling compared to base.

I insufflated a couple more 100mg lines during the course of the afternoon, bringing the grand total to 350mg. There was no major urge to redose, but I chose to push a little further out of curiosity. The effects tapered off during the evening.

At these levels this won't blow your socks off. It isn't stimulating and doesn't lift you to the clouds. I do not say this negatively, just factually. The biggest problem this chemical faces is going to be expectation, due to its marketing alignment with 4-MMC. Further, it just isn't very strong.

I can see why some people suggest similarity to MDAI, but I found it to subtly different, with a little more clarity of mind, and significantly less empathy.

I liked the short duration: for my current lifestyle, writing off a full day, and potentially a night's sleep, is difficult. For recreation, this can be slipped in for just a few hours, and is totally functional in social situations.

Contrary to my expectation, the night's sleep was not the best, and this morning I could still feel that I had recently consumed a chemical. This wasn't terrible, but it was noticeable. Perhaps there was some (latent) stimulation in this after all.

Mexedrone was one of those releases which attracted undue positivity; partly because it was legally and easily available, and partly due to the hype. It wasn't even close to being a mephedrone replacement, and its mild effects were such that I would seriously question its value in terms of a risk/benefit (much of the risk being that it was a new untested chemical). It certainly isn't one which I would ever use again.

2.8. CANNABINOIDS

Textbook Definition: *Cannabinoids are synthetic substances that act upon cannabinoid receptors, creating effects which can be perceived as similar to the cannabis genus in one or more respects.*

The following chemicals have been sampled and researched for inclusion within this section:

2.8.1 5F-AKB48
2.8.2 AM-2201
2.8.3 AM-694
2.8.4 JWH-018
2.8.5 JWH-073

Note that in December 2016 all commonly used synthetic cannabinoids were classified in the UK under the Misuse of Drugs Act, thus making possession a criminal offence.

The definition printed above isn't the usual single sentence description that is presented across the media, and frequently online. I have chosen those words particularly carefully.

More common and less precise forms imply that these chemicals closely mimic or replicate cannabis, often using the term "*synthetic marijuana*", or similar. This is extremely misleading. Under influence, some aspects of the cannabis experience are present, with emphasis on *some*, but the overall effect is distinctly removed.

The picture on the ground, the real situation, is far more complex than is often understood. It is steeped in the social and political history of cannabinoids as a whole, and has been sculpted largely via legislation. Indeed, this class of drug would never have emerged had cannabis been legally available.

My own first port of call was JWH-018. This was procured from head shops, was sealed in bright glossy packets, and was marketed under the original *Spice* brand. The smoke itself wasn't too bad in most respects, and inhaling material that smelled like flowers and tasted scented was novel. It seemed harmless enough.

The effects; yes, they were cannabis-like, but with facets missing, and significantly, there was a rougher edge to proceedings. There was also an artificial type aura to it, which was subtle, but present.

When this fell foul of legislation, other chemicals emerged. These tended to be harsher. Perhaps stating that they were one-step removed from JWH-018, and several steps further from cannabis, is a reasonable way of describing them.

As this cycle of creeping legislation continued, the cannabinoids became stronger and stronger, and further and further removed from the real deal. Many of them eventually became highly addictive and dangerous.

Simultaneously, hidden dose fluctuations often occurred due to the irregular concentration of the chemicals on the smoking materials they had been sprayed upon. This was another contributory factor to the significant increase in the number of overdoses and fatalities.

In terms of personal research, despite what I considered to be due diligence at the time, I nonetheless endured a couple of harrowing experiences. Following the second, I stopped researching this class of chemical completely and permanently.

I will make my advice with respect to synthetic cannabinoids as clear and unambiguous as I can: stay away from them.

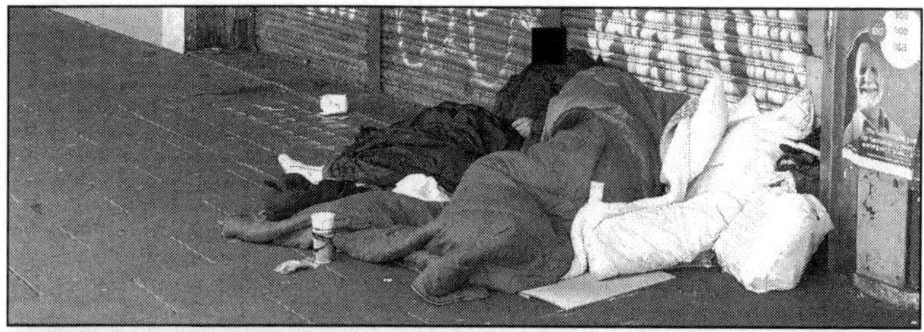

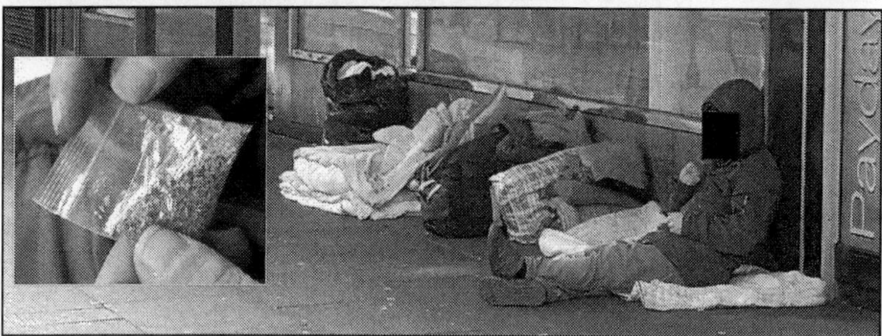

Shortly after legislation forced the sale of cannabinoids underground, an epidemic of addiction took hold amongst the homeless in the UK. The photographs above were amongst a set taken by the author in the centre of Manchester. An interview was attempted for the purposes of this book, but the desperate and unfortunate user was barely able to talk. He was living a hell.
A few days earlier, the local newspaper, quoting the charity *Lifeshare*, had stated that "*95 per cent of young homeless people are on Spice*" and cited 26 related ambulance calls in a single day. Meanwhile, in Westminsiter, politicians were preening over their latest successes in hardening their *war on drugs*. Their allies in the media continued to blame and besmirch the broken victims.

A civilised society would be helping these tortured souls, not punishing them.

2.8.1 5F-AKB48

Common Nomenclature	5F-APINACA
Street & Reference Names	Magic Dragon
Reference Dosage	Threshold <0.5mg; Light 0.5mg+; Common1mg+; Strong 2mg+; Heavy 4mg+ [Psychonautwiki]
Anticipated: Onset / Duration	20 Seconds / 2 Hours
Maximum Dose Experienced	Unknown
Form	Smoking Mixture
RoA	Smoked
Source / Jurisdiction	Head Shop / UK

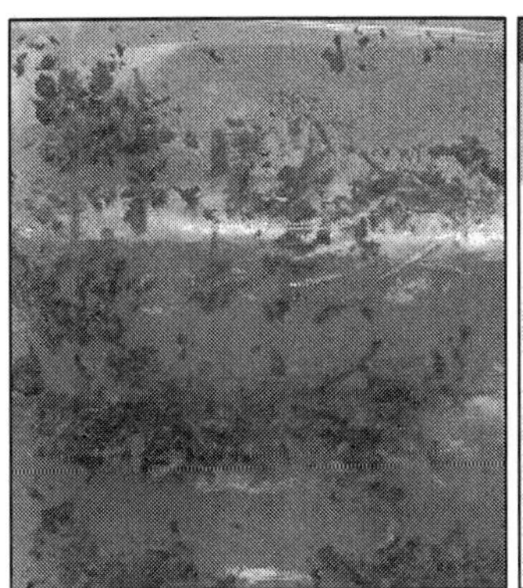

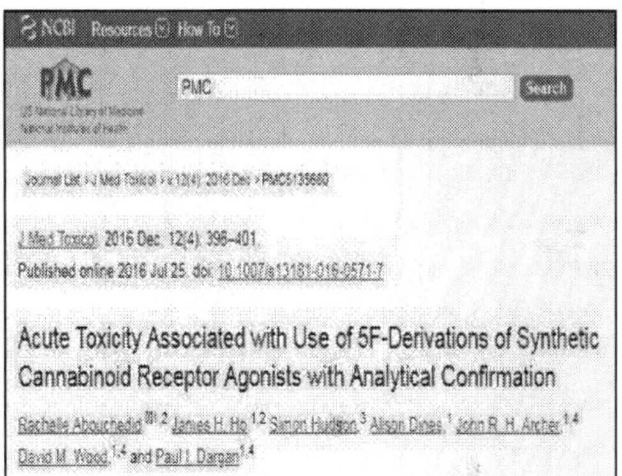

NCBI Resources How To

PMC

J Med Toxicol. 2016 Dec; 12(4): 396–401.
Published online 2016 Jul 25. doi: 10.1007/s13181-016-0571-7

Acute Toxicity Associated with Use of 5F-Derivations of Synthetic Cannabinoid Receptor Agonists with Analytical Confirmation

Rachelle Abouchedid, James H. Ho, Simon Hudson, Alison Dines, John R. H. Archer, David M. Wood, and Paul I. Dargan

SUBJECTIVE EXPERIENCE
As with all the compounds in this class, I purchased this under a brand name; on this occasion, *Magic Dragon*. The plant material it was infused with was much the same as every other brand I had encountered.

To say that this induced a bad experience dramatically understates it. To reflect this, and to urge caution, I posted the following words on an Internet forum at the time:

> I'm firmly in the *must-avoid* camp on this one.
>
> Acute anxiety, extreme fear, sheer panic?
>
> Whatever words are chosen to describe my distress, 5F-AKB48 produced the worst cannabinoid experience of my life, and possibly the worst drug related experience.

> Fortunately, I wasn't in a social situation and I managed to stumble upstairs to lie down. After perhaps an hour the horror eventually passed. It was at that point that I decided that synthetic cannabinoid brands and blends were off my menu for ever.
>
> In the past, cannabinoids like CP47 and JWH-018 had occasionally caused a degree of unpleasantness and discomfort, usually in the form of stress or anxiety. However, they were never like this. They were neither on the same scale nor even in the same ballpark.
>
> I should also stress that this trauma unfolded from just a couple of hits, rather than repeated deep inhalation. There was nothing abnormal about my usage.
>
> Take it easy and take the utmost care.
>
> Better still, don't take it at all.

There is no doubt in my mind that this was a lesson never to be forgotten. It induced a combination of gut wrenching dread and unbounded paranoia. In a Shulgin scale +++ state of mind, I fumbled my way into the bedroom and lay on the bed in foetal position.

It really was that bad.

Fortunately, I was still aware that I was under the influence of a drug. This helped a great deal, but it didn't fully mitigate the depth of terror I was embroiled in. I recall repeatedly telling myself that it would end soon, and that I would return to normal; a process which gave me light at the end of the tunnel.

For the inexperienced drug user, or for the uninitiated, I cannot begin to imagine how bad it could get.

I had in fact smoked this material on a couple of previous occasions. Neither of these episodes was particularly pleasant, but they were nothing like as intense as this third and final experience.

I suspect that this was a good example of what can happen when an amateur chemist mixes these types of compound in such a manner that the chemical is unevenly distributed across the material. This was presumably a contributing factor, and on this basis, it could have been worse; much worse.

I wasn't at all surprised to subsequently read media reports of tragic incidents associated with some of the blends which emerged around this chemical. This was many miles removed from even a pretext of being a legal substitute for cannabis itself.

Avoid it, like the plague.

2.8.2 AM-2201

Common Nomenclature	1-(5-fluoropentyl)-3-(1-naphthoyl)indole
Street & Reference Names	Black Mamba
Reference Dosage	Light 250ug+; Moderate 500ug+; Heavy 1mg+ [Drugs-Forum]
Anticipated: Onset / Duration	20 Seconds / 2 Hours
Maximum Dose Experienced	Unknown
Form	Smoking Mixture
RoA	Smoked
Source / Jurisdiction	Head Shop / UK

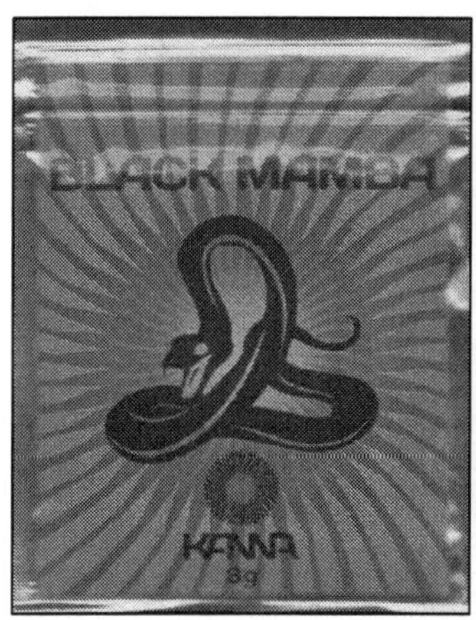

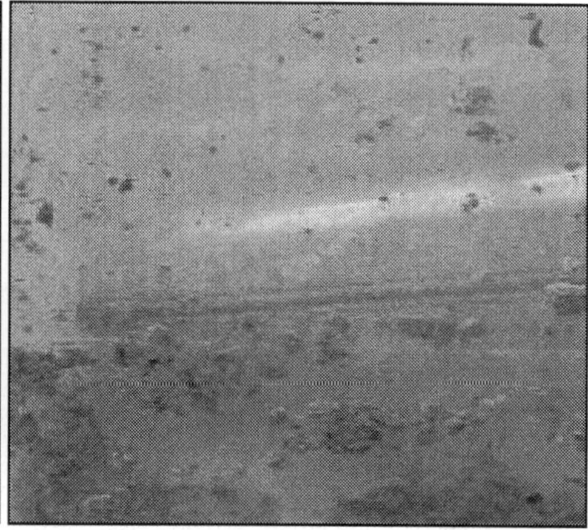

SUBJECTIVE EXPERIENCE

Like spice, the brand name *Black Mamba* was eventually to be misappropriated to become a generic name for all sorts of materials infused with a strong cannabinoid or combinations of strong cannabinoids. Originally, however, it appeared in a green and black glossy packet, infused with just AM-2201.

It was a monster.

In 2014 I posted the following on an Internet forum, as a response to a member who had articulated his own terrible story with the same compound:

> I had a very similar experience with this chemical, which I bought as an incense blend from a head shop. I tested it twice, optimistically and foolishly assuming that the first bad hit was a fluke.

> I felt the sort of anxiety that is possible via certain cannabis strains; but multiplied by a factor of 100. It was almost overwhelming: acute fear and intense paranoia are good words to describe it.
>
> After this second lesson, I flushed the rest of the bag. I still struggle to explain how it took two trips to the abyss to do this.
>
> The other cannabinoid that freaked me out was 5F-AKB48, which was also smoked courtesy of a head-shop procured blend. After the nightmare with that one, that was it: no more synthetic cannabinoids, ever.
>
> The sheer terror I endured with these two is hard to articulate, and I didn't even consume them in vast quantities.

On each occasion, the intensity of the dread eventually subsided, and the experience plateaued into a more regular cannabinoid-type state. Each had been a +++ on the Shulgin scale and an absolutely horrendous ride.

I have in fact held true to my forum comment above: I have not sampled an artificial cannabinoid since that particular day.

Don't even think about trying this one.

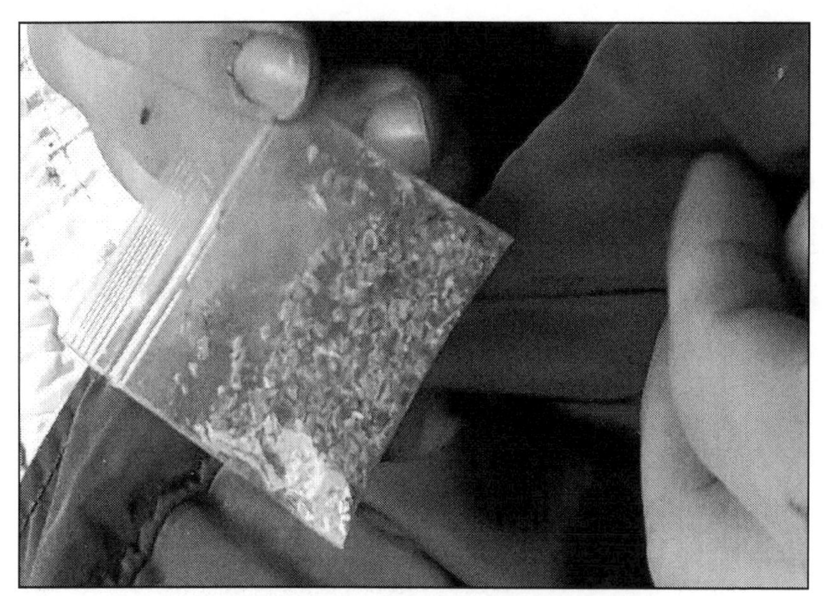

This was one of the cannabinoids which was central to the surge of addiction amongst the homeless in British cities circa 2017

2.8.3 AM-694

Common Nomenclature	1-(5-fluoropentyl)-3-(2-iodobenzoyl)indole
Street & Reference Names	Warrior Ultimate; Pulse Ultra; Shamrock
Reference Dosage	Unknown
Anticipated: Onset / Duration	5 Minutes / 2 Hours
Maximum Dose Experienced	N/A
Form	Smoking Mixture
RoA	Smoked
Source / Jurisdiction	Head Shop / UK

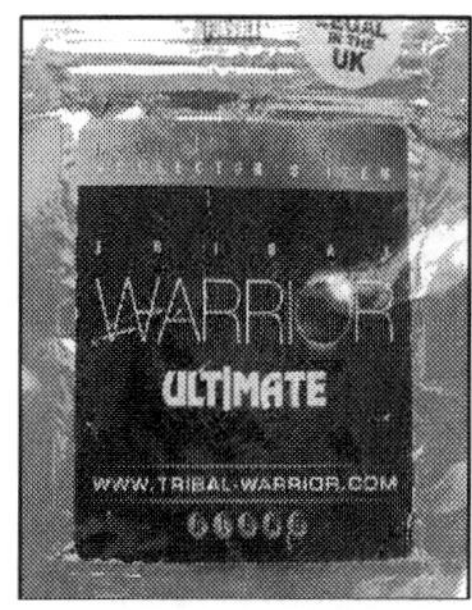

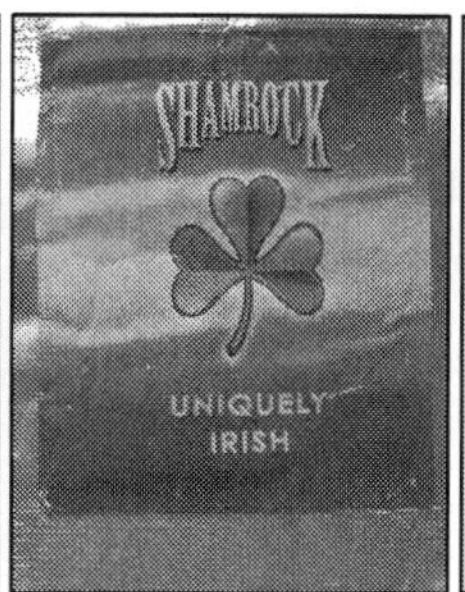

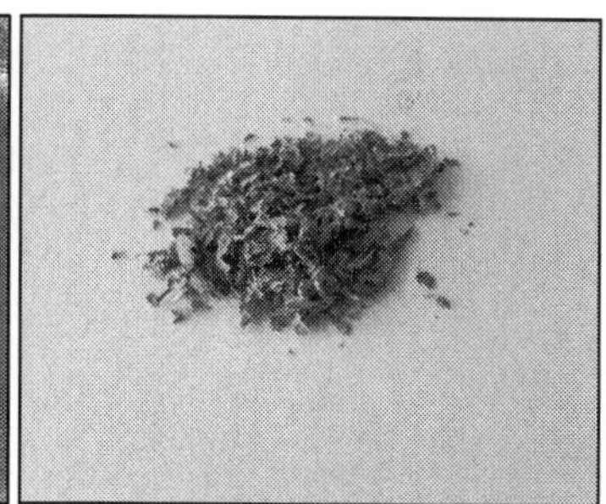

SUBJECTIVE EXPERIENCE
Plant materials infused with AM-694 appeared on the market shortly after the demise of the original spice (typically JWH-018 and JWH-073), circa 2010.

I sampled two such brands, and contrary to the usual flow of synthetic cannabinoid development, which is to create stronger and stronger compounds, I found these to be weaker and more benign.

They were psychoactive, certainly, but there was less of a punch. That isn't to say that they were necessarily inferior, but were instead, less intense on initial consumption.

I should note that I didn't redose with this or any other cannabinoid. My *modus operandi* was to toke the material once and once only, rather than to top-up over a prolonged period.

Finally, some recent reports suggest that AM-694 may metabolise into the highly toxic fluoroacetic acid when consumed orally. This RoA should therefore be strictly avoided.

2.8.4 JWH-018

Common Nomenclature	1-pentyl-3-(1-naphthoyl)indole;
Street & Reference Names	Spice; AM-678
Reference Dosage	Threshold <1mg; Light 1mg+; Common 2mg+; Strong 5mg+; Heavy 5mg+ [Psychonautwiki]
Anticipated: Onset / Duration	30 Seconds / 2 Hours
Maximum Dose Experienced	Unknown
Form	Smoking Mixture
RoA	Smoked
Source / Jurisdiction	Head Shop / UK

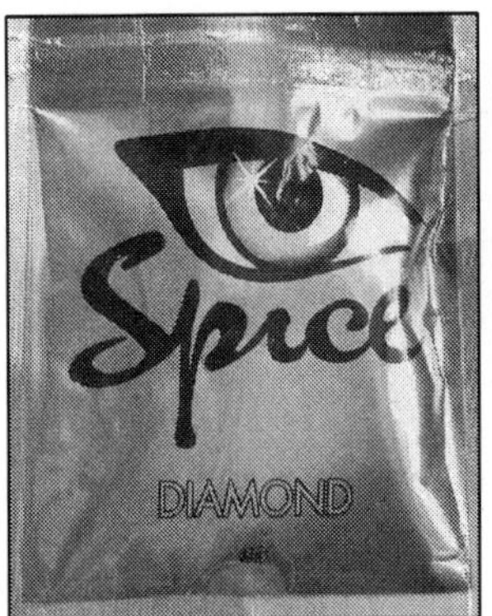

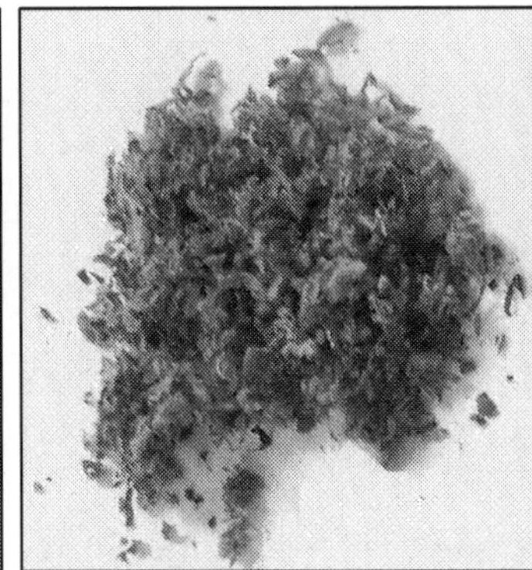
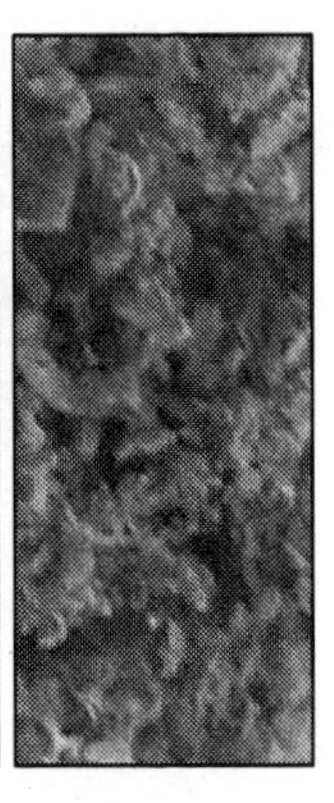

SUBJECTIVE EXPERIENCE
JWH-018 was the first artificial cannabinoid I sampled, and was procured under the original brand name of *Spice*. This was sold under the auspices of potpourri, and marked clearly as *"Not for human consumption"*.

From 2006 onwards, the spice brand became increasingly well known. The manufacturers leveraged this advantage with an entire family of related products: *Spice Gold*, *Spice Arctic Synergy*, *Spice Diamond*, *Spice Tropical Synergy*, and so forth.

The active cannabinoids used also varied. Along with JWH-018, I sampled JWH-073, and I believe, CP-47.

So dominant was this brand that spice was eventually to be used by many as a generic term for all artificial cannabinoids.

At the time, such compounds had a fairly unblemished reputation, with little or no association with the sort of horror stories which would eventually emerge. In relative terms, JWH-018 was also to prove to be one of the less harmful chemicals in this class. That is not to say, of course, that it wasn't corrosive in its own right. It was.

On face value, it was an attractive proposition: a cannabis type experience, via a smokable herb, with a pleasant non-cannabis type odour, making it suitable for consumption in public. Its bright packaging and obvious popularity enhanced the illusion of safety, and I naively consumed far too much of it.

For all the positives, there was always the feeling of artificiality: that this was a chemical and not a natural plant. That feeling was never far away.

In addition, the wealth of subtlety and variation that came with the infinite number of cannabis strains was absent. The experience was fairly standard, at least during those early years.

From my perspective, it was close enough to meeting certain demands, but not engaging enough to become a constant or frequent habit. Unfortunately this did not apply to everyone.

JWH-018 was classified in the UK under the *Misuse of Drugs Act* at the end of 2009, and in the United States during the summer of 2012. What was to replace it, however, was a slippery slope of ever stronger, ever more toxic chemicals, with the inevitable consequences for public safety.

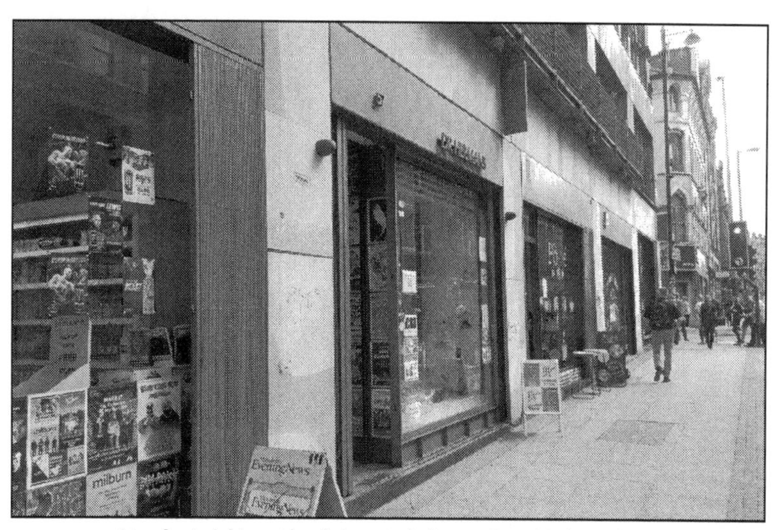

Manchester's biggest head shop stocked a number of *Spice* variants

2.8.5 JWH-073

Common Nomenclature	JWH-073
Street & Reference Names	Spice
Reference Dosage	Light 3mg+; Common 5mg+; Strong 10mg+; Heavy 15mg+ [Psychonautwiki]
Anticipated: Onset / Duration	30 Seconds / 2 Hours
Maximum Dose Experienced	Unknown
Form	Smoking Mixture
RoA	Smoked
Source / Jurisdiction	Head Shop / UK

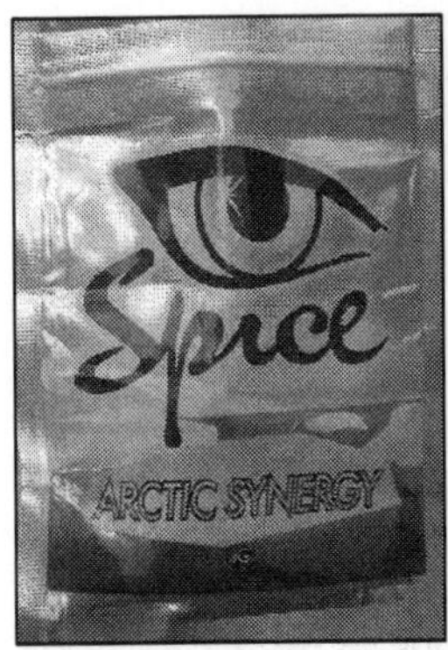

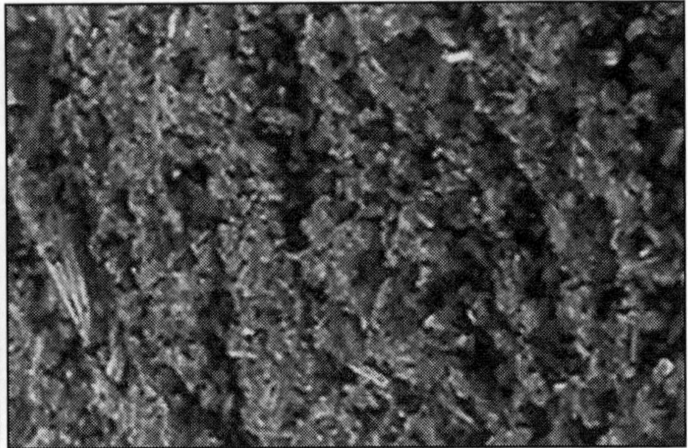

SUBJECTIVE EXPERIENCE
This was launched under the authentic *Spice* brand, and as far as I can recall, was the first variation from JWH-018 in the original series. As a novice, the difference between them was difficult to establish.

Again, certain elements of the experience were cannabis-like, but only to a limited extent. Some aspects were absent, and others were somewhat distorted. However, at the time it offered a decent enough experience to repeatedly engage.

On the face of it, this chemical seemed to have a similar safety profile to its earlier cousin. Given what was eventually to emerge in terms of synthetic cannabinoids, this was probably a positive.

The spice brand itself disappeared not far down the track, before most of the stronger cannabinoids became available under a huge variety of different labels and names. Its legacy, however, including the misappropriation of its name, remained.

2.9. NOOTROPICS

Textbook Definition: *Also referred to as smart drugs, nootropics are substances that improve or enhance cognitive function, including memory and creativity.*

The following chemicals have been sampled and researched for inclusion within this section:

2.9.1 Aniracetam + Citicoline
2.9.2 Armodafinil
2.9.3 L-Theanine
2.9.4 Modafiendz
2.9.5 Noopept
2.9.6 NSI 189
2.9.7 Phenibut
2.9.8 Picamilon
2.9.9 PRL-8-53

It wasn't just scepticism that caused me to tread slowly and carefully with this class of chemical. It was the fact that most of the users I encountered online ingested a cocktail of these drugs everyday. In nootropic lingo such a combination is known as a *stack.*

My hesitancy wasn't only driven by the fear of addiction, but by the very idea of putting a relatively untested chemical into my body with regular frequency and habit. The potential rewards never appeared to balance the risks.

Instead, my approach was one which is possibly blasphemous to aficionados: to take an average to strong dose once. Possibly, if sufficient evidence or large scale use indicated relative safety, I might indulge twice or more, albeit on one single day.

Thereafter I waited and hoped for some sort of effect; a suggestion of enhanced memory, an example of improved mental sharpness, enhanced focus or concentration, or some similar manifestation.

Usually, I was to be disappointed. However, on occasion, there was indeed some detectable psychoactivity, hence the presence of this section in this book.

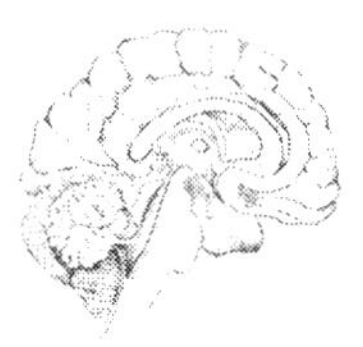
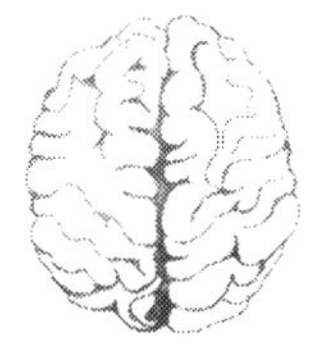
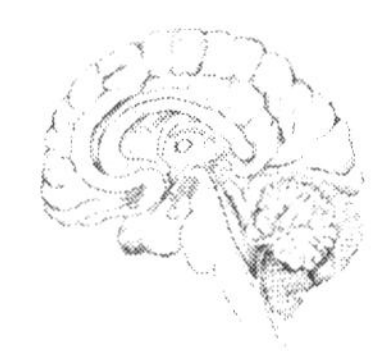

2.9.1 Aniracetam (+ Citicoline)

Common Nomenclature	N-anisoyl-2-pyrrolidinone
Street & Reference Names	N/A
Reference Dosage	N/A
Maximum Dose Experienced	Not Known
Form	Capsules
RoA	Oral
Source / Jurisdiction	Internet / UK

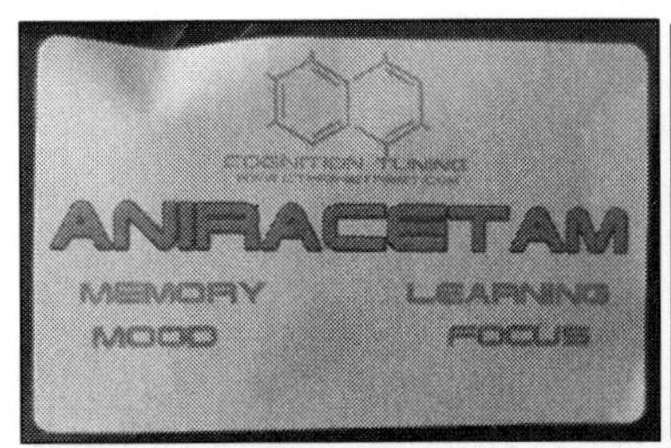

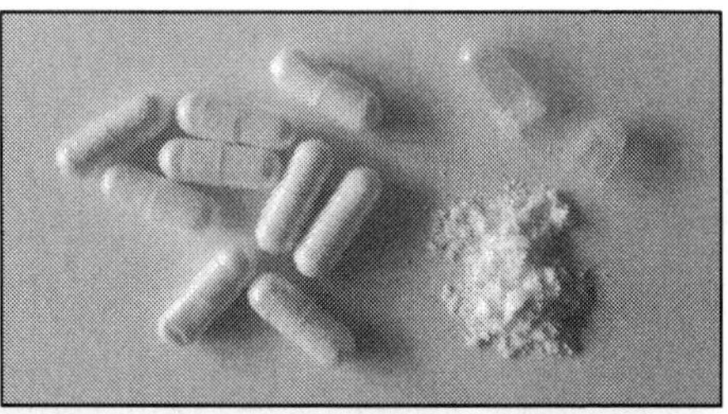

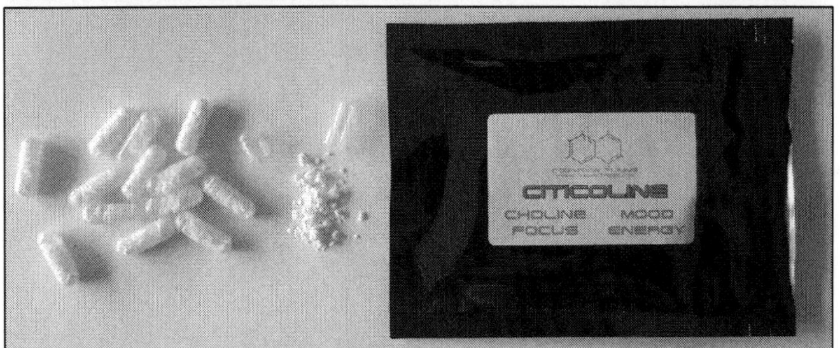

SUBJECTIVE EXPERIENCE
Welcome to the world of nootropic *stacks*. A stack is a combination of two or more *supplements* that have a synergistic effect on cognitive functionality and/or motivation. *Stacking* is a widely practised approach to nootropic medication.

This particular combination was highly cited at the time of testing, but was generally used as part of a daily or regular regime, which is outside the parameters I set for my personal safety. As a single dose experience, it was hard to distinguish its effects. In other words, it invoked a mild stimulation, with a possible clarity that could easily have been a placebo effect.

2.9.2 Armodafinil

Common Nomenclature	Armodafinil
Street & Reference Names	Waklert, Provigil; Modavigil; Nuvigil; Acronite
Reference Dosage	N/A
Maximum Dose Experienced	150mg
Form	Pill
RoA	Oral
Source / Jurisdiction	Internet / UK

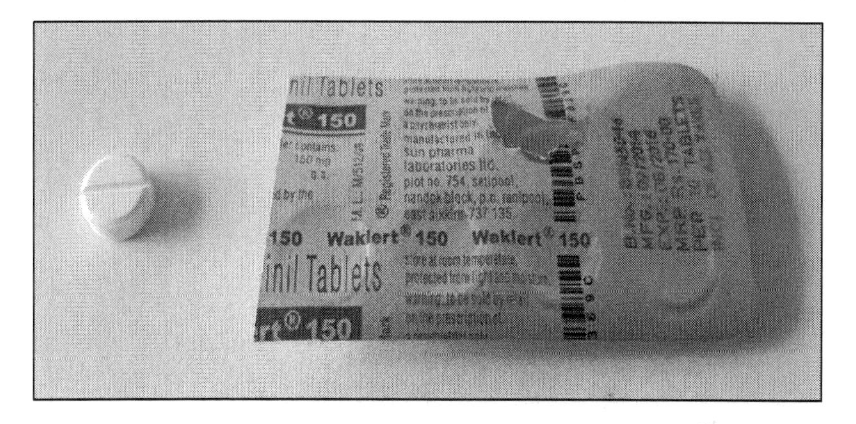

SUBJECTIVE EXPERIENCE
Armodafinil is a widely available wakefulness promoting agent, and is sold under a variety of trade names. I sampled it a couple of times, specifically on occasions on which I was feeling drowsy and mentally tired.

A 150mg dose taken in the morning did the job, in that it fought off fatigue and sleepiness. In this sense it did exactly what is claimed on the packet.

There was nothing particularly recreational about it: it was entirely functional. Equally, there was nothing markedly uncomfortable either. I didn't feel particularly stimulated; just not tired.

I should add that it is probably wise to consume this early in the morning. On the occasion on which I sampled it during the afternoon (2pm), I was unable to properly sleep during the night. The following day I was even more tired and drowsy than I had been at the onset of the experiment.

2.9.3 L-Theanine

Common Nomenclature	5-N-Ethyl-Glutamine
Street & Reference Names	Theanine
Reference Dosage	Common 100mg-200mg [TripSit] Threshold 50mg+;Light 75mg+; Common 175mg+; Strong 300mg+ [Psychonautwiki]
Maximum Dose Experienced	300mg + 300mg
From	Powder
RoA	Oral
Source / Jurisdiction	UK

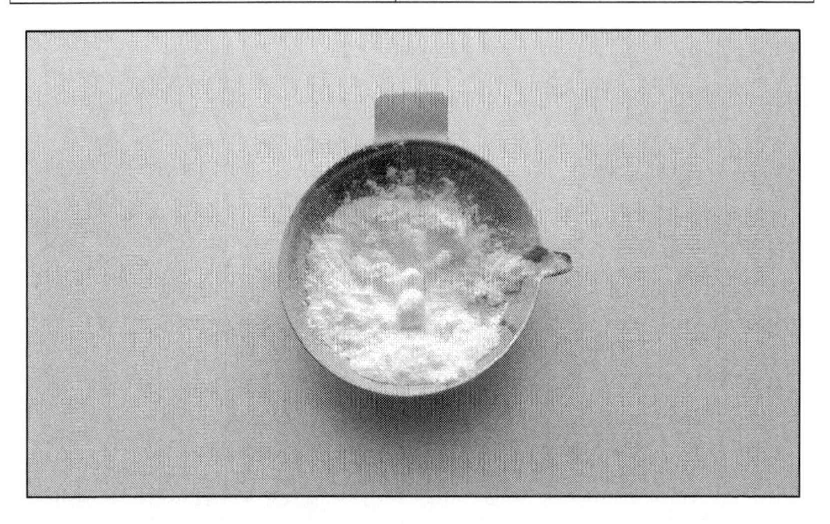

SUBJECTIVE EXPERIENCE
Discovered as a component of green tea in 1949, theanine is usually presented as a neutralizer for mood or anxiety, and sometimes, as an enhancer of cognitive performance. It is also frequently claimed to be synergistic with caffeine. For this reason I will initially take it with my morning tea.

I never have high expectations of materials which are sold as *supplements*, nor in fact of nootropics in general, so this isn't an exercise that I am particularly looking forward to. Having stated this, it has plenty of positive reviews, including on a number of drug related websites.

From the research, I anticipate an onset of about 30 minutes, and a duration of perhaps 3 hours or so.

I open the packet, freshly (and legally) purchased from Amazon, to reveal a very fluffy white powder. So light is its constitution that some of it puffs out of the bag, making a bit of a mess of my desk.

> T+0:00 I weigh 300mg on the scales and pour it into my now half-empty cup of green tea. I slowly drink this over the next 5 minutes. [09.15am]
>
> T+0:10 The mild caffeine jump is emerging and it does seem to have a slightly different character to usual. This isn't the easiest to assess, as it is somewhat on the margins, but it does align with claims that it takes some of the edge from caffeine stimulation.
>
> In addition, I was tired this morning, and although I still am, I am less inclined to want to sleep (although simultaneously I am not buzzing, jittery or fuzzy). Is there a sense of increased clarity? It is subtle, but perhaps there is.
>
> T+0:30 I have seen theanine described as relaxing but not sedating and I wouldn't disagree with this assessment. What I can also state confidently at this point is that it has had an impact on the effects of the caffeine, making it smoother and noticeably mellower.
>
> T+1:00 There have been no major developments since the last note, with the calmative effect on the caffeine-high still in play, and a perception of greater clarity of mind still present.
>
> I should stress that this is all in the shallow end in terms of impact, but there is definitely something to it, and it is pleasant.

These effects gently faded during the course of the morning, delivering a very soft landing and enabling my early afternoon nap to proceed as usual.

At 5:30pm I decided to take another 300mg, but this time without the caffeine. Would this have any effect at a time I was feeling a little stressed? Surprisingly, it did. It removed anxiety and induced a relaxed disposition for some hours. I was a little worn and tired at times, but I cannot deny the existence of psychoactivity.

The following morning I awoke normally and I felt fine. I did experience a little stomach upset overnight but this could be attributed to the substantial meal I ate during the previous evening, rather than the large (possibly excessive) doses I experimented with. With respect to this I would use significantly less on any future theanine expeditions.

Finally, I subsequently discovered both historical and contemporary accounts of monks drinking green tea because it aids meditation. Bearing in mind that green tea is higher in theanine content than other teas, from my experiences above I can certainly see why it would lend itself to this. Mindfulness, calmness and alertness are indeed words that align well with what was a gentle and pleasing sojourn.

2.9.4 Modafiendz

Common Nomenclature	Dehydroxyfluorafinil
Street & Reference Names	Fiendz
Reference Dosage	Light 50mg+; Common 100mg+; Strong 100mg+ [TripSit]
Maximum Dose Experienced	100mg
Form	Pill
RoA	Oral
Source / Jurisdiction	Internet / UK

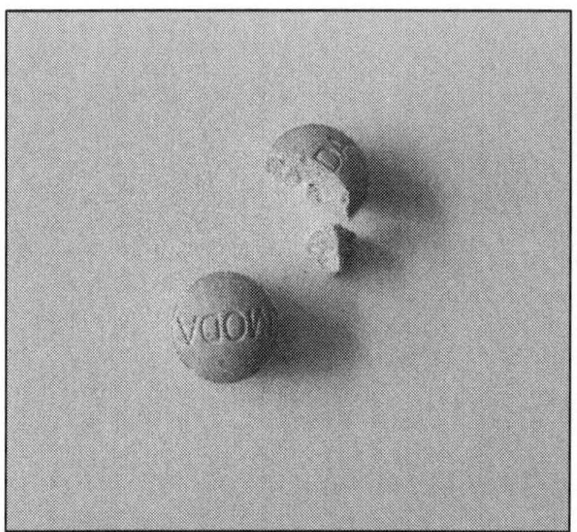

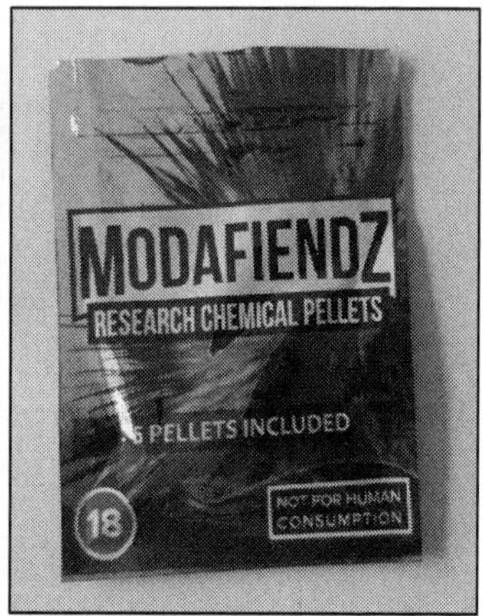

SUBJECTIVE EXPERIENCE
This legally available non-prescription *stay-awake* product was moderately popular circa 2015, and was purchased via a research chemical vendor.

Ingested, it produced an unremarkable functional experience, in that I felt sharp, a little stimulated, and awake, but distinctly under the influence of a chemical.

Generally, I didn't feel that this gave me as smooth a ride as the more commercially established armodafinil (see earlier) and it felt a little more like a stimulant than a wakefulness or alertness agent. This impression was re-enforced by occasional Internet reports of side-effects like jitters and vasoconstriction.

Whilst it was effective in terms of combating drowsiness and sleep, it wasn't particularly pleasant and was not one I would return to.

2.9.5 Noopept

Common Nomenclature	GVS-111
Street & Reference Names	N/A
Reference Dosage	Light 5mg+; Common 10mg+; Strong 20mg+; Heavy 40mg+ [Psychonautwiki] Light 5mg+; Common 10mg+; Strong 10mg+ [TripSit]
Maximum Dose Experienced	20mg+10mg+10mg+10mg
Form	Pill
RoA	Oral
Source / Jurisdiction	Internet / UK

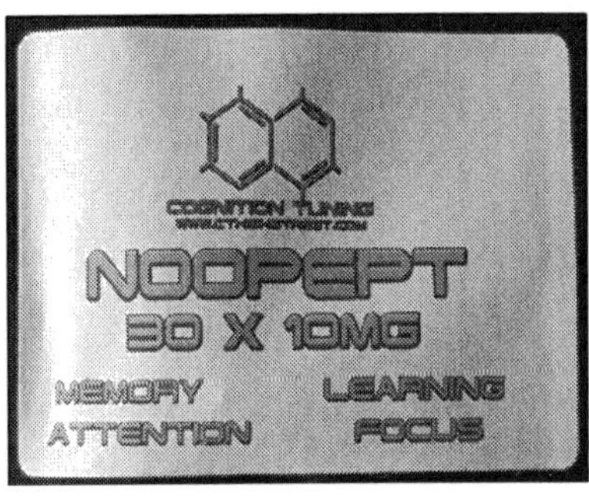

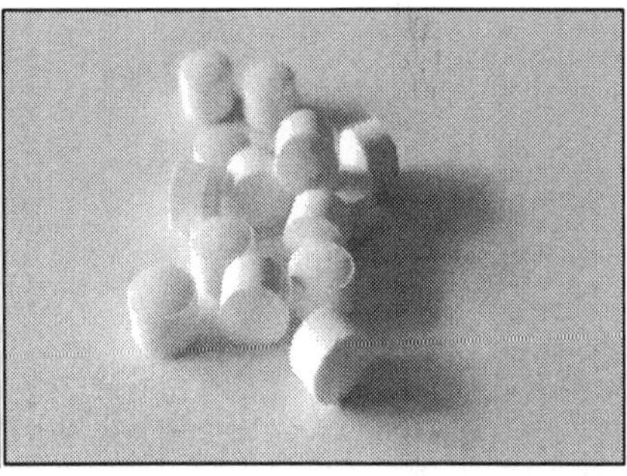

SUBJECTIVE EXPERIENCE
Noopept was developed by a Russian pharmaceutical company in the 1970s, and is a prescription drug in that country.

In recent years it has emerged as one of the most commonly used drugs in this class. Its profile and popularity has been such that it has repeatedly attracted the attention of the mainstream media.

This experiment was, in fact, my first experience with a formally recognised nootropic. Given again that I purposely refrain from ever taking the same chemical on a regular basis, it was a one-off exercise, which is counter to the usual *modus operandi* for this class of drug.

> T+0:00 I take two 10mg pills
>
> T+0:20 A light head tingle is now developing. There is no body-load or any other physical effect.

T +1:00 I am experiencing a low level buzz, but no blur. There is no euphoria or significant mood shift, but my disposition is generally good. I simply feel content, so if a mood-shift is in play at all, it is slightly positive. There is certainly no anxiety.

T +4:00 I take my afternoon power-nap, and I am able to sleep normally. Note as background that last night was a late night.

T+5:00 I take another 10mg.

T+6:00 It is easy to forget that I have consumed a chemical, but at the same time, I am aware of its effects when I do actually think about it.

Subjectively I believe that am experiencing some mental clarity and focus, but the accompanying buzz is extremely mild.

T+7:00 At this point I swallow another 10mg pill, bringing the overall dose for the day to 40mg.

In one respect this feels like the opposite of alcohol, with which vision (along with perception) tends to be hazy. Vision under the influence of this chemical seems to be clearer than usual, and if the experience itself is focused upon, I feel a certain strangeness, which is not unpleasant.

Also unlike post-alcohol consumption, I am also able to work well, with lucidity and a clear head.

T+8:00 I take a final 10mg, and continue to feel more or less as I have for the last couple of hours.

At 50mg my total intake over the last 8 hours has been a somewhat heavy, and is not recommended. To some degree curiosity rather than compulsion has got the better of me.

Do I have the slight hint of a headache? Perhaps I have, but it is mild, and it passes.

From here, I drift slowly back to normality, before retiring to bed.

Noopept probably does more or less what is described in the script. There is a strange background feel about it, with visible clarity, and there is at least the perception of a positive effect on mental functionality.

This is not really a stimulant, sedative or psychedelic, in the traditional sense, but there is a distinct experience in play, albeit a mild one.

Notwithstanding its subtle nature, I found noopept to be one of the more noticeable chemicals in this class.

2.9.6 NSI-189

Common Nomenclature	NSI-189
Street & Reference Names	N/A
Reference Dosage	N/A
Maximum Dose Experienced	40mg+20mg
Form	Pill
RoA	Oral
Source / Jurisdiction	Internet / UK

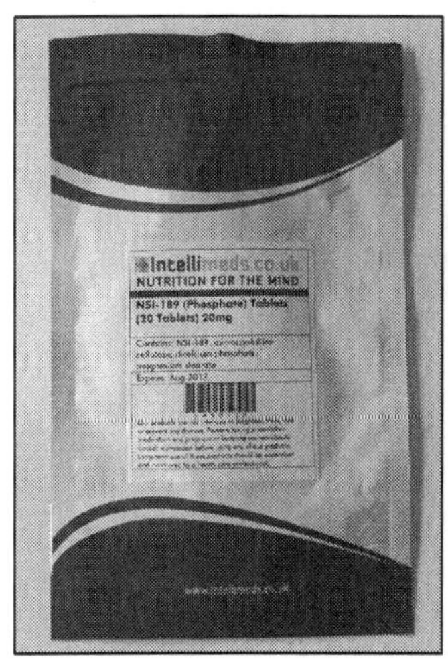

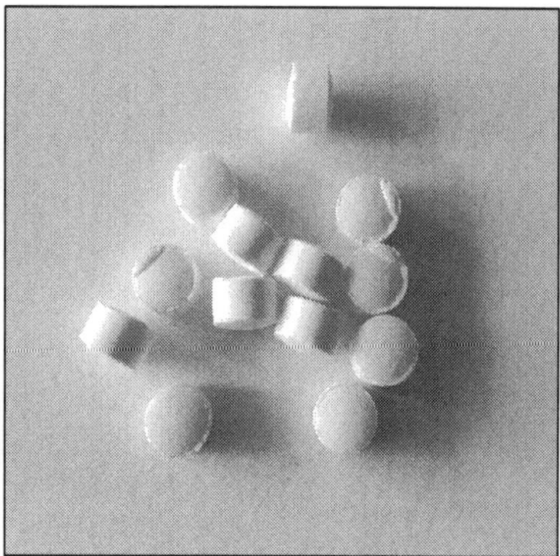

SUBJECTIVE EXPERIENCE
NSI-189 has been researched and investigated as a potential antidepressant, and as an agent for the treatment of cognitive impairment and neurodegeneration. Its efficacy has been vigorously debated over a number of years.

I pursued and sampled it following positive reports across a couple of specialist Internet forums.

Hardly surprisingly from a single experiment, I noticed very little. Like most nootropics it isn't geared for recreational use.

Whilst I experienced no ill or negative effects, it is unlikely that I will return to it for any further testing.

2.9.7 Phenibut

Common Nomenclature	β-phenyl-γ-aminobutyric acid
Street & Reference Names	Noofen; Citrocard;
Reference Dosage	Light 300mg+; Common 600mg+; Strong 1200mg+ [TripSit] Threshold 250mg+; Light 500mg+; Common 1g+; Strong 1g+; Heavy 3.5g+ [Psychonautwiki]
Maximum Dose Experienced	700mg
Form	Capsules
RoA	Oral
Source / Jurisdiction	Internet / UK

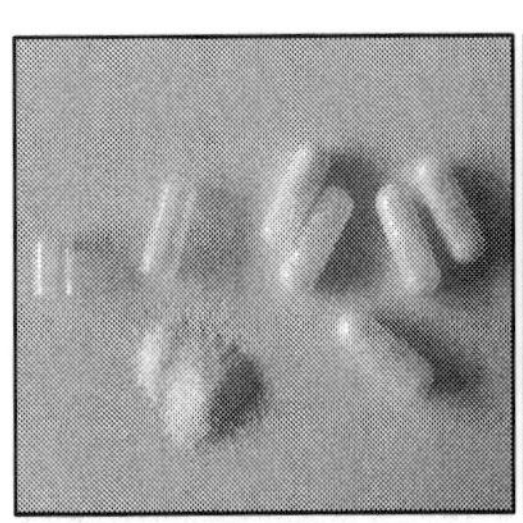

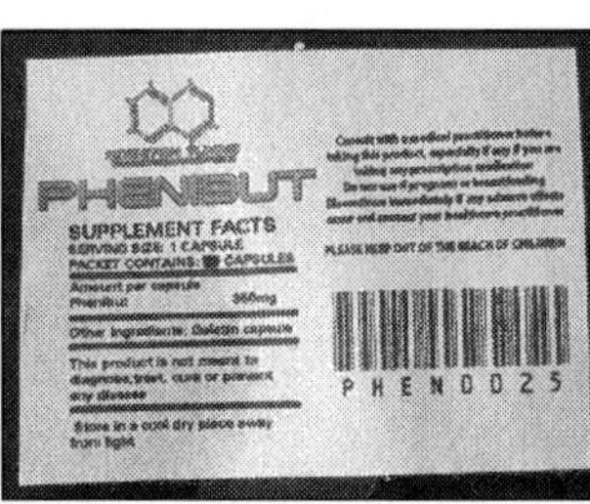

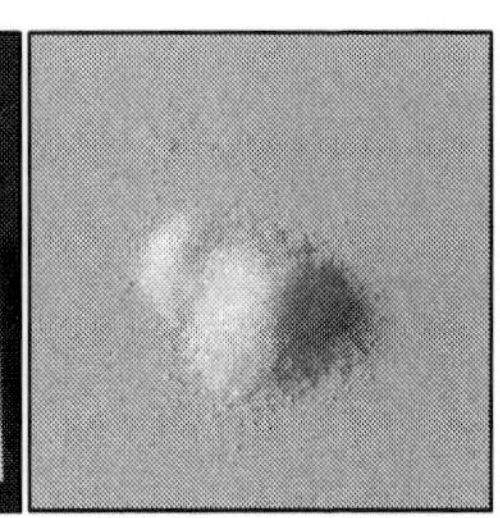

SUBJECTIVE EXPERIENCE
This is a well known and popular chemical, having been developed in the former Soviet Union. One claim to fame is that it is mandated for inclusion in a cosmonaut's medical kit.

It is used as a tranquilliser and an anxiolytic, but is prescribed for a wide range of ailments, including depression, PTSD and alcoholism. It is sometimes suggested that it causes less drowsiness than some of the more common remedies.

Whilst its nootropic related properties are less widely documented, it has had a presence in this field for many years, with claims that it enhances motivation, focus and concentration being commonplace. Again, however, it is positioned for use within a regular dosing regime.

On my single experiment, there were definite anxiolytic effects, with something of a clear headiness also present. I felt a strange artificial sort of well being, and a mood lift which lasted some hours.

Overall this proved to be one of the most active of the chemical nootropics I sampled, and one which I may re-test at some point in the future.

2.9.8 Picamilon

Common Nomenclature	N-nicotinoyl-GABA
Street & Reference Names	N/A
Reference Dosage	Light 40mg+; Common 80mg+; Strong 140mg+ [TripSit]
Maximum Dose Experienced	80mg
Form	Capsule
RoA	Oral
Source / Jurisdiction	Internet / UK

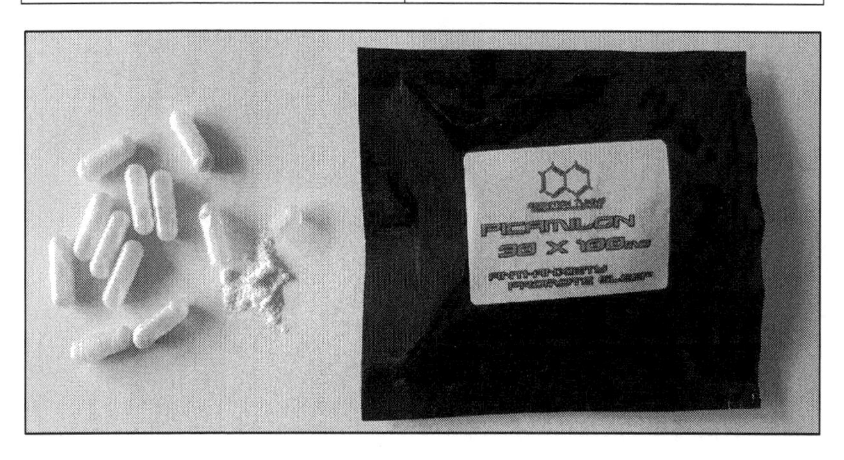

SUBJECTIVE EXPERIENCE
First developed in 1969, this is another chemical which is sold as a prescription drug in Russia. It is used as an anxiolytic, but does have a following for its nootropic properties.

Dose was difficult to pitch, but at 80mg I did feel an effect. This was a slight uplift, and minor change of headspace. However, this was minimal, making it impossible to document any further delineation.

There are a number of enthusiastic reports dotted around the Internet, many of which compare it to phenibut, and discuss its merits with respect to inclusion in a stack. As a one-off recreational drug, however, it has never gained significant traction.

Like phenibut, it could be worth pursuing further research at a later date.

2.9.9 PRL-8-53

Common Nomenclature	PRL-8-53
Street & Reference Names	N/A
Reference Dosage	N/A
Maximum Dose Experienced	5mg
Form	Powder
RoA	Oral
Source / Jurisdiction	Internet / UK

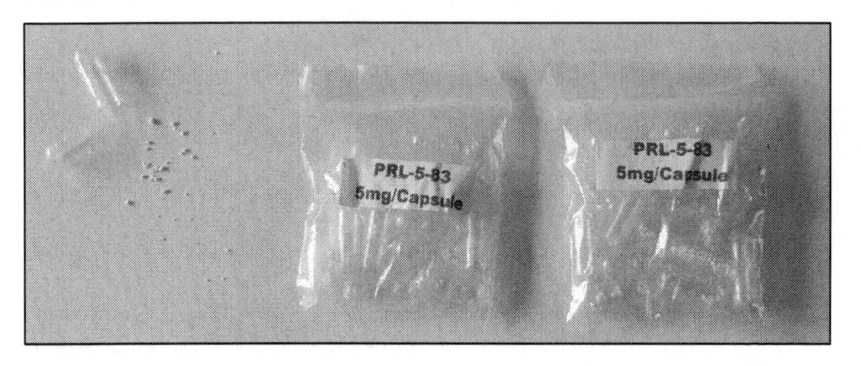

SUBJECTIVE EXPERIENCE
PRL-8-53 is purported to improve short term memory, a claim which has been supported via limited trial data:

> *"A single study in humans was reported in 1978. The double-blind trial of PRL-8-53 in 47 healthy volunteers measured its effects on a variety of cognitive measures. 5 mg of the drug was administered orally 2–2.5 hours before the study tasks. Overall improvements in recollection differed based on how many words were recalled under placebo, with the poor performers (six words or fewer) experiencing a 87.5-105% increase in recollection and the high performers (eight or more words) a 7.9-14% increase which failed to reach statistical significance; when controlling for subjects over the age of 30 only, a 108-152% increase was noted. No side effects were reported during the trial."* ~ Wikipedia

Short of engaging a formal testing regime it is impossible to substantiate this. There are, however, many online reports by nootropic enthusiasts to peruse.

I can confirm that I felt no ill effects from the experiment. In terms of positive recreational value, this was minor, and could easily have been a placebo effect. Additional commentary is therefore not justified.

3

A BOTANICAL JOURNEY

3. A BOTANICAL JOURNEY

3.1 INTRODUCTION

A vast array of plants and fungi can be used to induce psychedelic states, stimulation, sedation, empathogenic or entactogenic episodes, and indeed the full spectrum of psychoactive experiences commonly associated with chemical or drug use. Many of these are deeply entrenched in history and pre-history, being central to cultures and civilizations across the world.

Terminologically, however, Western society appears to struggle with the issues and concepts raised by these matters. The following are the closest related terms I could find to cover this field, as documented by Wikipedia:

> *"Ethnobotany (from ethnology, study of culture, and botany, study of plants) is the scientific study of the relationships that exist between peoples and plants."*
>
> *"An entheogen ("generating the divine within") is a chemical substance used in a religious, shamanic, or spiritual context that may be synthesised or obtained from natural species"*

Neither of these seems to place much focus on the study of the psychoactivity of botanicals in itself. Neither fully articulates the qualities and richness of the actual experiences that can be induced.

Whilst the study of the use of botanical materials purely for psychoactive purposes is not new, direct reports covering all but the most renowned and well known species tend to be sparse. There are exceptions, however.

The most comprehensive source I found during my research was Christian Rätsch's *The Encyclopaedia of Psychoactive Plants*. This is a hugely impressive work, spanning almost the full gamut of psychoactivity, and with a depth of historical research which is second to none. It is expensive, although as Rätsch himself states in the preface, it is his first "*life work*".

For hallucinogens, '*Plants of the Gods*', by Richard Evans Schultes, Albert Hoffman & Christian Rätsch, is unparalleled. This studies the major botanical psychedelics inclusive of their history and ritual use, and it presents them in superbly illustrated bite sized chunks.

Another major source of information came from the books and lectures of the most famed psychonaut, Terence McKenna. These again were largely limited to psychedelics, but were very much focused upon the experience itself.

McKenna's insights, and his own botanical research, provide invaluable knowledge and illumination to anyone willing to spend some time in this field.

These were the primary guides used to support the research which is documented within this section. Along with the Internet, I used these to navigate a path through the psycho-botanical realm, obtaining and experimenting with whatever samples I could acquire. They provided a roadmap for the overall adventure.

If necessary, due to either difficulty with sourcing or UK prohibition, I would travel. These individual journeys tended to deliver a richer and more fulfilling experience than any other. They also enabled an insight and understanding which underpinned the wider initiative.

Finally, like others who have worked with psychoactive plants, I feel that there is a depth and quality to this field which is of fundamental importance. There is profound knowledge to be gleaned from these experiences, particularly with the hallucinogens, which could address many of the most serious issues facing our species. This is ignored at our peril.

A NOTE ON SOURCING

Not all sources are equal. If a botanical sample isn't active, it could well be the case that the vendor has provided a product which has been in stock for too long, or which has dried out too much, or which is simply in poor condition. I have experienced this on a number of occasions, and have often persevered using alternative sources to finally find the requisite quality.

Note also that assumption can be dangerous. If you are testing material in indigenous surroundings, do not assume that the dose being consumed by the locals is safe for you. Tolerance applies as much to botanicals as it does to research chemicals. Tread slowly and carefully: and always research well, prior to experimentation.

BOTANICAL CLASSIFICATION

To facilitate reference, the botanicals sampled on my journey have been ordered into the following sub-sections:

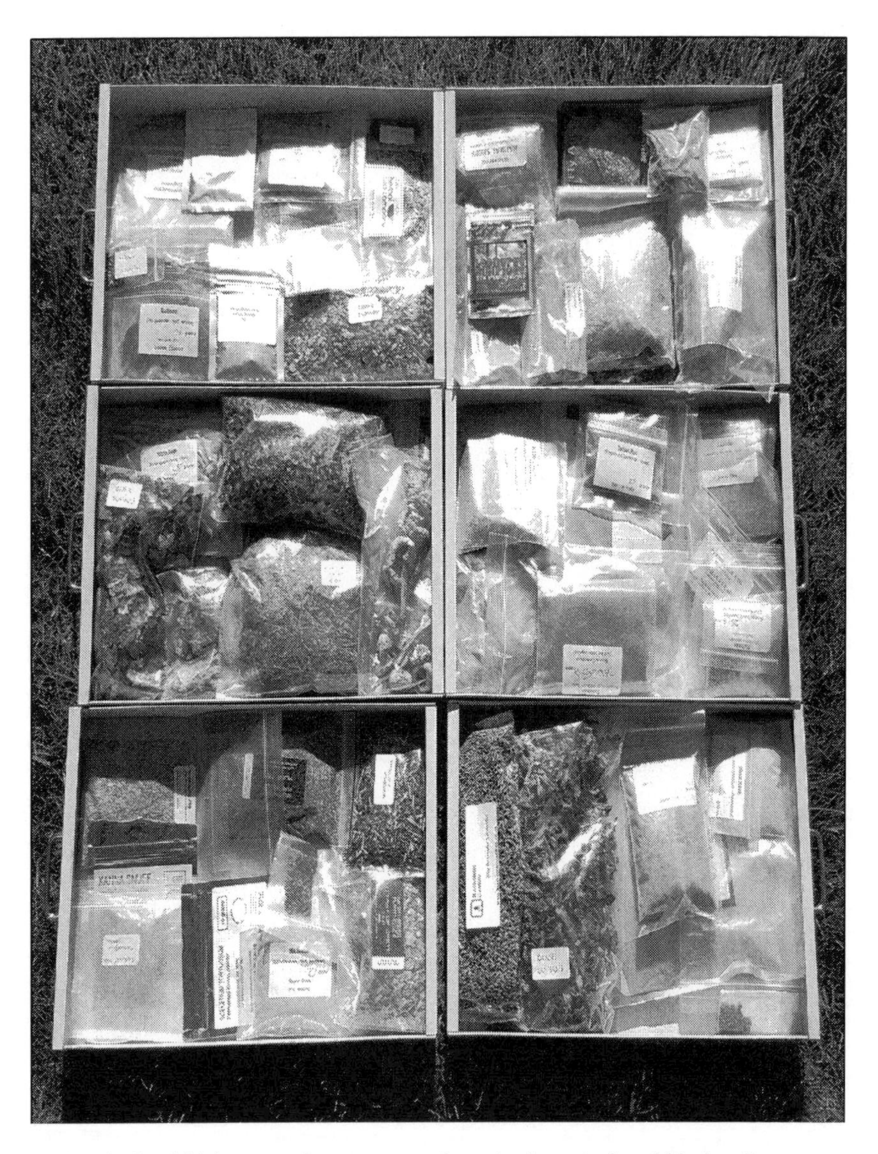

During the legal high years, almost any psychoactive botanical could be legally imported into the UK. A substantial number could be purchased online via the click of a mouse.

3.2 PSYCHEDELICS

Textbook Definition: *Psychedelics alter perception and cognition, creating an experience which is different to ordinary consciousness. The psychedelic state is often related to forms such as meditation, dreaming, yoga, near-death or out-of-body experiences, and even break through to other realms or dimensions of reality.*

The following botanicals have been sampled and researched for inclusion within this section:

3.2.1 Ayahuasca
3.2.2 Cebil
3.2.3 Chaliponga Leaves
3.2.4 Fly Agaric
3.2.5 HBWS
3.2.6 Iboga
3.2.7 Magic Mushrooms
3.2.8 Magic Truffles
3.2.9 Morning Glory Seeds
3.2.10 Ololiuqui
3.2.11 Salvia
3.2.12 San Pedro Cactus
3.2.13 Sensory Deprivation
3.2.14 Shirodhara
3.2.15 Sinicuichi
3.2.16 Syrian Rue
3.2.17 Yopo

The use of hallucinogenic plants dates back to human pre-history. Indeed, there is evidence to support the theoretical proposition that consciousness itself was perturbed and invoked via long term exposure to the psilocybe cubensis mushroom.

The intrinsic importance of these botanicals is recorded and depicted across human civilisations in a wide variety of forms, including cave paintings, hieroglyphs, ancient art and stone carvings. Often they took centre stage in terms of cultural influence, with the Mixtecs of central Mexico, for example, worshipping a god for hallucinatory plants.

Frequently, their ritual use was believed to summon the most divine of experiences, spiritual in nature, and capable of opening a mystical conduit to sacred visions and realms.

This rich history of use and appreciation is a huge topic in its own right.

In the modern era, a number of proponents have emerged to raise awareness of these remarkable plants. Amongst these, none has been more prominent than Terence McKenna.

Through the Internet, his lectures have provided the source of countless YouTube videos, and his books continue to sell, despite his death in 2000. My own journey, in fact, may not have started without exposure to these materials.

Others have since taken up the challenge of emphasizing the importance of hallucinogenic botanicals, not just in terms of individual exploration and proven value to medicine, but potentially, for the future of mankind itself.

Finally, McKenna offered the following advice to potential explorers:

> *"These are bizarre dimensions of extraordinary power and beauty. There is no set rule to avoid being overwhelmed, but move carefully, reflect a great deal, and always try to map experiences back onto the history of the race and the philosophical and religious accomplishments of the species"*

Consistent with this, some of the botanicals listed on the following pages have provided some of the most profound experiences of my life. Like others before me, these led me to consider them not to be mere drugs, but doorways, at the very least to knowledge, greater understanding, and higher levels of consciousness.

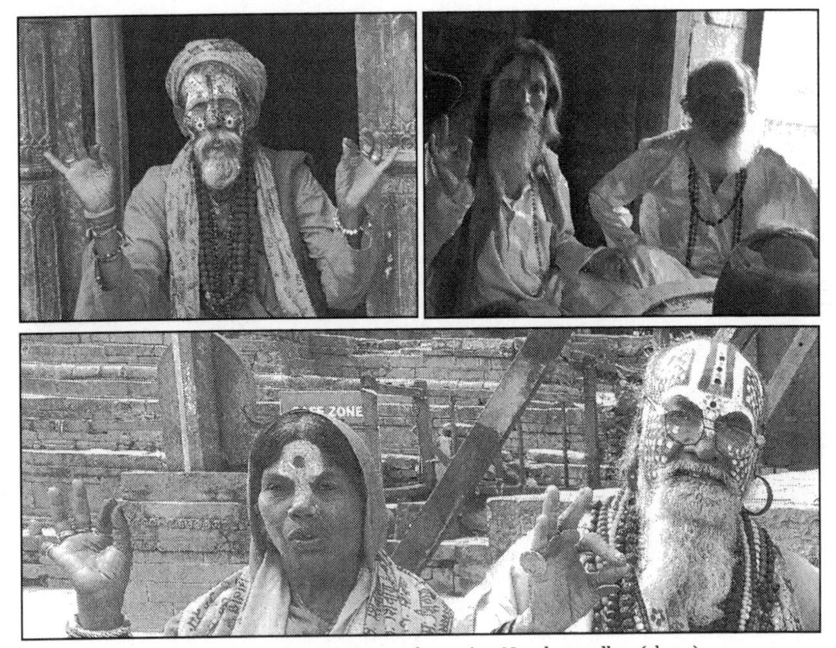

From Peruvian shamans (see ayahuasca) to Nepalese sadhus (above), botanicals are intrinsic to spirituality and higher states of consciousness

TERENCE MCKENNA'S THREE WAY TEST
Despite all the words written about his "*heroic dose*" (five grams of dried mushrooms) and relating to his breakthrough adventures using a variety of hallucinogens and psychedelics, Terence McKenna was in fact safety conscious. He didn't just drop any old drug into his body and then blindly run with the consequences.

Less known than many of his trademark propositions and theories is his "*Three Way Test*". This is a simple guide: questions to ask yourself if you are considering the use of a plant or compound.

The three test questions are:

1. Does It Occur In Nature?

   In his own words: "*Does it have some tangentiality to what is already existing? Because obviously what exists, that's nature, has undergone some vast winnowing process out of the set of all things which might exist.*"

2. Does it have a history of human usage?

   In his own words: "*That is your FDA approval, because if you can point to a tribe of people who have been taking this plant or mushroom or whatever it is for millennia, and they don't have miscarriages, tumours, cataracts, blindness, Down's syndrome, eight fingers on the left hand or whatever it is, then you can be fairly confident that this thing is benign.*"

3. Does it have an affinity to ordinary brain chemistry?

   In his own words: "*We don't want to launch something on your brain that it can't recognize at all, that it has no bio-synthetic pathways to degrade, that it has no receptors for, just some crazy thing, you know, 5-amino-3-triethyl-finphio-anaxidine or something. We don't want that.*"

If a compound or plant met these conditions, he considered it to be an excellent candidate for providing "*spiritual gain at low physiological impact*". In other words, he believed that the potential benefits of using a sacred plant that passed these checks might be worth the potential risks presented.

He referred to this test on a number of occasions, notably during a workshop at Claremont College, Southern California in 1991 (quotes above), the video of which is currently available on YouTube. It is also described in his book, *The Archaic Revival (Speculations on Psychedelic Mushrooms, the Amazon, Virtual Reality, UFOs, Evolution, Shamanism, the Rebirth of the Goddess)* on pages 15-16.

Note that this process covers only candidate selection, which is self-evidently not the same as the adoption of safety procedures as employed in the use of a specific plant or chemical.

3.2.1 Ayahuasca

Binomial / Botanical Name	Ayahuasca
Street Names	Huasca; Yagé; Brew; Daime; La Purga
Major Active Compound	DMT
Indigenous Source	Peru, Ecuador
Form	Beverage
RoA	Oral
Personal Rating On Shulgin Scale	+++

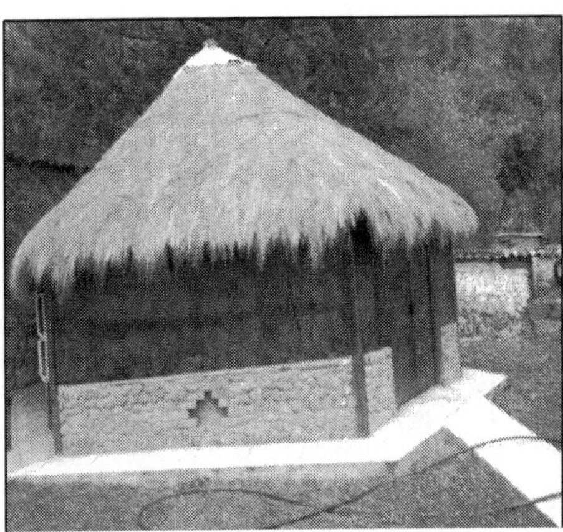

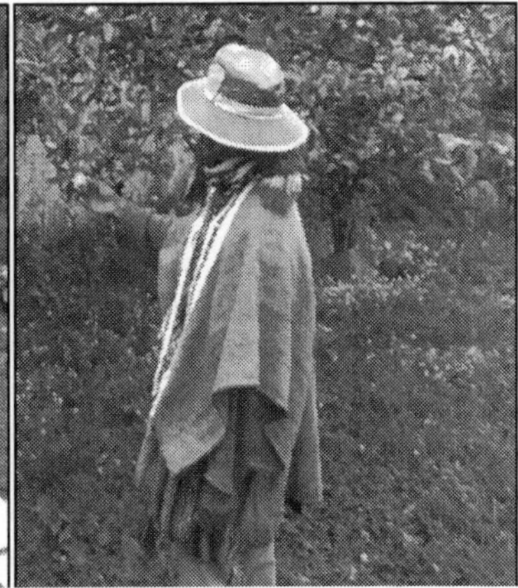

SUBJECTIVE EXPERIENCE
Ayahuasca is a brew, which is used as a spiritual medicine in traditional ceremonies amongst the indigenous peoples of the Amazon. Its ingredients include the banisteriopsis caapi vine and the leaves of a DMT containing plant, such as psychotria viridis or diplopterys cabrerana. Its preparation takes at least a number of hours, and sometimes one or more days.

The story behind ayahuasca, both factual and mystical, is extraordinary, and I was fascinated from the moment I first heard reference to its properties and potential. It was only a matter of time before I embarked upon a mission to experience it.

However, when I eventually arrived in Cusco I was suffering from jet lag, altitude sickness, and some sort of head cold, which I had imported from the UK. I was in no condition to engage what is frequently presented as a life changing experience.

The very next morning a nurse arrived at my hotel to *purge* me. This exercise comprised the drinking of cup after cup of rather unpleasant tasting volcanic water.

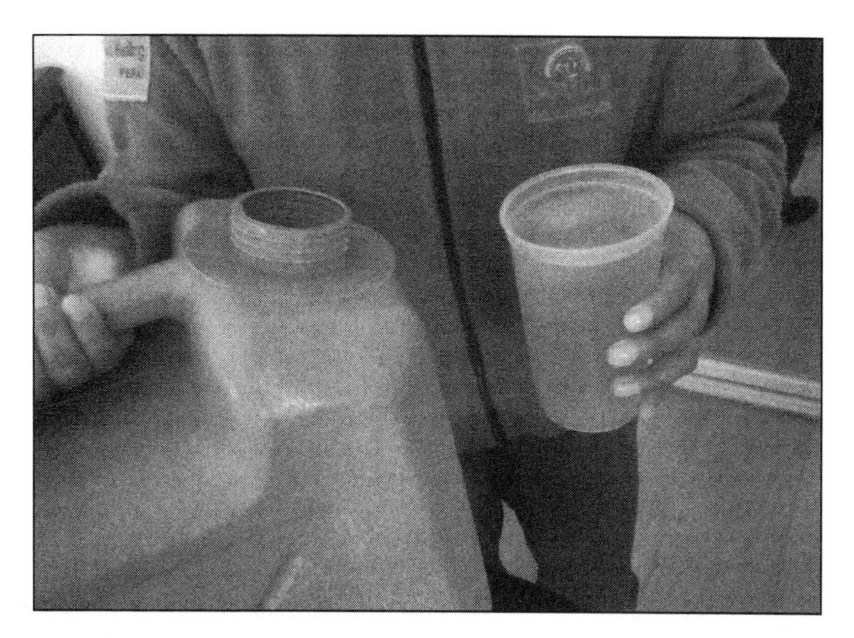

This continued mercilessly, to the point at which the resultant diarrhoea became fluid.

8. For a complete purge or cleansing of the system it is necessary to ingest 18 to 30 glasses depending on one's system.
9. When going to the toilet, do not force yourself to avoid undue strain to the rectum.
10. Drink the water until the liquid from your rectum is clear of feces. At this point you should stop drinking the water.

When the water torture was over I was provided with details of my permitted diet for the day (vegan), and told I would be collected at 7am in the morning (1st May, 2015).

This is what I had paid for and what, despite my pitiful state, I was still looking forward to. I wasn't to be disappointed.

Ayahuasca is widely considered to be the *Holy Grail* of the ethnobotanical sphere. It is seen by many as invoking the ultimate psychedelic experience and by others as a doorway to a spiritual nirvana, or even to a rebirth.

The retreat itself was beautiful. On the edge of a small village, it was surrounded by hills, and was tranquil and peaceful. I was allowed to wander within its boundaries and make myself at home.

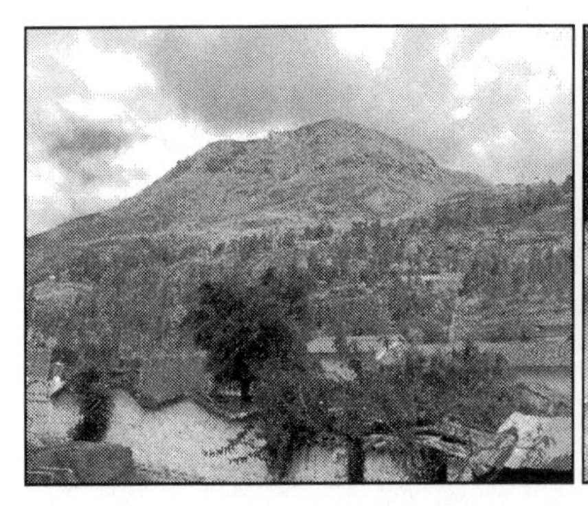
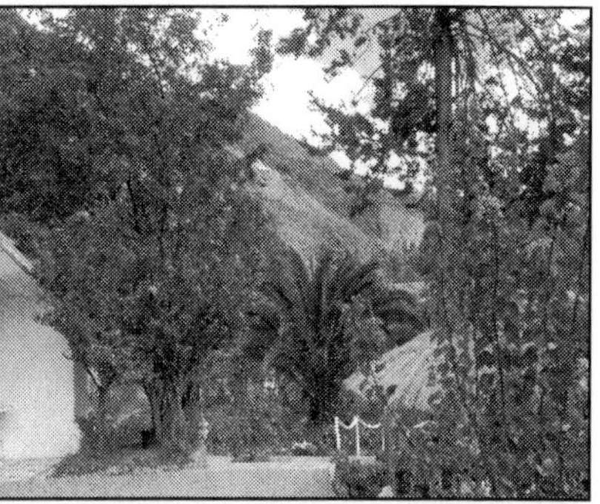

For psychedelics, *set and setting* are of vital importance, and this wasn't lost on me as the shamanic ceremonies unfolded. Here I was, relaxing into an authentic and age old theatre of experience, which itself must have evolved over the eons to support the journey.

These weren't for show: they fulfilled an extremely important purpose. They were supplemented with a private consultation with the shaman, and a personal reading of coca leaves.

By the time I was led into the darkened room for the ayahuasca drinking itself, I was feeling confident in the people around me, and comfortable with what lay ahead. I was ready.

This was well structured. I sat on my mattress with my two litres of water, and was provided with a bucket, into which I would vomit in due course. In front of me sat the shaman, a ceremony master, a facilitator, and a nurse.

The dark brown thick fluid was poured from a plastic bottle into a beaker and handed to me. I drank deeply, non-stop, realizing that the taste was foul and the smell was most likely to be revolting. When it was down I lay on the mattress waiting for something to happen.

The shaman engaged largely with the master. He also sang the icaros at periodic intervals, which was strangely haunting, but reassuring. It came across as natural and melodic: in fact, quite lovely.

Occasionally, the facilitator would approach and whisper encouragement into my ear. He would ask how I was, tell me all was well, and on one occasion rubbed a beautifully smelling fragrance into the back of my neck, which added to the ambiance.

I was aware that I was ill and that my digestive system wasn't at its best. I was thus concerned about the possibility of diarrhoea. I really wanted to avoid having to go to the toilet under the influence, for either function.

I lay there waiting impatiently for hallucinations of some sort to occur, to hopefully distract my focus from my ailing body.

Time passed with a headspace but little else. I heard the other traveller in the room vomiting, struggling, and even being helped to the toilet before vomiting again, and finally being settled by the nurse.

Why wasn't I vomiting? I knew that the real journey would not begin until I had. The discomfort of my prior ailments persisted, and I was feeling somewhat wretched.

Shortly thereafter, the master approached offering more ayahuasca. I accepted, expecting a top-up of maybe a quarter of a cup. A full beaker arrived again, so I drank it. The co-traveller didn't need or consume any more.

Perhaps five minutes or so later, I vomited. I purged, and out it came. I intentionally avoided looking into the bucket, as I had read that this wasn't a good idea. It can apparently appear to be some sort of toxic vortex, which was the last thing I needed to fall into.

I lay down and waited. There was no significant change initially, but I felt physically more comfortable and more positive. I scanned the inside of my eyelids looking for CEVs or some sort of hallucinogenic sign.

Then I found it. It was strangely like tuning in to some sort of wavelength.

Having got there, I could partially exit and tune in again almost at will.

In there were the colours and the visuals: much like you may imagine from the art representations of psychedelic hallucinations. However, there was more. There seemed to be some form of intelligence: a friendly benign other.

So apparent was this that I sought to communicate with it.

I asked myself what I wanted: what did I want to know? Did I want to explore myself, the personal issues from my own past? Not really, partly because I felt that I had already overcome most of the debris from my background, but also, there was a degree of fear.

I knew that I wanted to learn. I wanted to learn about reality, the world, the universe, as this would help me in itself. These were the questions I presented to the other.

I would think about a scenario, sometimes a serious real-world situation that I may have been involved with, and then ask what I should do. What was the solution? I got answers, and they always related to love in some way. It was within me.

Love was the answer, and that answer was presented rationally and in an appropriate way to each proposition, whether personal or external. This was beautiful. The entity, the other, was beautiful. The realisation was almost overwhelming.

I was able to look at an issue, any issue, however painful, almost from a third party perspective, without fear, without anger, without any negative emotion at all. I can fully understand how this can help to heal the deepest seated of personal trauma, and indeed, addiction.

I came out of that realm to the physical world and then returned to it with no fear whatsoever. In the distance the icaros drifted in and out, and was supportive and re-enforcing. I felt love for everything and everyone. I felt a healing.

After what must have been 4 or 5 hours, the ceremony ended and I was taken to my room. I was still very heavily under the influence as I lay on my bed. I vomited again. I realised that this must have been the second dose, and that much of what I had experienced thus far was likely to have manifested from the first.

I fell deep into it again on the bed. I may have dropped asleep or drifted away, as I was exhausted after days struggling under the weather.

About an hour later I was summoned to share my experience with the master, facilitator, and the other traveller. I was almost overcome with gratitude and love, as I articulated my experience. They listened intently.

More ceremonies followed, with the final one held under the stars, around a fire. It was absolutely magnificent: the canopy and clarity of the heavens, the setting, the entirety.

The journey was far from over.

For several days following everything seemed to be beautiful, everyone was incredibly friendly, and all seemed to flow so positively and kindly towards me.

This positivity followed me back to the UK and lasted for weeks and to a lesser degree, for months. Life seemed to be as it was supposed to be, and it always had a nice vibe.

Was this a life transforming experience?

Yes.

Was I glad I did it?

Yes, absolutely. I felt that it bestowed perspective, tolerance, wisdom, and so many other gifts upon me.

Would I recommend it to others?

Yes again. It was one of the most significant experiences of my life.

3.2.2 Cebil

Binomial / Botanical Name	Anadenanthera Colubrina
Street Names	N/A
Major Active Compound	Bufotenin
Indigenous Source	South America
Form	Seeds
RoA	Insufflated / Smoked
Personal Rating On Shulgin Scale	++ / +*

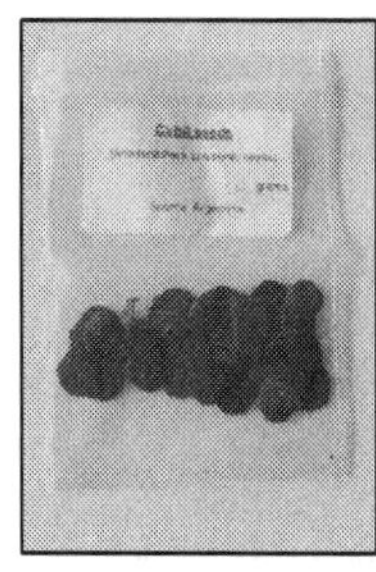
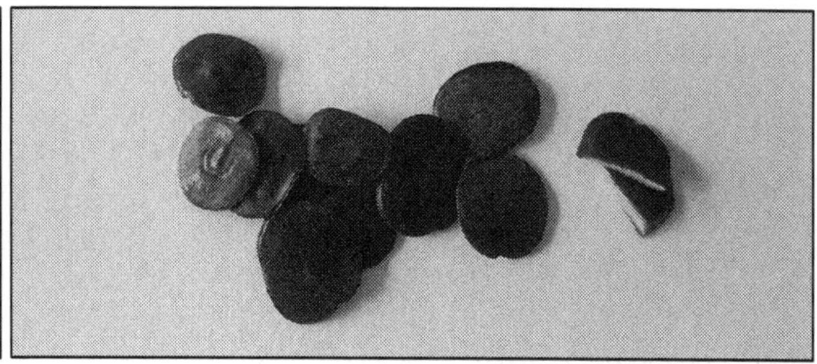

SUBJECTIVE EXPERIENCE
Cebil seeds have been used ritually as a hallucinogen in South America for at least 4,500 years, with some astonishing historical finds having been uncovered indicating a rich and profound cultural influence.

The seeds are generally used as snuff, although they can be smoked. For the former, the procedure to produce the requisite powder is relatively straight forward, and I followed the widely cited instructions as closely as possible.

I toasted half-a-dozen in a pan until they snapped like popcorn. I then removed the brittle shells and pulverised the kernel. I sampled this raw, and also, mixed it with some lime powder.

Make no mistake about it, the snort was painful. Indeed, it was eye wateringly painful. However, the psychedelic headspace which this induced was real, and simple line based CEV patterns and constructs were very evident. Disappointingly, this was fleeting and short lived.

I also tried smoking, via a pipe, but the outcome proved to be even less intense.

I feel that this deserves a lot more experimentation, and given the time, I fully intend to revisit.

3.2.3 Chaliponga Leaves

Binomial / Botanical Name	Diplopterys Cabrerana
Street Names	Chagropanga
Major Active Compound	DMT
Indigenous Source	Amazon Basin
Form	Leaves
RoA	Quidded
Personal Rating On Shulgin Scale	+

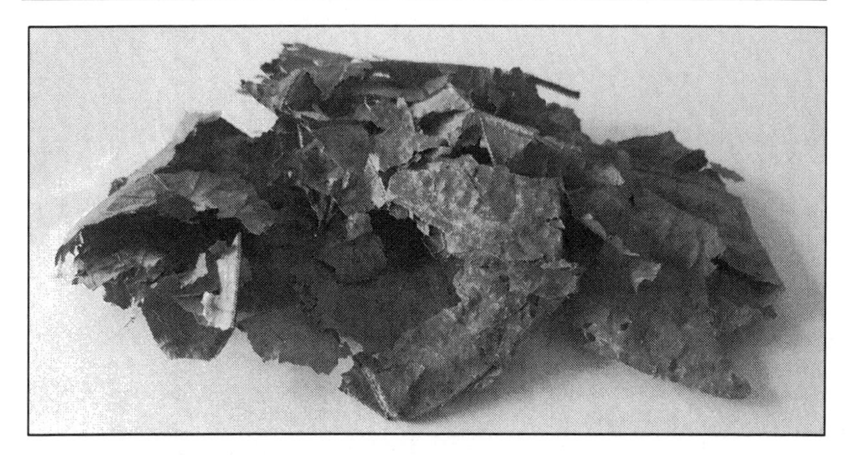

SUBJECTIVE EXPERIENCE
Whilst chaliponga is generally used as an ingredient of ayahuasca, I have occasionally encountered reports which claimed a degree of success via the route of quidding.

Whilst this sounded unlikely, I decided to experiment regardless, and procured the requisite material from an online vendor.

I placed the leaves into my cheeks, and held them there whilst they dampened. I held them and held them, for what seemed to be an eternity. I found it to be extremely difficult to forget that this stuff was there.

I got little. Perhaps a minor change in headspace materialised but perhaps not. However, as the leaves are supposed to be fresh, and mine were quite old, the chance of significant success was always going to be minimal.

This one was filed in the basket: *try again if you ever obtain fresh leaves*

3.2.4 Fly Agaric

Binomial / Botanical Name	Amanita Muscaria
Street Names	Beni Tengutake
Major Active Compound	Ibotenic Acid & Muscimol
Indigenous Source	Northern Hemisphere
Form	Fungus
RoA	Oral / Smoked
Personal Rating On Shulgin Scale	+ / +*

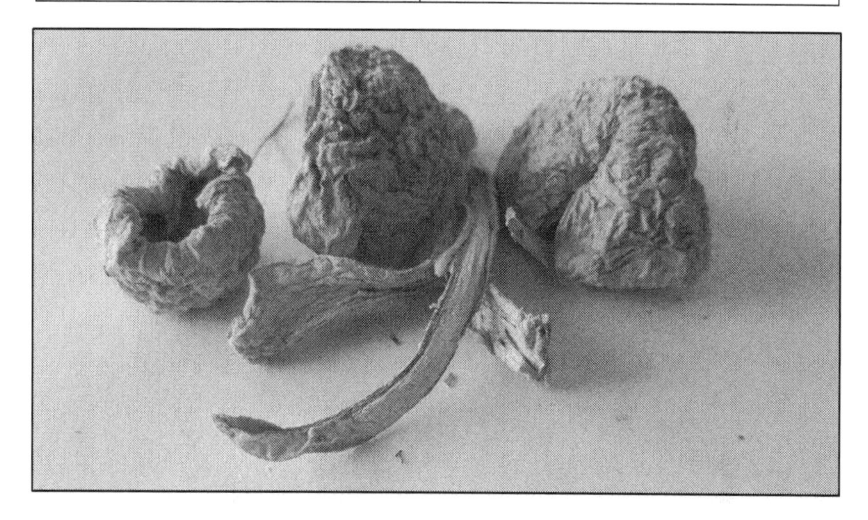

SUBJECTIVE EXPERIENCE
Visibly, amanita muscaria is probably the most famed psychedelic mushroom. Almost all readers of this book will have seen the bright red cap with white dots adorning children's books, cartoons, and a vast array of both serious and fantasy imagery. Usually there is no reference to its psychedelic properties, although often there are hints, couched in terms of magic or myth.

Its use as an hallucinogen has a long and varied history, sometimes embedded in folklore, but in many cases, carefully recorded in word or image.

A rather hideous chapter of its history stems from the fact that, subsequent to its ingestion, its psychoactive components remain potent when expelled in urine, whilst the more noxious chemicals tend to be metabolised. I am aware of two variants of this particular story.

The first is that in Lapland and northern Europe herders engaged in the practice of drinking reindeer urine as a means of inducing hallucinogenic intoxication. It has been mooted that this habit was actually the source of the trip-like fable of Santa Clause flying through the air with his reindeers.

The second is that, particularly at Christmas, the poor folks of both Lapland and Siberia would collect and drink the urine of the intoxicated wealthy, either by recovering it from the snow or by other means. Indeed, it is suggested by a number of historians that this was the original source of the term "*to get pissed*".

I think we can now move on.

My own experiments bore relatively disappointing results. Having secured a 5g sample, I dosed low, partly because, at the time, there were a handful of stories in circulation which warned of a degree of toxicity, and partly because of related suggestions of a high body load.

I chewed 2-3g and swallowed. In due course there was a reaction, a mild reaction, which was limited to a change of headspace. It was there, and it was of a psychedelic nature, but it bore no remarkable or compelling features. Eventually it faded, and that was that.

At a later date I decided to grind some of the material and smoke it via a bong, having seen this recommended in a variety of Internet forum posts. This came on more quickly, as would be expected, and was more intense. Again, however, it comprised largely of a mild headspace and a broad psychedelic feel.

I had hoped for more, but I believe that a combination of my reluctance to dose ambitiously, and the age and condition of the fungus itself, eliminated the prospect of an intense experience.

Whilst there is absolutely no doubt that this mushroom is a strong psychedelic, this outcome is fairly common. Inducing the requisite reaction appears to be easier said than done. Should the opportunity arise at some point in the future, I will revisit.

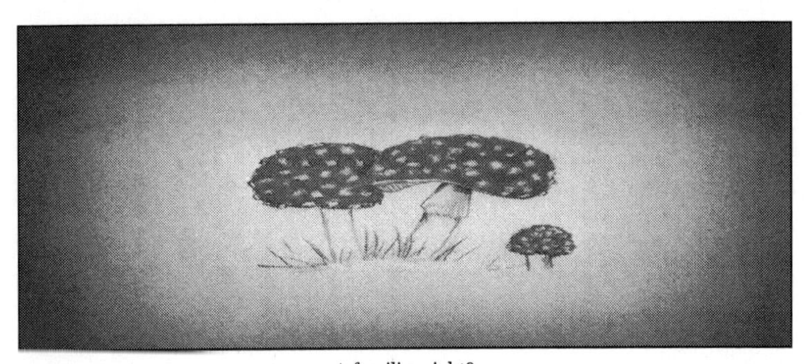

A familiar sight?

3.2.5 HBWS

Binomial / Botanical Name	Argyreia Nervosa
Street Names	Hawaiian Baby Woodrose
Major Active Compound	LSA
Indigenous Source	Indian Subcontinent
Form	Seeds
RoA	Oral
Personal Rating On Shulgin Scale	++

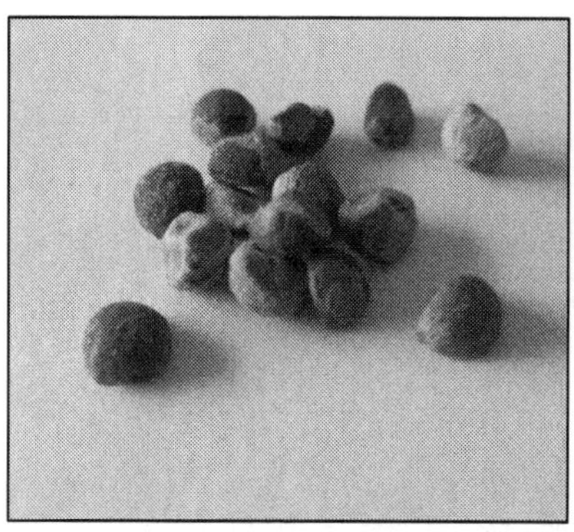
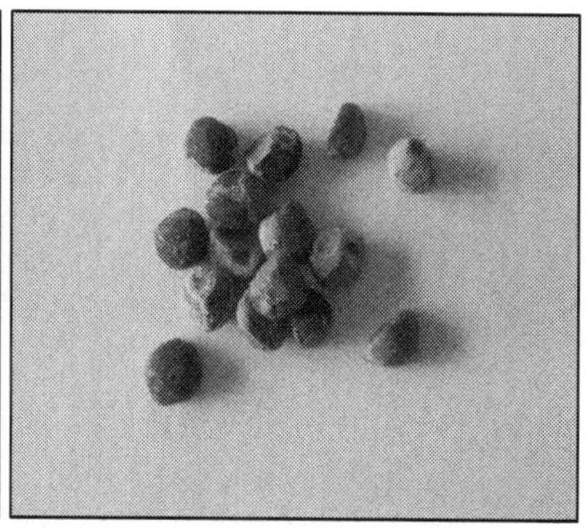

SUBJECTIVE EXPERIENCE
Argyreia Nervosa has a rich history of traditional use, including in ayurvedic medicine. It is referenced in a spiritual and ritual context in cultures as geographically dispersed as Hawaii and Nepal.

Its seeds provided one of my biggest surprises in terms of psychoactive strength. Contrary to the impression created by many Internet reports, just three were sufficient to take me into Shulgin ++ territory. This was even more surprising given that I had prepared a concoction, which for me, usually spells abject failure.

For the preparation I found that a number of approaches were suggested. In the end the formula I adopted was to scrape the worst of the darkest colouration from each seed, crush them with mortar and pestle, stir the powder into a glass of cold water (not tap water), place this into the fridge overnight (keeping it covered), and finally add a bit of shredded clove for the last hour or so, stirring every now and again.

This was quite an operation, but the outcome was a solid psychedelic experience, similar to LSD, but with variation in headspace, and perhaps fewer visuals. It was extremely pleasant, and without the nausea often reported. It faded after a few hours, with no hangover or disagreeable residue.

3.2.6 Iboga

Binomial / Botanical Name	Tabernanthe Iboga
Street Names	N/A
Major Active Compound	Ibogaine
Indigenous Source	Cameroon, Gabon, Congo, Central & West Africa
Form	Root bark
RoA	Oral
Personal Rating On Shulgin Scale	+

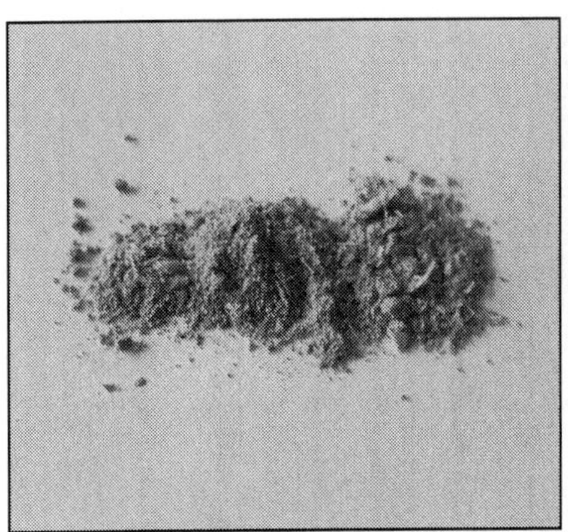

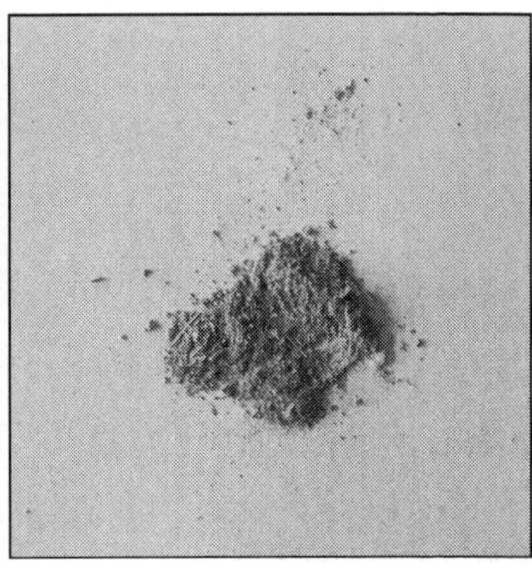

SUBJECTIVE EXPERIENCE
Iboga is used ceremonially in Gabon and other Central and West African states, and is fundamental and central to the Bwiti cult. It is used for rites of passage, spiritual communion, resolution of pathological problems, communication with ancestors, and many other intrinsic aspects of this indigenous society.

So respected is this plant that in 2000 the Council of Ministers of the Republic of Gabon declared it to be a national treasure.

Beyond this region, its primary alkaloid, ibogaine, is used therapeutically to address addiction. Clinics have been established in nations across the world. It is also claimed to be a true aphrodisiac, when used in the correct circumstance.

However, reports suggest that due to a variety of pressures, including over-harvesting, the plant population is now under threat, despite a number of conservation efforts.

Iboga had been on my must-do list for a long time before I finally dipped my toe into the water, one Saturday afternoon.

I had procured 5g from a well known vendor for initial testing: the idea being to start low and to ditch the experiment if the substance was totally inactive, or was nightmarish in some way. The duration, generally cited to be in excess of 24 hours, and for which Erowid stated that "*a user may be immobilised*", further promoted caution.

For the first experiment I therefore consumed 1g, intending to take perhaps 2g or 3g as a second pitch, and possibly go for the a more immersive experience sometime thereafter. The mid-range did appear to be commonly suggested across specialist Internet forums.

Although the 1g had been chosen primarily for safety reasons (containing about 25-50mg of ibogaine), many commentators considered it to be a sufficient dose with which to experience at least some psychoactivity. The following, for example, is reported on Erowid:

> "*Even at this small dose, the effect was noticeable. I wasn't completely sure about attributing the shift in my mental state to the impact of the drug (Shulgin calls this +1, I think), but my later trial with a larger dose reproduced a very similar state much more vividly (and dramatically).*
>
> *There were no perceptual changes, but the mood would be best described as tranquil lucidity. At this small dose, it was quite pleasant and kind. The mental effect formed clearly approximately 2 hours after the ingestion, and lasted for a few hours subsiding gradually in waves*"

At pre-threshold and threshold levels like this, detailed commentary is difficult, but I felt broadly as described in those notes. I felt serene, with a strange background headiness, and physically I was a little tingly. I certainly felt that there was at least some sort of effect in play, albeit minor.

I also noted that I wasn't ill, and that there was no body load. After a few hours, I thought that was that.

But it wasn't.

On the Saturday, Sunday and Monday I had dreams. These were far more lucid than normal. I didn't connect them to the iboga at all, particularly as on the Sunday I had consumed alcohol.

It was the Monday night dreams that made me stop and take stock. What was causing this? Was it something I had consumed last week?

I recalled that my entire intake comprised a few experimental bong hits of powdered acacia confusa root on the Wednesday, which seemed a rather unlikely candidate.

Nonetheless I Googled, using search words of *dream* and *acacia*. There was nothing to suggest any connection.

I performed a second search, but this time using *iboga* and *dream*.

Bingo!

There was a multitude of reports suggesting that iboga is an oneirogen. The following, for example, was posted on the *BlueLight* forum:

> "*Also I forgot to mention, I have been having super intense, vivid, varied dreams every single night. Sometimes really bizarre ones. Before the ibogaine it was incredibly rare for me to remember a dream, much less be present in my dreams, but lately I've had a number of dreams bordering on lucid.*" ~ Xorkoth

There could be a degree of confusion here because large doses of ibogaine apparently cause an awake dreamlike state. Here, however, I refer to dreams, whilst asleep. Reports on the Internet seem to cover both of these states, and often, in a confusing manner.

I should also note that I woke feeling refreshed and rested on each occasion.

This experience, of course, influenced my plans, as I felt that a period of contemplation was sensible, prior to diving deeper. I fully intend to return to this strange plant when I am able to find the time to do justice to it.

[*Shulgin Reference for ibogaine: TiHKAL #25, p487*]

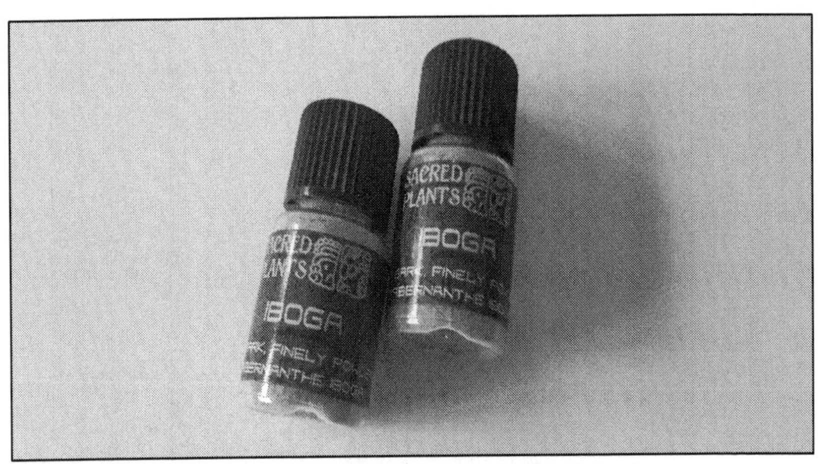

Iboga is embraced for both spiritual purposes and addiction therapy

3.2.7 Magic Mushrooms

Binomial / Botanical Name	Psilocybin Mushrooms
Street Names	Shrooms
Major Active Compound	Psilocybin
Indigenous Source	Widespread
Form	Fungus
RoA	Oral
Personal Rating On Shulgin Scale	++

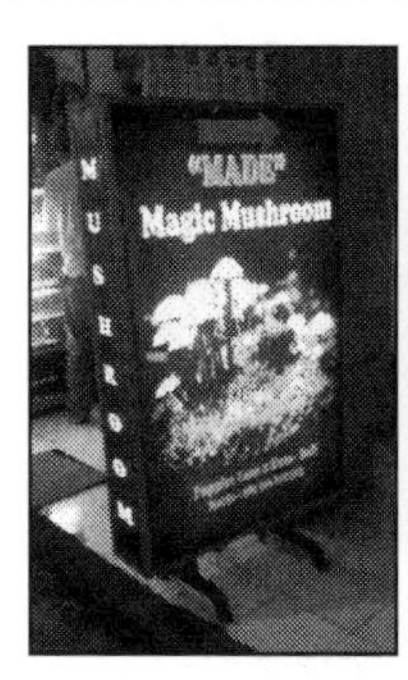

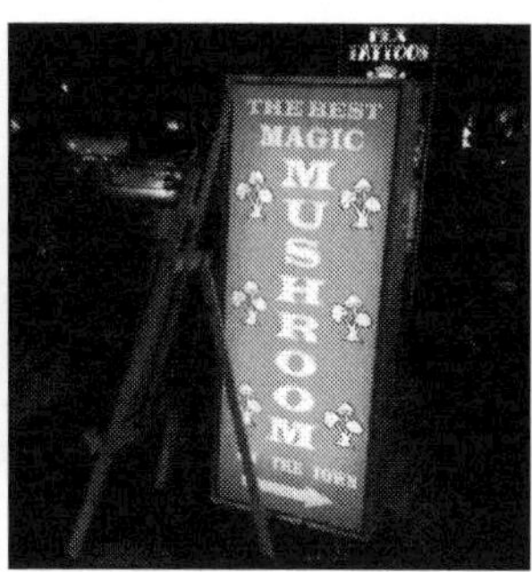

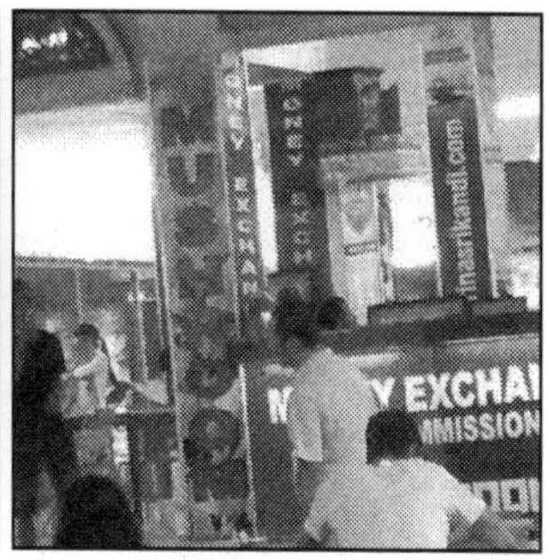

SUBJECTIVE EXPERIENCE
This was another trip which was undertaken in South East Asia, where at the time psilocybin mushrooms were legal and were openly on sale. It was also to be another group experience, shared with fellow travellers.

I recall that the vendor offered us a dose to "*take us to the moon*". How could we refuse an offer like that? The mushrooms themselves came in inflated transparent plastic bags, which he had stored in a fridge. He offered to serve them in milk shakes but given a degree of paranoia regarding the police, we preferred the idea of eating them raw in a hotel room.

They tasted, unsurprisingly, like raw mushrooms. They were edible but not exactly tasty. Being greedy I ate my bag, and almost a half of someone else's, who was rather more circumspect. Perhaps I would get beyond the moon, possibly to mars.

The ride didn't take too long to start; perhaps half an hour to an hour. As the headspace emerged, the paintings on the walls became more noticeable, and the colours more vibrant. Essentially, the traditional experience was emerging.

In actual fact, it didn't go too far, so the dose was not as high as the vendor had implied. Having stated this, there was the television incident.

We became immersed in, of all things, *BBC World News*. The stories were fascinating, and I found myself providing non-stop commentary and narrative to my non-British colleagues. I have no idea why, but it seemed to be appropriate.

We were also engrossed by the visuals. There was a sort of heavy drifting and double vision going on, and it was constant. Remarkably, we all shared it.

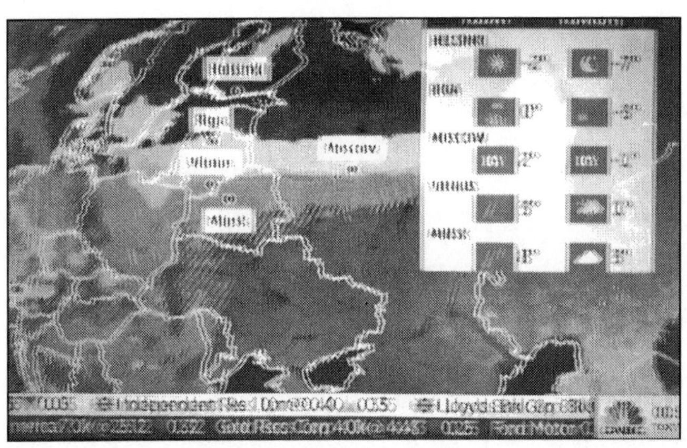

The OEVs were particularly groovy

I lost track of how long this continued for, but it must have been for close to an hour. Then someone changed the channel. Wallop! It suddenly struck us. We had been watching a 3D channel without the glasses, and hadn't even realised. We had simply assumed that the blurry edges were a manifestation of the psilocybin.

At this point we grasped that maybe we weren't as far gone as we thought we were. However, colours were still enhanced, and the headspace was still there. There was overall warmth, empathy, and a great vibe.

This continued into the night, as we slowly came down. It had, in fact, been an extremely enjoyable and memorable experience.

Such frivolity, however, grossly misrepresents a picture that includes the potential to embark upon journeys of incredible discovery and self-reflection. Shrooms are also commonly known to address ailments such as depression and addiction.

The former aspect is certainly on my agenda for the future, and will be reported in this book should I fulfil this objective in time for publication.

Despite their benign safety profile, and incredible potential, fresh magic mushrooms were classified in the UK as a *Class A* drug in 2005. In the United States psilocybin (and thus magic mushrooms) had fallen foul of the *Controlled Substances Act* in 1970.

GENERAL SPECIFICATIONS
The intensity of the magic mushroom experience varies from the barely perceptible effects of a micro-dose (often used as part of a routine) to the complete immersion of Terence Mckenna's favoured "*heroic dose*" (++++ on the Shulgin scale), which was 5 dried grams in total darkness. In establishing dose, it is also important to note that there is significant variance in potency between species and batches.

When I first acquired the most widely known species, psilocybin cubensis, which Erowid cites as medium strength, I was provided with the following guide:

< 1g Light
1-2g Common
2-4g Strong
4-5g Heavy
5g + Heroic

This broadly aligns with most of the established online sources.

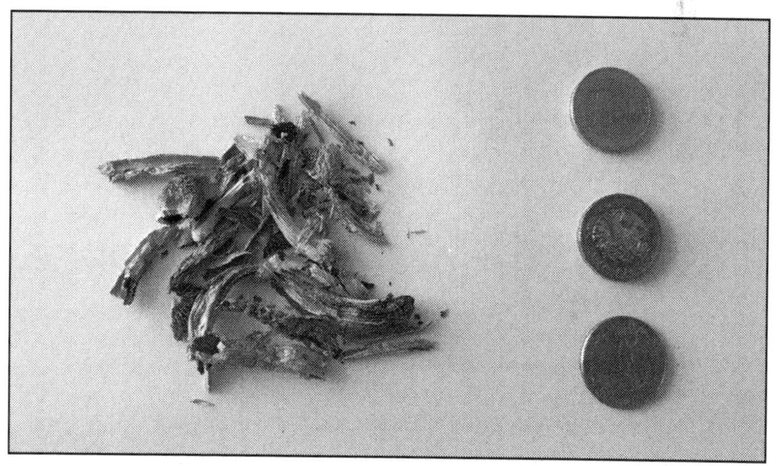

2g of dried psilocybin cubensis with 1€, 1£ and 25 cents

Again with shrooms of average potency, it is commonly suggested that a dose under 1g will usually create a light socially compatible experience, 1-2g will invoke a moderate psychedelic ride, 2-3g will produce a classic trip, 3-4g may send you flying (with loss of social functionality), and above 4g may render a full-on hallucinogenic state, with total loss of normal *reality* and distortion of perception.

It is extremely important to consider the appropriate set and setting for the dose and to dose responsibly, particularly if you are inexperienced. I cannot stress this enough.

Finally, onset time is usually half an hour to an hour, and the main part of the experience will typically last 4 to 5 hours or so, often with quite a long tail.

3.2.8 Magic Truffles

Binomial / Botanical Name	Psilocybe Tampanensis
Street Names	Sclerotia, Philosophers Stone
Major Active Compound	Psilocybin
Indigenous Source	Widespread
Form	Fungus
RoA	Oral
Personal Rating On Shulgin Scale	+++

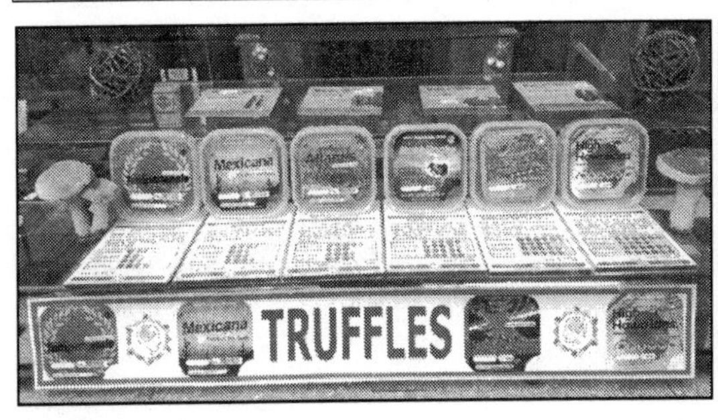

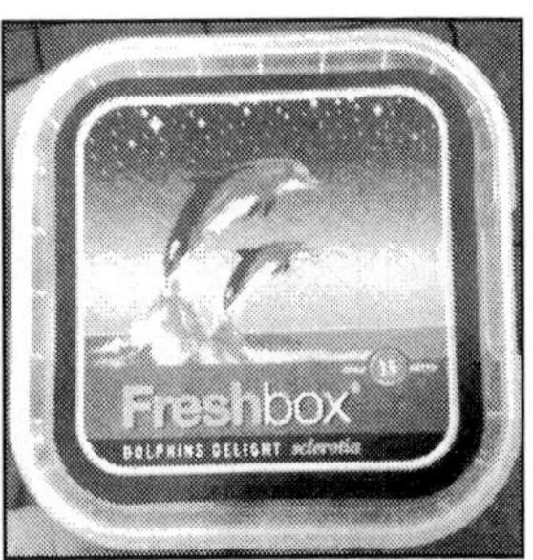

SUBJECTIVE EXPERIENCE
Truffles broadly comprise the underground hardening of a mushroom's mycelium, and are part of the fungus itself. Hardly surprisingly, therefore, magic truffles provide the same effects as regular magic mushrooms. When the Dutch government banned magic mushrooms in 2008, but left truffles unaffected, the latter exploded in popularity, particularly in Amsterdam.

My first truffle experience was planned well in advance, as a group expedition, although it didn't unfold exactly as anticipated or intended. Having previously tested psilocybin mushrooms, I was fully aware of the type of headspace I was about to engage, although perhaps not its intensity or the impact of the setting.

We procured the truffles from the Kokopelli smart shop, not far from Centraal Station. The idea was to consume the classic *museum dose*, and then stroll to and through the gallery itself, about a mile away.

Given my previous experience, the vendor suggested that I go for *Dolphins Delight*, which was one of the stronger of those on offer.

As we walked towards our destination, I slowly chewed and swallowed my way through the entire 15g, which was memorable only due to its strong earthy taste. As we entered the museum the effects had already started to be felt.

I was becoming warmer, and the familiar psychedelic headspace was fast emerging. It soon felt strong, and the standard visuals were manifesting, to the extent of the classic phenomenon of breathing walls. They were not yet at full throttle, but they were far from stable.

As occasionally experienced on certain psychedelics, we were but 10 minutes into the museum when I desperately needed to use the toilets. It was something of a challenge to find them, and I was grateful for the assistance of my fellow travellers in this respect.

Having relieved myself, I felt a little better, and set about enjoying the ride. Well; that was the intention.

As expected, colour was vivid, and the art and artefacts were significantly more engaging than normal. Yes, cool, at least until we reached the section which displayed portraits of the well-heeled from the Dutch Golden Era (circa 17th century).

The problem here was that they were more *alive* than usual, and the past era setting was occasionally dark. I found that they looked increasingly like.... pigs. Before long I considered them to be threatening.

We quickly moved along, but by now I was a little up and down, and unsettled. I knew that I was tripping hard, and that I was in a public place, full of strangers. I also knew that I had consumed far more than a museum dose.

Despite a little anxiety the rest of the visit passed relatively uneventfully, with various levels of engagement. Had I not perturbed myself I am sure it would have qualified as being rather exciting, but regardless, it wasn't so terrible and it did have elements of fun.

Outside the museum we wandered around the pleasant gardens and side streets, which surrounded the grand old building. However, I was again becoming slightly uncomfortable. My stomach was churning somewhat, with a hint of nausea, and the crowds were becoming increasingly difficult to handle.

Whilst I was fully aware that I was flying high, well into +++ territory, I was feeling a little claustrophobic as the streets seemed to become busier and busier; so much so that we had to weave in and out of people to make progress.

Given the location, the centre of a major European city, this was hardly a surprise. The hot weather also didn't help, nor did the sound of the hustle and bustle.

Eventually, I sounded the distress signal: I needed to get back to the hotel to lie down.

Achieving this was easier said than done, given that it was the best part of a mile away, and that the most tenable route was through the main shopping district.

Despite throngs of shoppers of every shape and size, kids that reminded me of aliens, and the almost overwhelming noise they collectively produced, we managed to get back without incident. My relief was palpable.

Lying on the bed I closed my eyes. Wow!

The CEVs were intense; as intense as I had experienced to that point. I was seeing the quintessential picture of colourful patterned snake-like bodies intertwining and moving. This was compelling, but given my current mindset, was slightly disturbing at the same time.

I should state clearly that this was by no means a traumatic experience. I knew at every stage that I was psychoactively immersed and that it would come to an end. It was, however, difficult, as the situation wasn't conducive to a heavy trip and I had allowed myself to go down a more challenging route than I should have.

Something like an hour later the peak had passed, and I was good to go again. The headspace lingered for some hours, but I had completely recovered my composure and I basked in the afterglow.

Overall, it was a memorable experience with some lessons learned, the main one being that 15g of strongish truffle was far too much for this sort of agenda. I feel that 10g would have been more like it, and would have had the desired outcome.

Maybe next time.

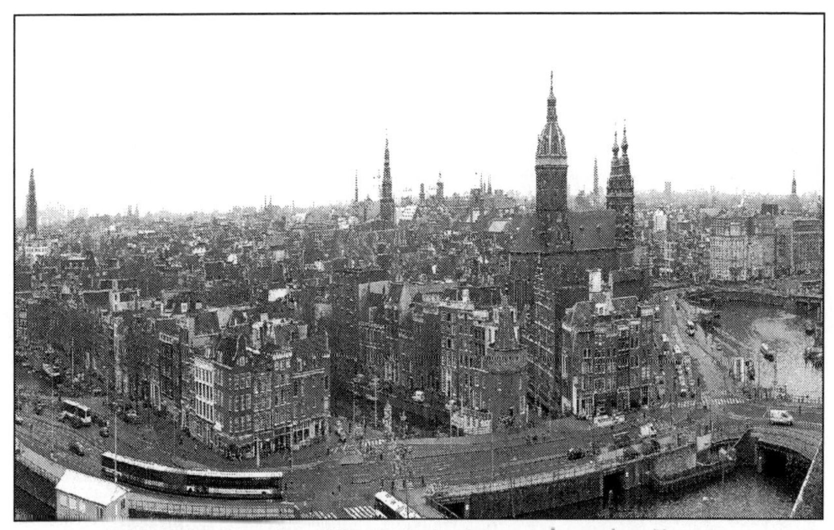

Traversing Amsterdam whilst tripping hard presented a number of issues

3.2.9 Morning Glory Seeds

Binomial / Botanical Name	Ipomoea Violacea
Street Names	Morning Glory; Badoh Negro; Tlitliltzin; La'aja Shnash; Xha'il
Major Active Compound	LSA
Indigenous Source	Mexico, S America
Form	Seeds
RoA	Oral
Personal Rating On Shulgin Scale	+**

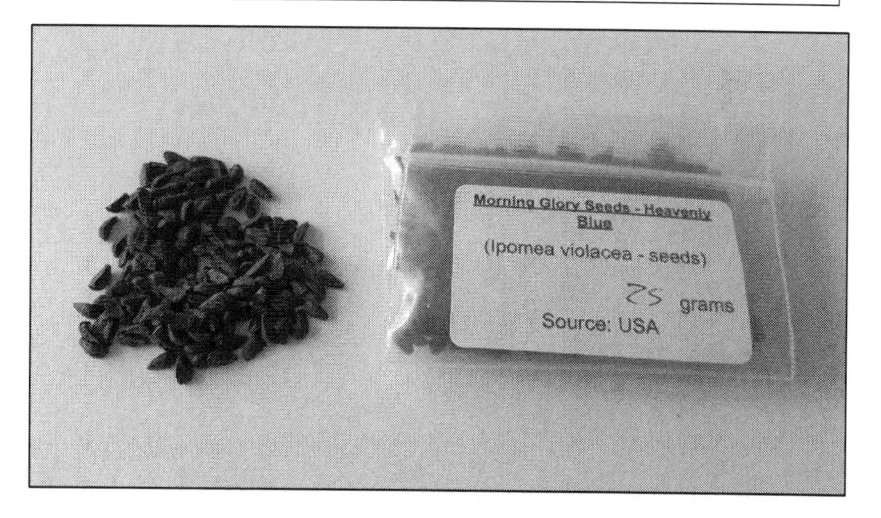

SUBJECTIVE EXPERIENCE
Ipomoea Violacea has a lengthy history of sacred and divinatory use, including by the Aztecs, the Chontal Indians and the Zapotec. In fact, in the Oaxaca region of Mexico, it continues to be held in high esteem for its visionary properties to this day.

Regarding preparation, the consensus seems to be that the seeds should be pulverised and added to water, with the resultant concoction being occasionally stirred and then refrigerated or left in a cool place at least overnight. Thereafter, the liquid is strained and drunk.

In his *Encyclopedia of Psychoactive* Plants, Rätsch broadly concurs "*The fewest side effects result from ingesting a cold-water extract of the ground or crushed seeds. Cold-water extracts have distinct hallucinogenic effects that are, however, not exactly the same as those of LSD.*"

The obvious question which arises, of course, is how many seeds should be used in this process? My research indicates that 50-100 is generally considered to be a light dose, 100-250 to be common, with anything over 400 to be heavy.

I opt to sample a relatively mild 100, partly because I am not drawn to the idea of eating so many seeds, and partly on account of having previously experienced HBWS and ololiuqui, both of which are also powered by LSA. I should note, however, that some Internet commentary equates this to about 100mcg of LSD, so in theory at least it should induce a solid experience. I expect an onset of about an hour, with perhaps a duration of around eight hours.

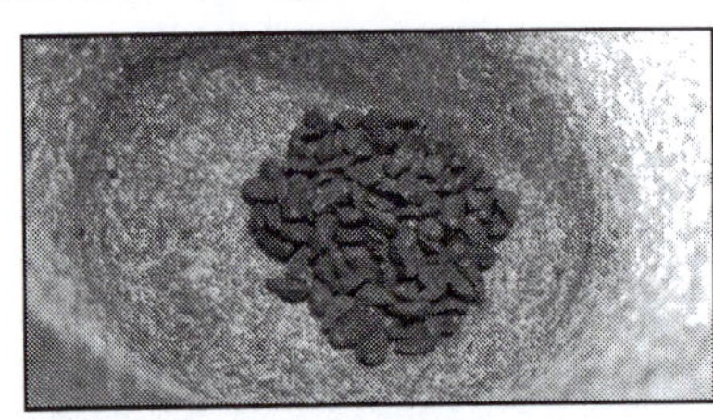

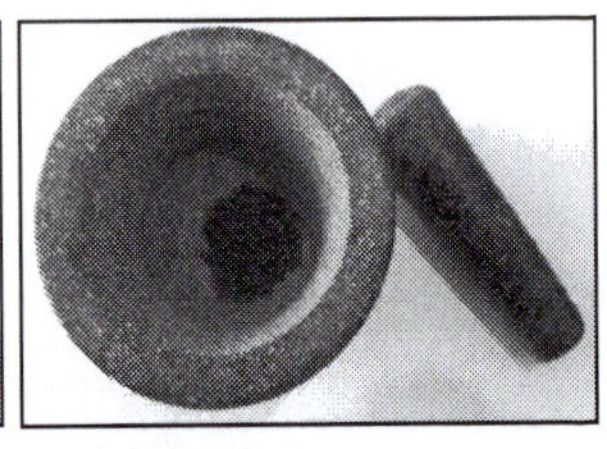

I begin the operation by mercilessly battering the 100 seeds with mortar and pestle. I then tip the wreckage into a half-full bottle of water, and occasionally swish this around. I place this into the fridge, returning occasionally during the day to swish again. I leave the bottle undisturbed overnight, shaking again the next day and then leave it for a second night. The following lunchtime, I strain my concoction into a glass through a scrap from an old shirt. I am ready to go.

> T+0:00 I swig the fluid down quickly. It doesn't taste so bad, although it does feel a little strange to the extent that my normal *modus operandi* with seeds is to swallow everything, including all the debris. [1:20pm]

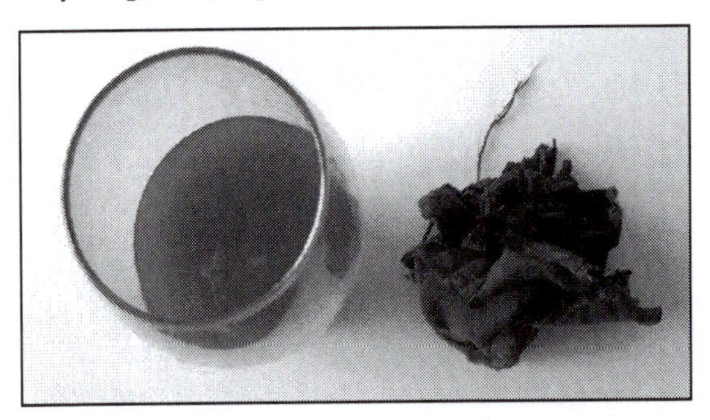

> T+0:30 Assuming that the concoction worked and the dose was sufficient the ride should soon commence. I already have the impression of a drifting psychedelic headiness, and I am warmer than earlier. Perhaps there is a hint of enhanced coloration in terms of vision. This is all very marginal but there is clearly something there.

T+1:00 There have been no major developments, although the headiness is now more intense. There is a hint of nausea rolling in and out, but only a hint. I feel like I am in the early stages of a trip, but an hour into the experience I do have doubts that it will actually take off and go anywhere.

On the upside, I feel that I have got at least something out of those seeds, which given my less than impressive record for preparations is a positive. With the mildly nauseous edge in the background, I could also, if I was really looking for silver-linings, consider that I have escaped some unpleasantness. I am definitely stretching it here though.

Remaining positive, yes, there is a psychedelic aura here, which ebbs and flows. If this was an LSD trip, at this point I would probably take a little more to intensify proceedings.

T+2:00 Whilst there are no OEVs or CEVS, a mild haze on vision is in play, with a familiar lazy drift as I turn my head. Behind this is the headspace, which has now solidified.

Overall this is reasonably nice, although nothing more. The uplift has been sufficient to remove prior anxieties, and it has created a fairly agreeable ambience.

Comparing it to an LSD dose, I would probably pitch it at around 50mcg. It is not too far away from the mark, and is certainly providing a psychedelic type vibe. Had I crushed the seeds to powder, and attended the concoction more conscientiously, it may have been pushing towards the 100mcg referred to earlier. These seeds have also been lying around for a few years, which may have had an impact on their efficacy.

T +3:00 Unexpectedly, the intensity has faded over the last hour. I ate a light meal 20 minutes ago, but I was already back on the way to base by then. The dying embers are still around, which largely comprise a positive mood and a slight headiness, but the main show appears to be over. Purely speculatively, could the fact that I drank this rather than ate it have played a role in the faster than anticipated turnover?

T+4:00 I am now very much in the afterglow phase.

Eight or so hours after ingestion, I settled into a good night's sleep, but perhaps with more vivid and recallable dreams than usual. In the morning I still felt some afterglow and headiness, but I was generally fine.

This was nice enough overall, and pretty solid for a while, without reaching any significant heights. It most definitely qualified as light rather than common on the generic scales, which is not to say that it wasn't pleasant.

A final note on supply: unless you are sure of the source, wash (soapy water) and dry the seeds prior to use, as some suppliers allegedly coat them with chemicals (such as fungicides).

3.2.10 Ololiuqui

Binomial / Botanical Name	Rivea Corymbosa
Street Names	N/A
Major Active Compound	LSA
Indigenous Source	Mexico, Latin America
Form	Seeds
RoA	Oral
Personal Rating On Shulgin Scale	++

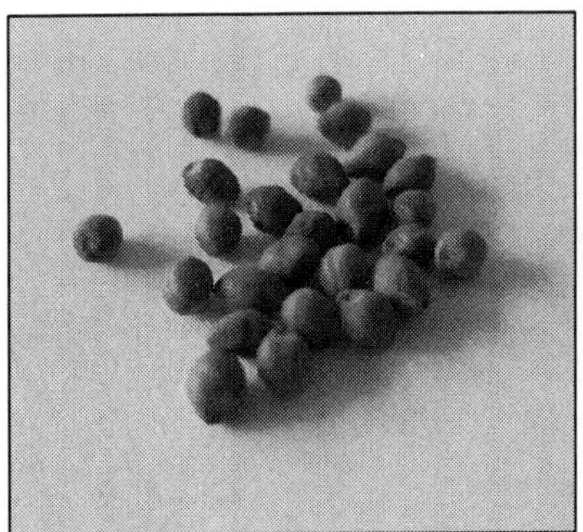

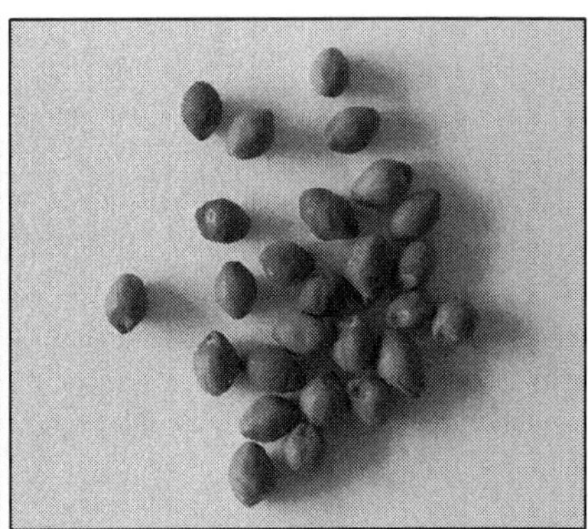

SUBJECTIVE EXPERIENCE
Ololiuqui seeds are known to have been ritually used by Indian groups in southern Mexico dating well back into the pre-Hispanic period. Their use amongst the Aztecs was subsequently documented by the Spanish, and they continue to be used to this day by various peoples of this region.

A variety of decoctions and preparations are recorded, most specifying the ingestion of between 10 and 15 seeds, but with the occasional outlier quoting a multiple of this. The most common form of concoction is to suffuse with water, with the following being quoted in *Plants of the Gods: "Thirteen seeds are usually ground up and drunk with water"*.

I sampled these about two years ago, broadly along the same lines. I prepared and consumed ten seeds, and still feeling fine after an hour, rapidly repeated the exercise with another five. I didn't take extensive notes, but did record a heavy + or light ++ on the adapted Shulgin scale.

This was certainly a psychedelic trip, but was neither immersive nor profound at this particular dose.

On this second occasion I consumed the same number, but in a single sitting. I used a mortar and pestle to crush the seeds more vigorously than the first time and placed the resultant compound into half a cup of water.

> T+0:00 I stir and swig the lot down in one. [11:30am]
>
> T+0:15 Earlier than expected I sense the slightest change of headspace. I momentarily focused upon my mindset immediately prior to the experiment, to provide a marker, and it is certainly in a different zone now. Accompanying this I feel some body chill and have cold hands, so I add a layer of clothes.
>
> T+0:30 There have been no significant developments during the last 15 minutes. The mind-play is still present, and vision is mildly softened. I have a marginally better sense of well-being than prior to initiation.
>
> T+0:45 The headspace is now solid at a gentle and relatively unobtrusive level, vision is still mellowed via the presence of a minor psychedelic sheen, and a general contentedness is clear. I would be happy if this went deeper, but this seems to be unlikely.
>
> T+1:00 At this point, the visual element has increased in intensity, as I detect the hint of a double-visioned haze. The breathing of objects in my peripheral vision is also evident (to a minor degree) as I dreamily stare. The headspace dwells within a comfortable but familiar psychedelic aura. There is no significant dilation of my pupils.
>
> T+1:45 I feel that the effects have weakened somewhat at this point. Although still present most facets of the experience have reduced in intensity. With the change, I notice a slight enhancement in visual acuity.
>
> T+3:00 I am now almost back to base. A drifting ambience remains, as does the mood lift and afterglow, but to all other intents and purposes the journey is over.

That mood lift and afterglow, and the dying embers of the general headspace, lingered for quite a few hours. This in itself was somewhat relaxing and provided a very gentle comedown. The night's sleep was good, other than being awakened via a third party disturbance.

This was an interesting and pleasant psychedelic ride, albeit flowing at a relatively modest level. Throughout, it intuitively felt like the consumption of more seeds would have induced a much stronger and sustained response.

Regarding body load, I felt no adverse reaction, other than some chilliness.

All things being equal I may well return to these seeds and dose a little higher on some future occasion.

3.2.11 Salvia Divinorum

Binomial / Botanical Name	*Salvia Divinorum*
Street Names	Salvia; Sally; SallyD
Major Active Compound	*Salvinorin A.*
Indigenous Source	Sierra Mazatec Region of Mexico
Form	Plant Material Extract
RoA	Smoked
Personal Rating On Shulgin Scale	+++

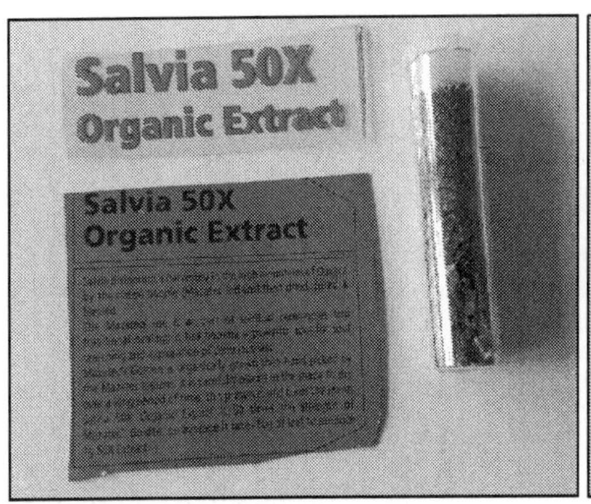

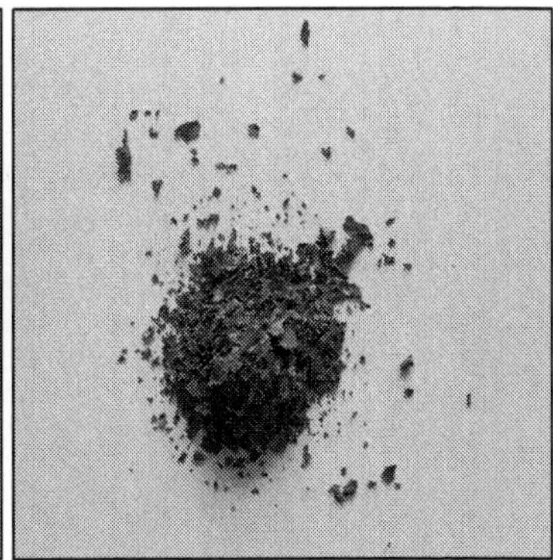

SUBJECTIVE EXPERIENCE
My experiences with salvia divinorum bear little resemblance to those of the shamans, as reported in literature. This is surely due to the fact that they chewed, whilst I smoked. Indeed, I smoked *extracts* on each of my three trips, rather than the raw plant itself, and these were of the order of 50x.

These forays were not pleasant. Each time I was overwhelmed, largely by fear. This was despite the fact that on the last two occasions I thought I had it nailed.

The first trip took me completely by surprise: I do mean completely, given that I thought I had purchased some sort of cannabinoid. For the second I was better prepared: I lay on a bed in the dark to contemplate. For the third, I had a sitter. Regardless of circumstance, however, I felt myself leaving my bodily existence and hanging on, or trying to hang on, in abject terror.

Colour became bright, edges became extremely sharp, and everything seemed to be morphing in a terrifying manner, stacking into an infinity of two dimensional layers. None of this was helped by the fact that I was inexperienced: these were amongst my earliest expeditions into the deliriant /psychedelic world

During each trip I had the curious notion that I was in a realm from which I could see different timelines unfolding and inviting in front of me. Also, that there was some form of intelligence there, which was aloof, and which was not necessarily benign. Indeed, the undertones were sinister.

I felt at the time that I got nothing out of these, at least in a positive sense. I now realise that the long-term value of the insights and perspectives I gained from them was in fact significant, even if the experiences themselves were traumatic.

The three trips were recorded as follows:

> TRIP #1
> I took a single hit of my apparent cannabinoid in the garden, from my small portable bong. I then walked slowly through the kitchen towards my office, when it struck me: suddenly.
>
> Rather than a mellowing and glowing relaxation, there was sharpness to edges, and there was a transposed repetition of objects like they were stacked behind each other multiple times. There was the immediate understanding that I was gripped by something and it wasn't a cannabinoid!
>
> Yes, I was terrified, as I stumbled into the office. Sinking to my hands and knees I crawled, and somehow pulled myself up into my chair.
>
> Everything on the computer screen presented the same stacked manifestation, with each window being repeated behind itself into the distance. I hit the keyboard in panic, obviously to no effect.
>
> How long would this last? Had I permanently damaged myself? Had I really done it this time?
>
> I was overcome by the fear that I might never return to normality.
>
> Eventually, I did start to return, to my enormous gratitude and relief. I managed to walk back into the kitchen. As I stood I felt something very strange. I felt connected to others, not through memory but through some strange sense; a sense that was in fact focused through a lens of compassion. This passed quickly, and could have been related to the overwhelming sense of relief that I was still feeling, but I distinctly recall it to this day.
>
> Of course, as soon as I was able, I researched *salvia divinorum* via the Internet, and the cause of this apparent derangement became clear.
>
> TRIP #2
> On the second occasion I planned the experience carefully, and I thought I was ready. I drew the curtains in my bedroom and lay on the bed. I was fearful of walking and hurting myself so I blocked the door.

Unfortunately, the preparation and anticipation did not mitigate the shock. It was still harrowing. The same sliced manifestation of reality occurred, with the same infinity of 2D layers morphing before me.

I sensed some other entity, possibly hostile, and had to suppress the urge to negotiate and plead for my safe return.

The experience was again other-worldly. I felt as though I was being sucked out of this reality, into some other. Perhaps this is why some of the people in those YouTube trip videos appear to pull against some invisible non-existent force.

This feeling induced panic. I didn't want to go, and I sensed that the anomalous presence was not benevolent. I swore myself to be a force for good, as I felt like I was bargaining for my life.

Fearing that I was leaving this realm for ever, I thought about my family, and all that I valued. I felt a primal need to fight to stay: I got off the bed and pushed my way out of the door.

As I lurched onto the landing, I thought momentarily that I was recovering, but I wasn't.

I found myself looking up the stairs to the third floor, and again, the notion occurred that I was looking at alternative timelines, or parallel worlds. The thought that I might return to the wrong one suddenly struck me, as my usual surroundings felt so alien and unfamiliar. In some of those worlds, it seemed that the house even had the wrong number of floors.

Things still didn't seem to be right as I shuffled down the stairs, but I was slowly emerging and returning to normality. When I came round sufficiently, I called family and friends, just to connect and to make sure that all was well and that I had found my way back into the correct slice of the continuum.

TRIP #3
This was a chicken trip; meaning that I barely inhaled. I did, however, smoke enough to skirt around the experience and semi immerse.

The same feelings were prevalent, but having someone present gave me a firmer anchor of this reality. I was still scared, very scared, as I stared into the threatening space which enveloped me, and I recall that again I tried to open dialogue, through panic.

As this slowly wore off I swore that I wouldn't put myself through it again.

Despite all this, if I ever find the opportunity to engage this interesting plant through its traditional and shamanic oral route, I will probably take it. Otherwise: no chance!

AN ANECDOTAL TALE (THE BLAST)
As I approached the counter in the head shop, a young man, perhaps 20 years of age, was stood directly in front of me, dithering. He pointed at a colourful packet which sat on the display, and mumbled words to the effect that he and his friends wanted to have "*a blast*".

The sales attendant couldn't help or advise, and would only respond to his questions with the legally prescribed mantra: "*It's not for human consumption*".

I then noticed that our young test pilot was pointing at a sachet of salvia divinorum (60x extract).

This rang alarm bells: his mates were clearly hiding around the corner outside, and they were likely to smoke this stuff somewhere in the street, with no idea at all of the effect they would be inducing.

Salvia wouldn't give them a *blast*; it would detonate the unexpected trauma of an out-of-body experience, potentially in a packed street, potentially on a busy road. I felt compelled to intervene.

I tried to explain, but the guy had clearly been drinking alcohol.

What to do?

I looked for the safest bet on offer on the presentation stand, and referred him to a well known stimulant. I explained that this was a terrible idea (given his alcohol consumption), but that snorting a stim would on balance be more likely to give him a good time, and less likely to lead to a nasty accident in the middle of the city.

He bought my logic, and purchased.

The assistant then smiled at me and said "*Well done. Are you his dad or just a good Samaritan?*"

Then it took a turn for the worse.

The kid returned, and asked for the salvia instead. It appeared that the scare story had appealed to his foolhardy mates. So off he went, armed with his *blast*, to take him directly to la-la land.

I am pretty certain that one toke on the salvia joint (which is how they planned to smoke it) will have demonstrated that my every word had been correct. I sincerely hope that their lesson was learned in a park or somewhere quiet, rather than in a place of potentially fatal danger.

You can't win 'em all.

3.2.12 San Pedro Cactus

Binomial / Botanical Name	Echinopsis Pachanoi
Street Names	San Pedro
Major Active Compound	Mescaline
Indigenous Source	Ecuador
Form	Powdered Plant Matter
RoA	Oral
Personal Rating On Shulgin Scale	+++

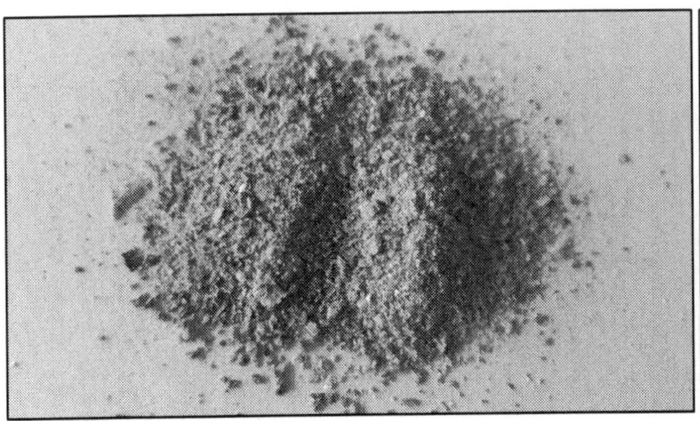

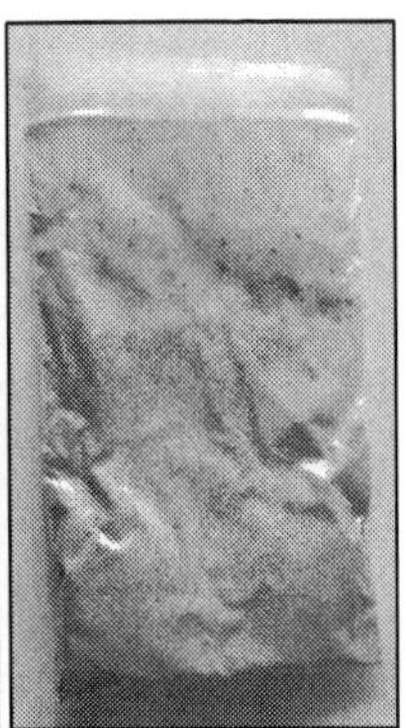

SUBJECTIVE EXPERIENCE

The san pedro cactus has been in continuous spiritual and medicinal use in Peru for over 3,000 years. This even survived post Spanish Conquest attempts to suppress it.

I had originally booked a *San Pedro Experience* whilst I was on my ayahuasca mission, but I was far too ill to proceed (due to a mixture of altitude sickness and a bug I imported from the UK). I did, however, benefit from a detailed introduction to this remarkable cactus, and its shamanic use, as the organizer was generous enough to spend time with me and provide a degree of education.

The psychoactive part of the cactus is layered just inside the skin. Apparently, this is scraped off, and then dried and turned to powder. I have also seen this sold on the markets as "chips", which are simply cut from the plant.

Regarding dosage, I researched this heavily, particularly online, but with little joy. To put it mildly, the forums were all over the place: some posters cited modest amounts; others suggested doses which bordered on the ludicrous. It was very hard to find any real consensus.

I therefore asked the vendor, which was tricky given that this was sold as "*not for human consumption*". However, through various coded messages, I eventually got there: 25g should be sufficient for a first dose.

This did seem to be sensible, and looking at toxicity data for mescaline, it wouldn't create undue risk. I therefore placed this measure into a large mug, and poured boiling water upon it. I stirred occasionally.

Over the next half hour I sipped this slowly. It was revolting, but I had tasted worse. I then sat back and waited, not really expecting too much. My pessimism was wholly misplaced.

Soon, I was flying high, and I knew that I was still coming-up. At one point I felt momentary alarm, wondering how far this would go. Fortunately this passed as the mescaline pulled me along with a significant mood lift. I knew I was tripping hard.

My expectation had been set by the many posts across social media, and substantially by those who claimed similarity with LSD. So was it really like LSD?

Yes and no. It was certainly LSD*ish* in broad terms, with similar visuals, general headspace and so forth, but there were real differences. It did seem to be more natural although I have to accept that knowing that this was a botanical could have influenced this perception. The wave I felt myself riding felt richer in nature, and the euphoric edge felt more intense.

The nausea I had anticipated didn't materialize, which was a bonus. The bottom line was that I really enjoyed it. It was intense, it was compelling, and it was profound. It was a ride I was not expecting. I was floating for hours, well into +++ territory.

In terms of recording the trip I was ill prepared, as I had expected merely to scratch the surface: hence the brevity of this report. This in no way does justice to this remarkable cactus.

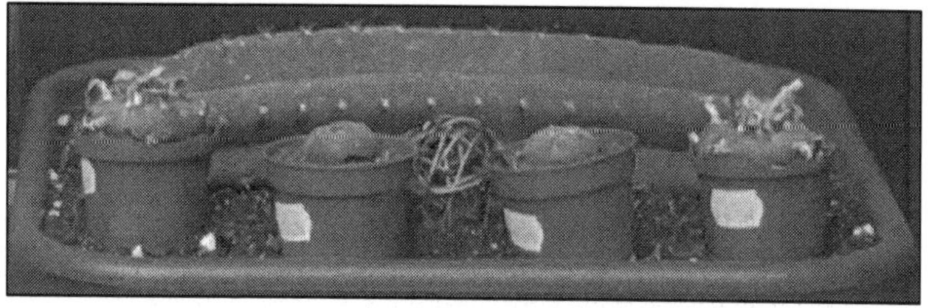

A nice fat chunk of san pedro sitting behind some peyote buttons

I fully intend to repeat this exercise, as I feel certain that it has much to offer in terms of personal development.

3.2.13 Sensory Deprivation

After my remarkable experience with shirodhara, my mind was well and truly open to the possibility of another hallucinogenic episode without using drugs, although I didn't actually expect to encounter anything. Indeed I didn't, until some years later, when I heard Robert Anton Wilson refer to floatation tanks in a YouTube lecture. These are also known as isolation tanks and sensory deprivation tanks and enable a silent darkness float in skin-temperature salted water.

Researching this further I found all sorts of people claiming psychedelic-like experiences and deep meditative states. Even Wikipedia chimed in:

> *"Short-term sessions of sensory deprivation are described as relaxing and conducive to meditation; however, extended or forced sensory deprivation can result in extreme anxiety, hallucinations, bizarre thoughts, temporary senselessness and depression."*

Subsequently, an opportunity to engage arose courtesy of Koan Float in Amsterdam. On arrival I was shown to my float-room, where I stepped into the tank. I chose silence as the audio option (as opposed to supportive music), closed my eyes, and floated. I waited, expectantly, for something to happen.

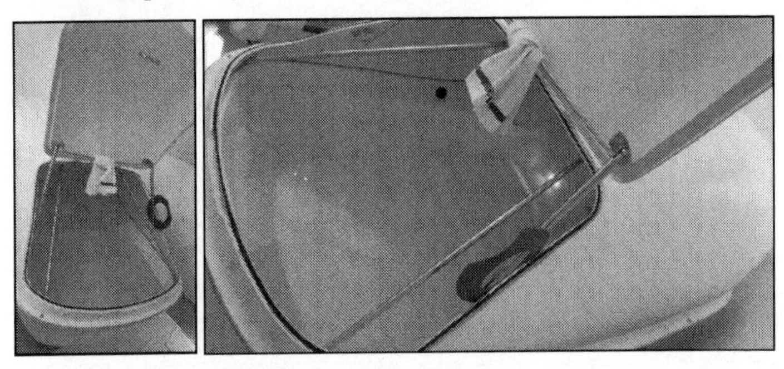

This was certainly relaxing, if somewhat fidgety and unexciting; which was probably caused by an active state of mind and my inability to meditate properly. I did find some interesting thought patterns but little else. I also lost track of time and somehow missed the end-buzzer, such that when the tank started to drain I thought that this was some sort of water massage. Eventually a voice came over the speaker to ask if I was okay. I suspect that I made a bit of an idiot of myself.

I should add here that others who were there at the same time claimed awake-dream-states and a variety of other manifestations, which added to my frustration.

Overall it was a glorious failure. Certainly, on reflection I should have selected music to carry me along, I should have approached the exercise relaxed and not hyped, and I should have done more research. However, I am told that success rates are higher the second time, so should another opportunity arise, I will give it another go.

3.2.14 Shirodhara

Binomial / Botanical Name	Various Herbal Oils
Street Names	Shirodhara
Major Active Compound	N/A
Indigenous Source	India
Form	External Therapy
RoA	N/A
Personal Rating On Shulgin Scale	++

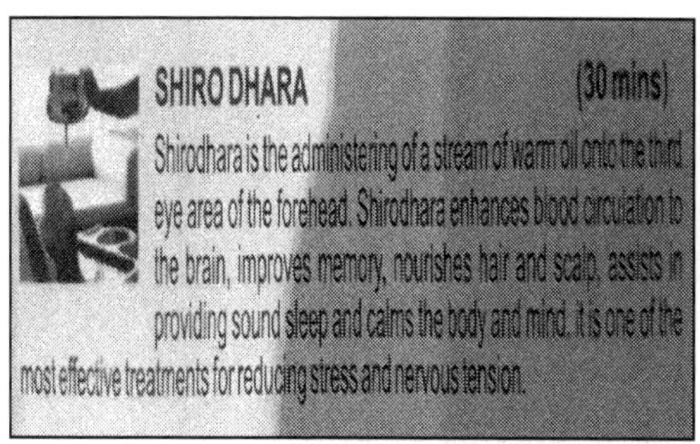

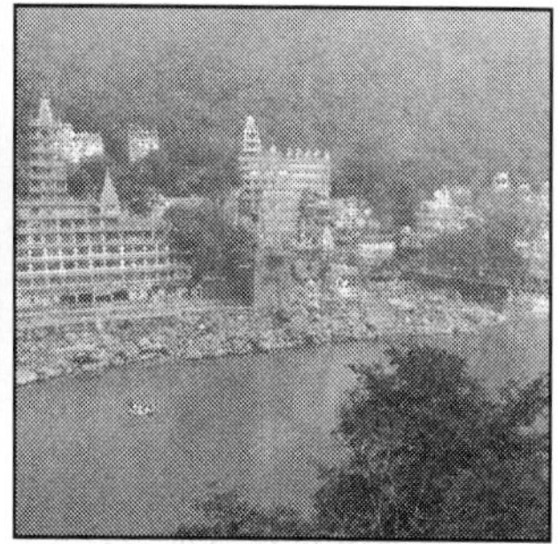

SUBJECTIVE EXPERIENCE
I know how this will sound to some people; largely because I may have been one of them had I not been the subject of the experience. It sounds wacky and unscientific, and I may come across as an unhinged freak (assuming I haven't done so already). Nonetheless, the story, which is true, unfolded as described below.

In December 2015 I visited Rishikesh, India, in the foothills of the Himalayas. This is famed as part of the 60's hippy trail, as the Maharishi Mahesh guru retreat of the Beatles, and as a world centre for yoga. This region is also at the heart of an ancient medicinal practice called *ayurveda*, historical variants of which dispense medicines containing opium and other psychoactive substances.

The tale I am about to impart, however, does not directly relate to consumption of a substance or the compelling beauty of the place itself, but rather, a totally unexpected aspect of the ayurvedic tradition.

Whilst talking to someone who had been there for a while, I was referred to a remedy called *shirodhara*. This wasn't a drug, but a treatment, which involved the pouring of hot oils onto the forehead. The interesting aspect of this is that these are poured directly on the spot behind which the *third eye* sits (commonly considered to be the pineal gland). I was told it would clear the mind and help me to relax.

Although this sounded like a glorified head massage, I duly attended, expecting the equivalent of a nice head rub and a rest. I lay flat on the bed, with pads covering my eyes, and the oils gently flowed: hot cool, hot cool, hot cool, with an occasional gentle massage. The hot was very hot; almost scalding.

Rather surprisingly I entered what felt like a pre-psychedelic headspace. This was nothing to write home about: it was the sort of feeling experienced when a trip is about to commence, but before it actually has. I put this down to some sort of meditative auto-suggestion and a possible pre-disposition due to fatigue.

However, then came a flash: an image of an African woman's head. Whoa! This was hallucinogenic! Disappointingly, this disappeared as quickly as it came, but shortly thereafter I had another, similar vision, involving a steam train. Then the overall experience faded as I mentally sought to compose and re-establish myself.

The picture was there for an instant, and then it was gone, but it was clear and distinct. Moments later there was a repeat, with a different picture. This took me entirely by surprise, and I spent the rest of the session coming to terms with it. The shock of this unexpected manifestation was somewhat unnerving.

Outside, I sought my hippie friend. She got in first "*What did you see? Did you see it?*" I most certainly did. She then described her own visions, which were more lucid and longer lasting than mine.

After this I rushed back to my accommodation and searched the Internet. Sure enough I found a variety of references. The following were typical:

> "*And the renowned Shirodhara treatment where they drip oil on your forehead, causing you to have wild dreams and hallucinations*"
>
> "*The rhythm of the oil trickling onto the third eye, which is the seat of our cognitive vision*" "*awakens the cognitive vision*",
>
> "*To say that I was in an altered state is an understatement. During the session, I had unusual pictures coming constantly into my vision*"

I even found claims (unsubstantiated) that shirodhara causes the brain to release pinoline and DMT.

Whatever the cause, it was as real as any other psychedelic manifestation I have experienced, before or since. Its validity was also verified by an independent third party.

Despite knowing that this actually happened, I still find it difficult to assimilate, given that nothing had entered my body. However, it isn't something I will ever forget, and it certainly opened my mind to a new frontier of possibilities.

3.2.15 Sinicuichi

Binomial / Botanical Name	Heimia Salicifolia
Street Names	Sun Opener; Shrubby Yellowcrest
Major Active Compound	Unknown
Indigenous Source	The Americas
Form	Leaves
RoA	Oral
Personal Rating On Shulgin Scale	±

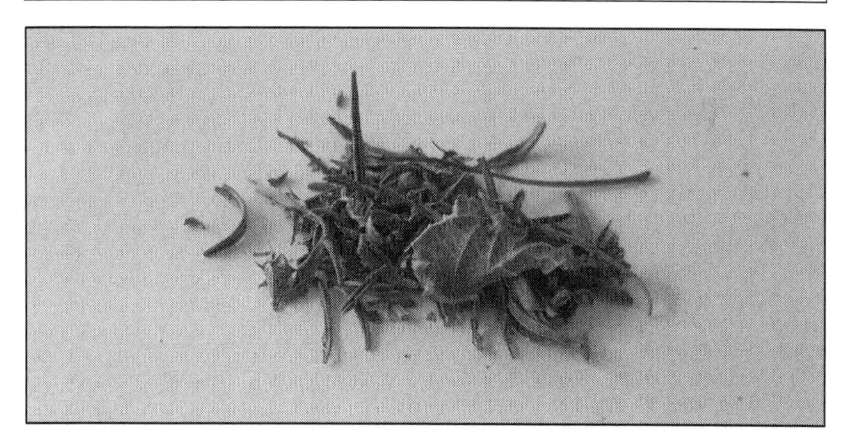

SUBJECTIVE EXPERIENCE
Although it isn't saying a lot, this experiment entailed one of the most convoluted preparations I have ever performed. It was a glorious failure.

I had created the decoction by mixing the material with water in a jar, placing it in the sun, maintaining it at the appropriate temperature, and tending it regularly and carefully.

The next day, when I eventually drank it: absolutely nothing.

To be fair, I knew the risks. Field reports of success are very few and far between, and its psychoactivity is disputed. However, the temptation of a unique form of psychedelic experience, including auditory hallucinations, proved too much for me, and I went for it.

Notwithstanding this, sinicuichi is documented in *Plants of the Gods*, including reference to its indigenous use, so I may well have missed a trick.

3.2.16 Syrian Rue

Binomial / Botanical Name	Peganum Harmala
Street Names	Esfand; Aspand; Harmel
Major Active Compound	Misc (Incl Harmaline and Harmine)
Indigenous Source	India, Pakistan, S Asia, Middle East
Form	Seeds
RoA	Oral
Personal Rating On Shulgin Scale	++

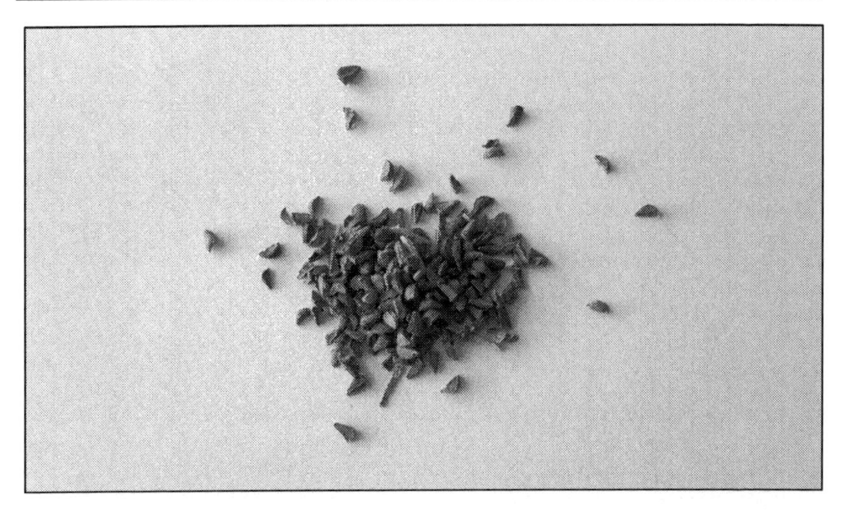

SUBJECTIVE EXPERIENCE
Often used as a component of ayahuasca analogues, Syrian rue is an MAOI which induces psychedelic effects in its own right. Its seeds have been in continual use in rites and ceremonies across various cultures for thousands of years, and indeed, it has been cited as a possible ingredient of the legendry Vedic brew, *soma*.

Online, a number of different preparations are suggested, usually involving boiling in acidified water (for example, water with lemon juice). However, whilst it does seem to be generally agreed that this reduces instances of nausea, I found there to be a great deal of contradiction in terms of it diminishing or increasing psychoactive effectiveness.

As I was not able to reach a firm conclusion on this matter, I elected to consume the raw seeds, as documented by sources such as Azarius.com:

"There are many ways to consume Syrian rue. The easiest way is to just chew upon the seeds. You have to hold them in your mouth for about two minutes, chew well and make sure they get in touch with your saliva as much as possible before you swallow them. Unfortunately, the taste is very bitter. It's, therefore, more comfortable to grind the seeds (for example with a pester and mortar or in a coffee grinder).

Regarding dosage, 2g-5g is widely suggested across forums and websites alike, with 3g being most commonly proposed for a first time encounter. I decide to heed this advice, which by most accounts will be effective but won't blow me away.

Before proceeding I revisit my own research on the use of MAOIs, which is referred to in other parts of this book. Wider afield, on Syrian rue specific threads I notice that multiple sources cite problematic examples which include aged cheese, various preservatives, red wine, and fermented foods. Exercising caution, I will maintain a very strict plain diet for at least 12 hours before and a day after ingestion. [NOTE: If in doubt on what foods to avoid it is worth consulting one of the many lists published on the Internet.]

Regarding duration this is not particularly well documented, but I anticipate a ride lasting 5 hours or so, and an onset of about 45 minutes.

With all preparations completed, I am finally ready to go.

T+0.00 I carefully weigh my seeds and crush them mercilessly with mortar and pestle.

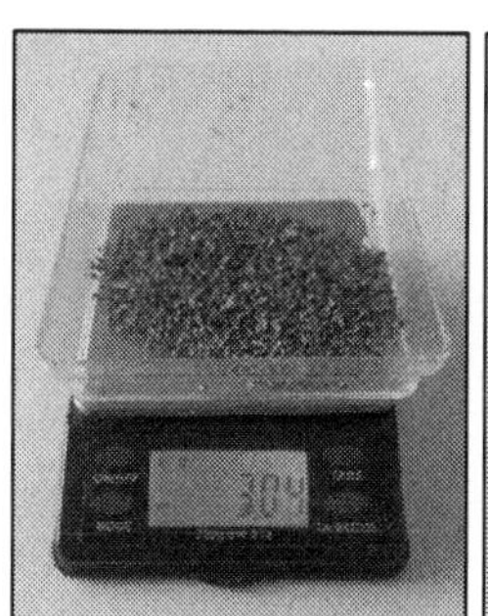

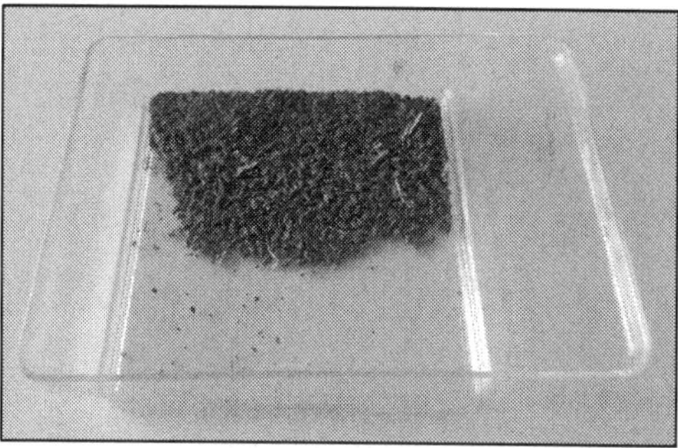

I now pour the resultant compound, which is more half-ground than powder, on to a large spoon and attempt to chew. This doesn't last very long as it is dry and pretty unpleasant. After a few moments I swill everything down the hatch with fresh orange juice. [2:15pm]

T+0:15 I am beginning to notice a change in my body temperature, with the familiar hint of a pre-psychedelic headspace there or thereabouts.

T+0:30 There is certainly a drifting headiness in play and something is starting to happen to my vision: nothing intense but not placebo driven either.

T+1:00 The mild psychedelic aura is now unmistakeable, with a lazy visual tracing impression to accompany it when I turn my head.

I am mentally in a reasonable place, and physically I feel well, with no indication of nausea, other than perhaps a heavy stomach.

T+1:45 Somewhat disappointingly the ride appears to have stabilised. There is definitely an established presence, manifested largely through the headspace and that gentle hazy vision. Physically there is some warmth, accompanied by slightly cold and clammy hands. My mood is good and there are no real negatives thus far.

T+2:00 There are no fireworks, but I do feel content and mellow, with the misty mindset ebbing and flowing gently in the background. Pleasant it is, spectacular it isn't.

T+3:00 Although I am still in the same zone, at this point I feel a little flatter. This is not uncomfortable; it is simply a sense that the main event is winding down. I eat a slice of toast and take in some fruit.

T+4:00 I am now heading back to base, wallowing amongst the dying embers of the trip. A dreamy sense of well-being is still present, but it hovers at a relatively low level

T+7:45 As expected, the effects faded during the previous hours and I retire to bed at about 10pm.

The night's sleep was fairly standard, but I had a slightly off-key heady feel when I awoke in the morning: not a headache or anything uncomfortable, but something lurking there in the background.

Whilst this ride didn't light any fires, it was nonetheless fairly decent. I was certainly playing in the shallow end but the vibe was a fairly positive one.

A fair assessment is that I hoped for more, but I got at least something. Were these limitations down to dosage, or the preparation, or the age of the seeds? Or was it simply that I now expect too much, due to other stronger psychedelic experiences? I suspect more of the latter, as I do know that Syrian rue has its enthusiasts, and not only as an MAOI.

On this note I will stress one final time the need for research and caution with respect to food, and anything else you may be tempted to indulge in when using these seeds. This is a powerful botanical, and must always be used with care and common sense.

3.2.17 Yopo

Binomial / Botanical Name	Anadenanthera Peregrina
Street Names	Yopo
Major Active Compound	Bufotenin
Indigenous Source	South America
Form	Seeds
RoA	Insufflated
Personal Rating On Shulgin Scale	++

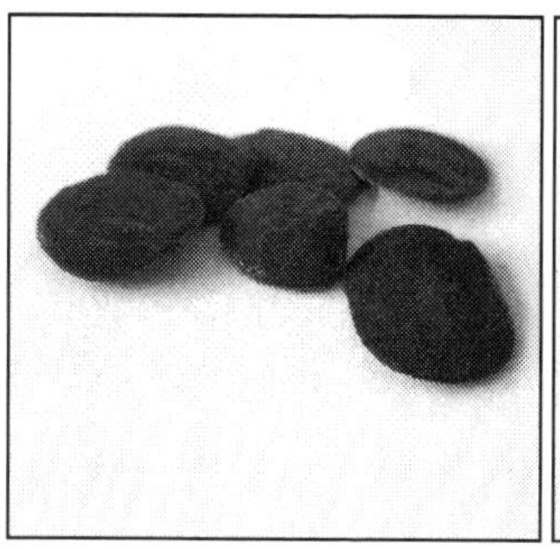

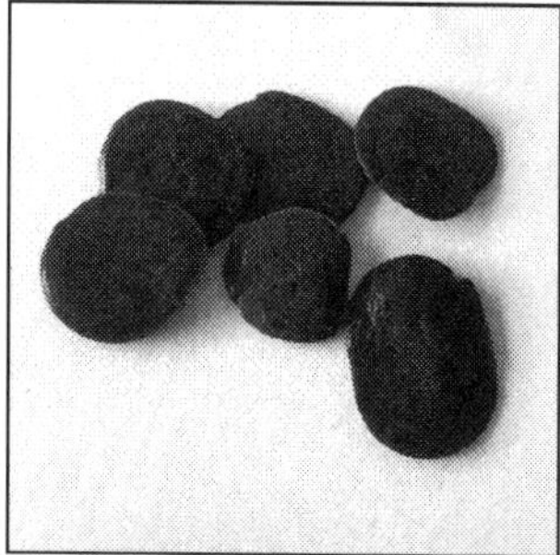

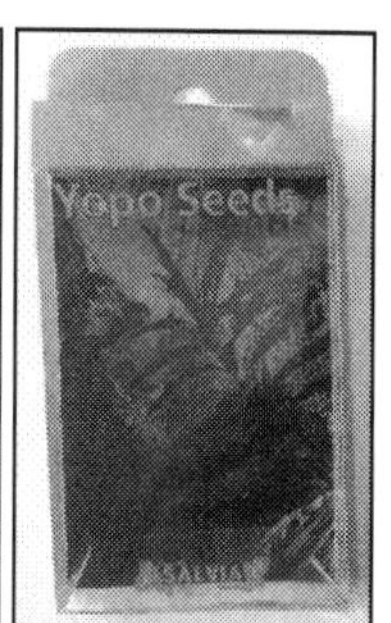

SUBJECTIVE EXPERIENCE
Yopo seeds are sometimes confused with cebil seeds, presumably because they look similar, and are both generally insufflated. They are not the same, either in terms of chemical composition, or with respect to the experience itself.

Having stated this, I did prepare them both in the same manner: I toasted half-a-dozen in a pan until they snapped like popcorn. Removing the shells, I then pulverised the kernel. I sampled this raw, and also, mixed it with some lime powder.

I had anticipated pain largely due to descriptions of authentic use: one member of the tribe blows it forcibly up the nostril of a colleague via a long pipe, who in some accounts, then rolls around on the ground in agony. Self administered, I found that it did indeed hurt: a lot!

The headspace emerged within seconds, and simple CEVs quickly followed. There was no significant complexity but they were there, and they were fluid. The downer was that the experience faded within 5 minutes or so. The afterglow lingered for some hours.

Undoubtedly, I have plenty more work to do with these seeds, assuming that I can overcome the enduring memory of the nasal pain.

3.3. STIMULANTS

Textbook Definition: *Stimulants improve mental and/or physical capability or functions. Manifestations of this can include alertness, wakefulness, focus, and apparent increased energy.*

The following botanicals have been sampled and researched for inclusion within this section:

Most people are aware, via consumption of tea and coffee, that some botanicals can produce stimulation. A smaller number understand that cocaine is derived from the coca plant. However, whilst these are the standard bearers in terms of public perception, they barely scratch the surface.

Each individual stimulant comes with its own character, and many have a rich heritage in terms of cultural and historical use. A number are multi-faceted, inducing a variety of psychoactive effects.

Whilst these were not the easiest of materials to source and experience, they were certainly worth the effort.

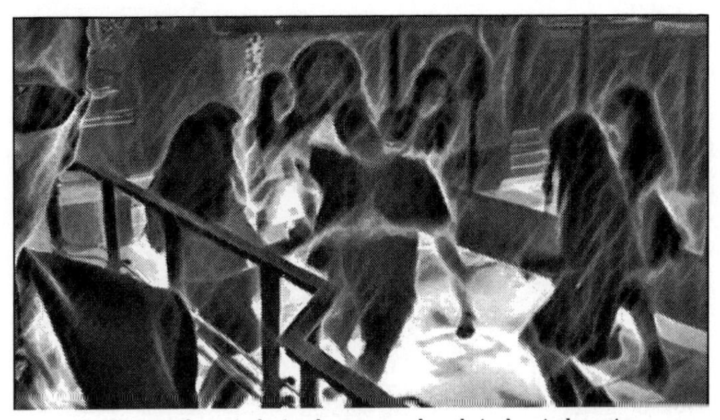

Don't expect botanical stimulants to emulate their chemical cousins

3.3.1 Betel Nut

Binomial / Botanical Name	Areca Catechu
Street Names	Betel
Major Active Compound	Arecoline
Indigenous Source	Tropical Pacific, Asia, East Africa
Form	Nut
RoA	Chewed/Quidded
Personal Rating On Shulgin Scale	+**

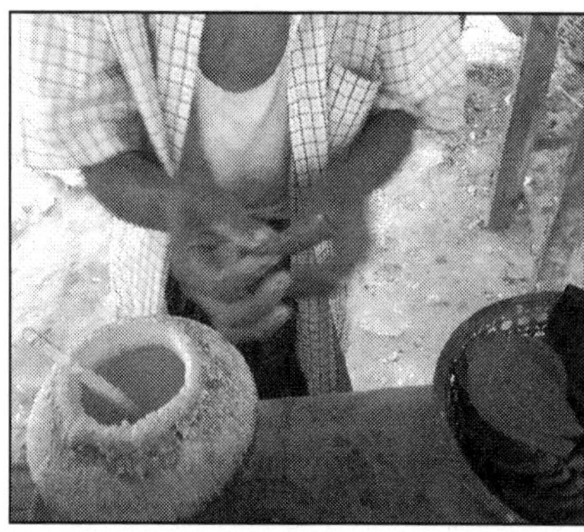
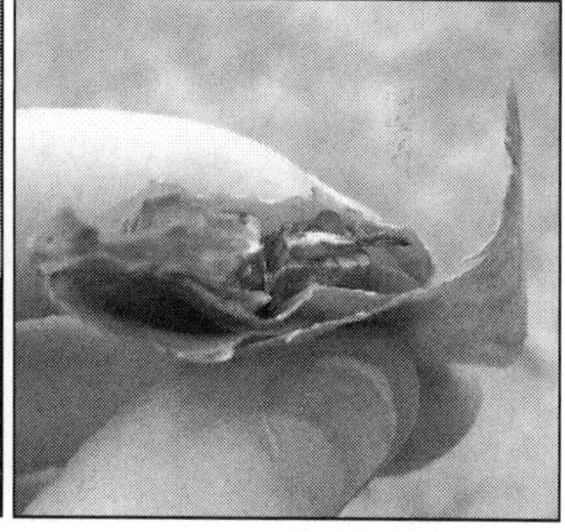

SUBJECTIVE EXPERIENCE
Betel nuts have traditionally been chewed across a number of Asian and Oceanic countries, and in some they remain extremely popular. I obtained my samples via the Internet, from two different sources, only to be disappointed. They were like lumps of concrete, and were totally useless. This equally applied to a third sample which was pre-sliced on delivery.

Eventually, I experienced the real deal in the more ethnic setting of Mandalay, in Myanmar. These were sold from portable stalls, which were dotted around the city, and chewed by locals of every shape and size.

The nuts themselves were crushed, mixed with some sort of slaked lime type powder, and wrapped in leaves. As a foreigner I was given one such treat *on the house* by a friendly street vendor.

The nuts were still hard, but I chewed and sucked as instructed. The effects came on quite quickly.

I would describe the stimulation as caffeine-like, but cleaner, with more clarity and with no jittery edge. As I walked around the pagoda district I was consciously aware that I was stimulated. What appeared to be slightly enhanced visual acuity was another reminder.

This was in fact quite pleasant, and it lasted for several hours.

Would I sample it again should the opportunity arise? Yes, certainly, provided that it was in a similarly authentic setting.

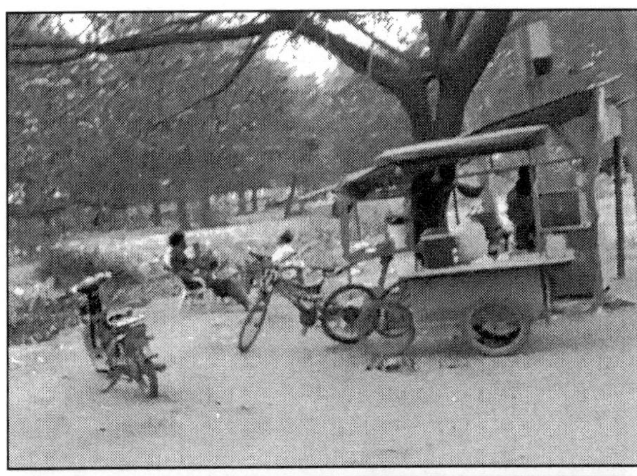

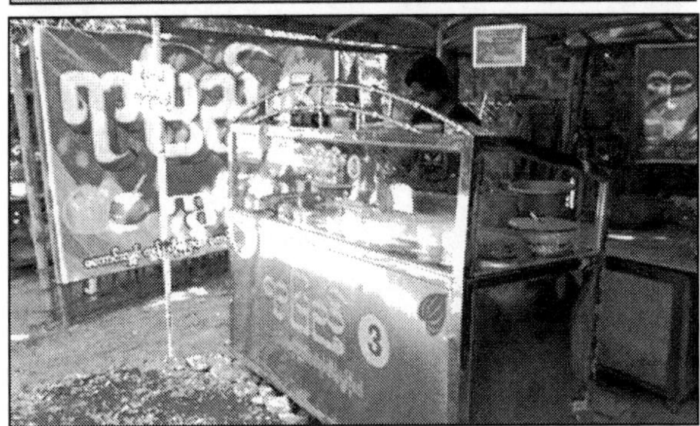

Typical betel nut stalls in Mandalay
[Bottom photo courtesy of C Brown]

Note that, contrary to the headline name of *betel nut*, the nuts are actually areca nuts, although the leaves are betel leaves (piper betel). As an interesting aside, it is sometimes claimed that areca nut is the fourth most commonly used psychoactive substance in the world (following caffeine, nicotine and alcohol).

3.3.2 Coca

Binomial / Botanical Name	Coca
Street Names	Coca de Java
Major Active Compound	Cocaine
Indigenous Source	South America (High Altitude)
Form	Leaves
RoA	Oral
Personal Rating On Shulgin Scale	+

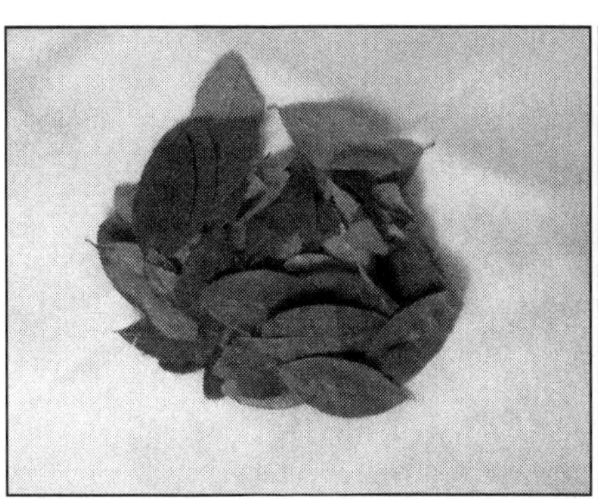

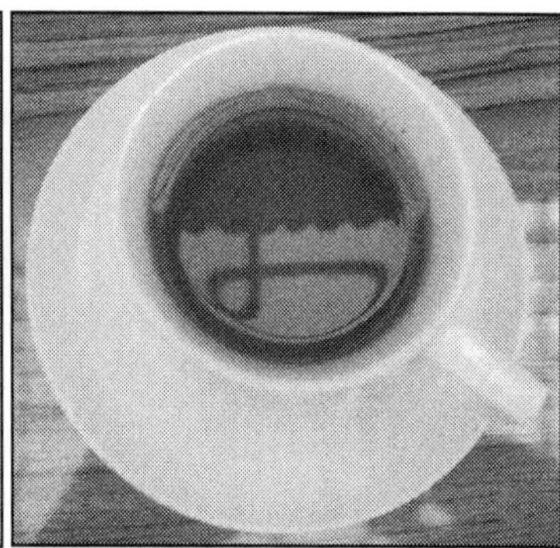

SUBJECTIVE EXPERIENCE
I tested coca in its native Peru, whilst on my ayahuasca mission. It was always my intention to sample this, although perhaps not as intensively as I was compelled to when I actually arrived.

Whilst in Cusco, at 11,000 feet, I quickly succumbed to what seemed to be altitude sickness. The local remedy for such a condition, as proffered by hotel staff, shop keepers and other tourists, was to chew coca leaves, and drink coca tea. I did both, in great abundance.

It did appear to induce a mild but clean feeling of stimulation. I am slightly hesitant in stating this categorically because my condition was poor and deteriorating: a general malaise and severe headache made it a difficult reaction to measure. All I really wanted was for the leaves to make me feel a little better. They didn't.

Of course, I cannot state with any certainty that they didn't stop me feeling even worse, but the stimulation was quite minor, considering what is often derived from it (cocaine). I should add that, regardless, it was quite pleasant to drink.

3.3.3 Ephedra

Binomial / Botanical Name	Ephedra Sinica;
Street Names	Ma Huang; Chinese Ephedra
Major Active Compound	Ephedrine
Indigenous Source	Northern China
Form	Powdered leaves
RoA	Oral
Personal Rating On Shulgin Scale	+*

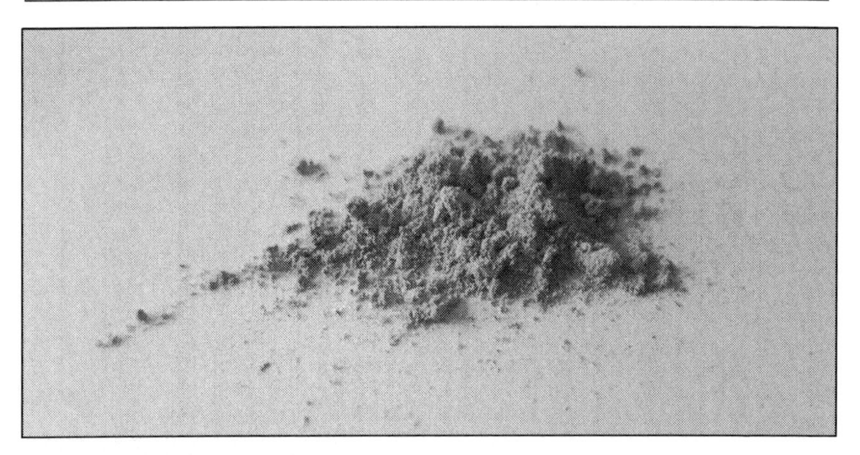

SUBJECTIVE EXPERIENCE
Ephedra sinica has been used in China as a herbal medicine for thousands of years. Independent use by indigenous peoples in various parts of the world has also been documented.

Wikipedia describes its history as follows:

> "*Ephedra sinica (also known as Chinese ephedra or Ma Huang) is a plant species native to Mongolia, Russia (Buryatiya, Chita, Primorye), and northeastern China. Ephedra is a medicinal preparation from the plant Ephedra sinica. Several additional species belonging to the genus ephedra have traditionally been used for a variety of medicinal purposes, and are a possible candidate for the Soma plant of Indo-Iranian religion. It has been used in traditional Chinese medicine for more than 2,000 years*"

With respect to its psychoactivity, the same article states that:

> "*Of the six ephedrine-type ingredients found in ephedra (at concentrations of 0.02-3.4%), the most common are ephedrine and pseudoephedrine. The stimulant and thermogenic effects of Ephedra sinica and other ephedra species are due to the presence of the alkaloids ephedrine and pseudoephedrine. These compounds stimulate the brain, increase heart rate, constrict blood vessels (increasing blood pressure), and expand bronchial tubes (making breathing easier). Their thermogenic properties cause an increase in metabolism, as evidenced by an increase in body heat*"

In terms of its use as a recreational stimulant, ephedra sinica is traditionally consumed as a tea. Regarding dose, there are few guidelines, although the following blog-comment seems to represent a fair reflection of general Internet opinion:

> "*So, Ephedra tea requires between 0.5 – 2.5 grams of Ephedra tea preparation per person on average to start feeling any effect at all. And the maximum dosage should never exceed 3 – 7.5 grams per person on average*"
> ~ simonsblogpark.com

Comforted by its long term indigenous use, I decided to go for 2.5g. I boiled the kettle and poured the water directly on to the powdered plant, making an average sized cup.

I waited for this to cool and then sipped for the next 20 minutes. The effects slowly emerged over the following 10-15 minutes, reaching a peak after around 2 hours, and maintaining a general plateau for perhaps 3-4 hours.

There was a definite stimulation, which was nothing like caffeine. It bore more resemblance to some of the chemical stimulants described in the previous section of this book, but was milder in nature.

An increase in focus was also apparent, and at times a tiny hint of euphoria, although this was certainly very minor.

There was perhaps a slight jittery feeling at times, possibly with an increased heart rate (although I cannot confirm). It is worth sounding a note of caution with respect to this: there are numerous comments posted around the Internet citing this as an issue, so it is something to bear in mind.

I tried to take my usual afternoon nap after 6 or so hours, but with no joy. This was almost certainly due to consumption of this tea.

Overall, I found this to be an enjoyable, albeit mild, experience. It was almost entirely functional, and it certainly enhanced my alertness on a day upon which I was quite tired.

Whilst confirming its effectiveness as a stimulant, I would equally stress the need for prudence, particularly with reference to dose.

3.3.4 Guarana

Binomial / Botanical Name	Paullinia Cupana
Street Names	Guarana
Major Active Compound	Caffeine; Theophylline; Theobromine
Indigenous Source	S America
Form	Powdered Berries/Seeds
RoA	Oral
Personal Rating On Shulgin Scale	+*

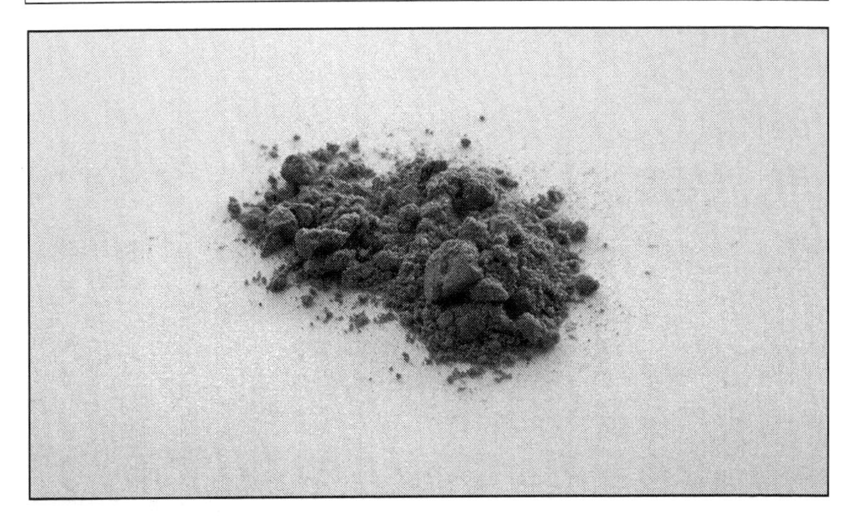

SUBJECTIVE EXPERIENCE

As a caffeine containing stimulant, guarana is well known as an ingredient of a number of popular energy drinks. Stand-alone, rather like coffee (and unlike regular tea) the seeds/fruit from the plant are brewed rather than the leaves. The plant itself is native to the Amazon basin and is particularly common in Brazil.

My brown paper packet, as delivered by Amazon (Inc), states that "*its main ingredient is guaranine, chemically similar to caffeine*". On a similar theme, Erowid describes the plant as a rainforest shrub whose seeds contain "*high levels of caffeine and other xanthines*". Certainly, its caffeine content is known to be much higher than coffee, but will the other contents make a difference to its psychoactive effects?

On opening, the first thing I notice is the kratom-like smell: pungent and not particularly pleasant. The light brown powder is finely ground and falls easily out of the packet.

In terms of dosage the vendor suggests adding "*up to 3g per day to water, juice or a smoothie*". The *per day* is something of a moot point for my single sitting, as websites like Livestrong and RxList refer to individual doses of well under 1g, whilst Holland & Barrett capsules each contain 900mg.

I have seen some extremely high doses anecdotally cited on Internet forums (e.g. 10g), but given the caffeine content alone I believe this to be somewhat reckless. After consideration I elect to roll with 2g, which I expect will be more than enough.

T+0:00 I prepare a cup of hot water (not boiling) and weigh 2g of the powder. Pouring this into the cup I stir vigorously, and then start to sip. The earthy taste isn't wonderful but it is certainly tolerable. [9:20am]

T+ 0:10 As I drink the last of the residue I can already feel a mild head buzz coming on: it's not jittery but is a definite hit.

This does have the characteristics of caffeine but with less edge.

T+0:40 With an unsettled night I was tired this morning. Underneath the pleasant head buzz I still am, but this is no longer as intrusive as it was.

T+1:15 The stimulation has now settled, and manifests as a background awareness rather than an overt or obvious excitation. There is a presence in play, and I can feel a sense of clarity when I focus upon it, but this isn't noticeable if I engage in thought or activity.

How does it compare to a regular caffeine based tea or coffee? Whilst it is not substantial there is a subtle difference in mental acuity, and I do sense that focus may be easier to sustain. The stimulation itself does appear to be gentler.

Whilst much of this is no doubt subjective, given that I had quite a significant dose the lack of restlessness and jitter is certainly a positive.

T+3:30 The effects have now wound down to the extent that I am again tired and feeling the impact of that lack of sleep.

T+5:00 My return to base was sufficient such that my afternoon nap passed without problem. I am feeling well, and back to normal for this time of the day.

This was quite a refreshing change from my usual caffeine based drinks. It seemed smoother in some ways, even though it was stronger, and it didn't distract from my normal activities.

Would I drink it instead of tea or coffee? Convenience and habit say no. However, if it was offered as an option in a coffee shop, for example, I would select it, at least for a change.

3.3.5 Guayusa

Binomial / Botanical Name	Ilex Guayusa
Street Names	Guayusa
Major Active Compound	Caffeine (plus Catechins)
Indigenous Source	Ecuador
Form	Leaves
RoA	Oral
Personal Rating On Shulgin Scale	+**

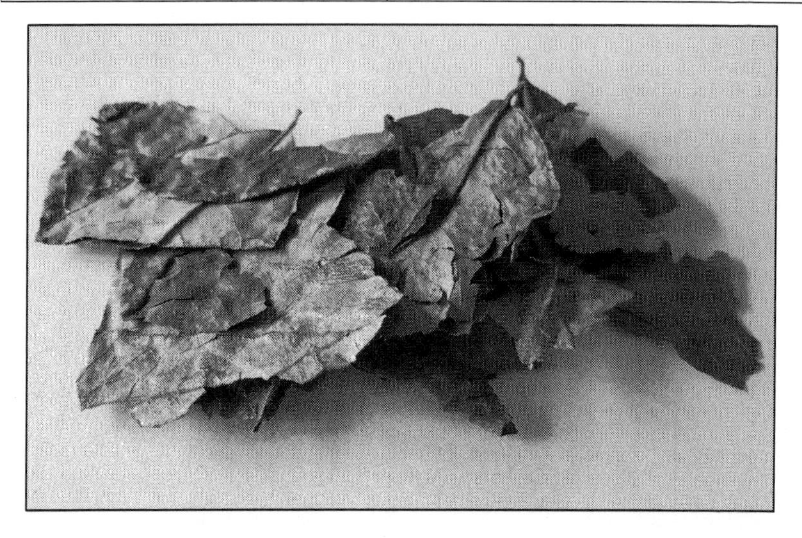

SUBJECTIVE EXPERIENCE
The ritual, ceremonial, and traditional use of guayusa in the western Amazon region dates back to at least 335 CE. As a stimulating tea it is known to have been used by a number of tribes, and as an ayahuasca additive by at least one. It remains popular in Ecuador to this day.

As I poured boiling water upon the large leaves sitting in the teapot, my expectations were not high. The exercise was undertaken on the back of a couple of unsuccessful experiments with other botanical teas, and I had no particular reason to be optimistic that this would be any different.

Whilst Wikipedia stated positively that "*the leaves of the guayusa tree are dried and brewed like a tea for their stimulative effects*", I was in a rather negative frame of mind, and I felt that I had heard it all before.

However, sipping on the second cup of the fairly strong brew I had produced, I suddenly began to notice a caffeine-like stimulation: caffeine-like, but much smoother and with a gentle feeling of lucidity.

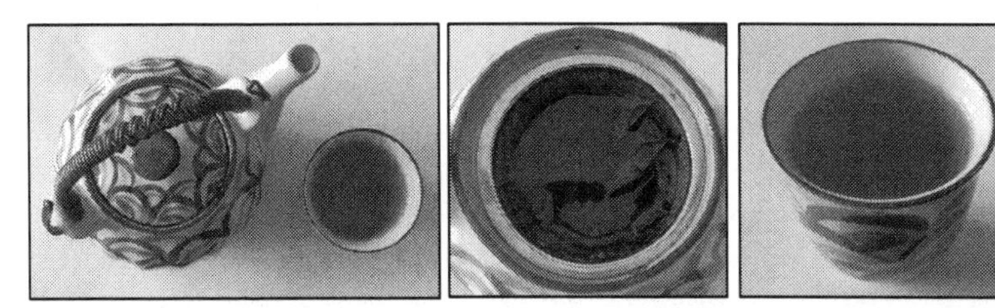

Somehow this seemed to be less jittery, which is the best word I can find. Its taste was actually quite pleasing, and there was also a clarity which is not present with the usual array of caffeine based teas.

I noted at the time that this was worth returning to, and drinking as an occasional and refreshing replacement for coffee. Further consumption downstream has not changed this opinion.

It is probably my favourite mild-stimulant tea.

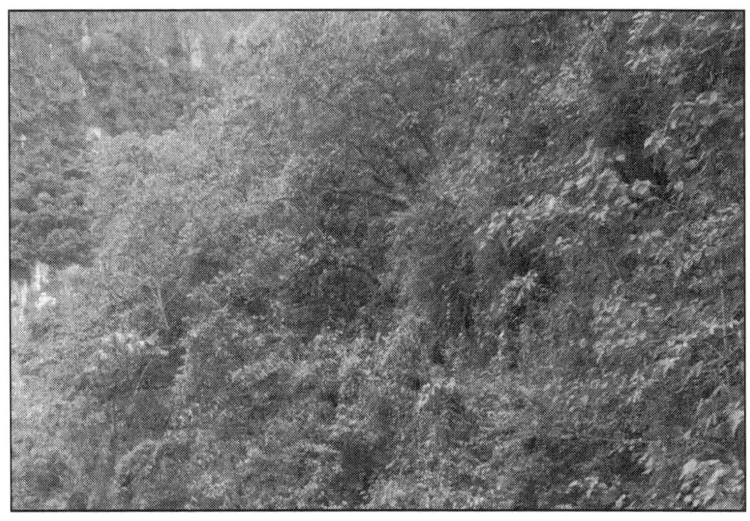

Legend has it that once guayusa is drunk, the visitor will always return to the Ecuadorian jungle

3.3.6 Khaini

Binomial / Botanical Name	Khaini
Street Names	Kaini? Paan Masala? Gutka?
Major Active Compound	Tobacco; Lime; Areca Catechu? Other?
Indigenous Source	India
Form	Plant Material & Powder
RoA	Chewed/Quidded
Personal Rating On Shulgin Scale	+**

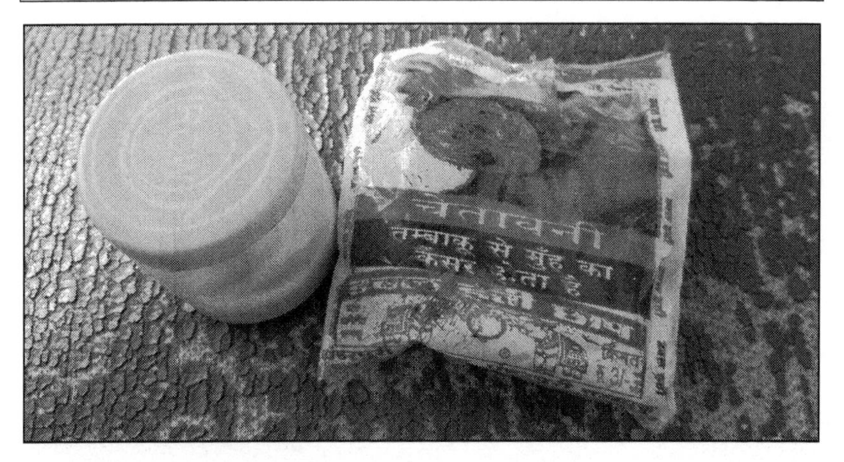

SUBJECTIVE EXPERIENCE
My encounter with khaini came in Goa, India. Whilst walking on the beach I noticed one of the local masseurs chewing some sort of plant material, and enquired accordingly. He described it as *masala* and was happy to display it. It comprised a small packet, containing tobacco-like ingredients, along with a green tub of a white clogged powder, which was presumably lime. The latter seemed familiar: on previous days I had occasionally spotted the odd discarded plastic capsule lying on the sand, which seemed to contain remnants of the same or similar powder.

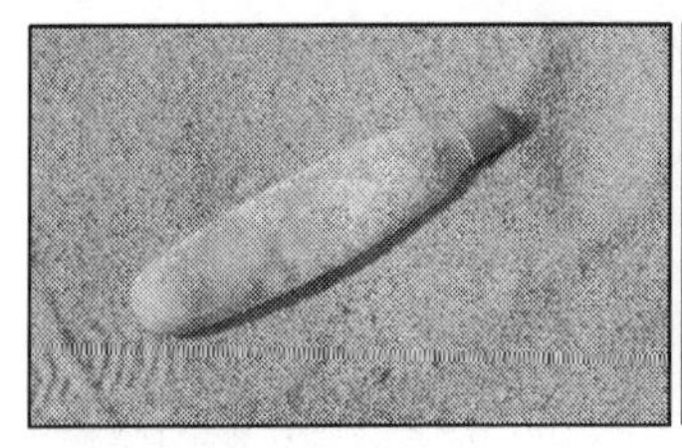

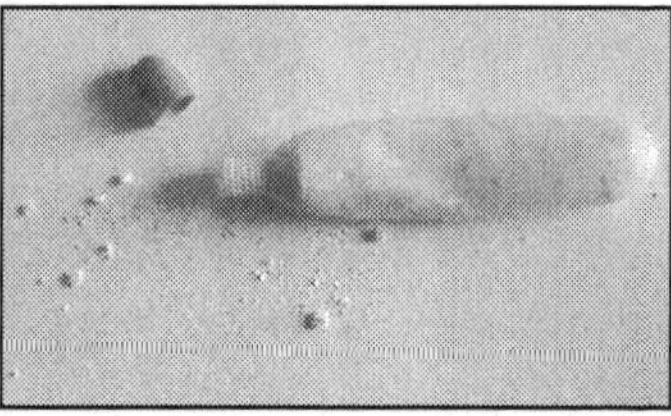

For a closer inspection, my friendly masseur tipped some of the tobacco substance onto his lounge bed, and peppered a little of the white powder onto it. I took a pinch and chewed. It was hot to taste, very hot.

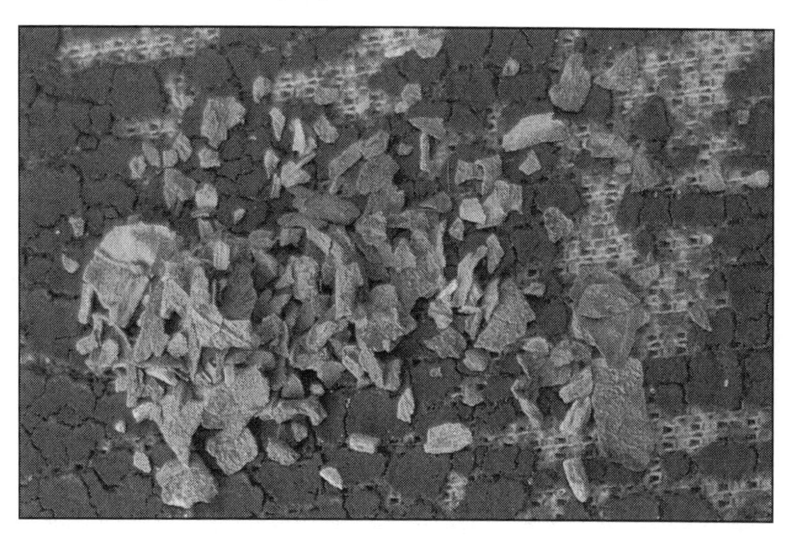

As I chewed he momentarily panicked, hastily telling me not to swallow, but to spit it out when finished. This was later amplified by a hotel receptionist, who explained that first-timers can be overwhelmed and can pass-out.

I wasn't overwhelmed, but I was definitely stimulated, with a clear change of headspace. It was a little uplifting, although not mind-blowing. The effects lasted for about an hour.

So what was this? Was it a variant of betel nut (see earlier), commonly known as *paan masala* in India? Or was it gutka, which Wikipedia describes as "a *preparation of crushed areca nut, tobacco, catechu, paraffin wax, slaked lime and sweet or savoury flavourings*"? Or was it something else?

When I returned home I enquired online, on an Indian *sub-Reddit*. I was informed that *paan masala* is in fact an extremely broad term that can be used for "*any of the stuff that goes into a paan*". Also, that the word *khaini* is used throughout India for chewing tobacco products, which usually contain catechu (from the areca tree) but not always.

This doesn't of course conclusively identify my mystery substance, although on balance it was probably tobacco, lime, plus, possibly, catechu or something else. Whatever this was, it was reasonably pleasant, but despite keeping my eyes open, another opportunity to test it didn't materialise.

SRI LANKA: BETELS
A couple of years later I came across a similar mix whilst in Sri Lanka. On this occasion I was very careful to establish the precise ingredients. These were areca nuts, betel leaves, raw tobacco leaves and lime paste. This was referred to locally as *betels*.

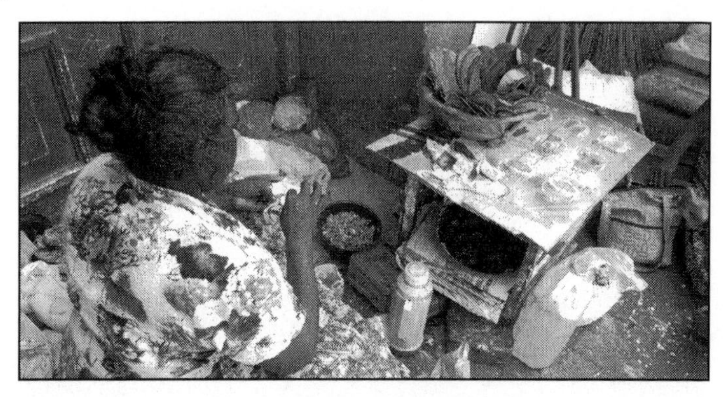

It was served as shown in the photograph below, with the large dab of lime wrapped in newspaper. I opened this and spread it over some of the tobacco leaf and areca nut, and chewed at this combination, adding some of the leaf for bulk.

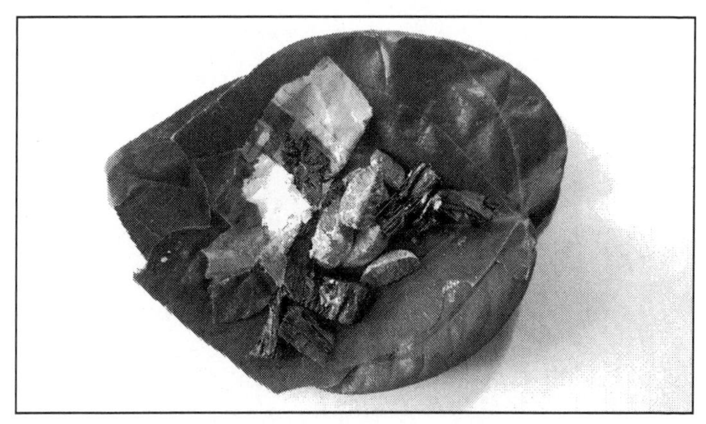

It was extremely hot to taste, and I experienced a rapid stimulation. This was less clean than that produced via the betel nuts I had sampled in Mandalay, presumably due to the presence of the tobacco. It was also far stronger than I had anticipated, and came with a touch of mapacho-like dizziness/nausea. Indeed, for a while I felt queasy and not particularly well, which was probably not helped by the fact that I swallowed some of it. This passed after a few hours, but was unpleasant enough for me to decide to bin the rest.

3.3.7 Kola Nut

Binomial / Botanical Name	Cola Nitida; Cola Acuminata
Street Names	Cola; Kola; Bitter Kola
Major Active Compound	Caffeine; Kolanin; Theobromine
Indigenous Source	West Africa
Form	Powdered Nuts
RoA	Oral
Personal Rating On Shulgin Scale	+

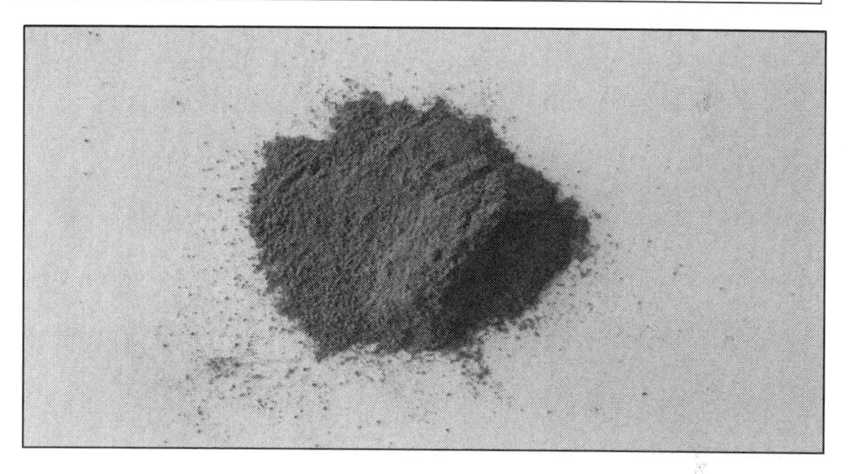

SUBJECTIVE EXPERIENCE
In terms of oral consumption, botanical powders are not my thing. More specifically, I tend to find that they frequently refuse to dissolve properly, and that their constitution is less than agreeable. Whilst I struggled a little with kola nut, at least it didn't taste revolting (à la kratom) as I swigged the fine woody-like powder down the hatch with water.

This is widely used in Africa, and it is claimed to increase both endurance and concentration, as well as act as a mild aphrodisiac.

It had a definite coffee-like kick to it. It was not overwhelming at the dose I used, but the strength was there. I felt clear, awake and a little energised, with a jittery edge. This lasted for some hours.

Note that I consumed in the morning, which I suspect was a good idea with respect to retaining a sensible sleep pattern.

3.3.8 Wormwood

Binomial / Botanical Name	Artemisia Absinthium
Street Names	Absinthe; Ambrosia
Major Active Compound	Thujone
Indigenous Source	Eurasia, North Africa, North America
Form	Shredded Herb
RoA	Oral / Smoked
Personal Rating On Shulgin Scale	+ / +

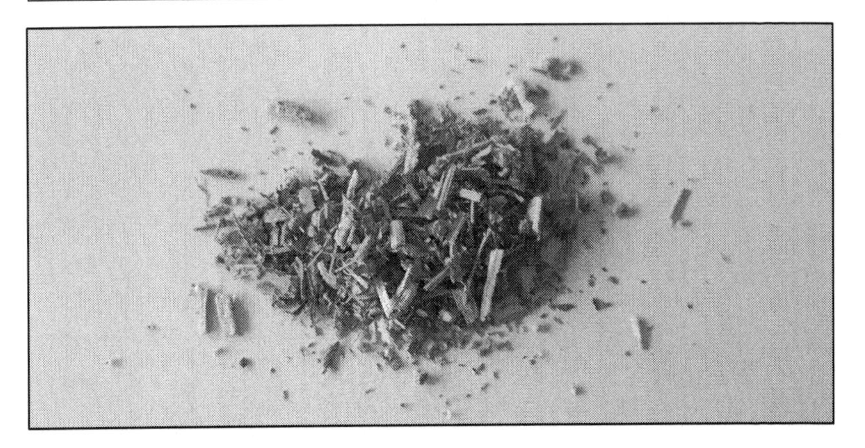

SUBJECTIVE EXPERIENCE
Wormwood is best known as the key ingredient of the alcoholic beverage, absinthe, with Erowid, for example, stating that:

> "*Artemisia absinthium is a silvery-green perennial herb growing up to 1.5 meters tall which contains the volatile oil thujone. It is added to distilled ethanol to create absinthe. Its effects alone are not well understood*"

For the purposes of this book I sampled wormwood in its own right, rather than as part of a mix with another material, or distilled with alcohol. In this context, the following descriptions are fairly typical:

> "*Wormwood is a mental stimulant. The effect of wormwood is narcotic, lightly anaesthetic, giving a peaceful and relaxing feeling*" ~ azarius.net

> "*Wormwood stimulates the brain to create a calming and relaxing effect.*" ~ smokableherbs.com

Whilst the usual approach to stand-alone use is to make a tea, there are some reports of use as a smoking herb. For example, smokableherbs.com makes the following observation:

> "*Those who want milder effects of Wormwood may smoke it instead of ingesting it. The effect is quicker but it is also shorter*"

I elected to test both methods, and wrote the following notes the day after the experiments:

> My 50g sample of a fresh-smelling shredded brown compound arrived double sealed in two transparent bags. Having made a couple of elementary checks on the contents, I was ready to go.
>
> I started with a few hits from a bong. Immediately there appeared to be an alleviation of anxiety, and perhaps more clarity of vision. However, this was marginal, and there was plenty of scope for a placebo influence. In this respect it should be noted that as I don't smoke tobacco, smoking any compound tends to register to some degree, if only via oxygen deprivation.
>
> Twenty minutes in, I could safely say that there was some effect. It was there, and by and large, it did fit the descriptions quoted above. It was extremely minor in nature.
>
> After half an hour I took my afternoon nap. It was a reasonable sleep, albeit with a slightly odd aura about it.
>
> On awakening I brewed a large cup of wormwood tea. I purposely didn't make this too strong, as during the preparatory research I had encountered occasional warnings along the following lines:
>
>> "*Wormwood is poisonous. Long and intensive use can lead to addiction*". ~ azarius.net
>
> The taste was bitter, but manageable.
>
> I had set my expectations low, as most accounts suggested that this would be a mild experience. And so it was. The effects were similar to the earlier smoking experiment, perhaps hinting at those described on Erowid:
>
>> "*The primary reported effects of wormwood ingestion are a mild, hazy disorientation accompanied by a dreamlike or surreal feeling sometimes called "the dollhouse effect". This refers to the appearance of things as though they are idealized copies of themselves, as if they are from a dollhouse. Other reported effects include a feeling of mental lucidity, stimulation, mild euphoria, and a sense of relaxation. Effects are frequently described as mild, and sometimes as "boring"*"

This was never strong, but it was evident, and it tapered off during the course of the day and evening.

Today, however, as I write these notes, I realize that I must have been under a pervasive sort of influence as my recollections of last night are a little odd and lacking.

There was also the matter of dreaming. I had previously read the following passage on the drugs-forum.com website:

> "*Wormwood seems to induce lucid dreaming, which is being asleep, and dreaming, yet consciously aware of your dreaming, and sometimes able to control it, dreams are usually pleasant, and aside from lucid dreams, it also seems to greatly promote normal dreaming, also pleasant.*" ~ Limpet Chicken

I did dream and the dreams were lucid. I woke several times. I wasn't able to control the dreams, and they were not particularly good dreams, but they were multiple, recallable, and vivid.

Regarding body load, when I woke during the night I was stiff, aching in places (particularly the lower side of the back) and my mouth was dry. I felt instinctively that this was as a result of consuming the wormwood. Perhaps it was, perhaps it wasn't, but it was sufficient to persuade me not to repeat this exercise in a hurry.

Overall, there was a definite psychoactive edge to this, which was noticeable but not intrusive. It was a little strange and slightly anxiolytic in nature. The dreaming, however, was of another order entirely.

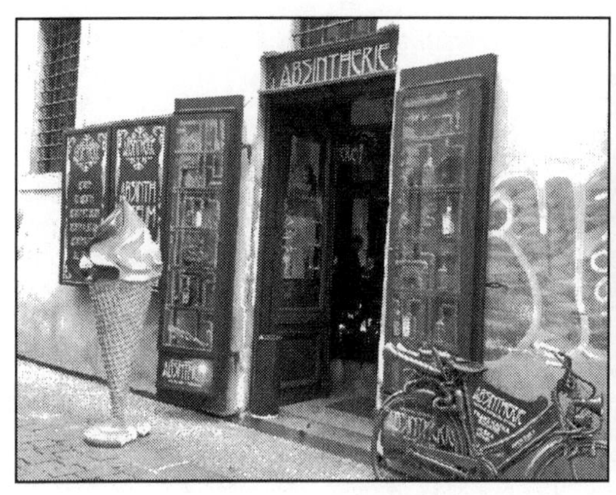

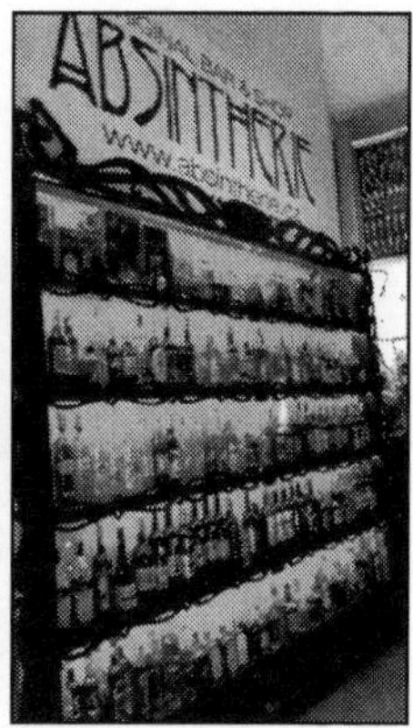

The Absintherie, Prague

3.3.9 Yohimbe

Binomial / Botanical Name	Pausinystalia Johimbe
Street Names	Johimbe
Major Active Compound	Yohimbine
Indigenous Source	Central & Western Africa
Form	Shredded Bark
RoA	Oral
Personal Rating On Shulgin Scale	++

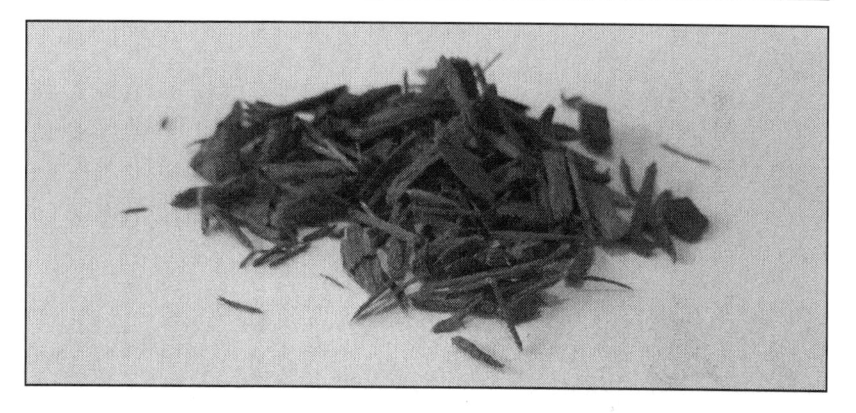

SUBJECTIVE EXPERIENCE
Classified by Erowid as a stimulant and vasodilator, yohimbe is a strange one, to say the least.

At lower and moderate doses it has been used as an aphrodisiac since ancient times. Consistent with this, it has latterly been employed in tantric based sexual rituals and to treat erectile dysfunction. At higher doses, however, it is widely reported to be hallucinogenic, and it is suggested that it has been used as an additive in iboga rituals.

However, scratching further below the surface uncovers another side to this coin. The ratio of effective dose to fatal dose is low. In other words, it is relatively easy to overdose, with tragic consequences. With this in mind, I tread particularly carefully.

For my first experiment, a couple of years ago, I brewed a tea using 3 grams of bark. I recall a very clear and specific stimulation, and accordingly, marked it as +** on the adapted Shulgin scale. I also noted some aphrodisiacal effects. As my notes were brief, however, I am repeating the exercise, using the same batch.

I again measure 3g, and immerse it in boiling water, using my handy-sized teapot with a built-in filter. I stir periodically until it is cool enough to drink.

> T+0:00 I pour the first cup and begin to sip the tea. It has a mild woody taste, with the lightest of tang. It is not at all unpleasant. [4:40pm]
>
> T+0:30 As I finish the last cup, I feel a light buzz about the head. A certain mental alertness is developing, inclusive of a gentle headspace that has a dreamlike recreational edge.
>
> Physically, I feel much warmer than earlier.
>
> Regarding its aphrodisiacal properties, there is certainly enhanced and sustained interest. I can also report that there is no stim-dick in play.
>
> T+1:00 I am now very warm and a little sweaty, which of course is a fairly typical reaction with respect to chemical stimulants. The head buzz has not dissipated at all during the last half an hour. The sexual aspect remains prominent too. This isn't debilitating in any way, and is quite pleasant.
>
> T+1:30 I feel more settled at this point: still nicely charged, but not as intensely. Physically, I remain warm, and I feel a little tingly and flushed.
>
> The effects, thus far, have been surprisingly distinct, and positive.
>
> T+2:00 The experience continues to roll, but is drifting down and slowly heading towards base.
>
> My blood pressure is 140/82. This is slightly above norm, as would be expected, but not significantly. Pulse is a fairly standard 56.
>
> T+3:00 After three hours I am lingering in a positive and energised place. This is a very nice comedown.

The comedown was indeed pleasant and gentle, and I remained invigorated until I retired to bed at about 11pm. The night's sleep was very good, and included significant dream time.

There is no doubt whatsoever that this is an aphrodisiac. This feature, along with the stimulation, was prolonged and clearly evident, and from my own personal journey is unsurpassed in the botanical field. The stimulation had a heady edge which made it recreational, and not merely functional.

What a pity about those dangers. Without this facet I would certainly be exploring this again, and at higher doses.

I thoroughly enjoyed this experience.

3.4. SEDATIVES

Textbook Definition: *Sedatives can produce a calming or relaxing effect, such that stress, irritability or agitation is reduced. In some cases they can produce hypnotic anticonvulsant, muscle relaxant and a range of other effects.*

The following botanicals have been sampled and researched for inclusion within this section:

3.4.1 Blue Lotus [incl: Pink Lotus Flower; Red Lily]
3.4.2 Catnip
3.4.3 Damiana
3.4.4 Frankincense
3.4.5 Imphepho
3.4.6 Indian Warrior
3.4.7 Kanna
3.4.8 Lavender
3.4.9 Maconha Brava
3.4.10 Marihuanilla
3.4.11 Mulungu
3.4.12 Passion Flower
3.4.13 Rhodiola
3.4.14 St. John's Wort
3.4.15 Skullcap
3.4.16 Valerian Root
3.4.17 White Sage
3.4.18 Wild Dagga
3.4.19 Wild Lettuce

That certain botanicals can be used to alleviate anxiety, sedate, or simply induce relaxation and mood chill, is hardly the best kept secret in the world. However, less well known are perhaps the often subtle variations of these states, their consequential and inherent nature, and the sheer number of plant species which can invoke them.

Those subtle variations can shape the entire character of the experience, adding edges which hint at or embrace other properties (e.g. psychedelic, oneirogenic). Whilst some are mild in nature, others are not, and for many, the chosen route of administration is a central matter.

Related to RoA is the set and setting of the occasion. As with other botanical classes, many have their roots in ancient practices, and mindset can be all-important in deriving the requisite ride.

With respect to this, I find that it helps to make an effort to relax and meditate into the experiment, and if possible, seek to engage in the authentic ritual itself, whether it is smoking, or brewing and sipping tea.

3.4.1 Blue Lotus

Binomial / Botanical Name	Nymphaea Caerulea
Street Names	Sacred Blue Lily; Blue Egyptian Water Lily
Major Active Compound	Unconfirmed: Nuciferine; Aporphin
Indigenous Source	Egypt and East Africa
Form	Dried Flowers
RoA	Oral / Smoked
Personal Rating On Shulgin Scale	+* / +**

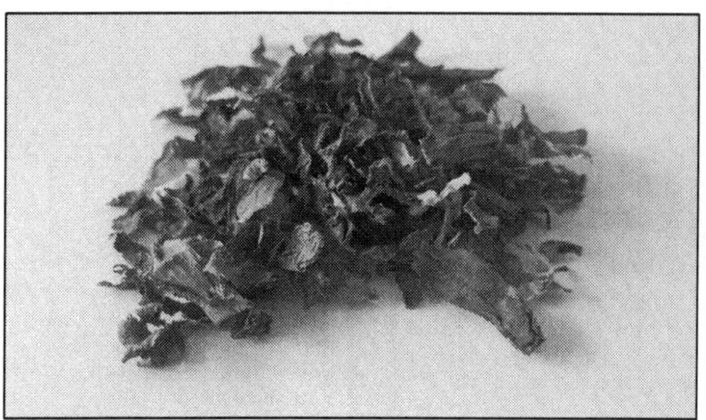

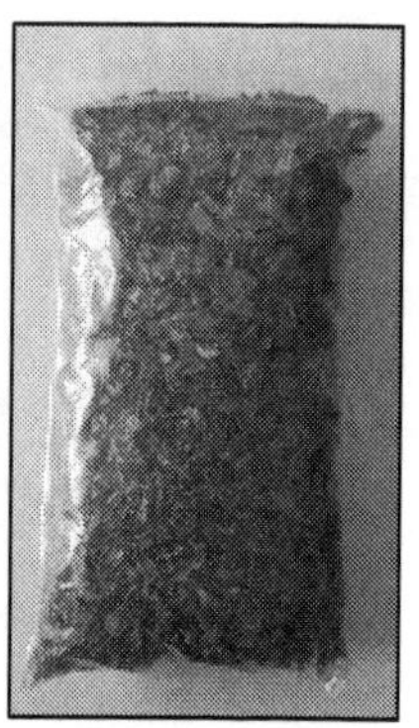

SUBJECTIVE EXPERIENCE
Given that it is so clearly embedded in ancient Egyptian hieroglyphs as a psychoactive sacrament, blue lotus's place in history is hugely impressive. Only recently, however, have historians provided the focus this strange plant deserves.

Whilst it is often suggested that the plant material is best experienced via a concoction created with wine, I have always sampled it stand-alone. This is invariably my practice, with both botanicals and chemicals.

My first forays were conducted exclusively via the brewing of tea. I experimented using varying strengths, and with material obtained from a variety of sources. This approach was largely undertaken on the basis that with so many historical references, oral consumption must surely produce the required outcome.

I found that this route tended to provide a calming or sedating effect: nothing exciting but definitely there. The frequently claimed euphoric and aphrodisiacal qualities were also present, but at a very low level. Accordingly, I marked it at the time as a +, meaning that I felt its effects, but these were not particularly noteworthy.

Some time later, whilst background researching a different but related species, I noticed that smoking was occasionally cited as an alternative RoA. As a number of users claimed that this was more effective, I decided to test this method as well.

Using this approach I found that the qualities referred to above were more pronounced, and the onset was predictably instant. I gave it a rating of +** to reflect this. It provided, at least if smoked rarely, a definite relaxing and anxiolytic feel, without a lingering intoxication or hangover. Again though, there was little evidence of a psychedelic edge.

I feel that there is significantly more to explore with this plant, but I can state with absolute certainty that it is psychoactive, although a little temperamental. I fully intend to return to this at some future date.

NYMPHAEA NUCIFERA & NYMPHAEA RUBRA

Subsequent to this investigation, I discovered that two other members of the same genus (nymphaea) were purported to be psychoactive. Accordingly, when the opportunity arose, I obtained samples and tested them.

PINK LOTUS

Binomial / Botanical Name	Nymphaea Nucifera
Street Names	Indian Lotus; Sacred Lotus; Bean of India
Major Active Compound	Unconfirmed: Nuciferine; Aporphin
Indigenous Source	Tropical Asia; Australia
Form	Flowers
RoA	Oral / Smoked
Personal Rating On Shulgin Scale	+ / +

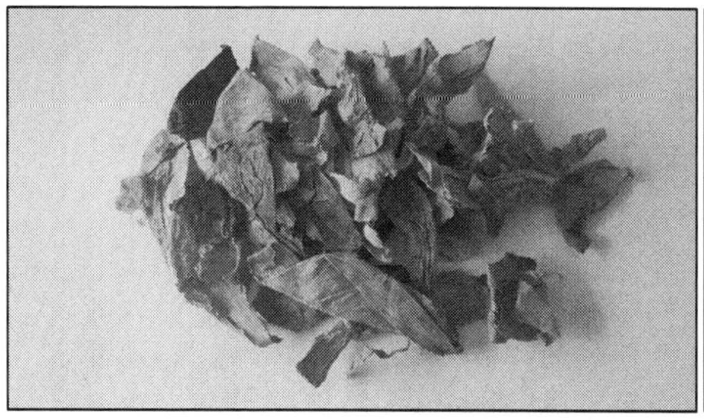
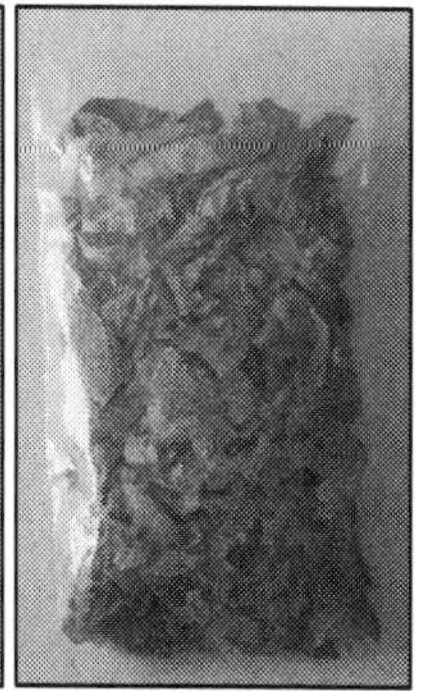

Given that I found far fewer references to this during research, it wasn't a surprise to discover that it was weaker than its more famous sister. Comments like the following (from the Shroomery forum) confirmed my own experience:

> *"Nymphaea Caerulea is better. They contain similar alkaloids, but Blue Lily, Nymphaea Caerulea, has more."* ~ rdnp2035

I tested it both brewed as a tea (5g) and by smoking it from a bong. The psychoactivity was there, and presented itself as a mild heady feeling with a degree of sedation, but it was relatively weak.

RED LILY

Binomial / Botanical Name	Nymphaea Rubra
Street Names	Red Water Lily
Major Active Compound	Unknown
Indigenous Source	Temperate & Tropical Asia; Australia; Papua New Guinea
Form	Flowers
RoA	Smoked
Personal Rating On Shulgin Scale	+

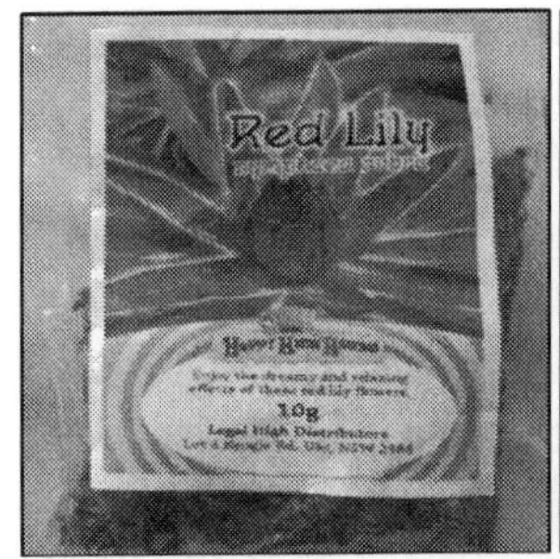

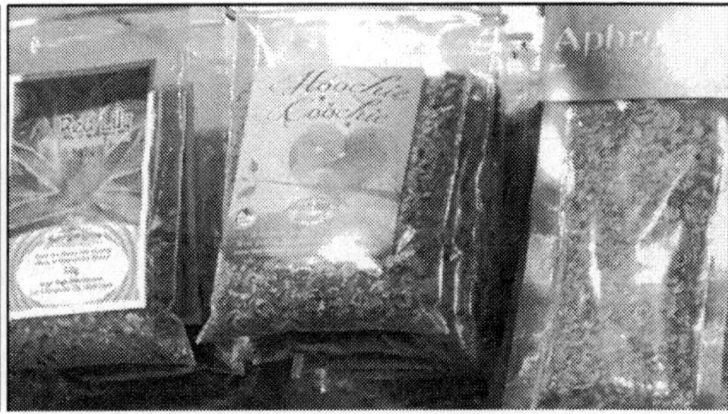

I purchased this from a head shop in its native Australia, in a desperate attempt to overcome jet lag. Sadly, this was to no avail, as I continued to struggle.

There was some psychoactivity in play, or perhaps more accurately, a hint of psychoactivity. However, to be fair, given my condition, this was always going to be difficult to distinguish from the general lassitude and tiredness.

This was the weakest of this trio, and has the fewest online references to historical psychoactive use.

3.4.2 Catnip

Binomial / Botanical Name	Nepeta Cataria
Street Names	Catswort; Catmint
Major Active Compound	Nepetalactone
Indigenous Source	S&E Europe, Middle East, Asia, China
Form	Plant Matter
RoA	Smoked / Oral
Personal Rating On Shulgin Scale	+ / ++

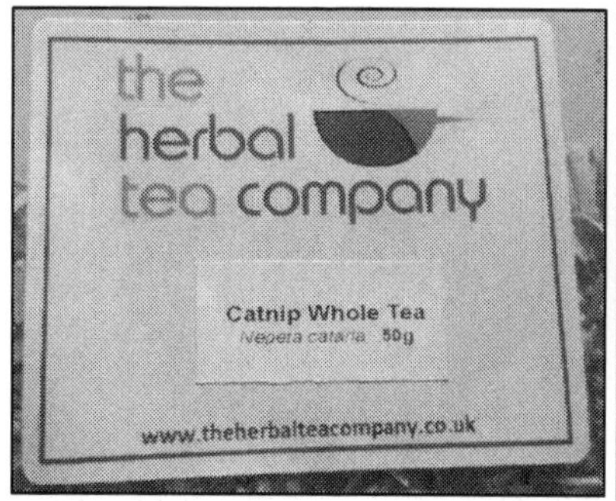

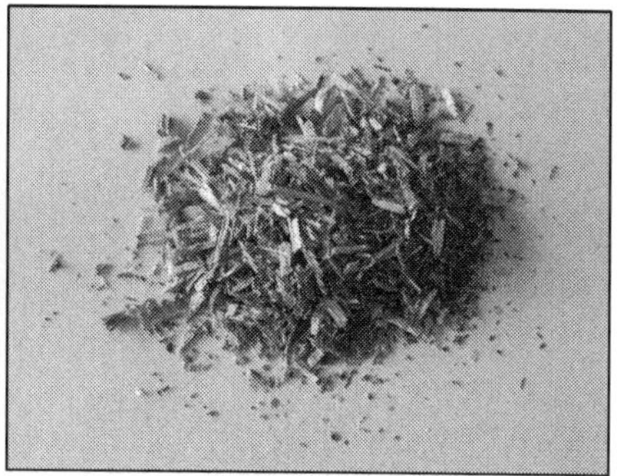

SUBJECTIVE EXPERIENCE

Best known for its behavioural effects on the cat family, catnip has also been used as a traditional home remedy for headaches, stomach and digestive pains, menstrual cramps, colds, fevers and a variety of other ailments. More relevant to this book are the suggestions that it is a cure for insomnia, and that it acts as a relaxant and a sedative.

For my first experiment I smoked it from a bong. It wasn't a particularly nice smoke, and the effect was somewhat disappointing. I felt that there was something there, but it could easily have been invoked through the act of smoking itself (oxygen deprivation), or via placebo, or both. At the mild end of the scale it is sometimes impossible to say, particularly if there is uncertainty about how clean (drug free) your body is. The catnip itself was also very dry, so could have lost potency through age.

Notwithstanding this, I decided to sample again, this time via the most widely recommended method: tea. On this occasion I made absolutely certain that I had no residue from other psychoactives in my system. I proceeded as follows:

> T+0:00 I boil some water. Given that it is frequently stated that boiling water destroys the active ingredients I allow it to stand for 10 minutes.

I then place 4 tablespoons of catnip into the teapot, pour the hot water over it, and leave it to steep for 10 minutes or so. I begin to sip slowly from a small cup. The taste isn't bad. There is no bitterness or particularly strong flavour or smell, and it goes down easily when it has cooled a little. [3:45pm]

At the start point I feel of fairly average disposition. I have had an afternoon nap, and I am fully awake. I am not particularly anxious or calm, but perhaps have a slight edge, although nothing more.

T+0:30 I have now drunk all the tea and refilled the teapot. I do feel slightly more relaxed. There's a minor headiness to it in the form of a mild dreamy buzz, and I am now warmer than I was. I feel calm and more content.

T+0:45 Whilst this isn't strong or overwhelming it is quite pleasing. I suspect that expectation would significantly impact the experience: expect a lot and you will be disappointed, but expect nothing and you will be pleasantly surprised. Pleasant is the operative word, because that is basically what it is.

T+1:00 The refilled teapot has now been polished off, and I am feeling generally sedated. My mind tends to drift with a relaxing aura, as I ease into a more positive ambiance and a gentle sense of well-being. This is definitely not a placebo effect.

As there are online suggestions that excessive dosing can cause nausea and vomiting, I won't consume any more, particularly as I have probably had quite a large dose already. Indeed, 2-3g is often cited as being adequate.

T+2:00 The effects are now wearing off somewhat. That slight tummy edge has returned, although mentally I still feel a buzz and some sedation.

I should note that a curious moment arose earlier, during which I felt that I entered some sort of collective unconscious in terms of thinking competitors' thoughts during a parlour game. This was fleeting and sounds irrational, but I document it partly as a marker for my own future research.

T+3:30 I now feel, more or less, back at base.

T+16:00 The anxiolytic properties dissipated as the evening progressed. The night's sleep was fairly standard, although I detected a mild headache and heaviness during the early hours. However, on rising this morning I feel completely normal.

This was quite a nice experience, which may have been better suited to an evening foray than late afternoon. It wore off after about three hours, leaving a bit of a void prior to bedtime. Had I consumed at perhaps 8pm, I may well have drifted off into a peaceful slumber as the effects waned.

Nonetheless, catnip was more interesting than I expected, and was worth the effort taken to conduct the experiment in a more determined manner.

3.4.3 Damiana

Binomial / Botanical Name	Turnera Diffusa
Street Names	Herba de la Pastora; Old Woman's Broom
Major Active Compound	Apigenin (Unconfirmed)
Indigenous Source	Central America, South America, Texas
Form	Plant Matter
RoA	Oral / Smoked
Personal Rating On Shulgin Scale	± / ++

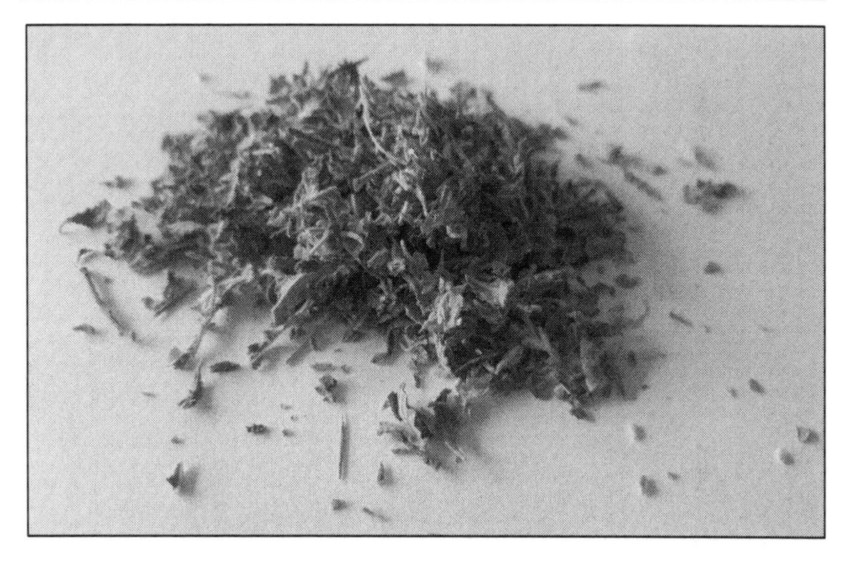

SUBJECTIVE EXPERIENCE
I had dabbled with damiana tea on a number of occasions, and had marked it firmly down as, at best, a slightly relaxing herbal drink. It was only after I had smoked it with hashish, as a filler, that I began to suspect that there may be more to it. Stand-alone experimentation via this RoA proved this to be the case.

The intensity of the first couple of smoking experiences came as a surprise, as reflected in one of my forum posts at the time:

> Damiana has been used traditionally in Central America and the northern parts of South America for many centuries. The Mayas and Aztecs, for example, used it as an aphrodisiac and a relaxant.

Strangely, identification of its active psychoactive content has proven to be problematic. Azarius.com describes this apparent conundrum in the following terms:

> "*Damiana contains from 0.5% to 1% of a complex volatile oil (thymol, alpha-copaene, 8cadinene, calamene, 1,8 cineole, alpha pinene, beta pinene, calamenene) that gives the plant its characteristic odor and flavor. It also contains the flavonoids and tannins. None of these ingredients are known to have psychoactive or aphrodisiac qualities. Hence there is no substantive data available to confirm the claimed effects.*"

Whilst this may imply that damiana is a psychoactive dud, studies with rats have demonstrated "*increased sexual activity in sexually exhausted or impotent males*" (Wikipedia, ref: sciencedirect.com, ncbi.nlm.nih.gov).

This is scant evidence, of course. More persuasive may be the number of *ad hoc* reports scattered around the Internet which unambiguously cite its effectiveness as a sedative, and indeed, its value as an aphrodisiac.

Some people will be familiar with this herb as the foliage used in spice and other cannabinoid brands, as sold in shiny packets from head shops. In this context however, any effect from damiana would be almost completely expunged by whatever chemical was sprayed upon to it.

Others have used it with cannabis, for which the same question applies: what effect is produced courtesy of the weed, and what effect is invoked via the damiana, if any? Most tokers assume everything stems from the former.

How many here have smoked damiana alone? Or taken it as a tea?

My first experiment was via the latter, which is the most common method of stand-alone use. The experience was underwhelming. A gentle relaxing aura emerged, but it was very mild. As an aphrodisiac, again, perhaps there was something there, but certainly not in comparison to serious stimulants or empathogens.

Smoking it, however, produced an entirely different outcome. Indeed, my initial expectation was such that its effects took me entirely by surprise.

Sedating? Relaxing? Yes. It wasn't in the same league of cannabis, but equally, it wasn't a placebo effect, nor was it barely noticeable. It actually worked: it was calming and there was a small mood life courtesy of an anxiolytic edge.

Was there any evidence that this could be used as an aphrodisiac? Yes, there was. This was not on the stim-binge level, but it was certainly there, and the phenomenon of stim-dick was entirely absent.

> The experience lasted perhaps a couple of hours or so, as I slowly worked through the joint. However, yet another effect emerged later, in the form of repeated and lucid dreaming.
>
> Since this experiment I have used damiana occasionally, and always on a dry day. In other words, when not under the influence of any other chemical or botanical, and usually when I am at a loose end, just wanting to chill. It is not mind blowing but it can be effective in certain circumstances.
>
> GENERAL CONSIDERATIONS
> I should make a couple of other points here. Firstly, not all damianas are the same: source matters. Fresh strong damiana may work, whereas old or substandard damiana won't have any real effect. Secondly, the effects seem to vary by person, with some individuals claiming no effect at all.
>
> Bear in mind that many of the latter group will have been under the influence of other materials, and that some will have procured bunk damiana, but there are enough people stating this to suggest that it is true in some cases.
>
> Why post such a long report at this point in time?
>
> One reason is the recent post regarding nicotine addiction: it struck me that a damiana joint might prove to be an aid for people who are trying to quit tobacco, or some other toxic substance.
>
> Another is that it doesn't yet appear to be on the radar for the UK's PSA legislation, perhaps because of the difficulty in isolating what occurs chemically or perhaps because it is so common. With this in mind, again, it might be useful as a route to legally ease cravings for substances which are no longer obtainable.
>
> One final point: although I haven't seen anything linking this to any serious side effects, smoking combustible material always comes with a certain degree of risk. Your lungs prefer fresh air, so anyone who samples it should take this on board. Consider it to be a *research herb* and act accordingly.

Following these initial smoking experiences, I found that damiana became more hit and miss. The effects were much less pronounced on subsequent experiments.

I have experienced this with other materials too: it is hard if not impossible to continue to reach the same intensity as that enjoyed on the first few occasions. Sometimes a gap of months or years may reset the body and mind, and sometimes not. In this case, on returning to damiana a year after these prior experiments the effects were once again solid.

Overall, it is surprising that such an interesting herb remains relatively unknown outside this niche. There is something to it, it is multi-faceted, and I didn't note any particularly strong negatives.

3.4.4 Frankincense

Binomial / Botanical Name	Boswellia Sacra
Street Names	Olibanum
Major Active Compound	Incensole Acetate
Indigenous Source	Arabian Peninsula; North Eastern Africa
Form	Resin
RoA	Quidded / Smoked
Personal Rating On Shulgin Scale	+*

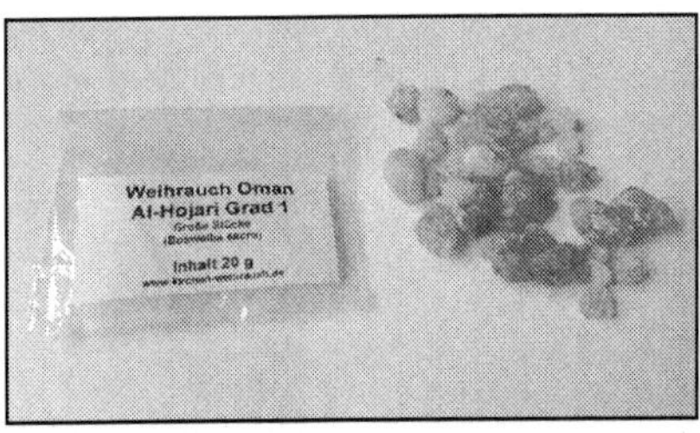

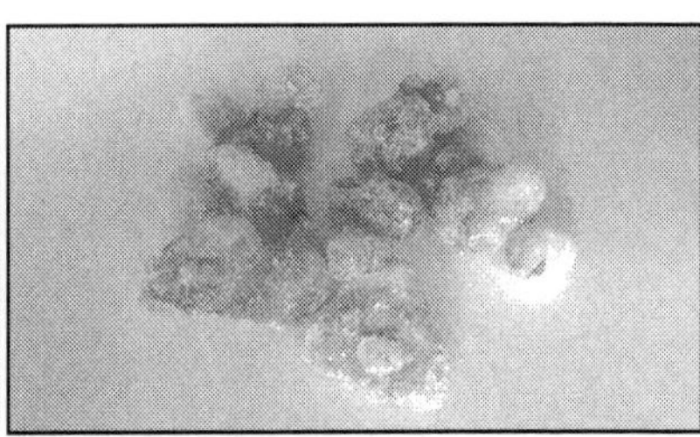

SUBJECTIVE EXPERIENCE
Frankincense is a resinous dried sap which is harvested from trees in the burseraceae family, particularly the boswellia sacra tree. Whilst not thoroughly documented, its mild psychoactivity is widely cited, including in a number of science journals.

Over the years I have occasionally used frankincense as incense. I always felt that it relaxed a little, but never assumed real psychoactivity. Eventually, however, I decided to explore this possibility.

The resin is available in various grades and qualities, which I found difficult to differentiate, largely because my purpose was untypical. I eventually procured 20g of "*the most exquisite pure frankincense from Oman*" courtesy of Amazon.co.uk. This was superficially hard but softened when pressure was applied, and was green in shade.

Regarding RoA both chewing (not swallowing) and smoking are referenced. I therefore elected to test both methods.

According to The Revisionsist (therevisionist.org), chewing on the highest grade resin creates significant psychoactive effect:

> *"It is quite relaxing, and it puts your mind at peace. You may work at a slightly slower pace, but that is because you feel more focused & more patient such that you actually take the time to comprehend what it is that you are doing. It's an awesome relaxant, with not a bit of sedation."*

> *"While I was chewing the Hojari frankincense tear, I noticed that it has a vision brightening effect, making colors more vibrant and pop out more."*

Whilst on the dmt-nexus.me forum smoking from a bowl was reported as follows:

> *"I found that 3-5 minutes after numerous inhalations that my mood was lifted quite a bit. I might even say a little euphoric. I closed my eyes and found that while i couldn't see anything, there was a definite depth to the blackness. When i covered my eyes and waited for something to emerge, flowing lights appeared which would sometimes form images of things i observed that day and then fade away. Another interesting thing was that i found myself forming sentences with much more ease. I was speaking before I knew what i was going to say, but the sentence was coherent."* ~ nickynack338

For the first experiment I separate approx 3g of the supply, pop it into my mouth, and masticate. Its constitution is chewy and it quickly softens into one large blob. I move it around my mouth waiting for something to happen.

The taste is a little perfumey with a slight cleansing-like tang, but it is not unpleasant. It soon begins to disintegrate, probably due to excessive saliva, which it seems to stimulate. It also sticks to my teeth. After about 15 minutes there is very little left.

I do sense that I am more relaxed and content, and generally more comfortable. There is no euphoria and there are no visuals, but perhaps a mild and gentle heady presence has slowly materialised.

After the resin has totally disappeared (apart from remnants still sticking to my teeth), my mind turns to smoking. Whilst still bathing in the mellow lingering ambiance I prepare a fresh clean bong and fill the bowl with broken pieces of the compound

After about an hour I take a few hits. It isn't the harshest smoke in the world but the resin itself soon catches fire, so the operation is far from flawless. In the background I light an incense burner, and occasionally hover above it and inhale.

I notice no sudden change in the complexion of the experience, but subjectively there is possibly a minor intensification of the headspace. This gradually dissipates but the soothing and subtle nature of the ride persists for an hour or two.

Overall this was quite pleasant. Noting that I have no idea of the quality of my supply, it wasn't mind blowing, but my change in disposition was evident, and I felt pacified without feeling sedated. Some of this could be placebo, but nonetheless this was certainly psychoactive.

I am unlikely to repeat the experiment, although as with other botanicals, should the opportunity arise to engage in an authentic Middle Eastern setting I will certainly take it.

3.4.5 Imphepho

Binomial / Botanical Name	Helichrysum Odoratissimum
Street Names	Silver Bush Everlasting Flower; Licorice Plant; Kooigoed; Trailing Dusty Miller
Major Active Compound	Diterpenes (Unconfirmed)
Indigenous Source	South Africa
Form	Plant Matter
RoA	Smoked
Personal Rating On Shulgin Scale	+**

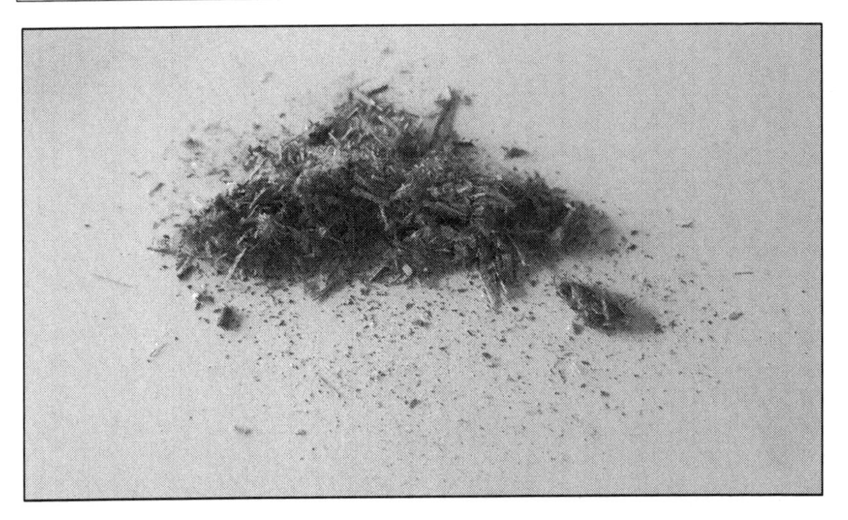

SUBJECTIVE EXPERIENCE
Helichrysum odoratissimum has been used for centuries in African rituals and ceremonies, for both medicinal purposes, and to help to induce visionary trance states. The contents of the latter are sometimes interpreted by shamans as communication with ancestors.

Traditionally, it has been used in smoking blends, drank in decoctions as tea, and burnt as incense. For my experiment, I elect to explore and investigate by smoking the stand-alone plant matter.

At time of testing, I am clean of all psychoactives, and as I have just had a mid-day nap, I feel quite fresh.

T+0:00 I take three large tokes on the bong. It is hot on the throat as I hold it in my mouth to cool, but it doesn't feel too bad on the lungs or trachea as I inhale. [3:40pm]

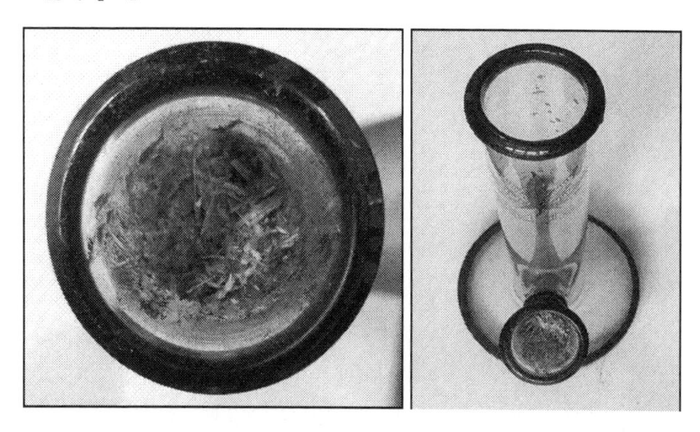

T+0:03 There is no instant intoxication or stoning. Perhaps though, there is a light headedness and a slight enhancement in clarity of vision.

T+0:05 I now feel a very mild intoxication. This comprises largely of a gradually changing headspace: a feeling of being a little distant. There is no tiredness or weariness to accompany it.

T+0:10 I am experiencing a general mood of contentedness, with a lucid type of head buzz. This is minor, but it is there.

T+0:20 I am calm and relaxed, with a clear but drifty heady feeling.

T+0:30 This is still quite pleasant, but is now floating down to a soft landing.

Referring to the book *'Muthi and Myths From the African Bush by Heather Dugmore and Ben-Erik van Wyk'*, Wikipedia states that:

> "*In order to experience the effects of Imphepho a lot of smoke must be breathed in for a long time*".

I wonder whether three hits, each held for about 15 seconds, qualify as *a long time*. I am reluctant to hold smoke in my lungs for too much longer than that.

Equally, Wikipedia's suggestion of *"Euphoria, ecstasy, uncontrolled giggling and sedation"* didn't materialize. However, at this intake it does provide a very gentle intoxication. This isn't on the level of a herb like cannabis, for example, but for the connoisseur it is well worthy of some attention.

3.4.6 Indian Warrior

Binomial / Botanical Name	Pedicularis Densiflora
Street Names	Warrior's Plume; Lousewort
Major Active Compound	Unknown
Indigenous Source	Western North America
Form	Flower Buds
RoA	Oral / Smoked
Personal Rating On Shulgin Scale	+* / +*

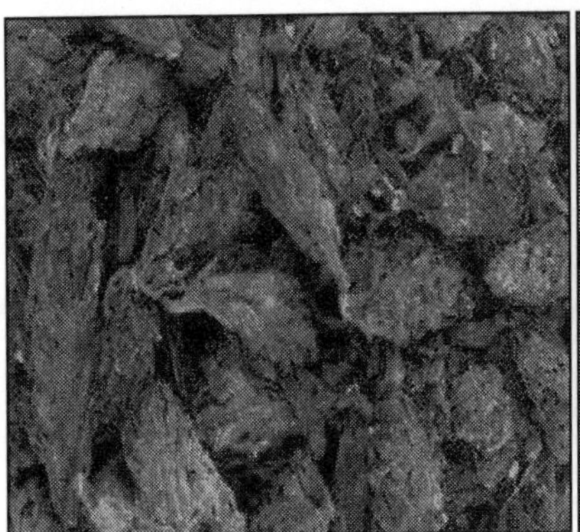
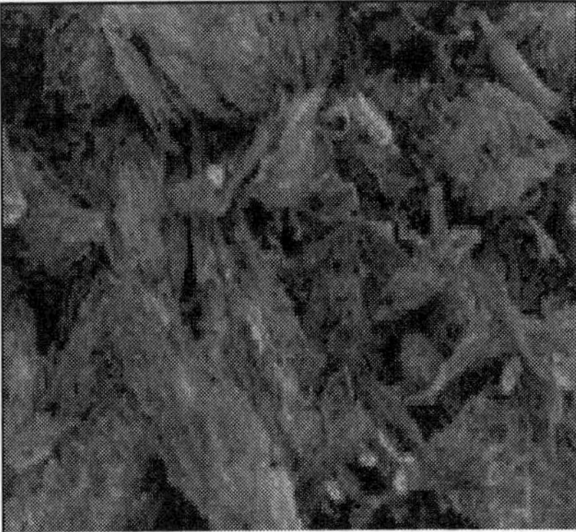

SUBJECTIVE EXPERIENCE
On reflection, I don't believe that I really did justice to this one, although this wasn't for a lack of will.

As always, I researched it well in advance. During the course of this, however, I found a variety of reports associating it with liver toxicity, tumours, and other serious conditions. This red light was re-enforced by the fact that I didn't find any references to indigenous or shamanic use, even in comprehensive sources like Rätsch.

This situation, of course, tended to act as a counter to the desired effects of the plant, which is cited as a relaxant and a sedative. Bluntly, with pictures of an agonising death in my mind, Indian warrior never had a chance.

Notwithstanding this, I can state factually that it is psychoactive, and that I did feel a calming effect, both orally (4g, tea) and smoked.

The fear factor will deter any further experimentation.

3.4.7 Kanna

Binomial / Botanical Name	Sceletium Tortuosum
Street Names	Canna; Channa; Kaugoed
Major Active Compound	Mesembrine; Mesembrenone; Mesembrenol; Tortuosamine
Indigenous Source	Hotentot Tribe, South Africa
Form	Plant Matter
RoA	Oral / Insufflated
Personal Rating On Shulgin Scale	+ / ++

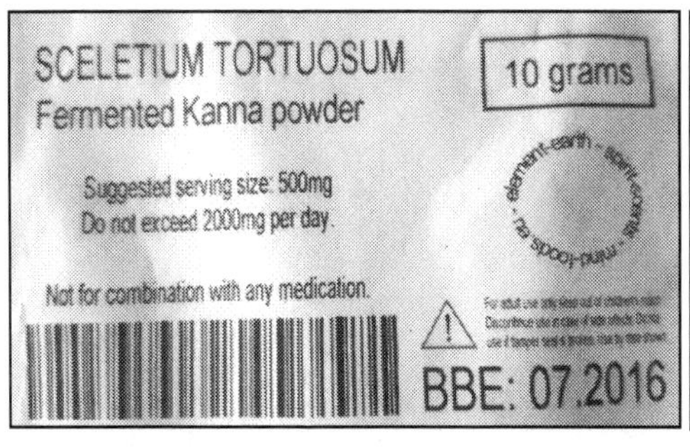

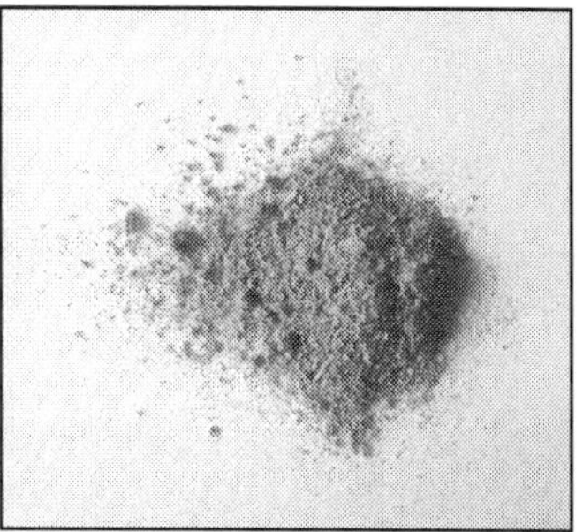

SUBJECTIVE EXPERIENCE
In its native Africa, sceletium tortuosum has traditionally been chewed as a *"vision-inducing entheogen and inebriant"* (ref: Erowid), notably by the Hotentot tribe. It can, however, also be smoked or consumed as tea.

I sampled it a handful on a handful of occasions, circa 2014/15, with perhaps a couple of months between each session. The reports below were written contemporaneously.

> INSUFFLATION TEST 1
> The package arrived in the post this morning. It contained 10g of brown powdered plant matter, almost sawdust in constitution, with a distinctive but not particularly pleasant odour.
>
> I set about testing by insufflating a single line. Wallop! It was awful, and brought tears to my eyes. Fortunately, this wasn't in vain.
>
> Despite harbouring doubts as to whether there would be anything to it there was a fairly immediate effect. Within seconds I felt a changing of headspace, and I was becoming strangely inebriated.

It was intoxicating in the sense of feeling slightly disorientated and a little drunk, but without the loss of clarity. The onset was rapid, and as it took hold I wondered how far it would go. However, the inebriation settled and it stabilised at the same level for approximately 20 minutes.

It then tapered into the promised sedation. The depth of this was difficult to measure as I was already quite chilled, but I was left feeling positively relaxed for some hours.

INSUFFLATION TEST 2
This sample was sold as '*Sceletium Tortuosum 40x extract'*, and was procured from the same source as the regular kanna I had tested earlier. I broadly followed the instructions printed on the packet: "*Serving size 10mg micros scoop, to be insufflated 1-3 times in divided doses*". As stated, there was a cute little scoop enclosed, which I piled high, thus reaching about 15mg.

A nice surprise was that there was no discomfort or serious sting, contrary to the excessive pain I had suffered when I snorted the raw leaves.

I experienced a very clean inebriating effect, perhaps lasting about 10 minutes. This then morphed into a distant sedation, but with a strange visual clarity. Overall it was quite pleasant.

This wasn't very long lasting, so I repeated the exercise, inducing a similar or perhaps stronger response. There was no nausea, and no body load.

As this does seem to be a nice way to fill a couple of hours, it is difficult to understand why this plant isn't more widely known and used.

Note that I was completely detoxed whilst undertaking these experiments.

ORAL TEST
I added half a teaspoon of plain kanna to a cup of coffee this morning, swigging it down quickly to avoid any unpleasant taste.

It certainly had a psychoactive effect, with the next few hours passing with a nice positive vibe. I spent much of the time enjoying the sort of ambient music I wouldn't normally listen to, whilst working on trivial tasks.

Overall this was a pleasant surprise. It was effective via each RoA I tested and in both its natural and extract form. Indeed, I would echo my earlier comment in wondering why this is not more popular.

One further aspect: there are a variety of credible reports stating that this has interesting synergistic properties with other psychoactives, including cannabis. This may well be another area worthy of study.

3.4.8 Lavender

Binomial / Botanical Name	Lavandula
Street Names	N/A
Major Active Compound	Linalool; Linalyl (Unconfirmed)
Indigenous Source	Africa, Europe, Asia
Form	Flowers
RoA	Vaped
Personal Rating On Shulgin Scale	+

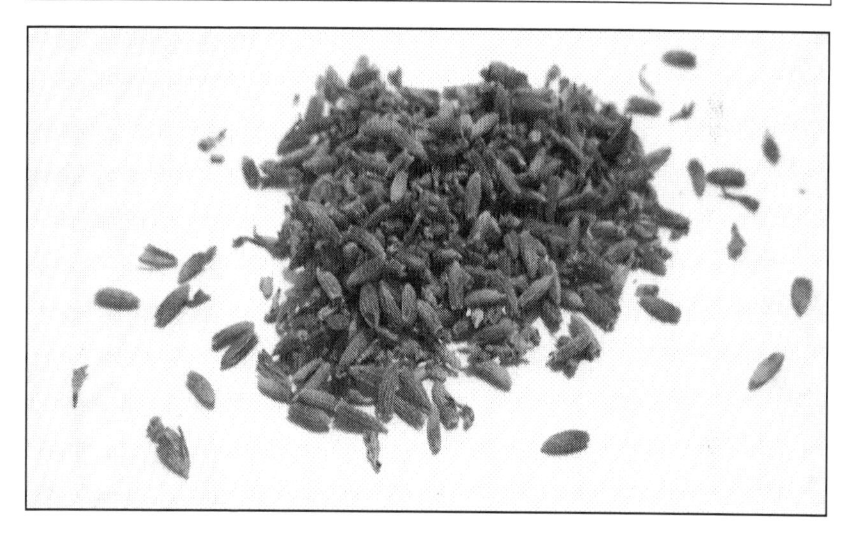

SUBJECTIVE EXPERIENCE
This is frequently used as a mix with cannabis, generally instead of tobacco. However, it is occasionally reported that when smoked alone it does have a gentle calmative effect.

Contrary to expectation, this was indeed my own experience. Although it was certainly nothing to write home about, there was a mild relaxing edge there, somewhere. I should stress that mild is the operative word.

SAFETY WARNING
I have encountered claims that lavender is sometimes *treated* with toxic chemicals by horticulturist vendors to preserve colour/odour. Particular care should therefore be taken with respect to sourcing.

3.4.9 Maconha Brava

Binomial / Botanical Name	Zornia Latifolia
Street Names	Koemataballi; Zornia; Tencilla; Barba De Burro
Major Active Compound	Unknown
Indigenous Source	South America; West Indies
Form	Extract (25x)
RoA	Oral / Smoked
Personal Rating On Shulgin Scale	+ / + [++ Oneirogenic]

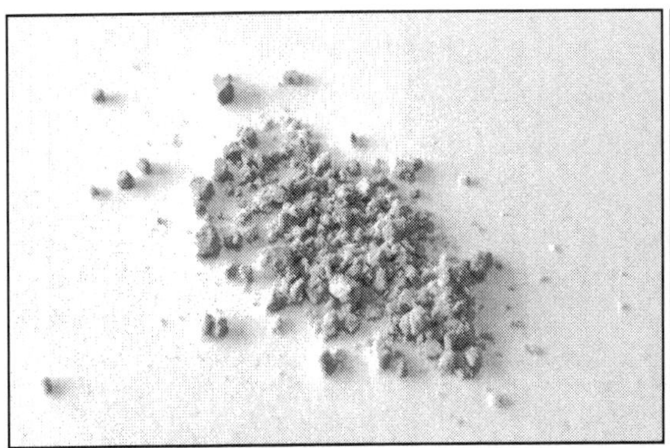

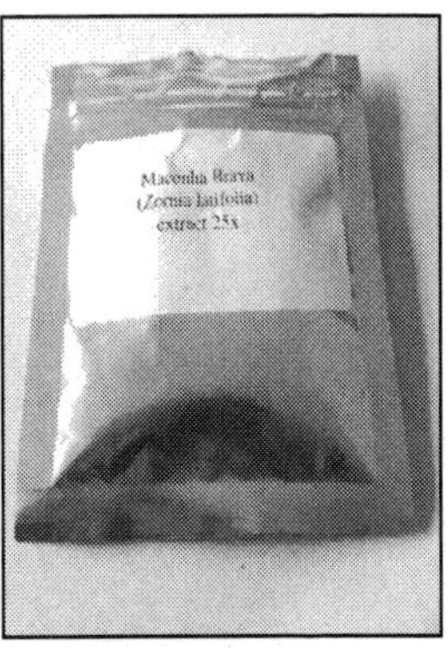

SUBJECTIVE EXPERIENCE

This is used in South America as a mild sedating psychedelic, and according to *Plants of the Gods*, is sometimes smoked as a substitute for cannabis. Internet references, however, were sparse, suggesting that I shouldn't raise my expectations too high.

I didn't, and I was correct not to. The 25x extract I purchased invoked the mildest of headspace, with no notable features.

I should add that the quality of the supplier may have been a relevant factor, particularly as the packet was marked *"Source: Thailand"* (where it is not indigenous). The style of the vendor's website didn't inspire confidence either.

The main effect came out of the blue: vivid dreams.

I hadn't noticed anything on this during research, but upon re-visiting, the reports were there, or at least some reports were there. This is, perhaps, an aspect worthy of further exploration, assuming a more reliable supply.

3.4.10 Marihuanilla

Binomial / Botanical Name	Leonurus Sibiricus
Street Names	Siberian Motherwort; Honeyweed
Major Active Compound	Unknown
Indigenous Source	SE Asia; Siberia; S America; Mexico
Form	Gritty Plant Matter
RoA	Smoked
Personal Rating On Shulgin Scale	+

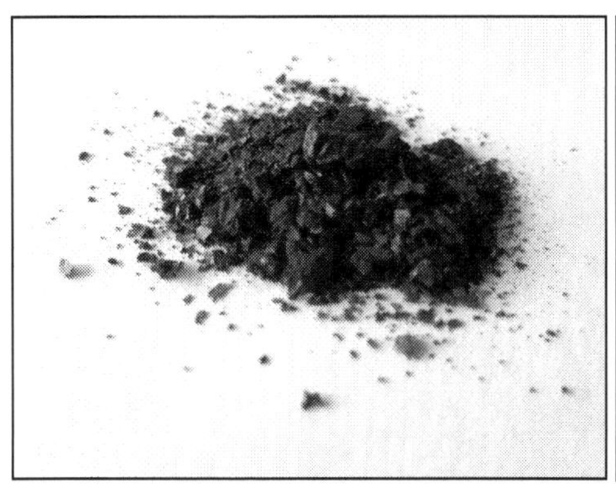

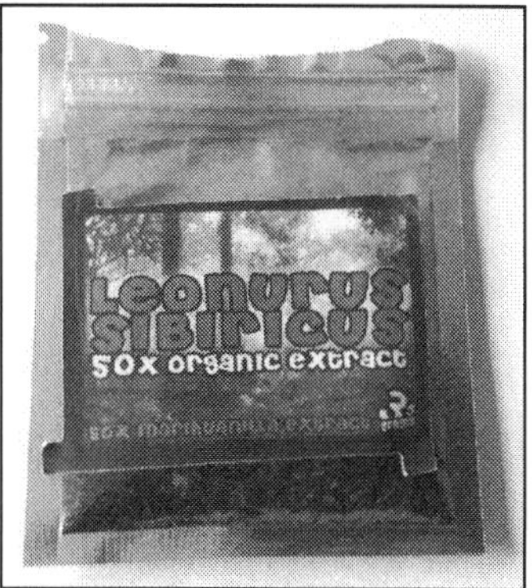

SUBJECTIVE EXPERIENCE
At the time of research, leonurus sibiricus was a widely available legal botanical, and was largely sold as a mild relaxant. Internet descriptions like the following were commonplace:

> *"Leonurus sibiricus, commonly known as Siberian motherwort or Marihuanilla, is an herbaceous plant native to Asia, including southern Siberia, China, Korea, Japan, and Vietnam. It grows wild in the coastal regions of Brazil as well as Chiapas (Hofmann et al. 1992, 47)"*
> ~ entheology.com

> *"In South-America and Mexico Leonurus sibiricus has been used as a substitute for cannabis. That's why the plant was nicknamed Marihuanilla ("little marijuana"). It induces a state of relaxation and has a pleasant taste"*
> ~ *herbsofthegods.nl*

> *"The effects of Marihuanilla can be described as mildly narcotic, though not especially pronounced; thus it is sometimes mixed with other herbs and smoking blends to heighten its potency"* ~ entheology.org

Despite these positive references, my expectations were not high, which is the reason this experiment had been hanging around on my *to-do* list for months.

The vendor I finally sourced from provided the following description:

> *"Leonurus Sibiricus (Marihuanilla) A popular herbal preparation in South America and Mexico. Famous for having a delicious flavor and a calming, full bodied relaxing effect. Mildly narcotic in effect, it is often used as a substitute for illegal drugs."* ~ potseeds.co.uk

With the promise:

> *"Each gram of our extract is equal to 50 Grams of dried herb. A lot of vendors offering 50x extract, but it's very common to take 50g of fresh material and sell it as 50x. Again, we use 50g of dried material to get 1g real 50x extract"* ~ potseeds.co.uk

The substance arrived in the small packet pictured on the previous page, and had a gritty quality to it. It had a distinctive odour, which is difficult to put a name to: a sort of stale fruity spicy smell, but not unpleasant.

I placed a large pinch of it into a bong, lit up, and inhaled.

There was no particular burn, and it was not especially unpleasant to smoke. I took three hits, and returned to my desk.

Almost immediately there was a noticeable psychoactive effect. It was absolutely nothing like as strong as cannabis, but nonetheless it was there. It was quite sedating, but I was in no way stoned.

As I had expected nothing at all, this was a pleasant surprise. It was mild, offered a strange mental clarity, and had a distinct calming effect. There was no nausea or anything of that nature.

I ought to add that I had not consumed any psychoactive materials for a week or two, so I was very detoxed. This probably helped, but regardless, the chilled feeling, which lasted an hour or so, wasn't a placebo effect.

One final observation is that this was followed by a restless night's sleep, during a period in which I had generally been sleeping well. This could be unconnected, but is worth bearing in mind.

ADDENDUM
Some of the sources I consulted during preliminary investigation referred to marihuanilla's use as a potentiator for cannabis and other substances. The general feel I experienced during the experiment suggested that this may indeed be an interesting area of exploration.

3.4.11 Mulungu

Binomial / Botanical Name	Erythrina Mulungu
Street Names	Coral Tree
Major Active Compound	Unknown
Indigenous Source	Brazil
Form	Shredded Bark
RoA	Oral (Decoction)
Personal Rating On Shulgin Scale	+** / Oneirogenic ++

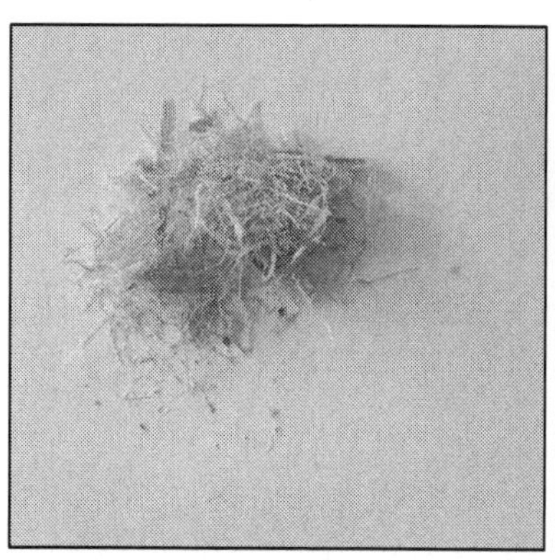

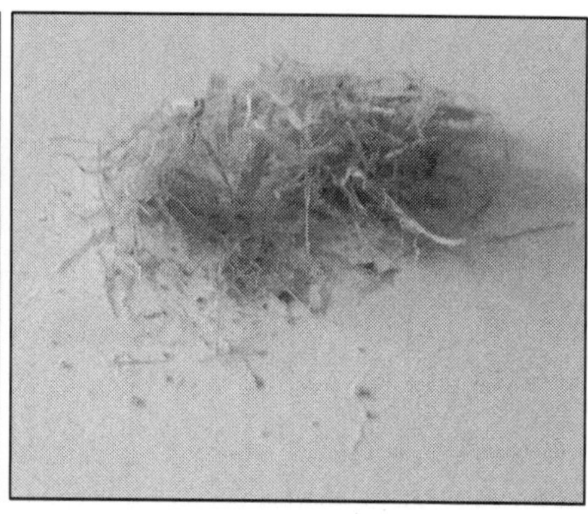

SUBJECTIVE EXPERIENCE
Mulungu has a long history of use as a remedy for stress, anxiety and insomnia in its native Brazil. It is a natural sedative, but it has also been used to treat a wide variety of other ailments.

It is certainly psychoactive, and this was an experiment I was looking forward to.

However, in the ethnobotanical world, the depth and strength of an experience is often determined by the quality of the source and the competence of the preparation. These are fundamental matters, and will often set the course of the experience, or non-experience. Many vendors do not stock fresh, and over a prolonged period botanicals can lose their potency and efficacy. Regarding preparation, this can be complicated, with some decoctions producing better results than others. Some methods simply don't work.

With mulungu I engaged in what was, for me, a complex decocting effort. I simmered 9g of root bark for 45 minutes, strained it, and then consumed the liquid as tea. It wasn't a bad taste.

It worked to a degree, as I felt moderately relaxed and light headed. I then had my usual afternoon nap, and slept in peace.

A distinct psychoactivity was in play, even though it was far from overwhelming. I also experienced dreams during the subsequent night which were slightly more persistent and vivid than usual.

Despite this minor success, I had a feeling that I could do better. Some months later I therefore experimented again, using an entirely different decoction.

On this occasion I used 5g to produce a tea via a more conventional method, but using piping hot rather than boiling water. I gently stirred the mulungu in the teapot and sipped the mild tasting fluid over a 15 minute period.

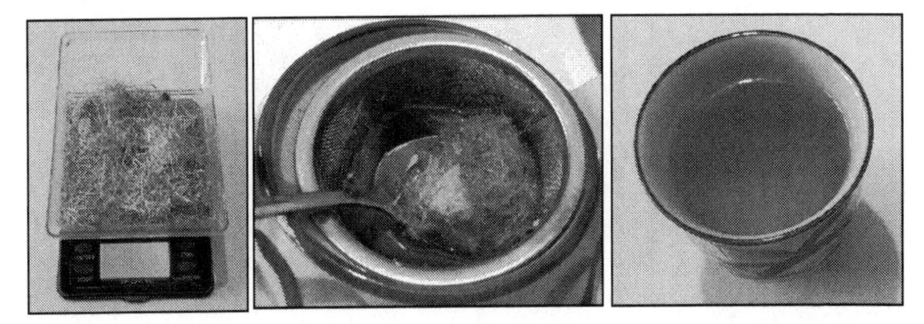

I consumed at 7:30pm, and sure enough, over then next few hours I experienced a heady sedation, which peaked somewhere around the two hour mark. To a lesser degree it was still in play when I retired to bed at 11pm.

During my sleep cycles the mulungu really did manifest itself. Dreams were abundant, and were again lucid and vivid, with the memory of the final lengthy episode still being clear well after I awoke.

This rather took me by surprise, so much so that I spent part of the following morning researching this aspect via the Internet. It does appear that this is indeed a serious dream herb, with similar reports appearing across a number of specialist forums.

My surprise was magnified given that I had procured this from a source which didn't always offer the freshest of materials.

This is an extremely interesting botanical. It invoked a range of sedating effects, and my overview of its oneirogenic properties is by no means exaggerated.

It is certainly one which I intend to return to in the future.

3.4.12 Passion Flower

Binomial / Botanical Name	Passiflora
Street Names	Passion Vines
Major Active Compound	Harmala Alkaloids
Indigenous Source	Pantropical
Form	Stems/Leaves/Flowers
RoA	Oral
Personal Rating On Shulgin Scale	+ [Oneirogenic +*]

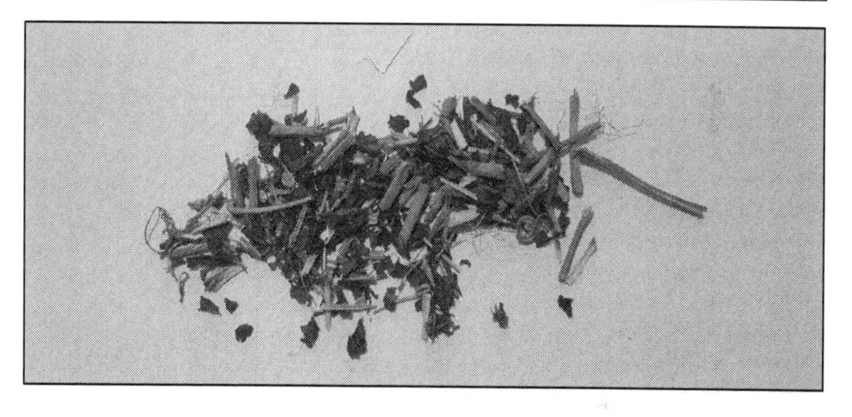

SUBJECTIVE EXPERIENCE
It should be noted at the outset that passiflora is an MAOI*, meaning that you should thoroughly research prior to its use with any other compound or botanical. Better still do not use it in the chronological proximity of any other drug use. Abstain for at least a few days before and after unless you really know what you are doing.

Passiflora is one of the most commonly used botanicals in this class, and is often sold as an aid to combat insomnia, including by major retail chains.

I have only used it a couple of times, primarily because I found it to be a little rough. It did seem to help induce sleep, but the sleep cycles were somewhat distinct, and I tended to consciously awake between them.

Did I dream? Yes, but due to the abruptness of the cycles, these were not particularly satisfying episodes. However, it could well be that knowledge of the above matters was a contributory factor to in the framing of this experience.

* See Section 4.8.1 and the entries for Changa and Syrian Rue for further information

3.4.13 Rhodiola

Binomial / Botanical Name	Rhodiola Rosea
Street Names	Golden Root; Rose Root; Aaron's Rod; King's Crown; Arctic Root
Major Active Compound	Rosavin; Salidroside
Indigenous Source	Europe; Asia; North America
Form	Powdered Root
RoA	Oral
Personal Rating On Shulgin Scale	+*

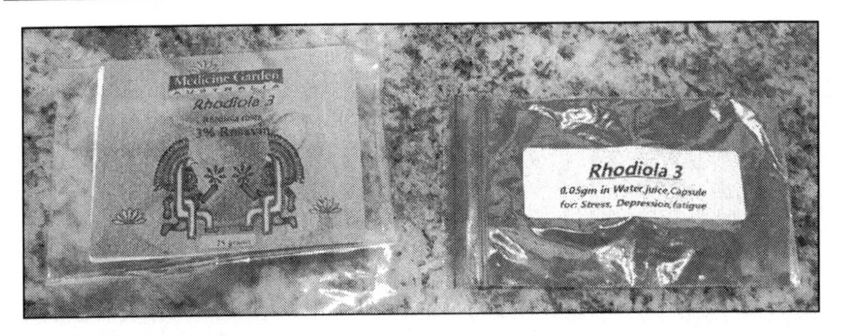

SUBJECTIVE EXPERIENCE
Rhodiola Rosea has been used in traditional medicine to treat a variety of disorders, but primarily with respect to this book, anxiety and depression. Its root contains about 140 chemical compounds although contemporaneously rosavin is often extracted for these purposes.

I sampled this on the second day of a visit to Australia, whilst (as usual) I was suffering from significant jet lag. The packet was labelled *Rhodiola 3*, and *3% Rosavin*, with *Super Concentrate* capitalized on the rear.

At about 1pm a colleague poured some of the powder into a gel cap. This wasn't a measured dose, but given my condition and that I was feeling wretched my judgement was impaired and I consumed it anyway.

By 2pm I was experiencing a mild heady sedation, which wasn't unpleasant. I was being driven down the M1 towards Brisbane, and it produced a generally relaxed blanket over the jet lag. At 3pm I noted the impression that if I was lying in a bed rather than sitting in a car this would have helped me to drop off. I generally felt sleepy and relaxed in a less jet-lagged and more positive sort of way.

Overall this was a mild but decent anxiolytic ride, which faded over the following hours.

3.4.14 St. John's Wort

Binomial / Botanical Name	Hypericum Perforatum
Street Names	Perforate St John's Wort
Major Active Compound	Hyperforin; Adhyperforin;
Indigenous Source	Europe; Asia
Form	Shredded Leaves & Plant Matter
RoA	Oral
Personal Rating On Shulgin Scale	+**

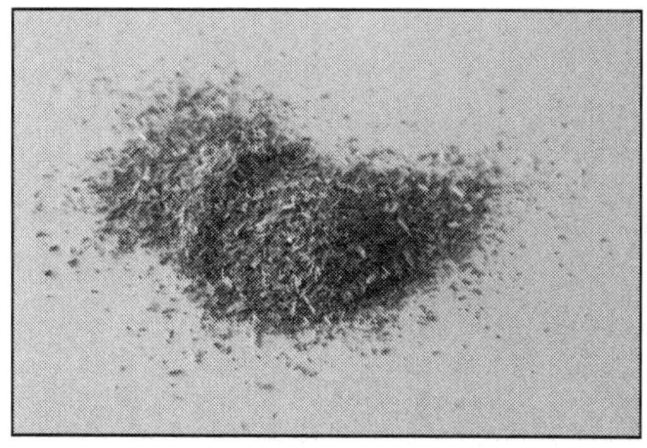

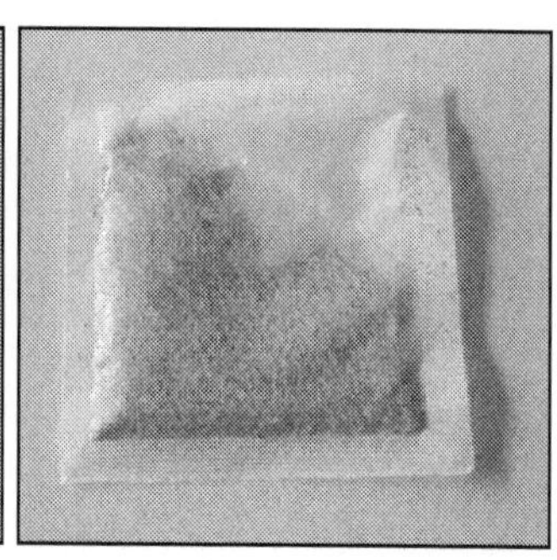

SUBJECTIVE EXPERIENCE
Whilst this is widely purported to alleviate depression, and is sometimes sold as a herbal remedy for insomnia, its effect upon healthy non-depressed individuals is occasionally called into question, including by Christian Rätsch, in his magnificent tome *The Encyclopaedia of Psychoactive Plants.*

Equally, whilst its Wikipedia page supports its efficacy, it continued to be sold via major retail chains in the UK following the implementation of the all-embracing *Psychoactive Substances Act.*

Despite these apparent contradictions, it appears to be undisputed that St John's Wort can interact with a significant number of drugs, sometimes dangerously. It may also reduce their effectiveness. In both cases I refer to prescription medicines as well as recreational psychoactives. For these reasons it is not a plant that I will be testing extensively or at large doses.

Instead of purchasing an extract, or a cocktail of herbs within a commercial remedy, I opted to acquire a box of tea bags, courtesy of Amazon, for a whopping £2.39. I was somewhat surprised when my purchase arrived just a few days later, directly from Bulgaria.

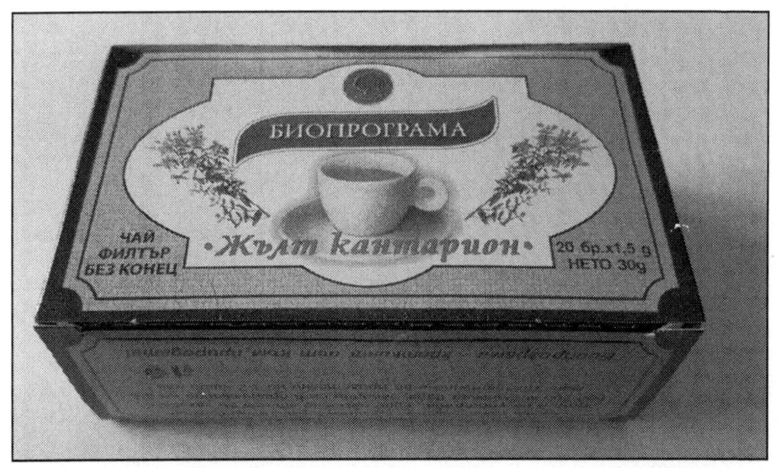

The advert stated "*Top Quality 100% Natural St John's Wort from the Balkans*"

Given the warnings just referred to, I decided to use just a single bag, containing 1.5g of tea. I did, however, soak this well in the cup of boiling water.

> T+0:00 I sip the tea slowly as it cools. It tastes fairly neutral, being neither unpalatable nor pleasant. [8pm]
>
> T+0:20 Having drunk the entire cup, I lean back in my chair, and wait. I begin to feel a mild warmth and an anxiolytic wave takes hold, but I muse that these could be placebo effects, given that I was not depressed at the outset. Undoubtedly, however, I do feel more relaxed at this point, and calmer.
>
> T+1:00 Whilst I expected nothing from this experiment, I feel rather heady and sedated. I have definitely wound down from earlier, and can confirm that, for me, this tea is certainly psychoactive.
>
> T+3:00 This has induced a very relaxed evening, with a nice background buzz, which is quite mild but rather pleasant. I retire to bed, sleepy, with a chilled and almost serene disposition.

The night's sleep was another surprise. I slept like a log for the first time in weeks. Given the conflicting reports, I didn't see this coming at all. This morning I felt a little drowsy but generally positive and well.

This was nice. The flip side is that if Christian Rätsch's reference is correct, I apparently have underlying *issues*.

Reminder: don't use this with other medicines or drugs.

3.4.15 Skullcap

Binomial / Botanical Name	Scutellaria Lateriflora
Street Names	Mad Dog Skullcap
Major Active Compound	Baicalin; Misc
Indigenous Source	North America
Form	Herb
RoA	Oral / Smoked
Personal Rating On Shulgin Scale	+ / +*, ++

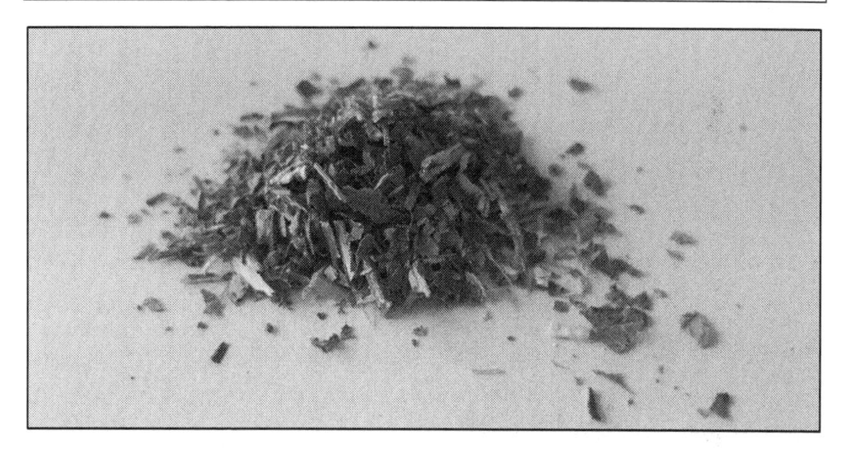

SUBJECTIVE EXPERIENCE
I had sampled skullcap a couple of years previously, but my notes were sparse. On the adapted Shulgin scale they indicated a + when drank as a tea, and a +* when smoked. Translating this, I felt a very minor effect, possibly too minor to articulate, but enjoyed slightly more potency when I smoked it.

This was contrary to most Internet reports, which claimed greater effect from tea than smoking. Regardless, I decided to re-test by smoking, as on the evening in question I had a full stomach, which could have reduced the efficacy of oral ingestion.

As I wasn't feeling at the top of my game, I was hoping for some sort of mood lift, or less optimistically, for an anxiolytic response. My expectations, however, were not at all high.

> T+0:00 Filling the bowl of a small bong, I take five large hits, in fairly quick succession. [7pm]

None of the hits are terrible in terms of taste, although they are perhaps slightly harsh. On the first hit, I feel a slight and momentary head rush. Thereafter, I don't feel any obvious response or any immediate form of intoxication.

T+0:03 Sitting down at my desk, perhaps I do feel slightly better. The stomach anxiety has diminished, and there is a slight fuzziness there or thereabouts.

I am not stoned, but I do feel a mild but marked reaction. There is nothing unpleasant about it, but it isn't a high or any form of euphoria. It is simply a more chilled heady feeling and accompanying state of mind.

T+0:10 Ten minutes in, these effects are still with me. I feel a gentle calmness, relative to where I was beforehand. There is a distinct headiness about this which is quite soothing.

T+0:20 I am still relaxed. Throughout I have retained mental clarity, and at no stage have I felt that my functionality has been impaired. It is a solid and reasonably interesting experience.

T+0:30 The ride is starting to subside a little, although I am still calm and chillaxed.

T+1:00 The effects are now less pronounced, and I am close to base, but certainly not at base. It strikes me that I could have been more deeply sedated earlier than I thought I was.

T+3:00 Most of the headiness has gone. I feel more or less back at baseline, although anxiety is still absent and I still feel calm in a naturally sedated way. I am wondering if there will be a knock-on effect for the night's sleep.

The night's sleep was a little strange. There were weird dreams, which could be unconnected, but the sleep tended to have the same skullcap headiness quality to it, and this was definitely there when I awoke in the morning. There was no discomfort but it was present and it only dissipated after an hour or so, with the help of a cup of filtered coffee.

Following this experiment, I am now left wondering about skullcap consumed as tea. Given that smoking touched a fairly pleasant ++ experience, this may well be worth another fling.

I should also state that the skullcap I used was very dry, and had been lying around for some time. This suggests that fresh skullcap might produce an even stronger ride. Bear in mind here that with a higher quality sample five bong hits may well be overdoing it.

Finally, it is worth noting that a number of species of *scutellaria* are cited as being psychoactive. Of these, *scutellaria nana* is sometimes claimed to be the most potent, although it may be difficult to procure.

3.4.16 Valerian Root

Binomial / Botanical Name	Valeriana Officinalis
Street Names	Garden Valerian; Garden Heliotrope; All-Heal
Major Active Compound	Miscellaneous
Indigenous Source	Europe; Asia
Form	Root
RoA	Oral
Personal Rating On Shulgin Scale	+*

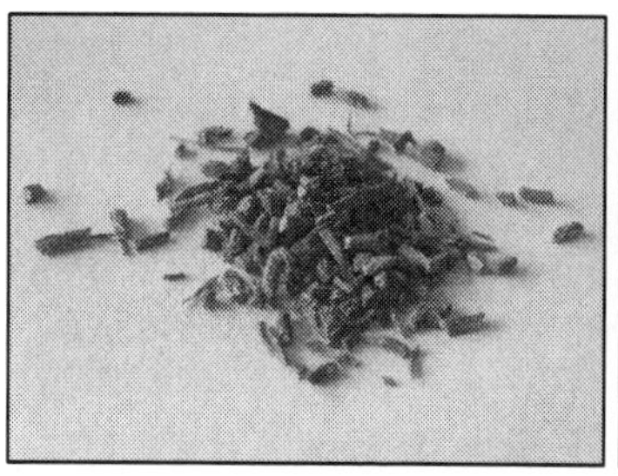

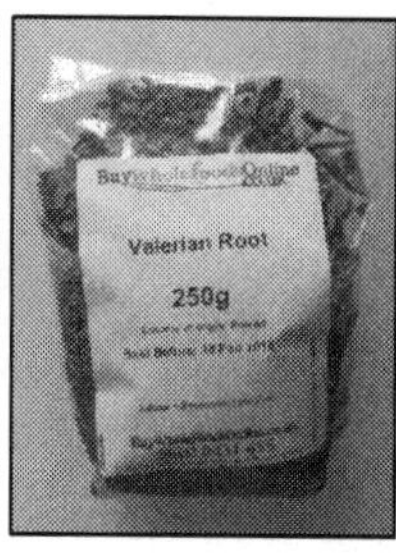

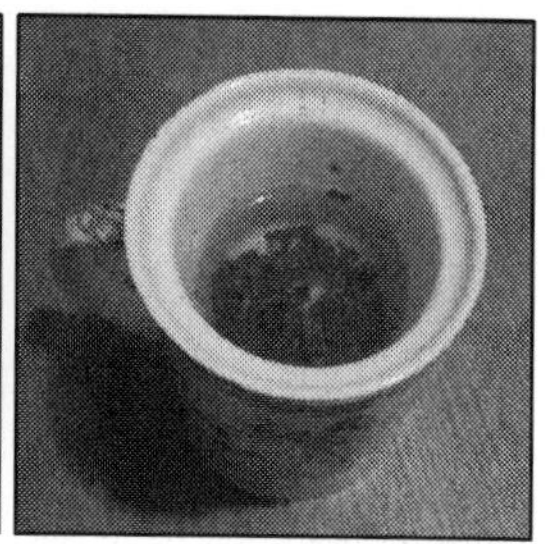

SUBJECTIVE EXPERIENCE
I have previously consumed valerian as an extract, within commercially sold herbal remedies for insomnia. I recall varying degrees of success, but on occasion, a headache if I over indulged. Due to its hit and miss nature, and possible side effects, I tended to avoid regular or even periodic use.

Establishing the appropriate dose for tea made solely from the natural root was not as straight forward as it might have been. During research, I found quite a few references to valerian, with the word *root* absent, which seemed to refer to the extracted form. For tea comprising the native root only, there were far fewer reports. The most common recommendations, however, seemed to cite 2-3 grams for an effective cup.

After due consideration, I went for 3 grams, and weighed this in the usual manner.

I boiled the water and left it to stand for five minutes, so that it was hot, but no longer boiling. I then poured it onto the root, which I had placed in the filter on top of a cup. I immersed the filter under the water line, so that I could stir the root and infuse as much as possible from it. I stirred several times over a period of about ten minutes.

T+0:00 I begin sipping the tea. This is not a bad flavour. It is slightly woody in nature, but with no bitterness, and with a reasonable aftertaste. [8:30pm]

T+0:10 I have finished the cup, and I chew and swallow the sediment at the bottom. Again it tastes mild and palatable.

T+0:30 I do feel a slight drowsiness about the head, and some sedation. It's very gentle, but there is something there. There also appears to be the hint of an anxiolytic undercurrent.

At this point the effects align with Erowid's classification, which lists it as a sedative, relaxant and anxiolytic.

T+1:00 I feel weary but relaxed. I lean back in my chair wondering how much is tiredness, and how much is the effect of the tea.

I note though that this is a subtly different sort of tiredness than the weary exhaustion of recent evenings. It could currently be described as a drowsy relaxing lethargy.

T+1:10 I can safely say that my earlier conclusions were correct. I am sedated and I feel more inclined to fall into a quality sleep than I have for a while. I should add that I haven't had enough sleep in recent days, so it is possible that this has released that need, rather than created it.

T+2:00 The initial effects have now run down a little, but I am still left with a heady relaxed sleepiness. I retire to bed. I feel no headache or negative effects thus far.

T+11:00 Surprisingly, I struggled to fall asleep. I wasn't uncomfortable and was still slightly sedated, but I couldn't drop off for quite a while. Neither did I achieve the full night's deep sleep I was hoping for. It was disturbed and I woke up periodically, as I have done for the last week or so.

On the other hand, as I type these notes in the morning, I still feel comfortable and fairly relaxed, which is quite a pleasant disposition.

Overall, this was calming during a stressful period, but as a sleep aid I noticed little on this occasion.

As a sedative it was surprisingly effective. I suffered no adverse side effects, but I did feel a certain heady sensation which suggested that a higher dose might induce a headache.

I suspect it is one to try again under different life-circumstances, and possibly at a lower dose.

3.4.17 White Sage

Binomial / Botanical Name	Salvia Apiana
Street Names	Bee Sage; Sacred Sage
Major Active Compound	Thujone
Indigenous Source	SW United States, NW Mexico
Form	Leaves & Twigs
RoA	Smoked
Personal Rating On Shulgin Scale	+**

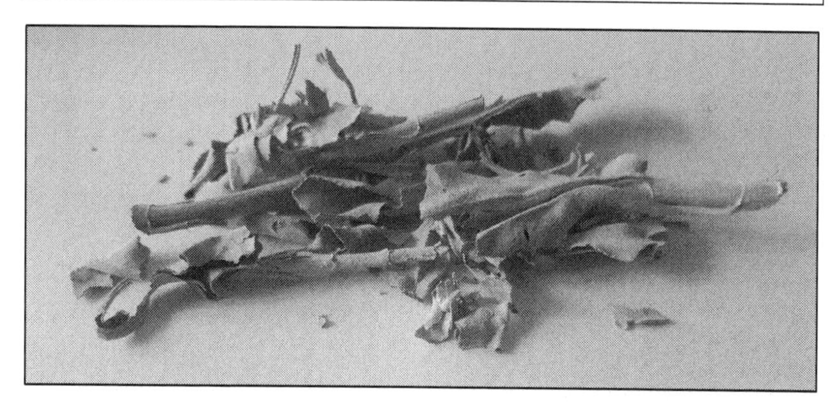

SUBJECTIVE EXPERIENCE
White sage has a lengthy history of use as a ceremonial plant, with Native Americans using it as incense to fend off evil spirits, to clear negative energy, and to create sacred spaces. It has also been used medicinally across a number of civilisations.

I had used it a year or so earlier and vaguely recalled a light sedation but a harsh uncomfortable smoke. I re-sampled it to document this more thoroughly for the purposes of this book.

I broke the dry and brittle leaves into the bowl of a large bong. The smell had a mint-like edge, but largely reminded me of the old *sage & onion* stuffing that used to arrive on my plate at Christmas. It certainly had a pungent and strong odour, at least prior to incineration.

> T+0:00 I take the first hit, which is not as harsh as I recall. Indeed, given that the smoke is thick and intense, it is quite mild. [8pm]
>
> T+0:01 My head has lightened already, and I do feel a relaxing effect, with a clear anxiolytic benefit. This is minor, but certain.

I repeat with two or three reasonably large hits. Via the large bong this isn't too bad to toke at all. It feels almost cleansing.

Strangely, the smoking ritual itself also feels pleasing, which could have something to do with the pre-reading I have just completed on ceremonial use.

T+0:05 I stop inhaling at this point, having taken maybe half a dozen hits over the last five minutes. The light-headedness remains, and there is a vague dreamy feel in play.

T+0:10 I was quite anxious at the start of this experiment, having endured a difficult day. At least for now, however, this has dissipated. The headiness is mild but present, and I can see how some people claim that this plant holds meditative qualities. Physically I feel quite tranquil.

T+0:15 A relaxed mood remains, as does a little of the general ataraxy. I continue to feel a background sedation and serenity, but expect this to slowly drift down from here.

T+0:30 I have indeed moved towards base, although a balmy and mellow ambience persists.

T+14:00 For the rest of the evening I felt relatively normal, but with muted anxiety and a calmer disposition. This is quite usual during the slow unwind from this sort of experience. The night's sleep was disturbed, but with some periods of deep sleep, and a period of vivid (or at least recalled) dreaming.

This morning I feel fairly standard, although perhaps a little off-key.

Whilst I found that this was not a ++ on the adapted Shulgin scale, as some members of this class have been, it certainly invoked a clear psychoactive response. Overall, it was quite pleasant for a one-off or rare occasion, but given that it contains thujone, which has been reported as toxic to the brain, kidney, and liver, it is not one to make a habit of.

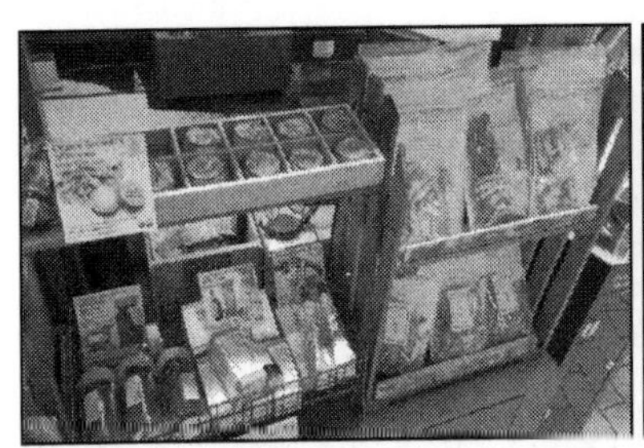
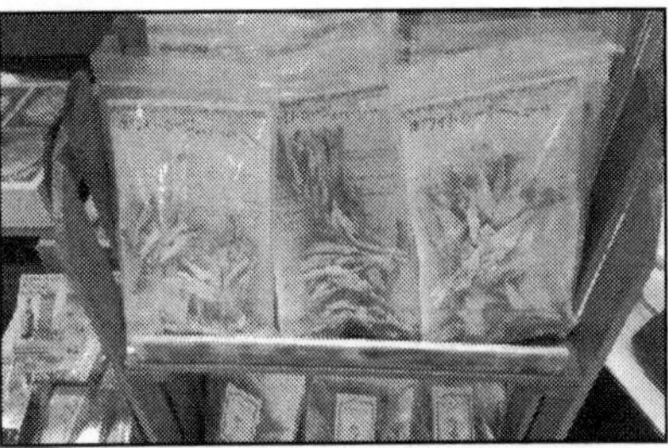

White sage as sold in a city centre tobacconist, Shinjuku, Tokyo, Japan

3.4.18 Wild Dagga

Binomial / Botanical Name	Leonotis Leonurus
Street Names	Lion's Tail
Major Active Compound	Leonurine
Indigenous Source	South Africa
Form	Petals
RoA	Oral /Smoked
Personal Rating On Shulgin Scale	+** / +

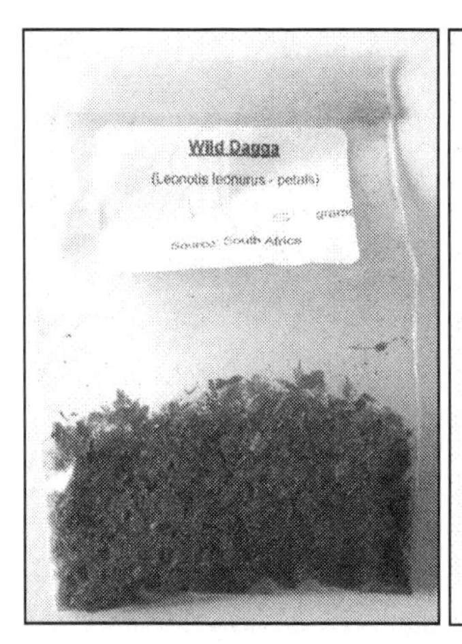

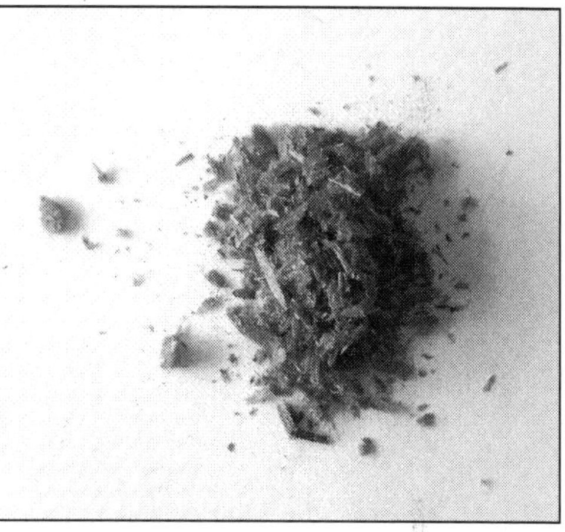

SUBJECTIVE EXPERIENCE
Wild dagga is one of the better known natural sedatives, particularly in southern Africa. It has been used as a remedy for a significant number of ailments, and recreationally, as an occasional substitute for cannabis. My notes at the time of testing were as follows:

> Also known as *Lion's Tail* and *Wild Dagga*, Erowid classifies this as a *Sedative; Intoxicant*, and it was my latest venture into the ethnobotanical arena. It was quite pricey, but did it work?
>
> Online reviews are mixed, but this seems to be the most common sentiment:
>
> > "*It is a nice smoking blend but don't buy it if you are looking to get high. It does have some calming effects but just slightly. It's nothing like pot is what I'm saying.*" ~ Danlennon3, shroomery.org

Last week I tried smoking it. It was a bit rough, and tasted pretty nasty. In terms of psychoactive effect, there was some, but nothing notable or particularly pleasing.

Unperturbed I decided to vape, having identified a couple of temperature recommendations [150°C to 175°C (302°F to 347°F)]. This produced a minor background effect, but not really what I was hoping for from my £10.

Smoking it in a bong, as opposed to rolling it into a joint, I found the effect to be a little stronger. It helped that it was more pleasing from an aesthetic perspective.

Tonight I tried wild dagga tea. I used about 14g over several cups. This was much better. There was no particular high; just a mellow buzz and a mild lifting of anxiety. I wouldn't describe it as being stoned, but the psychoactivity was definitely there, and was quite pleasant.

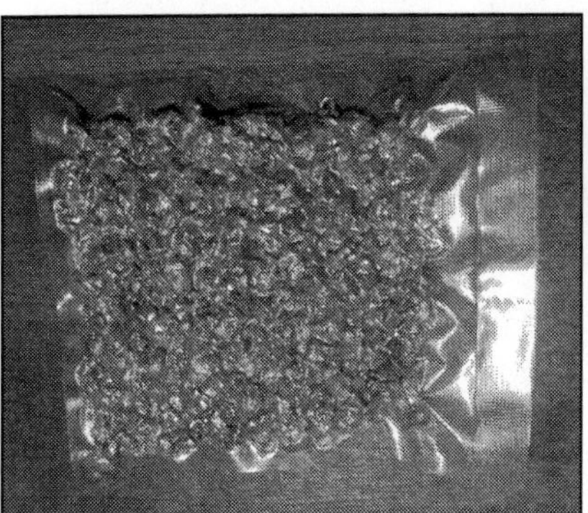

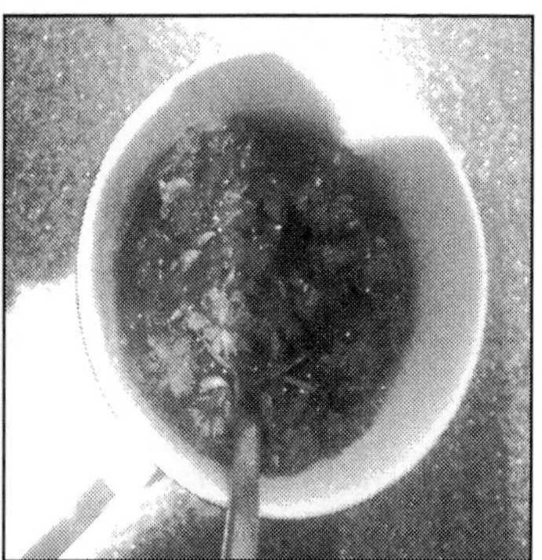

In making these observations I should note that most of the wild dagga I have seen for sale on the Internet is more colourful than mine. It is possible that it is more potent.

Overall, I found this to be more pleasing and sedating when taken as a tea, although nowhere near as active as, for example, kanna or kratom. It did, however, produce one final surprise: on retiring to bed I felt that there was some form of oneirogenic reaction, albeit minor.

At a later date I managed to obtain a fresher batch of this material. This felt cleaner, and I found smoking to be slightly more rewarding than described above.

This certainly creates a buzz-like sedation, at the lower end of the scale, but it is not a plant I am particularly drawn to return to.

3.4.19 Wild Lettuce

Binomial / Botanical Name	Lactuca Virosa
Street Names	Bitter Lettuce; Laitue Vireuse; Opium Lettuce
Major Active Compound	Lactucin; Lactucopicrin
Indigenous Source	Europe; Asia; Australia
Form	Leaves
RoA	Smoked / Oral
Personal Rating On Shulgin Scale	+ / +

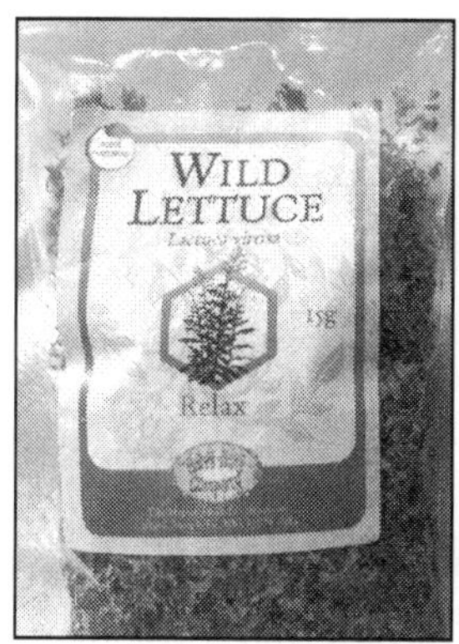

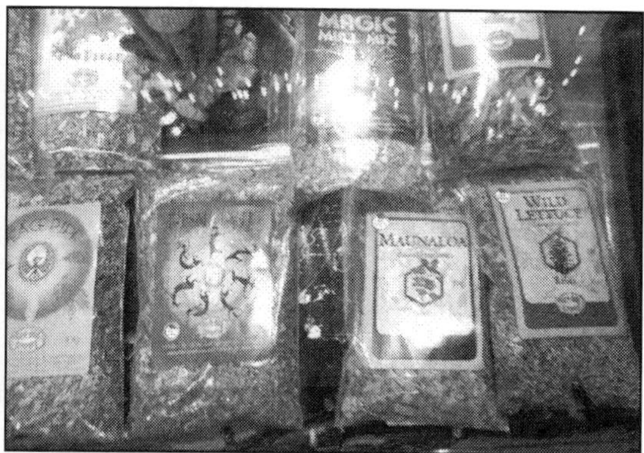

SUBJECTIVE EXPERIENCE
It is easy to confuse this with the common lettuce, as purchased from the supermarket. Whilst I should categorically state that it is a different member of the genus, I should add that there is more to the family itself than meets the eye.

I purchased a pack of wild lettuce in Australia, as a self-help remedy for jet lag. I simply couldn't sleep through the nights. My experiments with this were therefore undertaken at unconventional times: I smoked it from a small pipe at 3am and 4am respectively.

Did it work?

No, at least to the extent that it didn't send me to sleep. I continued to toss and turn hopelessly.

Was it psychoactive?

Yes. Even though I already felt rather strange, courtesy of the jet lag, this changed the complexion of the feeling slightly.

There was a definite sedation, as there was the following day when I consumed this as tea. It was more anxiolytic than sleep inducing, with a heady presence. Perhaps the latter is what causes some users to claim that it has an opium type feel; something which I didn't really notice.

Although minor, a background form of sedating psychoactivity was certainly in play, via both RoA's.

THE IMPULSE OF YOUTH

As an aside, this was not my first experiment with the lettuce family. Many years ago, I read somewhere that all lettuces were, to some degree, psychoactive.

Whether this was true or not, the impulse of youth drove me to purchase two whole lettuces, and eat them, or at least, eat as much as I possibly could. This amounted to approximately one lettuce and a half.

I have no idea which type of lettuce these were, but they were procured as normal lettuces from a normal grocer.

I ate them in the evening, and dropped into a deep and extremely long sleep (10+ hours) a few hours later. At the time I was astonished, and never saw the humble lettuce in the same light again.

During the research for this book, I discovered that perhaps there is something to it, as lettuce is often promoted as a natural remedy for insomnia.

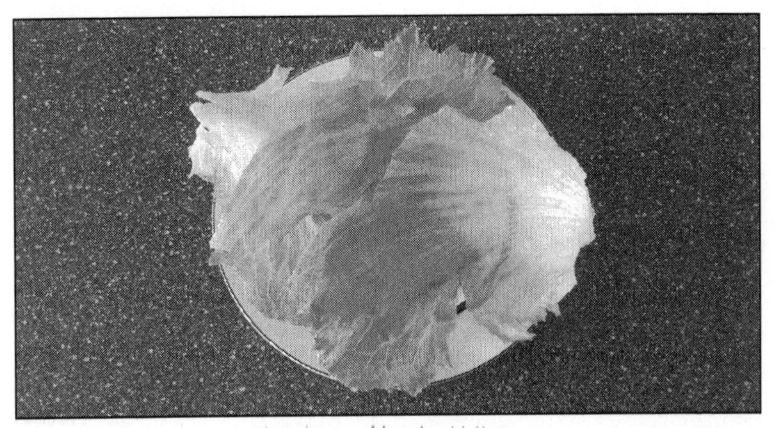

There is something about lettuce

3.5. NOOTROPICS

Textbook Definition: *Nootropics improve or enhance one or more cognitive functions, such as memory, focus and creativity.*

The following botanicals have been sampled and researched for inclusion within this section:

I was always sceptical about nootropics, having serious doubts that any of them were genuinely effective.

At time of writing this section, I had experimented with a handful of chemicals, but never in terms of repeated daily dosing, which tends to be the *modus operandi* for this class of substance. The effects of these was usually to invoke some sort of stimulation, but nothing to convince me that any measure of cognitive enhancement had actually occurred.

The jury remained out, and I wasn't prepared to take what I perceived to be risks with my safety and long term health by creating a regular dosing regime.

The idea that a botanical could produce nootropic effects didn't occur to me. Indeed, I wasn't aware that such properties were even claimed; until I saw celastrus paniculatus on sale, courtesy of a popular botanical website.

That this plant could actually produce a tangible nootropic experience, on a single dose, was the last thing I expected. But it did. Furthermore, it isn't the only botanical for which this sort of effect is claimed.

Again, given my self-imposed limitations, I cannot do justice to this particular field, other than to present details of my own introductory experimentation. However, it is certainly an area deserving of further research, which I will undertake if and when the opportunity arises.

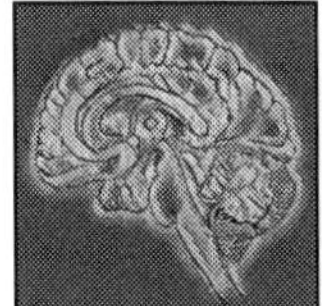
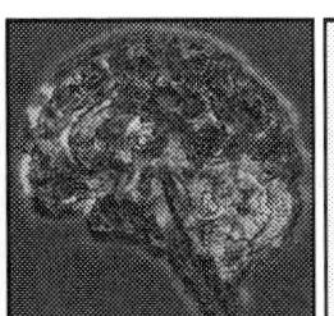
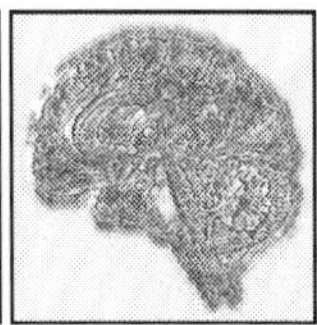
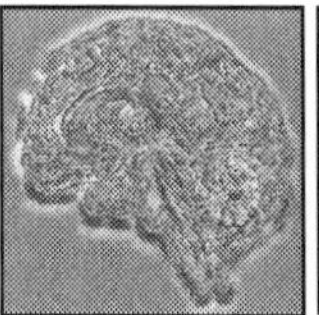
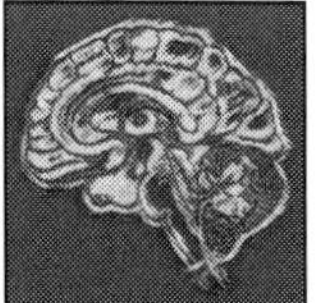

Botanical nootropics are worth far more than a scratch of the surface

3.5.1 Catuaba

Binomial / Botanical Name	Erythroxylum Catuaba
Street Names	Caramuru; Catagu;
Major Active Compound	Catuabine A/B/C/D
Indigenous Source	Brazil
Form	Shredded Bark
RoA	Oral
Personal Rating On Shulgin Scale	+**

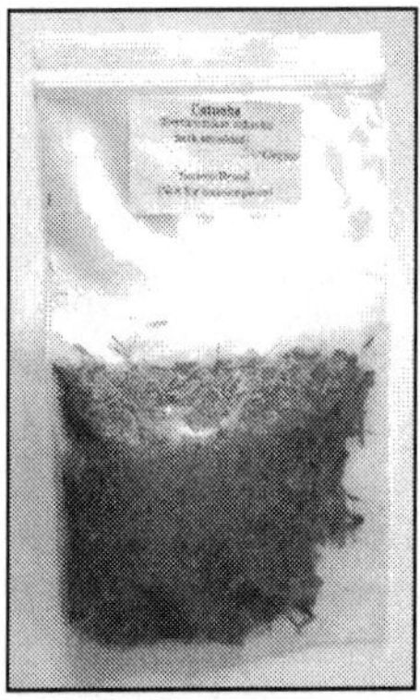
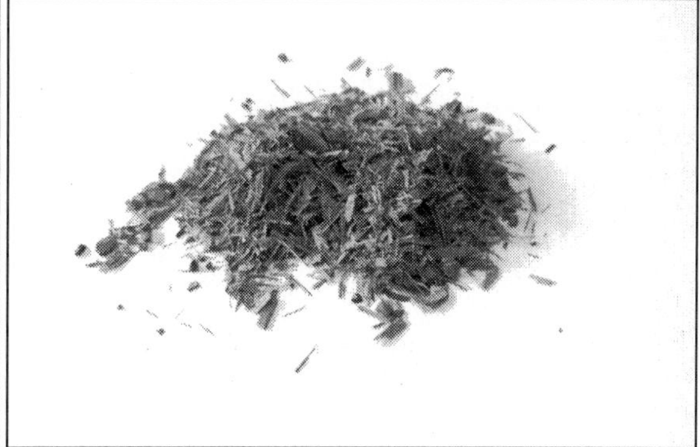

SUBJECTIVE EXPERIENCE
In its native South America, catuaba has traditionally been used as an aphrodisiac and a stimulant. However, with respect to the latter, there are occasional reports which appear to contradict this, suggesting that it also possesses calmative and anxiolytic properties. Regarding the former, references to this as a *love plant* and a *sex drink* are not uncommon.

In terms of its value as a nootropic I have frequently encountered claims that it is used to address poor memory and forgetfulness, and even that it has been used as a treatment for Alzheimer's disease and dementia.

I should add that many reports cite daily use as the route to accentuate these effects, an approach which is beyond my own *modus operandi* (largely for safety reasons).

For my original test I brewed 12g as a tea. The results were inconclusive, registering the mildest of body/head changes. For the more rigorous re-test, I have abstained from any other psychoactive for over a week to enable a more focused study.

The recommended dose is usually 1-2 tablespoons, with suggestions that higher doses can leave a headache. After due consideration, I scoop two generous spoonfuls from the transparent plastic bag, which equates to 8.2g, and steep this in a pot of hot but not boiling water for ten minutes.

> T+0:00 I pour the first cup and begin to slowly sip the tea. It is a pleasing red/brown colour and tastes a little woody and slightly bitter, but is quite palatable. [3:50pm].
>
> T+0:10 I am on to my second cup. Perhaps a slight head change and body warmth is emerging.
>
> T+0:30 The tea has now been consumed. I feel warm, with a mild head buzz within an overall calmness. There is certainly something of a simmering background stimulation in play.
>
> T+0:35 There is more of a feeling of being in a zone than perhaps with caffeine, with a slight physical response in terms of a moderately raised temperature.
>
> T+0:45 The buzz and general comfort are still there, and I am not feeling any of the fatigue I have endured over the last few days. In terms of a nootropic effect, I am able to concentrate and focus, although no more so than when using a mild functional stimulant. The claims regarding enhanced memory, of course, are impossible to verify without formal testing.
>
> Regarding its use as an aphrodisiac, there does seem to be something there. Compared to amphetamine, for example, this hardly registers. Unlike amphetamine, however, it does not seem to induce stim-dick, which probably supports the suggestion that it can be used to alleviate this symptom if combined with it (which is not something I recommend).
>
> T+1:10 The mild stimulation and heady feel continues on the same level as earlier. I should also add that I am no longer hungry, so there may be some appetite suppression in play.
>
> T+2:00 The effects are now slowly winding down.

Overall this provided a reasonably pleasant low level stimulation, with minor aphrodisiacal properties, and some appetite suppression, whilst wrapped in a background of gentle sedation. The only rough edge was a very minor pre-headache type feeling which I experienced during the evening (probably due to dose), and which persisted into a heavy headedness during sleep disturbances.

In terms of its use as a nootropic, I found that concentration was clear, but there was nothing exceptional to note. On a single experience I cannot comment sensibly with respect to memory and dementia.

3.5.2 Celastrus Paniculatus

Binomial / Botanical Name	Celastrus Paniculatus
Street Names	Black Oil Plant; Climbing Staff Tree; Intellect Tree
Major Active Compound	Unknown
Indigenous Source	India
Form	Seeds
RoA	Oral
Personal Rating On Shulgin Scale	++

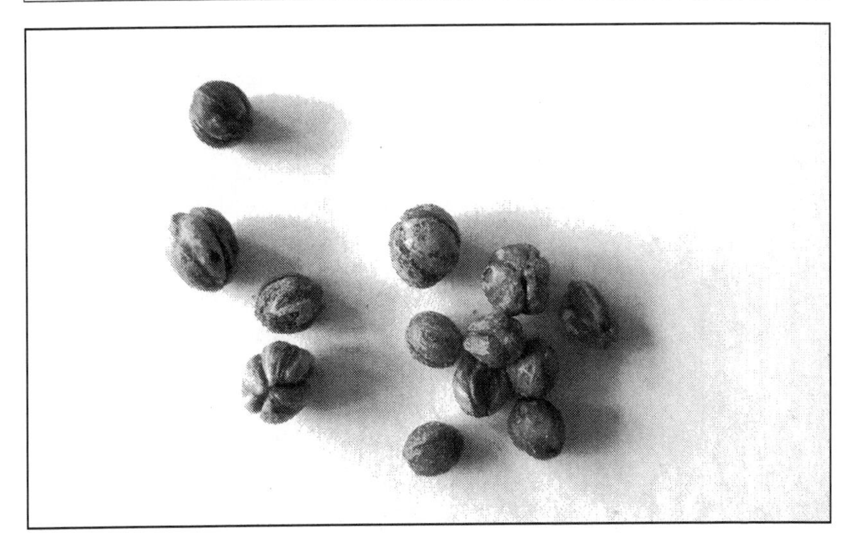

SUBJECTIVE EXPERIENCE
Celastrus Paniculatus has been used in traditional ayurvedic medicine for many centuries. It has long been considered to offer a variety of benefits and address a range of ailments, but it is most well known for the stimulation of both intellect and memory. Indeed, to this day, Indian students are known to use it prior to revision study and academic examinations.

My first experiment comprised the multi-dosing of 20+ 20+10 seeds over several hours. For my second, I consumed a single dose of 40 seeds. In each case I chewed the seeds for a few minutes and then swallowed with water.

On both occasions the outcome surprised me.

With nootropics generally, and certainly on a single dose, I usually feel that there might be something there, and often I believe that there is, but it is not clear enough to absolutely dismiss the chance that this is a placebo effect. It tends to be is borderline, at best.

Not with this.

I was absolutely certain that it was effective.

It induced an on focus clarity, and it delivered this the day after a fairly heavy night. I should have been feeling a little fuzzy, but having munched down the seeds, the opposite was the case.

The second exercise, which was undertaken some weeks after the first, confirmed its efficacy.

Celastrus Paniculatus has a positive reputation, and a wide variety of claims continue to be made about it. Here is just one list, which I found via a random search:

> *"appetizer, emetic expectorant, sodorific, liver tonic, aphrodisiac, stimulant, powerful brain tonic, stimulate intellect and sharpen memory, cure joint pain, paralysis, rheumatism, weakness; seed oil enriches the blood, cures abdominal complaints, stomachic, tonic, treats cough, asthma, leprosy, headaches, leucoderma"* ~ celastrus.com

Obviously I cannot confirm most of these, but I can state categorically that it is psychoactive. Within hours, on the specified dose, there was a clear, unambiguous and beneficial effect on my mental acuity.

There was no euphoria or obvious stimulation to it, as far as I could tell, but I felt confident and content whilst under its influence.

On retiring to bed I fell asleep without difficulty, and during the night I experienced a multitude of dreams. In some, the frequently claimed aphrodisiacal properties did in fact manifest themselves.

Repeat experiments yielded similar results to these first two encounters, certainly in terms of clarity, sharpened focus and cognitive enhancement.

It would appear that this is a nootropic that actually works, and is one which produces a return from a single dose. Continued research on the Internet, with reference to field reports, indicates that the same opinion is shared by a substantial number of individuals.

This again is a plant that is deserving of further experimentation. It isn't one which produces a high or a recreational trip, but it does provide considerable scope for intellectual exploration and research.

3.5.3 Ginkgo

Binomial / Botanical Name	Ginkgo Biloba
Street Names	Ginkgo; Maidenhair Tree
Major Active Compound	Flavonoids; Terpenes
Indigenous Source	China
Form	Powdered Leaves
RoA	Oral
Personal Rating On Shulgin Scale	+**

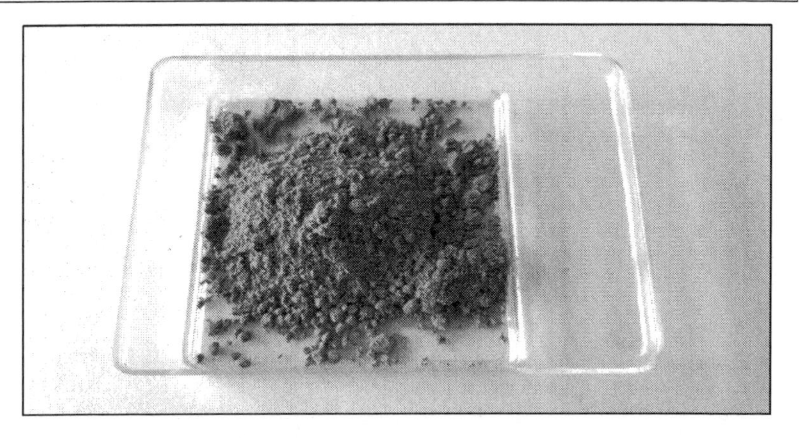

SUBJECTIVE EXPERIENCE
Found in fossils dating back 270 million years, ginkgo biloba is one of the oldest species of tree on earth. Its leaves have been used in traditional Chinese medicine for thousands of years, and more recently extracts have been sold as a dietary supplement. Despite this, its efficacy is disputed.

What isn't contested is that it can produce a number of adverse side effects, and consequently, should not be used unless in full health. Also, it should never be used by individuals with allergic reactions to alkylphenol-producing plants.

It is claimed that ginkgo improves mental alertness and clarity, as well as enhancing memory and overall brain functionality, particularly in older people. Other claims I have occasionally encountered include improved vision, increased energy and mood elevation.

Regarding dosage, I identified no universally agreed figures, although I did find numorous suggestions that a single 120mg-240mg dose would have an effect. Interestingly, many included advice that it should be taken with food.

I noted however that all these reports seemed to refer to standardized extracts, rather than to the raw leaves. Seeking information on the latter, I found a number of references to *ginkgo tea*, including brands which comprised solely of the leaves.

From the explorer's perspective, this does seem to be the way to go. Unfortunately though, my supply is of *powdered* leaf, meaning that I am likely to swallow some if not all of it. Furthermore, as with extracts, investigation into dosage in this form was not conclusive, with identified recommendations ranging from 2g-7g.

Due to the possible side effects referred to earlier, the potential to cause allergic reactions and suggestions of toxicity of certain leaf constituents*, I decide to temper my inclination to push too high.
[* "*However, the ginkgolic acid (GA) contained in GBE is proved to be highly allergenic and cytotoxic, even minimal residual could also cause severe adverse effects.*" ~ PMID: 22568222]

I measure a 6g dose, pour it into a teapot, and stir. Shortly thereafter I pour into a large cup. I notice that much of the powder has dissolved into the water, making it a muddy brown/green colour. A little sediment is left in the tea pot, which I discard.

> I begin to sip the tea (on an empty stomach) [9:30am]. Ten minutes later, some dark green sludge remains at the bottom of the cup, which again I discard.
>
> Almost straight away I actually feel something: a light head buzz. I'm not convinced that this is a nootropic type of enhancement, but rather, it is a light headedness with a strange quality to it, and some sensation behind the eyes.
>
> After an hour, a settled buzz remains in the background. It isn't unpleasant; just unexpected. Again, measuring a nootropic value is difficult, but this is definitely psychoactive. I feel fairly relaxed with it, and given that I remain tired from an unsettled night, I don't feel overly stimulated.
>
> The head presence still remains after a couple of hours, having evolved to possess a dreamy sort of aura. There is also a certain clarity in play when I choose to focus, which could now perhaps be defined as nootropic in nature. From a recreational perspective this is quite interesting.
>
> From here, the effects fade slowly during the next few hours.

Following this, whilst I noticed no adverse effects, the night's sleep did have a strange edge to it. Note here that claims of lucid dreaming are quite common.

Overall, ginkgo delivered far more than I expected. The buzz and tingly sensations about the head were unmistakable, and the later clarity came with a hard-to-define almost dreamy headiness.

This is probably worth further exploration for nootropic enthusiasts, although the warnings referred to above certainly need to be considered and taken on board.

3.6. ONEIROGENS

Textbook Definition: *An oneirogen is considered to induce, enhance or promote lucid or vivid dreaming. It is sometimes defined as a substance that produces dream-like states of consciousness. These can be profound, and can manifest as realistic or abstract.*

The following botanicals have been sampled and researched for inclusion within this section:

I wasn't really convinced that lucid dreams could be induced until I actually encountered them via experimentation. I was astonished.

They were not psychedelic or hallucinogenic in nature, but were regular dreaming cycles, enhanced by a certain clarity and sometimes by detailed recall. In some cases, there was also a hint that the direction of the unfolding dreams could be influenced.

Separately, I have found that a number of other psychoactives, particularly psychedelics, can also promote dreaming, although I have usually felt this to be background continuation: the dying embers of the main trip. The botanicals categorised in this section differ because their primary effect relates to the dream state.

I should note in stating this that there was a handful which I almost classified as oneirogens, as they unambiguously produced clear recallable and lucid dreams on each occasion I used them. They could have fit equally comfortably here or under their current designation. Examples include mulungu and wormwood.

Lucid and vivid dreaming is a huge subject in its own right, and not one I can really do justice to. However, the experiments I cover may serve as a brief introduction to this fascinating field.

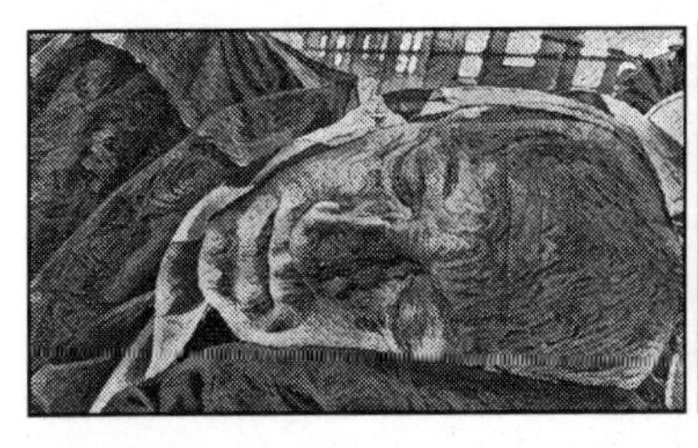

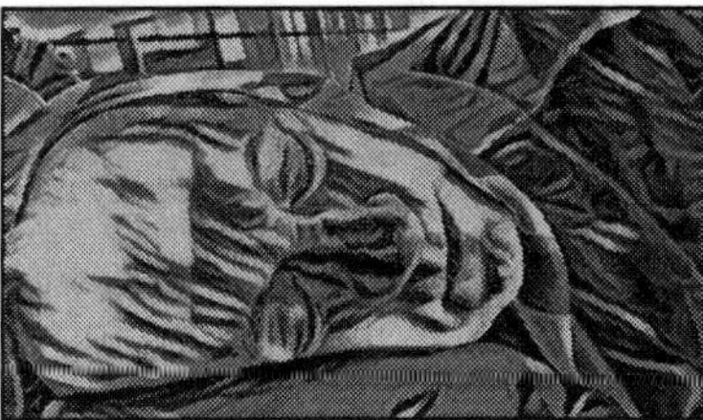

3.6.1 Calea

Binomial / Botanical Name	Calea Ternifolia; Calea Zacatechichi
Street Names	Dream Herb; Leaf of God; Bitter Grass
Major Active Compound	Unknown
Indigenous Source	Mexico and Central America
Form	Leaves
RoA	Oral / Smoked
Personal Rating On Shulgin Scale	+**

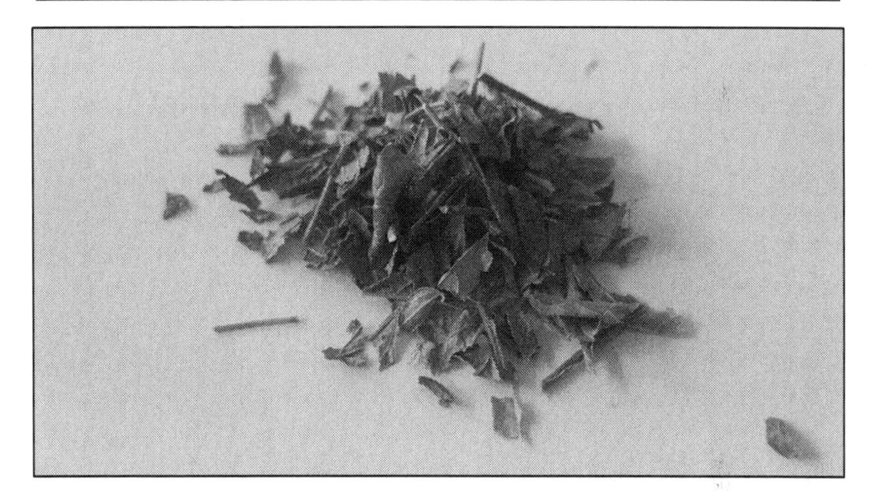

SUBJECTIVE EXPERIENCE
Traditionally used by the Chontal Indians of Mexico to induce visions in dreams, calea is possibly the most well known natural oneirogen. However, scattered amongst the reviews on various Internet forums and message boards, comments like the following are not uncommon:

> *"Crept up slowly to a moderate 'stoned but trippy' feeling, audio was certainly enhanced. Short duration though - 20 minutes and Im back to baseline."* ~ Mezza, Drugs-Forum.com

> *"Yea so i just vaporized some calea, and damn im really stoned, like this high is better than cannabis, i think its really euphoric cuz when you smoke it or drink it, its bitter and that counteracts the euphoria, but i straight up just got the chemicals"* ~ Zaltoa, dreamviews.com

These suggest that this is more than a dream herb, which of course, was an added attraction for my own experimentation.

Alarmingly, a respected poster introduced a different complexion:

> *"NO. Just fcking no. Never again. Ever. Don't fcking bother. I'd rather be stabbed in the eye with a pitchfork that try this again. After a gram taken in a brew of tea, I found myself sleeping in a world of looped, tormenting nightmares of morphing monstrous creatures with tentacles coming out of horses mouths on crab legs which would spawn mange wings with claws attached to piranhas...This went on for a week, I was scared to sleep after some days and had to resort to Diphenhydramine to get through it."*
> ~ Lolcat, ukchemicalresearch.org

This was not quite what I had in mind.

I decided to take it easy, so I made just one cup of calea zacatechichi tea, and took a single toke of it from a bong.

I had seen the abhorrent taste of calea tea mentioned in a few places, but dismissed it as exaggeration. However, it was genuinely revolting. I shuddered with each gulp, as I battled my way through it. It tasted absolutely foul.

I experienced some mild but real effects. Were these *stoned but trippy* as described above? To some degree they were, although not in a strong way. I was definitely chilled, and audio was indeed enhanced.

After an hour or two I went off to bed, hoping that the main course was yet to be served.

There was a lot of tossing and turning, but nothing much by the way of dreams until later on, during the early hours of the morning. I also recalled them, and they were slightly more lucid than usual.

Encouraged by this toe in the water, I decided to have another go a couple of nights later. This time I couldn't face the tea, so I *bonged* repeatedly.

Again, I definitely experienced a nice chill. It was not a knock-out stone, but quite pleasant in its own way. The night's sleep was good, and I woke refreshed, but without any noticeable dream lucidity or recall.

From my experience, therefore, tea would appear to be the route to take for dreaming, if the taste can be faced.

Overall, I feel that I have only scratched the surface of this one, and may well return at a future date.

3.6.2 Entada Rheedii

Binomial / Botanical Name	Entada Rheedii
Street Names	African Dream Herb; Snuff Box Sea Bean; Cacoon Vine; Dream Bean
Major Active Compound	Unclear
Indigenous Source	Indian Ocean Countries
Form	Dried Seeds
RoA	Smoked, Oral
Personal Rating On Shulgin Scale	++

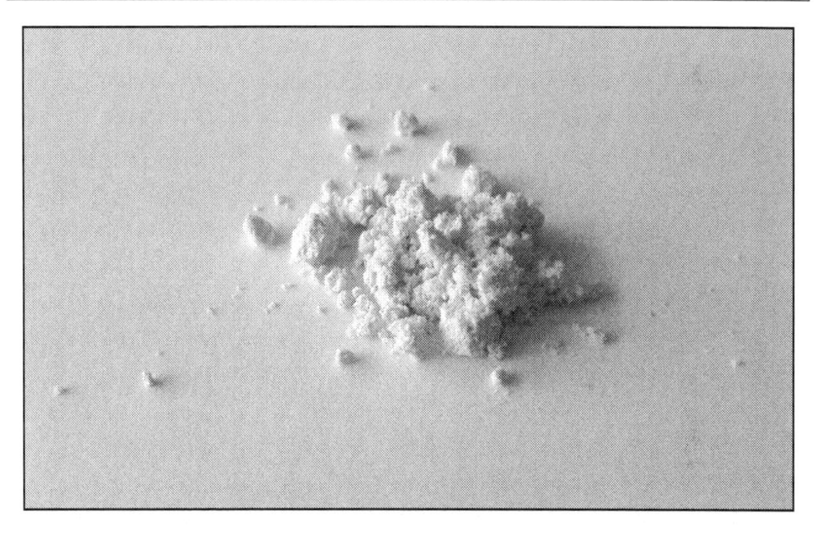

SUBJECTIVE EXPERIENCE
Entada Rheedii has a long history of use for a variety of purposes, but most notably by indigenous tribes in Africa to communicate with ancestors ('the spirit world') by inducing vivid or lucid dreams.

Entheology.com describes its traditional use thus: "*...the inner meat of the seed is either consumed directly, or chopped, dried, mixed with other herbs like tobacco, and smoked just before bedtime*" whilst the South African National Biodiversity Institute states simply that "*To induce these vivid dreams, dried seeds are powdered and smoked in a pipe before bedtime.*"

Not wishing to experience the effects of tobacco or other plants, I elect to smoke it stand-alone. I also elect to eat a small amount.

The exact source of my own supply is unknown. I purchased it from one of my usual online vendors some years ago, but I am unable to recall which. The sealed silver packet is clearly labelled and as I open it I find that the creamy coloured nut has been ground into an extremely fine almost fluffy powder.

Whilst I found no indications of toxicity or related issues during research, I did find a post referring to allergy. With this in mind I pre-test a small dab on my tongue. All is clear.

Regarding oral dosage, one bean is frequently cited as sufficient. Given the nature of my supply this really doesn't help me much: how big is a nut? After deliberation I decide to go for 1 gram.

I am in good condition, but do have a bit of a cold. For the record, I haven't been dreaming much recently.

At 9:30pm I weigh 1g and swill it down with water. It tastes a little odd, but not bad, and it morphs into a sort of slimy feel as I swallow it.

I now fill the bowl of my hand bong, step outside, and take a couple of large hits. This isn't so terrible, but it has a sort of woody tang as I inhale. I am smoking a nut after all, so I shouldn't be surprised at its slightly unusual quality.

On sitting back at my desk I immediately notice a mild sort of heady strangeness and possibly enhanced clarity of vision. I could be imagining this, as it is only a hint, but a minor change of disposition appears to be evident. I was tired, but this seems to have drifted into a more sedated dreamy and more pleasant sleepiness.

I retire to bed just before 10pm. On hitting the pillow I drop asleep quickly and easily.

I awoke at 7am. Did I dream? Indeed I did.

I dreamed constantly all night, waking (with a dry mouth) on at least three distinct occasions with dreams still spinning in my head. The dreams were lengthy, vivid and recallable, although not necessarily nice. For the periods during which I was half-awake I was aware that I was dreaming and allowed this to continue in something of a twilight zone.

This is a genuine oneirogen; possibly the most effective I have tested to date. A remaining question, however, is which RoA is most effective? As I used both methods (oral and smoking) I cannot answer this, although the fact that I was still dreaming early morning does tend to suggest oral was in play at that point.

Note that I encountered a number of sources which stated that for significant impact it is necessary to repeat the exercise over a number of nights. My experience runs counter to this, which is not to say that the dreams don't become even more vivid and lucid over subsequent occasions.

3.6.3 Mexican Tarragon

Binomial / Botanical Name	Tagetes Lucida
Street Names	Yauhtli; Psychoactive Marigold; Tagates
Major Active Compound	Unknown
Indigenous Source	Mexico, Central America
Form	Herb
RoA	Oral / Smoked
Personal Rating On Shulgin Scale	± / ++

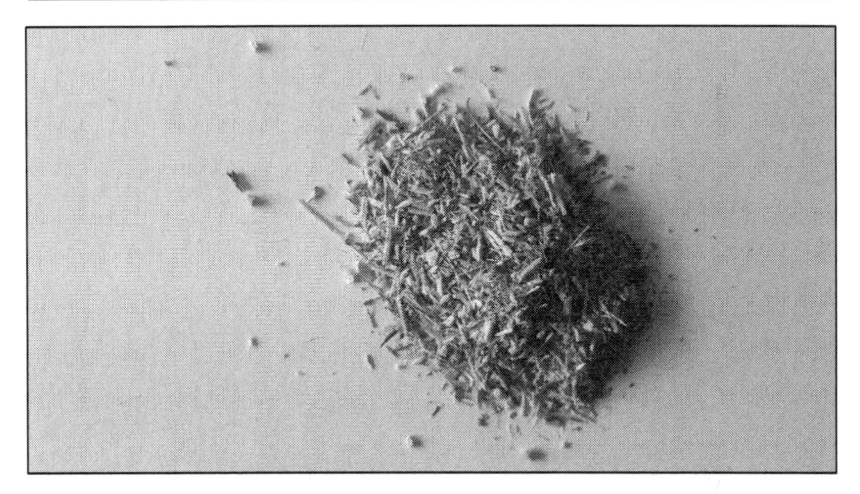

SUBJECTIVE EXPERIENCE
Used ritually by the Aztecs, this plant is contradictorily reported to be both a sedative and a stimulant. Of the two propositions, the former appears to be more widely adopted. It is also cited as being smoked with peyote (and other substances) to enhance visuals, and with nicotiana rustica as an aphrodisiac.

My experiments were originally undertaken during the evening, in the anticipation of sedation. The effects in this respect were mild, at best.

However, an unexpected outcome was vivid and lucid dreams. Subsequent research revealed that tagetes lucida has indeed been widely used as an oneirogen. It certainly worked as such in my case.

I should also note that I found smoking to have a significantly greater effect than oral ingestion.

3.6.4 Mugwort

Binomial / Botanical Name	Artemisia Vulgaris
Street Names	Felon Herb; Chrysanthemum Weed; Old Uncle Henry; Sailor's Tobacco; Naughty Man; Old Man; Wild Wormwood; Moxa
Major Active Compound	Thujone; Cineole
Indigenous Source	Europe; Asia; N Africa; Alaska
Form	Plant Matter
RoA	Oral
Personal Rating On Shulgin Scale	++

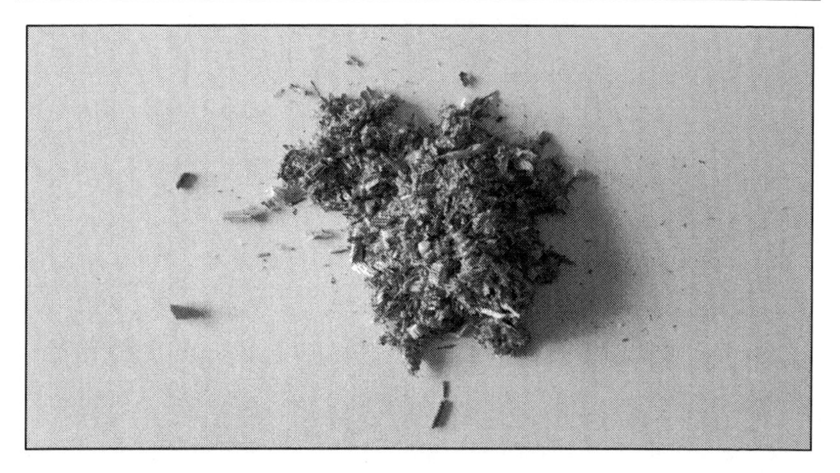

SUBJECTIVE EXPERIENCE
Mugwort has a lengthy history of herbal use, and is immersed in folk tradition, certainly in the UK, where it tends to grow as a weed. With respect to the latter, it is even present in my own garden.

Given this commonality, it can't be psychoactive, can it? The answer is yes it can.

As I wasn't proficient enough to identify it at the time of testing, I ordered from a well known online vendor. I made a huge pot of tea, and drank it over perhaps half an hour. It wasn't great to taste, but was manageable.

Lo and behold a mild sedation soon emerged. This was nothing to write home about, but it was strong enough to be sure that it wasn't a placebo effect. However, it was when my head hit the pillow that the action really started.

The dreams were lucid and vivid, particularly the last one. I recall the dream in question to this day. I existed on a Facebook page. This was neither exciting nor worrying: it was simply where I was in the dream.

What was different, however, was that when I awoke and went back to sleep, I was immediately back into Facebook, albeit on a different page. This repeated itself again and again, to the point at which I was no longer comfortable and wanted to escape.

Of course, escape I eventually did, and I awoke fully.

As this was my first *dream herb* experience it had taken me by surprise, particularly as I had no pre-conceived ideas regarding the nature of these manifestations and effects.

Another aspect I discovered was that it doesn't seem to be possible to chase the dreams, at least for me personally. I subsequently repeated the experiment several times, on each occasion with less effect.

There thus appears to be some sort of dream tolerance in play. I have no idea how long this lasts, or whether the vivid nature of the first mugwort dream can ever be repeated. The only way to determine this will be to rerun the exercise in a few months, which I will endeavour to do.

I should point out that this does not appear to apply to everyone, as there are many Internet reports which do claim success with frequent and regular use. It should also be noted that some people smoke it instead of making tea.

Overall, this is a very interesting plant, and well worthy of further exploration.

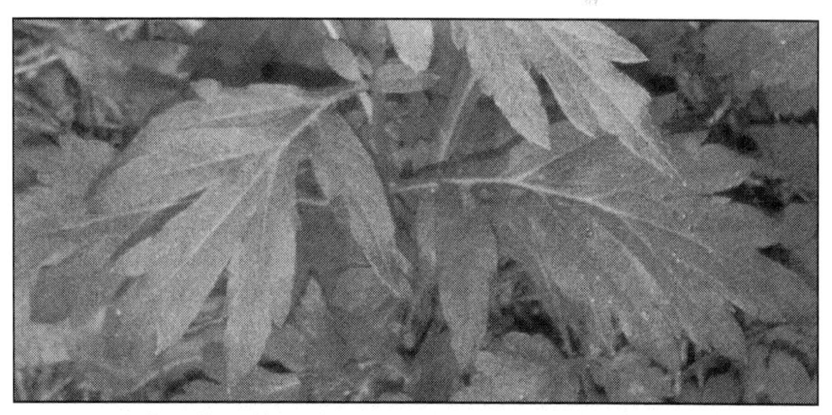

Traditionally used by witches for an array purposes, mugwort is sometimes considered to be a sacred herb which bestows magical or psychic powers

3.6.5 Ubulawu

Binomial / Botanical Name	Silene Capensis;
Street Names	African Dream Root; Xhosa Dream Root
Major Active Compound	Unknown
Indigenous Source	Eastern Cape of South Africa
Form	Root
RoA	Oral
Personal Rating On Shulgin Scale	±

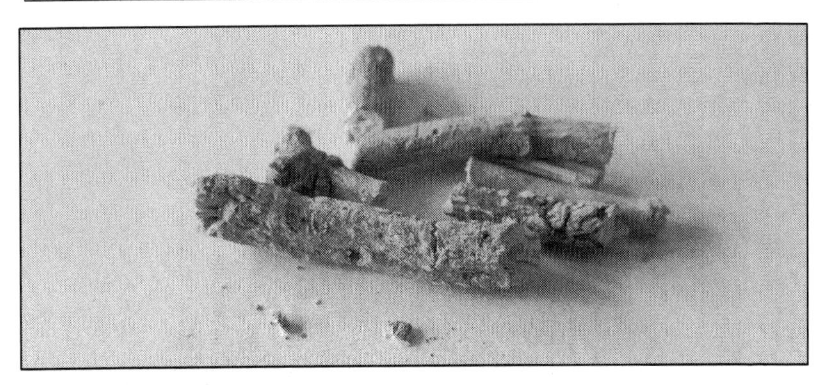

SUBJECTIVE EXPERIENCE

Enticed by stories of its ancient ritual use in Africa, I chose ubulawu for one of my first forays into the botanical arena.

I paid much attention to detail during the preparation, following authentic techniques as closely as I could. The procedure included crushing the root, shaking it in half a jar of water until froth appeared on the top, and spooning this into my mouth. This task was performed first thing in the morning, on an empty stomach.

Whilst it is often impossible to determine the difference between placebo and minimal, there were no wild or vivid dreams, or in fact, anything else. I experienced practically nothing.

In retrospect I can't necessarily draw too many general conclusions from this. I have stated elsewhere that the source of botanicals is usually vital. Here, the dried root perhaps gave the game away: it looked old; so old that it may have lost whatever psychoactivity it originally carried.

Internet reports suggest that this is worthy of further experimentation, which I will endeavour to undertake in the future, should the opportunity arise.

3.7. DELIRIANTS

Textbook Definition: *Deliriants invoke an acute confusional state. They are often toxic, and prone to expose the user to personal risks.*

The following botanicals have been sampled and researched for inclusion within this section:

Given the disturbed state of mind and overwhelming confusion of delirium, it is hard to understand why this class of botanical would ever be used for recreational purposes. Certainly, my personal experience with nutmeg was absolutely horrendous. It was only consumed courtesy of ignorance and naivety.

Quite apart from the unpleasant nature of the ride, and the accompanying risk of psychosis, many deliriants tend to have a degree of toxicity, with some commentators even referring to them as poisons. Death from consumption of high doses is not uncommon.

Make no mistake about it: deliriants are not psychedelics. The experience is disjointed, dysphoric, and terrifying, and the potential for disaster whilst under influence is absolutely real.

My general advice is hopefully unambiguous: give these a miss.

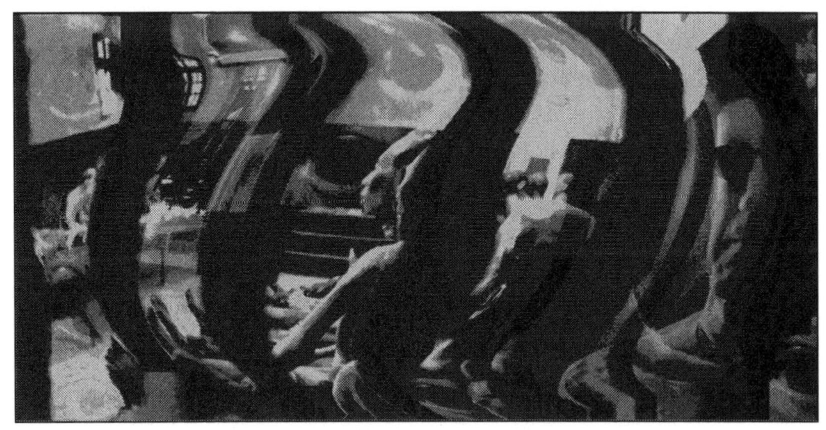

In addition to a dysphoric and terrifying mental state, deliriants tend to cause a host of dangerous and painful physical side effects, and in some cases death.

3.7.1 Datura

Binomial / Botanical Name	Datura
Street Names	Jimson Weed; Moonflower; Devil's Weed; Thorn Apple; Devil's Trumpets
Major Active Compound	Scopolamine, Hyoscyamine, Atropine
Indigenous Source	Temperate / Tropical Regions
Form	Seeds
RoA	Oral
Personal Rating On Shulgin Scale	++

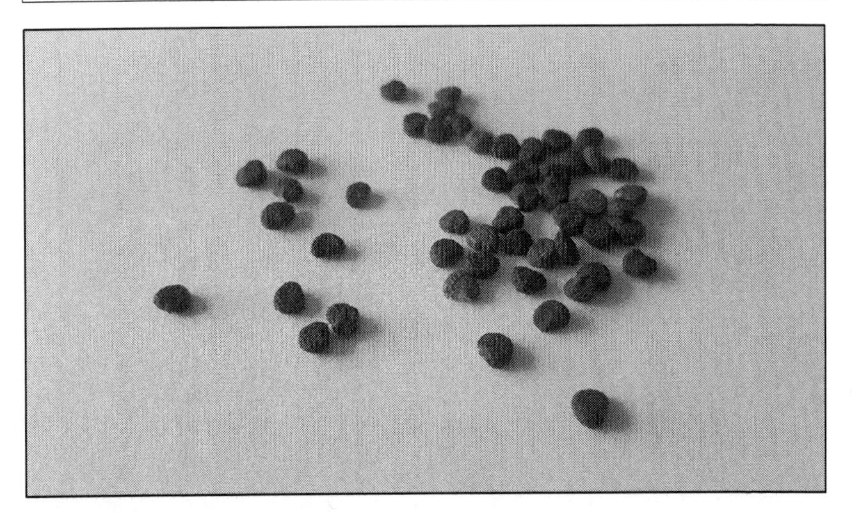

SUBJECTIVE EXPERIENCE
I wasn't going to include datura in this book, and I didn't include it the first edition. Having experienced delirium at the hands of nutmeg, I saw no sense whatsoever in exposing myself to it again, risking my life and my mental health in the process.

Why have I changed my mind? I would argue that I haven't. What I have decided to do is to go through the normal routine (research, document and record), but critically, using a minimal dose.

The idea is to more fully elaborate upon the dangers of this plant, and on deliriants in general, whilst limiting the threat of self-harm as far as I can. This is, after all, a book about drug safety, and on balance, given that most readers will already have heard of it, I feel that it would be remiss not to include datura in some form.

At the outset, I think it is worth stressing again what delirium actually is. A contributor to the *DMT-Nexus* forum described it in these terms:

> *"When a patient gets hallucinations from Datura alkaloids (hyoscyamine, atropine, or scopolamine), it is a medical sign of a near fatal dose."* ~ 69ron

On this basis, to experience delirium or hallucinations with this it is necessary to overdose, with risk of death. Hardly surprisingly, therefore, on sensible social media platforms the advice of experienced people is unambiguous in stating that datura should be avoided. This is usually expressed in stark and graphic terms.

Even Wikipedia joins the chorus:

> *"Most parts of the plants are toxic, and datura has a long history of use for causing delirious states and death."*

Medical papers are awash with details of the adverse effects, which can include seizures, hyperthermia, wide-complex dysrhythmias, cardiovascular collapse, failure of organ systems, rhabdomyolysis, and liver, kidney and brain damage. I hope that you are painting a picture from this.

For my own cautious experiment the question of dosage is obviously of paramount importance. However, it quickly emerges that dose measurement is far from a straight forward exercise. Online comments like these are not uncommon:

> *"There is no way to guess a reasonable dose, because potency of the plant material itself and appropriate dose for an individual appear to vary so much."* ~ Erowid

> *"A good dosage advise on Datura is not possible, as the alkaloid content varies so extreme. The seeds are recognised as the part of the plant with the least variation, but they can have anywhere from 0.1 to 0.7% tropane alkaloids."* ~ Ginkgo, DMT-Nexus.

On the premise of the latter comment, one seed could have seven times the potency of the next seed. This is a huge disparity, and it doesn't help to answer the fundamental question with respect to my own dose, which is: how much am I prepared to poison myself for the purpose of this experiment? The answer to this is as little as I can get away with whilst reaching a sufficient threshold to write about it in a credible way.

In view of the potential horror, and given the enormous dose variability, I decide to take a single seed. On this dose, of course, I don't anticipate delirium. However, some form of dream potentiation during sleep is perhaps a possibility.

Regarding duration, a moderate dose is generally considered to last around 8-12 hours, with higher doses persisting for perhaps 2-3 days. Effects can apparently be felt after an hour, give or take half an hour, with peak typically being reached at around 4 to 6 hours.

Ready to proceed, I select a *datura stramonium* seed from the small plastic baggy: one which looks relatively wholesome and alive. Aware of the potential for impaired judgement and lost memory under its influence, I dispose of the rest.

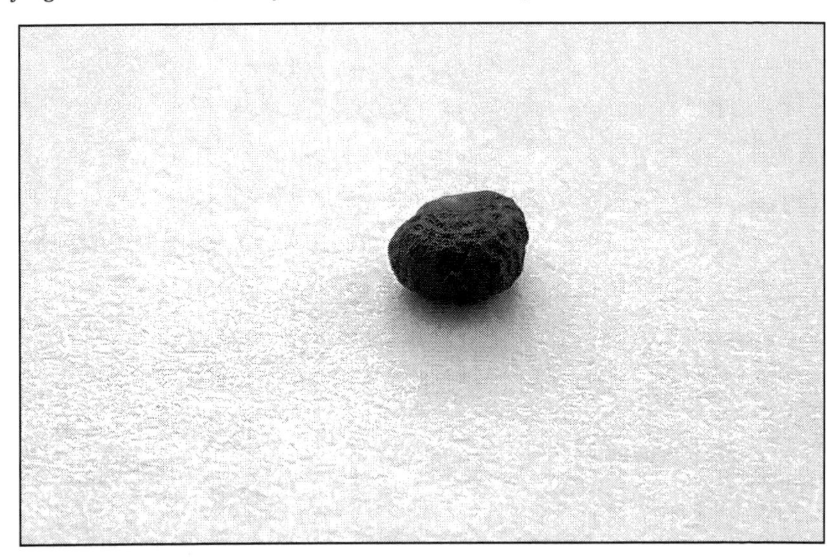

As I prepare to take the plunge, I cannot deny that part of me is hoping that the exercise fails, and that my supply is somehow deficient. Yes, my nutmeg experience really was that terrifying.

> T+0:00 I briefly chew the seed, breaking it with my teeth, and I swallow the debris with a glass of water. I have started the experiment at 5:00pm so that any effects will over-run into my sleeping hours.
>
> T+0:45 Unexpectedly, I do feel a little something. Placebo effects can be convincing, but there does seem to be a heady strangeness present. This is not debilitating in any way, but it manifests largely through a tendency to linger on thought-patterns. I am in a calm but slightly off-key space, aware of distinct sounds and sights, but fully rational. This apparent psychoactivity could of course have been initiated via buccal absorption whilst I chewed, in which case I would expect it to dissipate relatively quickly.
>
> T+2:00 The mild psychoactivity has stabilised, or perhaps I have come to terms with it. It is there in the background, but is not really intrusive, in that I could probably forget it if I was heavily engaged in an absorbing task. As it is not unpleasant I would in fact like it to persist, at least for a while longer.
>
> T+3:00 I feel quite close to base, but with a touch of headiness enduring. I have had a bite to eat and will now embark upon some light exercise.

T+4:00 *"The swim passed as standard. I find myself maybe a little more self-reflective than usual and possibly more neutral in mood. Apart from this I now feel normal. The self-reflection is interesting in that, given that this was induced via a single seed, it aligns with the idea that consuming many seeds would result in total withdrawal from the outside world."*

I scribbled the above paragraph on a scrap of paper at the pool, but on the way home I noticed a mild feeling of disconnection with the visible world around me, but inclusive of greater visual acuity. I again sensed a more distinct separation of sounds. Certainly, all of this was quite minor, but it was a sustained perception during the 10 minute walk.

T+5:00 I am now tiring and ready to retire. I retain that slightly strange heady feel, without uplift, but it is now tinged with fatigue. I head to bed hoping for easy sleep and pleasant dreams.

The night's sleep was not what I expected, bearing in mind that I had ONE seed. It delivered fairly vivid dreams, which were a little stronger than usual and perhaps more weird, but not crazily so. However, on each wake-up, about four of them, I was so dry-mouthed that I needed water. I also needed to urinate, although not through volume (the need was simply there).

During the course of the night the headspace of the evening before also turned heavier, and in the morning I had a headache. I won't over-egg this: it wasn't particularly painful but it was there, I was aware of it, and to some degree it lingered for some hours. Initially there was also a minor background buzz and a slight aura of strangeness.

The message was crystal clear. The experiences I outlined earlier were solidly psychoactive and one seed isn't the joke of a dose I thought it was. Thank goodness I only had the one. The potential for negative payload was obvious even at this level.

Finally, if you want some anecdotes to convince you further, read '*Datura 'Train Wrecks"* on Erowid. Often, delirious people do not know what they are doing: they are out of control whilst their body is fighting the poison. If the datura doesn't kill them, their real-world situation may well do so instead.

Trying to run through a wall or through a window to escape the demons, digging out the burrowing ants from your flesh with a sharp knife, cutting off your penis with shears because you are demented; anything is possible in this terrain. This is what delirium is: you lose the plot and you lose rationality, and not in a nice way.

I unashamedly repeat that this doesn't induce a psychedelic experience. Whilst datura can be used as an admixture by shamans, it is absolutely not a recreational drug. If you want to trip, or to hallucinate, use a tried and tested hallucinogen.

Finally, let's be clear: I skimmed the surface here. To some degree I have just gone through the motions, but by doing so hopefully the message is obvious: don't even think about it. Don't let curiosity kill you. Trust me on this: it's just not worth it.

3.7.2 Nutmeg

Binomial / Botanical Name	Myristica Fragrans
Street Names	N/A
Major Active Compound	Myristicin
Indigenous Source	Indonesia; New Guinea
Form	Nuts
RoA	Oral
Personal Rating On Shulgin Scale	+++

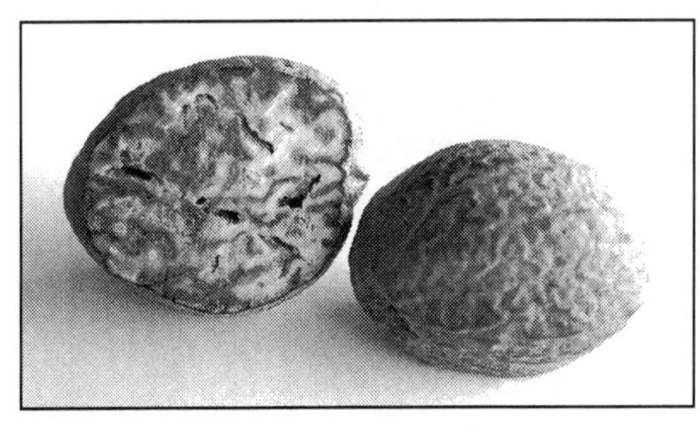

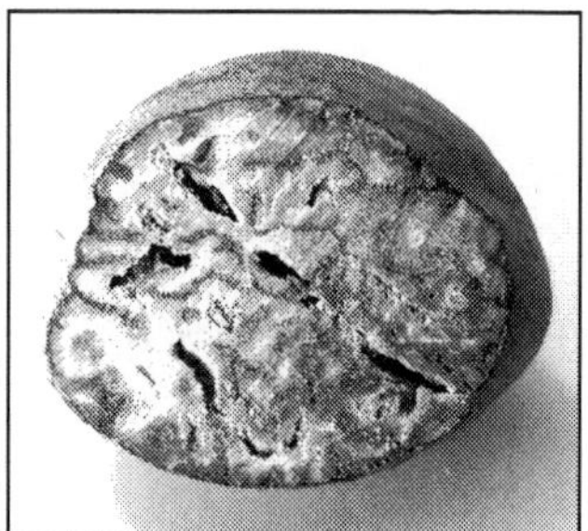

SUBJECTIVE EXPERIENCE
This is classified by Erowid as a *deliriant*. It most certainly is, but does anyone actually like being delirious? Is there any pleasure to be found in such a state? From my experience the answer is a categorical *no*.

I gnawed on a nutmeg and a half, or whatever amount it was, several decades ago. I won't even dignify its effects with the word *trip*. I was nauseous, dizzy, and unable to grasp solidity, whilst simultaneously suffering terrible head pain in totally unmitigated confusion. It was horrible in almost every conceivable way.

The next day it didn't end: dry mouth, hangover, hell on earth. I thought I would die. I was ill for days.

As I recall, it took so long to come-on that I thought I had eaten a dud. I waited several hours, maybe more, and eventually I went to bed still waiting.

I awoke in the night to go to the toilet, and had to literally crawl there on my hands and knees because I couldn't stand. The floor was all over the place: my hands went into it like they were going into thick glue and I had to pull them out with each lurch forwards. My head was spinning sickeningly, my ears were ringing, and I was struggling through a living dysphoric hell.

Quite apart from the nightmare of the ordeal, if you have too much this can easily kill you. It can damage vital organs, leave you with serious medical issues, and not care a hoot. I still shudder after all these years just thinking about it.

Don't even be tempted, because I can assure you there is no joy or knowledge to be found in it. All I learned was to avoid it like the plague.

There are some seriously good trips to experience, and this isn't one of them. It is a million miles removed.

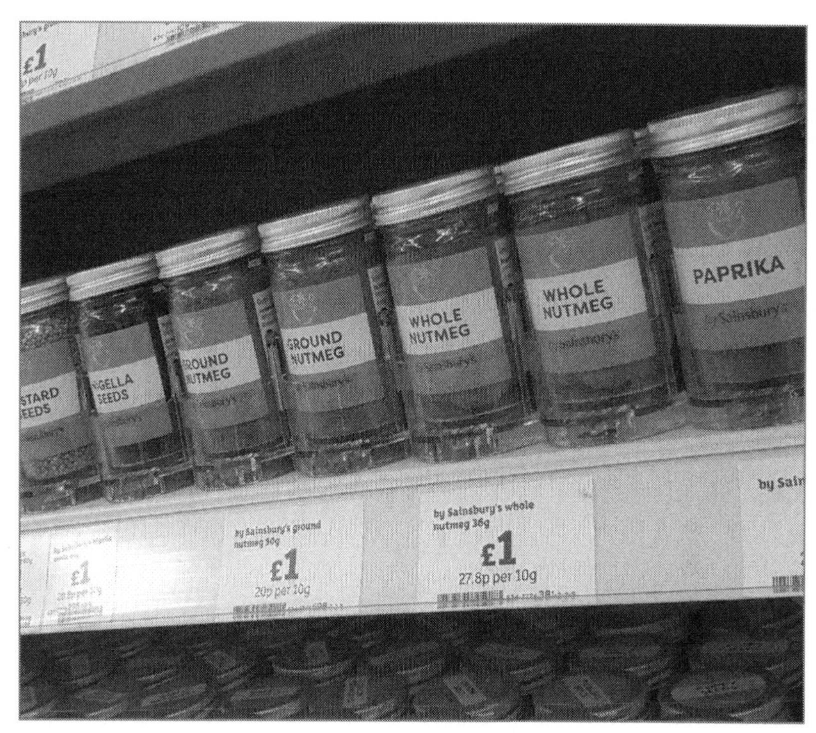

An innocent looking spice

I'd rather eat boot polish laced with rat poison than face this again, and I am not joking.

I would suggest that experimenting with nutmeg presents an entirely pointless risk, using your welfare and life as the stake, for a prize you don't want. My unwavering and sincere advice could not be clearer: don't do it.

3.8. UNCLASSIFIED

Textbook Definition: *A number of botanicals produce effects which do not fit comfortably into any of the previous categories. Some, for example, induce a combination of effects, providing a very distinct experience. Others create differing effects as the experience itself unfolds.*

The following botanicals have been sampled and researched for inclusion within this section:

How could you place a psychoactive plant like cannabis, with its huge diversity of effects, under a single classification? Erowid, for example, describes it thus: "*Intoxicant; Stimulant; Psychedelic; Depressant*".

What about mapacho, with its knock-out punch and eventual clarity?

What of the mood-lift, the semi-euphoria, and the eventual sedation of kratom?

These are examples of botanicals whose characteristics simply do not sit comfortably under the standard types of classification, as listed earlier in this book.

Those included are notable in terms of popularity, history, or with respect to the experience induced.

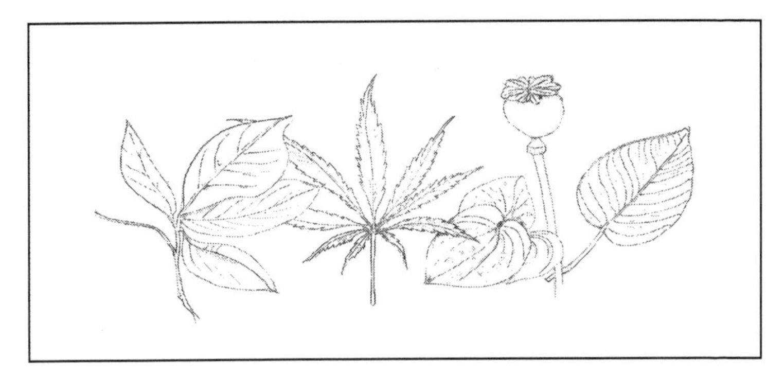

3.8.1 Cannabis

Binomial / Botanical Name	Cannabis Sativa; Cannabis Indica
Street Names	Marijuana; Mary Jane; Weed; Ganga; Pot; Grass; MJ; Green
Major Active Compounds	THC; CBD
Indigenous Source	Central and South Asia
Form	Plant Material
RoA	Oral / Smoked
Personal Rating On Shulgin Scale	++ / +++

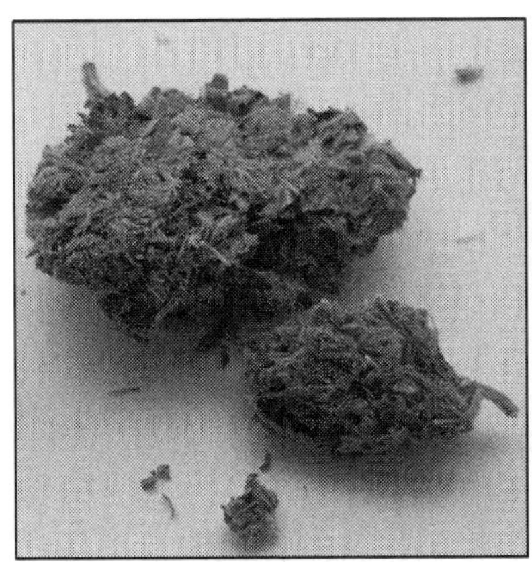

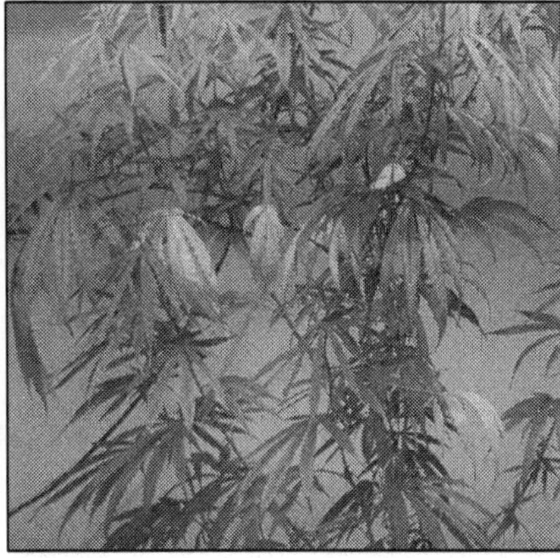

SUBJECTIVE EXPERIENCE
I was introduced to cannabis in my late teens. Back then, its primary form was hashish, a hard but malleable oil-based resin, from which smaller pieces could be broken off, sometimes with the aid of a lighted match to soften the compound. This tended to be sourced from Morocco, Lebanon or perhaps Afghanistan. There wasn't much delineation beyond this, at least in my locale.

As a non-smoker, mixing with tobacco, as was the norm, made me a little dizzy, so I tended to *hot-knife*. This dubious technique employed two kitchen knives and a plastic bottle. I would cut a small hole near the base, large enough to fit the ends of the two knives. The ends of the knives were then heated over a flame until almost red, and a small fragment of hash was placed between them, whilst they themselves were positioned through the hole in the bottle (with the top of the bottle bunged). The hash combusted into smoke as the knives were pressed together, filling the bottle. The knives were removed, the hole was quickly plugged with the palm, and the smoke was inhaled through the neck of the bottle.

The hit came on quickly, and was usually much deeper than that experienced via a spliff. This wasn't elegant, probably wasn't healthy, and most definitely wasn't a great idea, but from my young perspective at the time, it worked.

When I returned to cannabis many years later, the scene had changed dramatically, for the better. High quality cannabis was now widely available in bush form, and it was usually much stronger.

There was also a myriad of choice in terms of varieties and strains, which tended to have exotic names. I quickly learned that these were not simply marketing or packaging gimmicks: the differences between them were real.

The two species of the plant offer markedly different experiences. Broadly, sativa is well known for its cerebral high, and indica for its sedating body effects. Between these, a huge spectrum is available for the connoisseur, with each strain or hybrid having its own characteristics. Amnesia Haze, Silver Bubble, Sputnik, White Widow, Jack Herer, Kush, Super Lemon Haze - the list is endless. Over recent years I have been fortunate enough to sample these and countless others.

Perhaps predictably, my favourite city for this activity has been Amsterdam, where quality is almost assured, and the general atmosphere is tailor-made for a relaxing and pleasant sojourn. Dreamy sunny afternoons sat smoking on the lawns in Rembrandtplein, watching the world go by, or generally strolling and chilling in a plethora of coffeeshops, constitute precious and golden memories.

There is also a huge canopy of cannabis experience available via the oral route. Whilst hash cakes are famed, there are entire cookbooks dedicated to the production of carefully crafted edibles.

As is the norm for oral-versus-smoking, the former takes longer to come-on, but lasts longer. Variation between different cooking preparations and different varieties of cannabis again create significantly different effects.

With so many possibilities, it is simply impossible to describe one of them and state that it accurately reflects the cannabis experience. The diversity between strain, preparation and RoA is far too great.

What I can state is that no-one ever died from cannabis intoxication. It is not realistically possible to overdose. With this in mind, experimentation does at least carry certain assurances.

In terms of harm reduction I should perhaps mention anxiety, or panic attack. Some strains do induce this in some people, including in myself. The trick here is to use a different variety instead, or use less. Whilst in the midst of such an experience, however, try to relax, perhaps sing, think about pleasantries, do something rather than just sit, and bring to mind the fact that it will soon pass. Studies have also demonstrated that snorting or eating black pepper can help alleviate the problem.

TERMINOLOGY: CANNABIS
Cannabis is the formal botanical name for a genus of flowering plant, which includes its two most important species, cannabis sativa and cannabis indica. The terminology surrounding this, however, has taken a life of its own, with the psychoactive parts of the plant being referred to by a never ending list of terms, including cannabis, marijuana, pot, ganga, green, mary jane, grass, and weed.

Another word sometimes used is *skunk*, the meaning of which varies depending upon location and context. In the US this tends to refer to certain strong smelling strains (with reference to the mammal of the same name). In the UK, the media have frequently used the term generically, to describe all THC-strong strains, a misuse of the word which has been widely adopted. Notwithstanding this, skunk was and is an independent strain in its own right, variants of which are still available, and popular.

TERMINOLOGY: HASH & DABS
Wikipedia describes hashish (or hash) rather cumbersomely as "*an extracted cannabis product composed of compressed or purified preparations of stalked resin glands, called trichomes, from the plant*". These words basically mean that the trichomes from the flower-tops of the plant are collected and compressed/purified, with the resultant material yielding a higher concentration of psychoactive chemicals. Collection is usually performed by sifting or rubbing/scraping (Indian sub-continent), making it solid or resinous.

Finally, the most recently emerged form of cannabis goes by the name of *dabs*. These are concentrated (thus stronger) doses of cannabis, created by extracting THC (and other cannabinoids) via a process involving a solvent, such as butane. The oily substance produced via this technique tends to be vaporised or smoked (dabbing), and is known by a variety of terms, including BHO (butane hash oil), shatter, wax, honey oil, budder and of course, dabs.

TERMINOLOGY: JOINTS v BLUNTS v SPLIFFS
Whilst to some degree there is regional variation in the broad meaning of these words, the following generally holds true in the UK, US, and most western societies.

> A *joint* contains only cannabis. It is usually wrapped in normal cigarette paper, but can also be rolled with hemp or other material. More often than not the finished article is relatively small, reflecting the size of the standard paper.
>
> A *blunt* again contains only cannabis, but is wrapped in tobacco leaf or in tobacco paper. As a result, it is usually significantly larger than a joint.
>
> A *spliff* is the same as a joint, but contains a mix of tobacco and cannabis.

Whilst I have long understood these differences, I do have to confess that I have not always found smoking to be as straightforward as most. Fortunately, a chap by the name of Bob Marley eventually lent a metaphorical hand.

EDIBLES: BHANG LASSI
Whilst my trip to sample bhang lassi didn't go according to plan, it perhaps serves as a cautionary note regarding complacency with respect to edibles. With the best of intentions, and with significant experience, I made a number of wholly avoidable errors...

Lost In Varanasi
Within any study of the historical use of cannabis an Indian preparation known as *bhang* will be prominently listed. As an intrinsic part of the ancient Hindu tradition it has been used in food and drink dating back to at least 1000 BC.

The epicentre of its spiritual use is widely considered to be Varanasi. Sitting on the banks of the Ganges this is a place of spectacular classical beauty and for many westerners, a culture shock; a step back in time.

To this day bhang is openly available there, being sold through *lassi shops* as *bhang lassi*, a smooth and creamy milk-shake type drink. Prior to embarkation, I had identified three particular dispensaries, and of these, fate delivered me to *The Green Lassi Shop* shortly after 12 noon on a warm balmy afternoon.

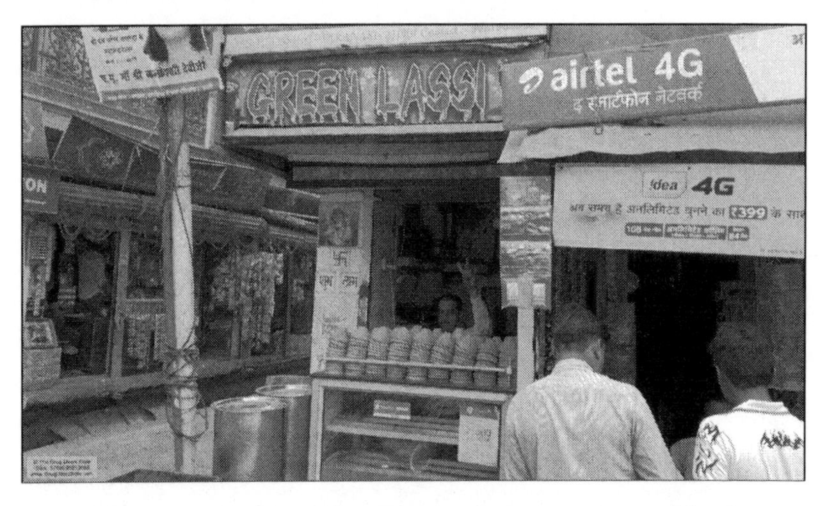

It was small, almost tucked away, but sitting on a busy street. Approaching the counter I specifically asked for bhang lassi *light:* I didn't really want to find myself entirely out of mind, as the day was still young.

In truth my expectations were not particularly high. During the 10 year period in which I wrote this book, it is fair to say that I consumed my fair share of cannabis edibles. I therefore approached this expedition with what turned out to be an entirely misplaced degree of complacency.

Let The Stoning Commence

The owner prepared the drink, pouring a heavy green fluid into the milky white contents of an earth coloured bowl. Plopping a dollop of cream on top he then handed it over, and I parted with a grand total of 150 rupees (about £1.50, or $2).

There was no interior to this place, just a bench in front of the counter, and he indicated that I should face inwards whilst drinking. A couple of others were milling around doing the same, but I sat down on the bench itself.

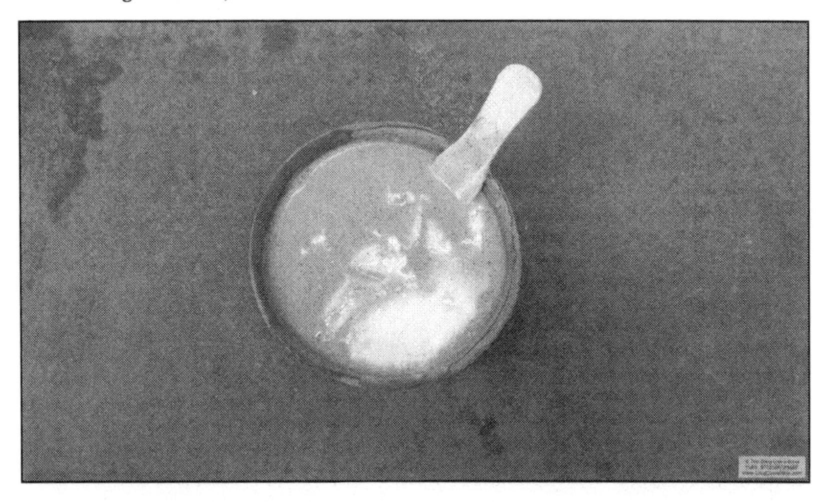

The taste was smooth and pleasant, and not cannabis-like at all. I sipped slowly, taking a few photographs as I relaxed. Finishing off, I dropped the empty bowl into the bin and continued my walk around the noisy, bustling and typically colourful Indian streets.

For perhaps the best part of an hour this remained a pleasant stroll. A mild buzz was emerging, and I slipped in and out of a gentle cannabis ambience. Soon, however, a somewhat sinister edge began to manifest with almost every passing thought.

From Groovy To Gruesome

Recognising the potential for a difficult ride I headed back to the ghats, by the water, where I hoped for some relative quiet. On arrival I encountered a Hindu burial ceremony, which under normal circumstances would have been a fascinating spectacle to witness. I edged around the periphery and found an inconspicuous place to sit and contemplate.

Although it now seems obvious, watching bodies being burned in my deteriorating condition was not the best idea. As might be expected, it was an extremely intense experience, but one which was increasingly disturbing to my stoned mind. Soon it was full-on gruesome.

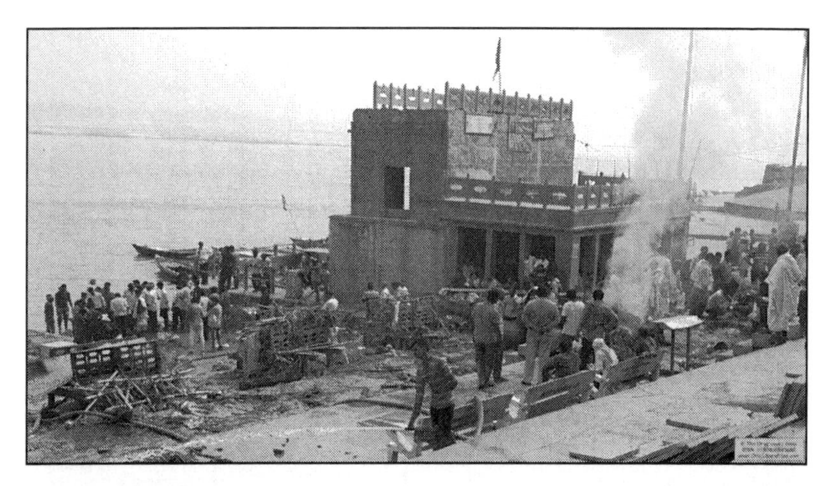

The Journey From Hell
Eventually I decided that I had to make an exit and head for the tranquillity of my hotel bedroom. This was easier said than done. The hotel was 40 minutes away, via the only tenable form of transport, tuk-tuk. I didn't relish the journey but had little choice, so rejecting an offer from a driver who appeared to be about 12 years old I grabbed a more mature sensible looking chap. So began the journey from hell.

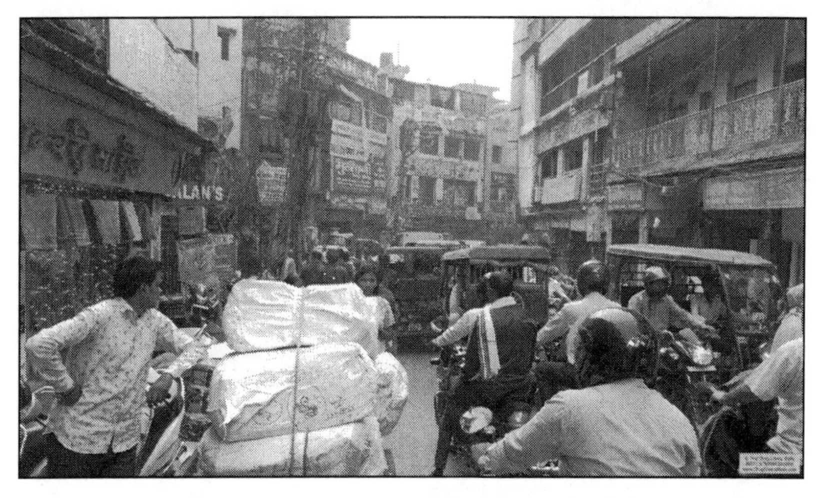

My normal contented acceptance of the craziness of Indian roads quickly evaporated. This was traumatic. With traffic attacking at speed from every direction, the noise and bedlam was now completely off the scale. I was literally hanging on with white knuckles, as the vehicle ducked and weaved. The drama seemed to continue forever, as I sought and failed to recognise anything which might indicate that I was close to base. When would it end? Would I survive it? Had I really done it this time?

Throughout this ordeal my mouth was so dry that I could hardly speak. I desperately needed water, but even more acutely I needed this horror show to stop. Eventually, after an eternity, it did.

Sanctuary & Slumber

I had survived, and I reached the sanctuary of my room with a feeling of almost overwhelming relief. I glugged a bottle of water, turned on the TV, lay on the bed, and reflected upon my folly. Still anxious, and seeking refuge through slumber, I closed my eyes and drifted.

I occasionally awoke, again with a parched dry mouth, to view the Indian version of MTV, which was astonishingly raunchy. This was India, and I couldn't comprehend how moves which would not beat the censor's cut in the US or UK were apparently routine here.

Some hours later I began to emerge from the morass and managed to eat a hearty vegetarian meal before bedtime proper. I slept like a log.

In the morning I was back to my usual self, albeit with a bit of heady strangeness. I felt a little drained, but generally sober, and was good to go again. I headed back to the ghats, this time as a regular tourist.

Lesson Learned

Clearly, the cannabis strain itself was not entirely one for me. The mix of THC and CBD is of course a defining factor of the cannabis experience, and under normal circumstances I am able to select a strain which will deliver what I am looking for. Here, this luxury was absent, and I had to take what was available. This was clearly high in THC and a high dose, creating the anxious edge which persisted throughout.

One thought that occurred after the event was: if this was *lassi light*, what on earth must the full-Monty be like? Perhaps the guy at the shop had misunderstood and served a heavy version, but regardless, this was an accident waiting to happen.

If you are going to *bhang lassi* anytime soon, take it easy. Start low, and double check that you are really starting low. Equally, be very aware of your *set and setting*, taking full cognisance of where you are. Make sure that a safe haven is in close proximity, and always be ready to remind yourself that you are under the influence of a drug and that it will end in due course.

Perhaps my story serves as an example of how not to do it, but I am profoundly aware that this is provided in Varanasi to aid a spiritual journey, rather than to pique the curiosity of an ageing European psychonaut.

Yes, I would do it again, as this could have been a rich and rewarding experience, but next time I would learn from these mistakes. Or perhaps I would adhere to the motto: when in India don't necessarily do as the Indians do.

A TRICK OF THE TRADE

A tour of Bob Marley's house and mausoleum in Jamaica was an opportunity I couldn't possibly refuse. Despite the hair-raising ride to the centre of the country, via elevated single track roads, it was an outstanding experience.

Outside the gate, members of the group were able to procure Jamaica's finest, including edibles, and the famed and quite exquisite *sensimilla*, which I simply couldn't resist.

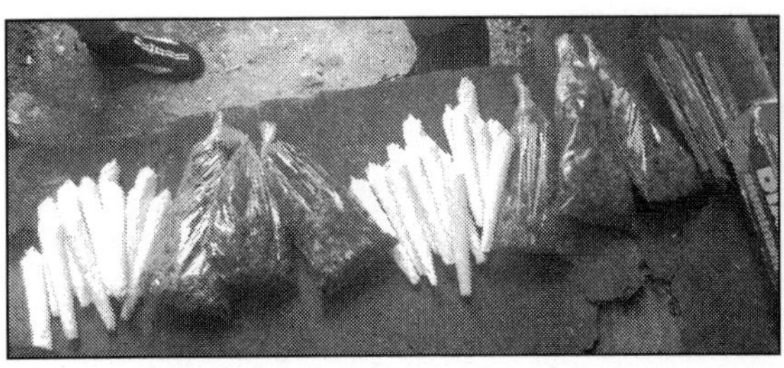

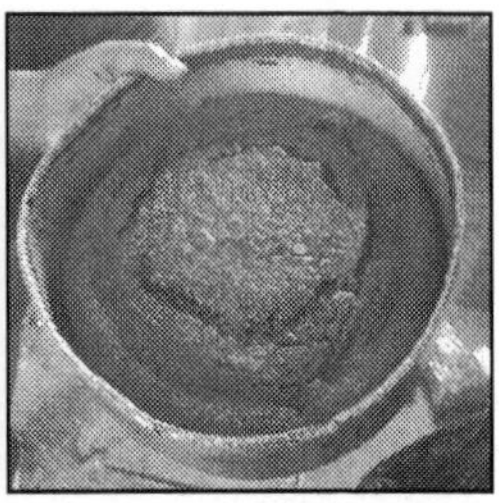

For one young woman, however, the strong cannabis, combined with the high altitude, was too much, and she collapsed with a crash behind me. She was helped away by the guide, Robert. It was when he returned that he was handed an exhibit, which she had landed upon and destroyed.

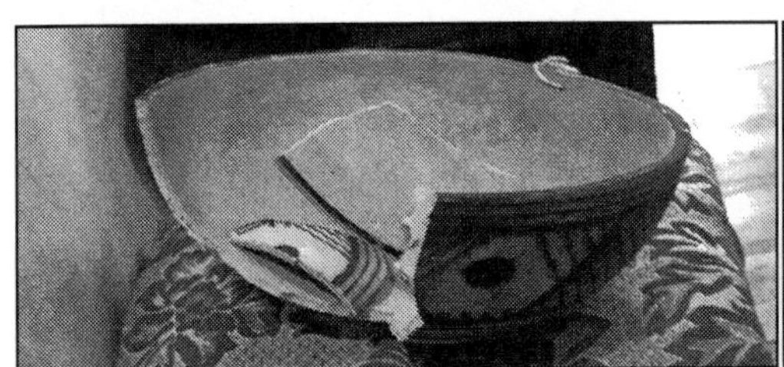

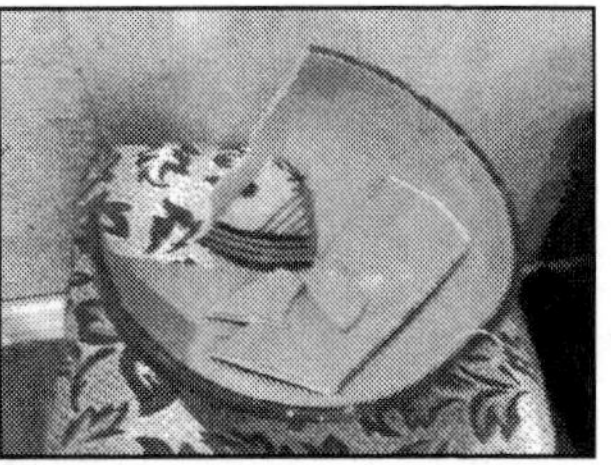

His response was memorable: "*Fck!*" He then immediately bust into hysterical laughter. Everyone else followed his lead.

At the end of the tour, I finally learned how to stop my weed dropping out of the end of a joint when smoking it pure, courtesy of the bus driver, Roy.

He had obviously watched my unsuccessful efforts to keep my big fat one intact as I puffed furiously at it, and took pity. The trick is to lightly wet the paper at the business-end before lighting up, so that it doesn't burn away more quickly than the contents.

I guess that this is pretty obvious, but after so many years of frustration, wasted weed, and embarrassment, I finally got there. D'oh!

AN ANECDOTAL TALE (TWO FACES OF CANNABIS)
A common effect of cannabis is to relax, to remove those sharp edges, and to create a bubble of anaesthetised comfort and cosiness. It can make you chilled and friendly.

So it was when I left the *Green House* coffeeshop in Amsterdam. Fatally, I also had my camera to hand.

Between the coffeeshop and the canal, to the left, was a public urinal. This was particularly prominent, due to the fact that it was a double, designed to enable two men to urinate at the same time, one at each end.

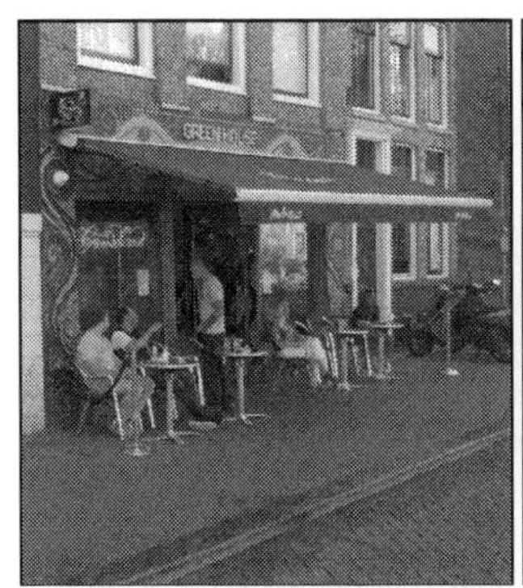

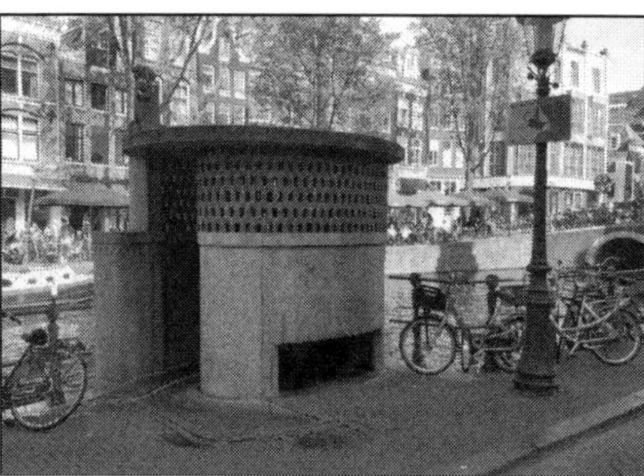

As these are not a common sight back in the UK, I took a few photos, and moved inside for a couple of interior shots. Mission accomplished, I then moved to use the facility for its intended purpose.

At this point, a young man appeared in the doorway. Somewhat stoned, I explained to him that "*I've been taking a few photographs*" and, "*There's room for two in here*".

His face reacted with an expression of horror. He turned around, and beat a hasty retreat.

It then occurred to me how he must have interpreted my friendly greeting, on the edge of the red light district, in the dark of the evening, in the doorway of a urinal.

Another occasional effect of cannabis suddenly took hold. This was anxiety and paranoia, as I envisioned him reporting me to the local police for some sort of solicitation in a men's lavatory. I shuddered at the prospect of the subsequent public shaming.

My face must have reacted with the same horror as my unfortunate victim, and it was my turn to beat a hasty retreat.

3.8.2 Kava Kava

Binomial / Botanical Name	Piper Methysticum
Street Names	Kawa; Awa; Waka; Lawena; Sakau; Yaqona; Kava
Major Active Compound	Kavalactones
Indigenous Source	Vanuatu
Form	Powdered Kava Root
RoA	Oral
Personal Rating On Shulgin Scale	++*

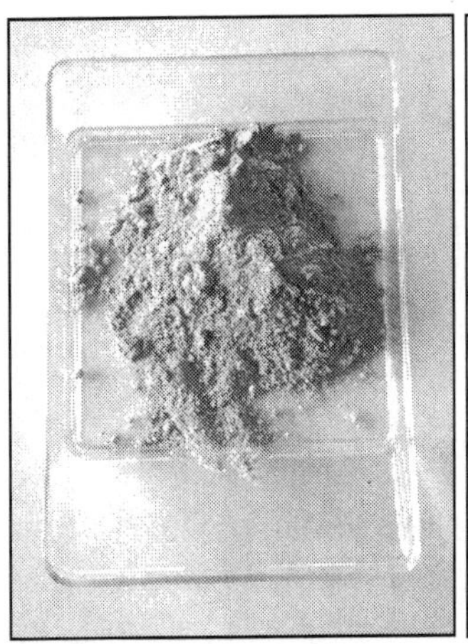

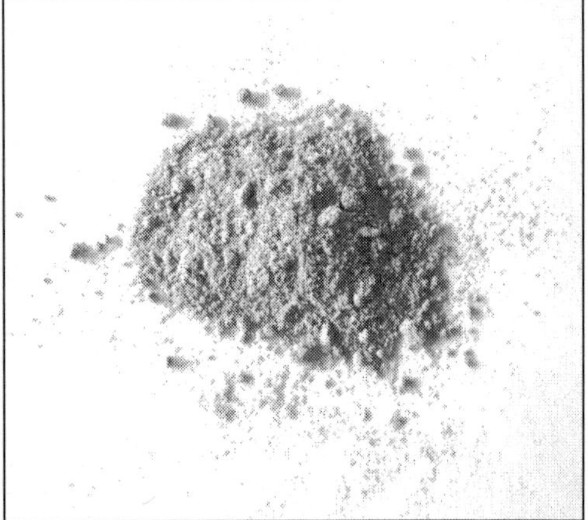

SUBJECTIVE EXPERIENCE
The use of kava root for social and ceremonial purposes dates back at least 3,000 years. It continues to be used in a social and recreational context across Pacific Polynesia to this day, and in recent years, thanks partly to the Internet, it has been adopted by increasing numbers across the world.

Many claims are made about its effects, particularly with respect to its properties as a relaxant, sedative and euphoriant. It is also sometimes cited as an aid to treat addiction to alcohol. Online, there are whole communities dedicated to this plant, so clearly there is something to it.

I sampled kava kava as a tea some years ago. Although vague, and to some degree lost in the past, I recall a sense of disappointment. I didn't really get off on it, and recorded it as only a + on my adapted Shulgin scale.

Returning to this recently, it is not hard to understand why I struggled. For new users in particular it appears to be temperamental. Factors such as reverse tolerance (the more often you drink, the less you need), variable break-in thresholds (*kavalactone* build up periods), and multiple preparations, are all in play.

I also found that a significant number of users stated that the quality of the powder itself was a critical factor. Hence, I purchased from one of the most reputable vendors, GKE (now defunct).

For the root itself, I went for what appeared to be the best bet for the passing user in terms the likelihood of success: *Quick Kava Powder*. I found a multitude of positive reports on this particular product, most of which recommended a dose of between 3g and 6g.

The most frequently quoted time for this to take effect was half an hour, and for duration, about four or five hours is generally cited.

When it finally arrived on my doormat, I found it to be a very fine powder, with a light earthy smell, but with a hint of that appalling kratom odour, which I absolutely abhor. As a consequence, I worried that this might not be the easiest substance to get down the hatch.

As a common recommendation is to consume this on an empty stomach, I abstained from breakfast. By lunch time I was ready to go.

> T+0:00 I weigh 6g of the powder. As some users recommend repeated doses throughout the day, I weigh another 5g for potential later use. [11:35am]
>
> I pour warm water into a glass and sprinkle the powder on to it whilst stirring furiously with a spoon. I slug it down in two large gulps. Job done!
>
> First surprise: it isn't too bad. Indeed, the taste is decent and nothing like kratom at all. It almost feels cleansing in some way, as though there is an antiseptic edge to it, which lingers in the mouth. Drinking it simply isn't a problem.
>
> I recall that in Vanuatu and dotted around the world there are *kava bars*, where users can drink this in a social setting. This no longer seems to be particularly strange. The powder I am using, in fact, is purported to have been made using the same process employed by these.
>
> T+0:15 There are minor changes taking place in terms of my headspace. I do feel a very slight buzz.
>
> Is there any body relaxation? I cannot rule this out, but at this stage the main thrust is driven from the head, and it is gentle and pleasant.

T+0:30 There has been no real change since the 15 minute mark, and it does seem to have settled, with no nausea (which is sometimes reported). I therefore consume the other dose (5g) in the same manner as above.

T+0:45 There is absolutely no doubt that there is a light headiness now, which is mildly relaxing.

Clarity of cognitive function remains, so this isn't an alcohol type of intoxication. It seems to be much gentler in nature.

It is probably a good idea to point out that I am not stoned, or inebriated, or high, in terms of the effects documented for many of the compounds in this book. I am, however, calm, relaxed and content. It seems to take the edge away from anxieties, whilst not clouding mental lucidity.

T+1:00 As I have not encountered any body load at all, and as this is a benign plant with a rich history of safe use, I decide to measure another dose (6g) to keep this rolling and to see where it goes. I gulp it down as described earlier. I have now consumed 17g in total.

By this point the head buzz is quite solid. I remain functionally unimpaired, and it is interesting that visual acuity and focus seem to be, if anything, enhanced, which is not usually the case for compounds which relax. There is no tiredness or drowsiness whatsoever.

T+1:30 I gulp down another 6g, taking the total to 23g. There is now almost nothing left in my 25g pack.

Erowid cites this as a "*Depressant; Intoxicant*", which is broadly how alcohol is sometimes described. I can see the similarity, as I do feel intoxicated. However, the operative word is *broadly*, as this ride is much more refined and subtle than that of alcohol, and to be blunt, it feels less damaging.

I am at ease and relaxed, both in my head and body. Regarding the latter, it also carries a certain physical numbness.

Walking around the feeling of intoxication is more apparent, but in a positive sense. My head has a warm strangeness about it, but there is no dulling of mind, and perceptually vision remains at least as sharp usual.

From my current perspective, its use as a social replacement for alcohol makes every sense.

This is a pleasant experience, and is much stronger than I anticipated. Whilst I stated earlier that I wasn't inebriated, I couldn't possibly argue the same now.

T+2:00 I drink the last 2g, so over the previous 2 hours I have consumed the full pack of 25g.

All anxieties are absent, and the tranquil mood lift continues to flow. I am not surprised in the least that this is so popular.

T+3:00 The experience has now settled a little, and has plateaued at a slightly lower level than earlier. I am still very much under the influence, but the effects have stabilised, remaining enjoyable and anxiolytic in nature.

T+4:00 I am slowly edging down towards base, although the general vibe lingers. As this drifts down, I am starting to feel a little tired and sleepy.

T+5:00 At 4:30pm I retire for a nap, as I often do at this time in the afternoon. I have a peaceful and deep sleep for the best part of an hour, and wake feeling refreshed, and, more or less, back to baseline.

Overall, this took me by surprise, largely because it actually delivered the effects which had been widely claimed, contrary to my earlier experience.

It was a nice relaxing but non-debilitating inebriation, which lasted for the hours I engaged, and tapered down in the background throughout the evening.

A picture I paint in my head is of drinking this in a social setting, instead of alcohol, making those kava bars a very attractive proposition indeed. I felt no ill effects, no hangover, and the ride itself of was positive and pleasing. It was well worth the effort I took to repeat the exercise.

This was a really enjoyable experience, and was an excellent way to spend a Sunday afternoon.

Weight: 250g
Contains: Ground Kava Root (Piper Methysticum)
Storage Instructions: Store in a cool dry place, keep out of direct sunlight
Best Before: Jan 2017

Product of Republic of Vanuatu
Packaged and shipped from the United Kingdom
Distributed by Kava Europe

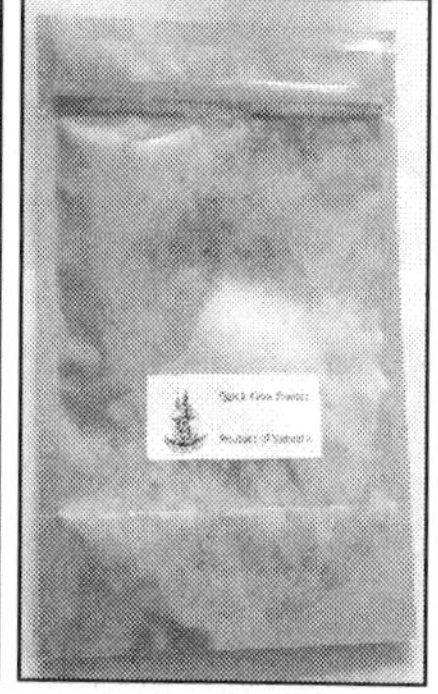

The Pacific island of Vanuatu has introduced legislation to regulate the quality of its kava exports

3.8.3 Kratom

Binomial / Botanical Name	Mitragyna Speciosa
Street Names	Ketum
Major Active Compound	Mitragynine; 7-hydroxymitragynine
Indigenous Source	Thailand and South-East Asia
Form	Powdered Plant Material
RoA	Oral
Personal Rating On Shulgin Scale	Standard (5g): ++ Extract (0.5g): ++

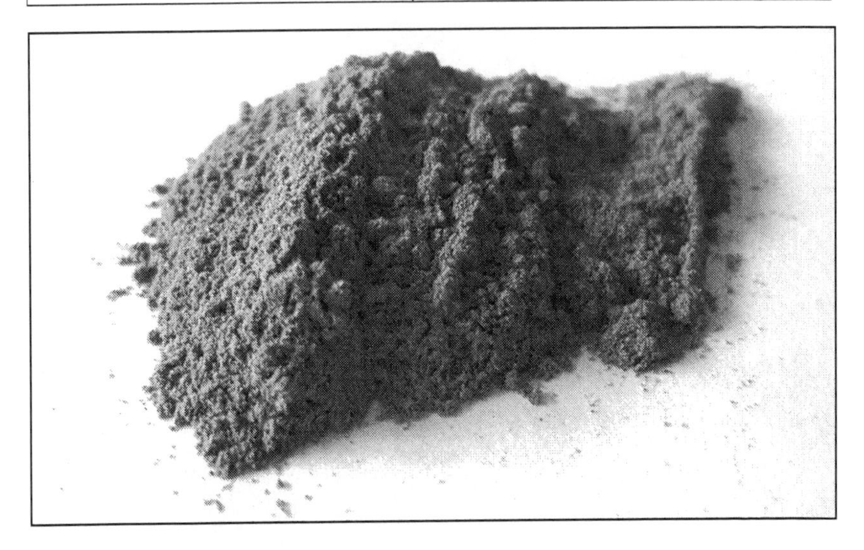

SUBJECTIVE EXPERIENCE
Kratom has long been used in its native South East Asia as a traditional medicine, and is known for its opiate-like effects. Given its wide scale use and general popularity, it was always going to be a candidate for early research. However, despite my best endeavours, it took over half a dozen attempts to finally hit the mark.

Early experiments were conducted with samples obtained from city centre head shops. These tended to be totally useless, despite ingestion via both tea, and toss & wash. I could have given up, but it was absolutely clear that significant numbers of people were successfully using kratom for recreational purposes; some of them regularly.

As is so often the case, source was the key, and I eventually found a reliable internet vendor who supplied a product of sufficient quality.

Rather like cannabis, a variety of strains are available. Each strain produces a different effect, an indication of which is provided by the colour of the vein, which is frequently referred to in its name. It is also common for the name to include the region of origin.

The five strains which were included in the selection pack I purchased for testing provide examples of this *ad hoc* naming convention: *White Sumatran; White Liang Teh Putih; Red Vein Borneo; Red Liang Teh Merah; Green Liang Teh Hijau.*

The effects also vary according to dose, particularly with respect to the pitch between sedating (higher doses) and energising (lower doses).

Connoisseurs are able to adjust these variables with a high degree of skill and sophistication, thereby inducing a specific kratom experience according to personal predilection. This impressive level of expertise was well beyond my own limited capabilities, however.

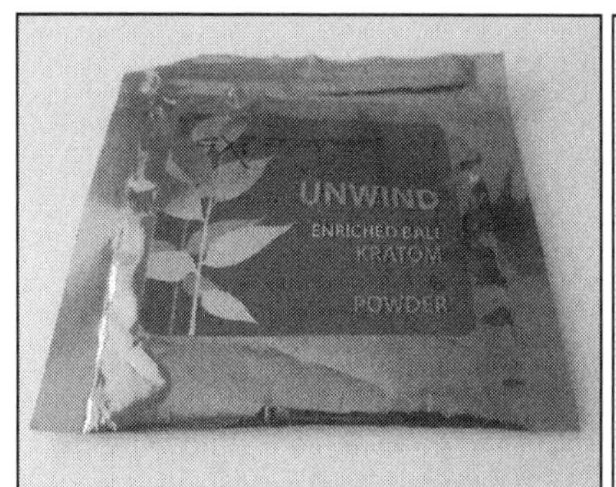

Kratom as purchased via a head shop.

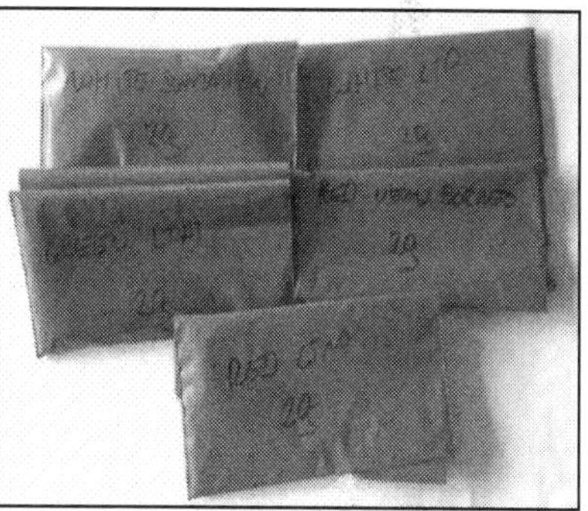
Kratom as supplied by an online vendor.

The taste of kratom was always absolutely revolting and, over time, even its odour became repugnant. To make matters worse, the fine powder would somehow manage to stick around in my mouth, however hard I tried to swallow.

In an effort to counter this problem I focused upon an extract to reduce the volume required to score. I obtained the material, which was named *Gold Standard*, from the same vendor. This proved to be my most successful foray, and it did indeed mitigate most of the horrors regarding taste.

The experience itself was indeed opiate-like, with a sense of well-being which was not quite euphoric, but was engulfing. Accompanying this was a strange yet pleasant aura of physical numbness. This started to emerge after perhaps 15 minutes, and lasted for four or five hours.

Kratom invariably turned a dull afternoon into a happy and contented one. It was a genuine anxiolytic and mood lifter.

I redosed on a couple of occasions, seeking to extend and intensify the session, but this wasn't particularly successful. However, I did learn from this that a kratom hangover is actually a real deal.

If I pushed the dose I awoke in the morning with a solid headache. This faded as the day progressed, but on each occasion I was absolutely certain that it was due to the previous evening's kratom binge.

Was there a longer term come-down during the following day or days? Perhaps there was, but this was not intrusively evident, at least on the doses I consumed.

For a period, testing different kratom strains offered a pleasant diversion, and was something I dabbled with when I was at a particularly loose end. However, given its very real addiction potential, it was a plant which required caution, and was thus one I would only turn to every blue moon.

KRATOM ADDENDUM

In subsequent years, via the remaining contents of the selection pack I refer to above, I learned to work with kratom more proficiently, and was able to produce a pleasant experience on demand. It never induced an enormous high in the traditional sense, but rather alleviated stress, eliminated cravings, and provided relief from any aches and pains I was carrying.

Unfortunately, during this time, efforts to ban this plant gathered pace, particularly in the US. Supply and import had already been prohibited in the UK, and I distinctly recall a Tory MP at the time glibly stating that "*We must be certain to capture kratom in this legislation*", referring to the draconian *Psychoactive Substances Act*, which was implemented in 2016.

What was particularly stark was the background against which these initiatives were developed. Kratom was and is used by many opioid addicts to ease withdrawal, and is occasionally cited as an aid to address acute alcohol dependency. Despite the enormous scale of these two social scourges, and the rapidly worsening opioid epidemic in the US, here was a situation in which politicians and authorities were openly undermining a potential recovery route for desperate victims.

Note that I am not making any bold claims here: I am simply stating factually that kratom has been used successfully by a significant number of former addicts. Rather than researching this with open minds, the opposite course was being pushed, and in the case of the UK, was legislated.

Finally, stating the obvious, if you are exploring this to taper or withdraw from a drug don't be rash or reckless. Replacing one addiction with another is not what you want, so research thoroughly and consider deeply before embarking.

Kratom is a remarkable botanical, but if you are going to use it, dose sensibly and be careful not to make a habit of it.

3.8.4 Mapacho

Binomial / Botanical Name	Nicotiana Rustica
Street Names	Aztec Tobacco; Wild Tobacco
Major Active Compound	Nicotine; Beta-Carbolines
Indigenous Source	Peru; Vietnam
Form	Leaves
RoA	Smoked
Personal Rating On Shulgin Scale	++*

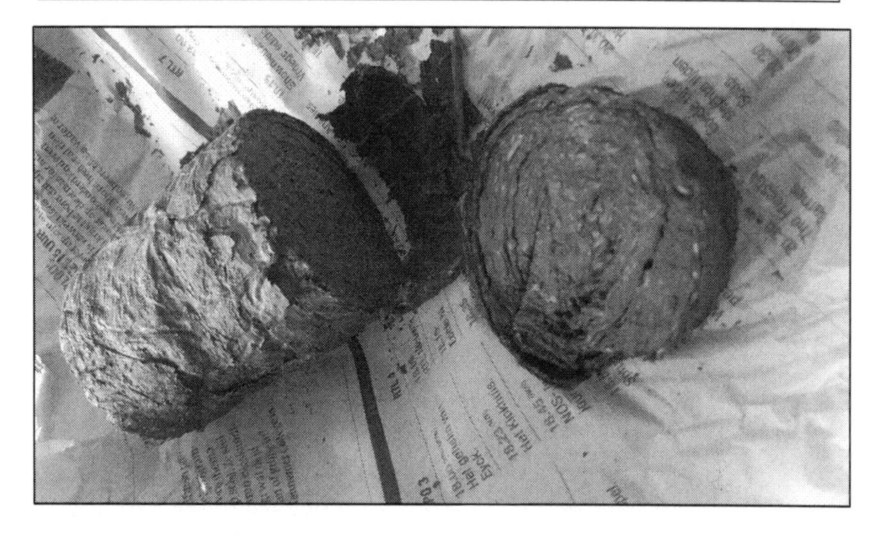

SUBJECTIVE EXPERIENCE
Mapacho (nicotiana rustica) has a rich history of entheogenic use, primarily amongst South American shamans, and sometimes during ayahuasca ceremonies. It is not to be confused with common tobacco (nicotiana tabacum), not least because its nicotine content is commonly stated to be about 20 times higher.

My experience with this was, shall we say, not successful. Perhaps being a non-smoker didn't help, but it was a sorry story.

> REPORT #1
> I undertook the experiment at about 6pm. I loaded the leaves, still pungent and fresh, into a large bong, and took two enormous hits. I'm not sure why I was so greedy: perhaps it was the foolish notion that it was *only tobacco*.

It was a pretty rough smoke, and then boom: I was suddenly dizzy and was almost falling over as I slumped towards a soft chair. I thought I might pass out, but I didn't.

I felt rough, very rough, with head spinning and a sense of nausea.

This gradually wore off and I returned to some sort of normality in about 15-20 minutes. I didn't fully recover until the next day, and I had a very poor night's sleep.

I was completely overwhelmed by it, and vowed never to smoke it again. It didn't feel healthy at all.

Did I actually use the words "*vowed never to smoke it again*"? I suspect that the following report, circa 2016, could fall under the heading "*he never learns*".

REPORT #2
Last week I was in Vietnam, and as I tend to whenever I am in a far flung country, I checked out the local (legal) psychoactive scene.

In this case, I found very little. Occasionally, however, I did notice small groups of men in the streets smoking something from huge bamboo pipes. I presumed this to be tobacco, although I hoped it was something else.

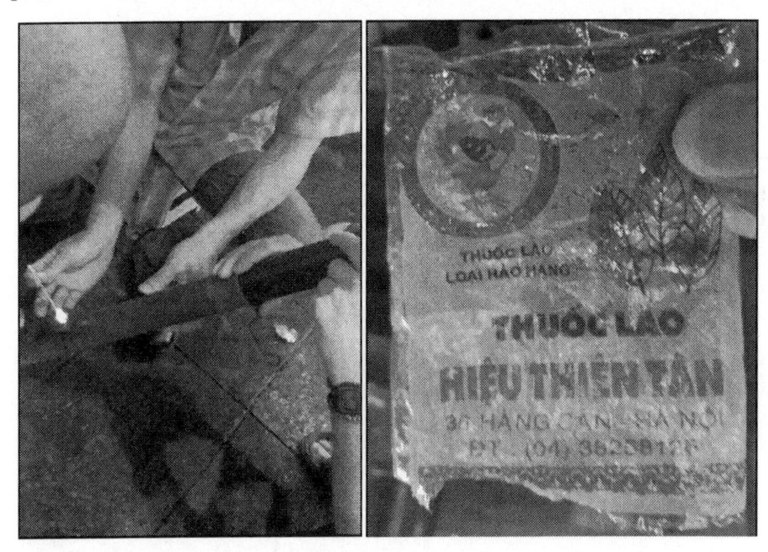

Naturally I couldn't resist, so I approached a couple of chaps, who looked friendly enough, and offered a few local shekels for a toke.

They refused the money but proffered the pipe freely. In fact, they urged me to sit down, an offer which I accepted.

Taking a large hit I immediately realized why.

I was hit for six. I was dizzy, I thought I was fainting, and I felt nausea coming-on. It wasn't nice. It felt very much like a re-run of my earlier nicotiana rustica ordeal.

I didn't slump into a heap this time, but I was close.

After a few minutes, and many deep breaths, I started to slowly get my head together, and I took a photograph of the packet.

On returning to the hotel, later in the evening, I asked the concierge if they could translate the front of this and explain what it was. Yes, it was indeed nicotiana rustica, which also bore the words *Aztec tobacco* and *wild tobacco*. I also discovered that its more formal name there was *thuoc lao*.

What did I deduce from this second slap in the face?

1. Perhaps this feeling is normal, and people get off on it. God knows how. By seating me the locals obviously knew what was coming.

2. I had consumed about 3 bottles of beer: the experience sobered me up instantly, and I remained so for the rest of the evening. Indeed, I didn't feel like engaging any further intoxicant of any type, and didn't drink for the rest of the night.

   After about half an hour, I felt half-decent and strangely clear-headed. Indeed, I felt quite good. Perhaps this phase is the attraction.

3. Like the first time, it felt rather toxic and unhealthy. It's hard to see how anyone could get used to this, but they do appear to. I have no idea what it does to the health of habitual users, but it certainly can't be good news.

Despite the flip side, I'm glad that I re-sampled, largely to have experienced it in a more authentic setting than my room. However, I don't see any scenario at all in which I will repeat it again.

This time I mean it.

ADDITIONAL SAFETY NOTE
It is reported that due to its high nicotine content large doses of mapacho can present the risk of acute poisoning and potentially death. Take it easy!

3.8.5 Opium

Binomial / Botanical Name	Lachryma Papaveris (Source Plant: Papaver Somniferum)
Street Names	Poppy Tears;
Major Active Compound	Morphine; Codeine; Thebaine; Papaverine; Noscapine
Indigenous Source	Uncertain. This sample: Australia
Form	Dried Sap
RoA	Oral / Smoked
Personal Rating On Shulgin Scale	++

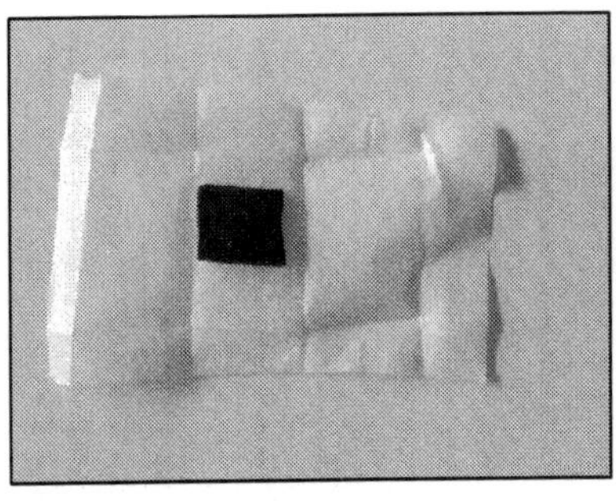

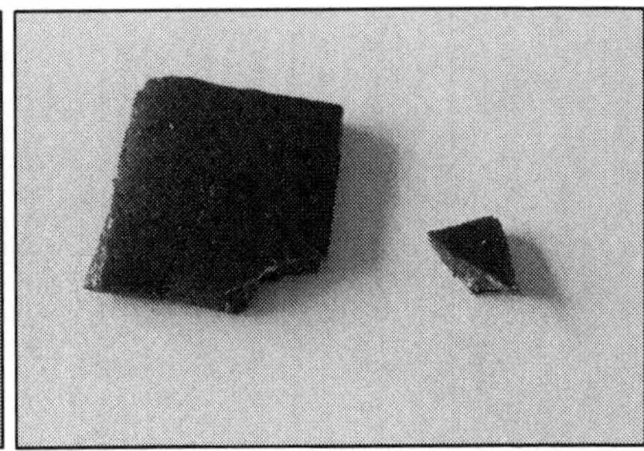

SUBJECTIVE EXPERIENCE
My sample of this most infamous of plant narcotics was offered as *raw dark brown opium*, and was purported to have been hand harvested from pharmaceutically grown Tasmanian white poppies. Its quality was reputed to be extremely high.

Despite its long historical use, I found that there was a distinct lack of information available, including via the Internet, regarding dosage. In the sense that this is a botanical and not an artificially produced substance, this might be expected, at least to some degree. However, I found virtually nothing of any real value.

As a non-opioid user, the vendor recommended that I should start with "*cautious oral use (just swallow a piece)*". Specifically he suggested that I should "*start at 50mg, i.e. half a point*". As his advice to seasoned users was to "*dose upwards from 100mg*" he was halving the dose on account of my lack of tolerance and experience.

He did appear to be reasonably genuine, and of course, had no motive to harm or kill his customers. Regardless, I elected to halve this again, and try 25mg. Given the obvious risks and the serious consequences of overdose, I felt that such caution was probably merited.

With respect to onset, there were a few references, which pitched this at anything between 30 and 90 minutes. I used this as a gauge, but as I had no intention of redosing, it was largely of academic interest.

Forum posts suggested that I should expect the duration to be of the order of 12 hours.

Regarding effects, my expectation was framed by both kratom and heroin, and I anticipated mild euphoria, contentedness, and possibly some nausea. I hoped for minimal hangover, at least on the dose I had chosen.

> T+0:00 I break a small corner off the square of the raw opium, which I believe is sometimes referred to as *dried latex*. I weigh this carefully: 32mg. I consider this to be close enough to my intended 25mg so I go with it. It smells of plant matter and is malleable.
>
> It has a strong taste, very strong in fact, and is quite bitter. I chew and suck this for a minute or so and it begins to dissolve in my mouth. I swig it down with water. The taste lingers so I suck on a clove to dissipate it.
>
> It is 11am, and all I have eaten this morning is a carrot, which I ate with a cup of coffee a couple of hours ago. My stomach is therefore empty and settled.
>
> T+0:30 I feel ever so slightly dreamy; so slightly that I can't at this stage rule out a placebo effect.
>
> Then again, perhaps I can, as I am certainly more tranquil than I was an hour ago.
>
> I should add at this point that I am not really into opioids per se. This relative lack of interest is purely on the basis of their effects: meaning that I don't find the high or quasi-euphoria to be particularly exciting or rewarding. At low doses I also tend to find it difficult to establish when I am actually under the influence, which was something that plagued my kratom experiences in particular.
>
> T+0:45 There has been no significant change thus far, although I do sense that dreamy headspace developing further. There is no pupil constriction or dilation or anything of that nature.
>
> T+1:15 I beginning to feel mentally relaxed. A good measure of sedation is now fairly obvious. Although the anxiolytic effects are clear, there is nothing that I would call euphoric.
>
> T+1:45 Whilst there has been no particular change, time is passing quite quickly. If I had to find a parallel with this at the moment, it would be that it was like a strong benzo, not that my benzo experience is at all prolific.

T+2:00 For no reason other than passing interest I take my blood pressure. It is 137/89, and a heart rate of 50bpm. The former is slightly high, but the latter is more or less within normal parameters.

I still feel sedated, relaxed, and generally fine.

T+2:15 Because the anxiolytic effect is so pleasant, I entertain the thought that this would be even better if I made it stronger: in other words, if I redosed and induced euphoria. I can understand from here how that slippery slope becomes hard to resist.

T+2:30 There is no sign of a come-down as yet. Standing up and walking around I still feel calm and chilled. There is a nice background feeling to it.

I will admit it: this is rather nice.

T+3:15 I am still chillaxed, and on the same contented plateau as earlier, but in a slightly more fatigued way.

T+3:45 I remain broadly the same place, but over the last half hour a weary edge has increasingly emerged. This is not to the level of any discomfort, but I am now a little tired.

I should emphasize that I am still in a very decent place. However, for the first time I feel like I am heading down from the peak.

As it is now closing in on 3pm, I order some (vegetarian) food, which duly arrives: a cheese and tomato sandwich. From this I deduce that there is no appetite suppression in play. I find that can eat normally.

T+4:15 I decide to take a nap, as I often do in the afternoons. I wonder if I will sleep normally.

T+5:15 I slept reasonably well. I have now come-down substantially, with the original effects now just lurking somewhere in the background.

I expect to land slowly and gently over the next few hours.

Overall, this was a very gentle ride: it was a smooth and positive experience. The 32mg dose produced a definite mood lift, with mild sedation and a clear presence. There was the occasional feel of nausea, but this was very slight, and it faded as quickly as it came. Perhaps there was a hint of a headache the following morning.

I may return to this, either for a smoke, or a slightly higher dose. If I do, it won't be until my body is fully reset from this experience, and given the risks with this class, I won't be overdoing it.

3.8.6 Rapé

Binomial / Botanical Name	Rapé
Street Names	Yawanawa; Katukina; Mapacho; Others
Major Active Compound	Nicotiana Rustica; Misc
Indigenous Source	Amazon Basin
Form	Snuff
RoA	Insufflated
Personal Rating On Shulgin Scale	++

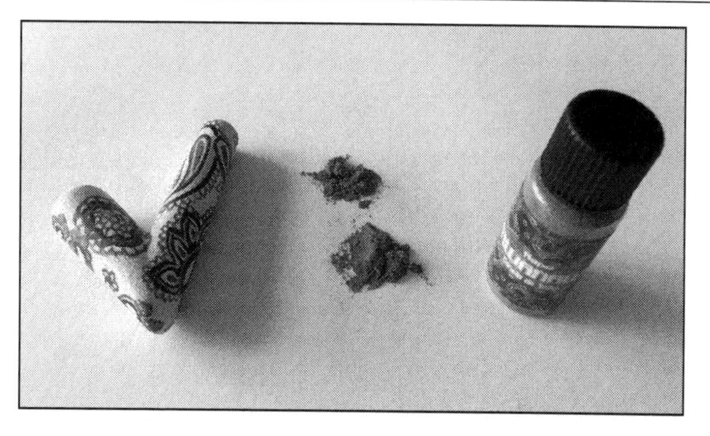

SUBJECTIVE EXPERIENCE
Rapé appeared on the UK market just a few months prior to the blanket ban on psychoactives in 2016. I wrote the following forum post at the time:

> In recent weeks I have noticed a couple of websites suddenly offering this in the UK. It is a type of snuff, which the most prominent vendor states is "*a complex blend of pulverized plants, which usually contain a strong tobacco*". Instead of regular tobacco (nicotiana tabacum) it tends to be based around a much stronger cousin, nicotiana rustica.
>
> Rapé is prevalent around the Amazon basin. It is used as a shamanic medicine, and is occasionally offered during ayahuasca and other sacred ceremonies.
>
> Independently, nicotiana rustica also has a very long history of ritual use. Its effects are rather different to those of the manufactured version of tobacco, as pimped on the high street. They broadly include a strong stimulation, a head rush, and greater focus, with a lengthy sedation occurring later.

The reason I post this now relates to timing. It speculatively occurs to me that these vending initiatives may be a direct or indirect response to the forthcoming ban on psychoactives: tobacco will remain legal, and these substances may therefore remain openly available.

Whether this is a positive or not, it is important that harm reduction is considered early in the fray. There is very little information available with respect to this, but hopefully this post can start the ball rolling.

I have experimented previously with both nicotiana rustica and a couple of rapé variants. They can certainly pack a punch, and not necessarily a positive one.

In the indigenous environment the snuff is blown into the nostril by a partner, in a similar manner to that practised for yopo seeds. However, self-administration tools are also available, in the form of a sort of V-shaped bamboo tubing, called a *kuripe:*

The effect can also be induced via a very strong snort. This is a central matter, as the intensity of the experience is closely linked to both the amount taken and the strength of the blow (or inhalation).

I have remained cautious with this substance partly because tobacco itself is addictive and harmful. I don't smoke, and don't want to. Bearing in mind that nicotiana rustica is frequently cited as being about 20 times more powerful than nicotiana tabacum you can probably see my point. It may or may not present a significantly higher risk of addiction, but I have never felt inclined to take the chance.

The other issue that concerns me is the recurrent claim that large doses (of nicotiana rustica) can cause acute nicotine poisoning and death. This sort of comment, found on drugs-forum.com, can't be ignored:

> *"I've never heard of anyone doing this outside of various Central/ South American tribal shamans. These people systematically addict themselves to tobacco and develop tolerances that are staggering, so that they are able to ingest what would be lethal doses for most people. And even these shamans have been known to OD and wind up dead as a sacrifice to their art."* ~ rawbeer

I'm not trying to put a damp cloth on this, or generally undermine it, but clearly, caution is advisable.

Also relevant is that it is usually extremely hard to uncover exactly what is in most of the rapé variants, including their actual nicotiana rustica content. Having stated all this, it should be noted that there are versions of rapè that don't contain nicotine, although I have not personally encountered them.

> If anyone can add to this starter in any way please do so. Rapé provides a definite and strong psychoactive effect, and my hunch is that it will become much more widely used in the short term.

Regarding content, the vendor of my particular samples stated that rapé can contain alkaloid ashes, which can be "*made from psychoactive plants*" and in some cases hallucinogens. Given its historical and ritual use this is undoubtedly true, although I cannot confirm this with respect to my own experiments.

In addition to the recreational aspects I have focused upon above, and as also stated in the post itself, rapé has long been used for medicinal purposes, usually in a traditional sacred context. Clearly, the specific plants used in a particular rapé variant will determine its individual effects. The scope is obviously enormous.

As for my experience, whilst hard hitting, with something of a head shock, rapé was similar to but nothing like as debilitating as standalone nicotiana rustica. However, with a strong enough snort/blow perhaps it could be. Further information on nicotiana rustica itself is provided under the heading of *Mapacho*, earlier in this section.

There are clearly certain subtleties with rapé in terms of its different versions and ingredients, but I suspect that for many these will only manifest themselves with repeated or prolonged exposure to the tobacco. For the tobacco smoker this may provide an interesting field of (cautious) research.

ADDENDUM

Some years subsequent to writing the above, and having read a couple of positive reports, I revisited rapé via another standalone experiment.

I prepared 2 pea sized doses of finely ground *yawanawa* powder and embarked at approximately 4:20 pm. In traditional style I blew the first up my left nostril using a kuripe, and despite gasping with watering eyes managed to repeat with the left.

I was hit immediately. Following on from the severe olfactory discomfort, heat quickly engulfed my brain/head, top down, and a debilitating and not very pleasant headspace emerged. The burning sensation drifted into what almost felt like an illness or flu. I tried to meditate into it and confront it but it was too unpleasant. It was overwhelming and I stumbled to bed, sweating profusely.

There were mapacho-like aspects to this, which was not surprising, although it was not quite as intense. Ten minutes passed and I lay there feeling poorly and quite wretched. After half an hour I was a little better but still unwell. An hour later I was finally able to rise. I slowly recovered but was not in a good condition for the rest of the day.

Clearly, such tobacco based materials are not for me, and I certainly won't be repeating this.

3.8.7 Sakae Naa

Binomial / Botanical Name	Combretum Quadrangulare
Street Names	Sakae Naa
Major Active Compound	Combretol
Indigenous Source	Vietnam, Cambodia, Laos, Myanmar, Thailand
Form	Dried Leaves
RoA	Oral / Vaporised / Smoked
Personal Rating On Shulgin Scale	+ / + / +*

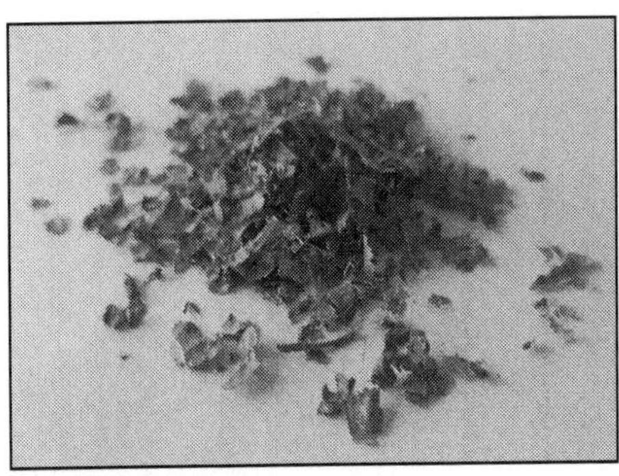
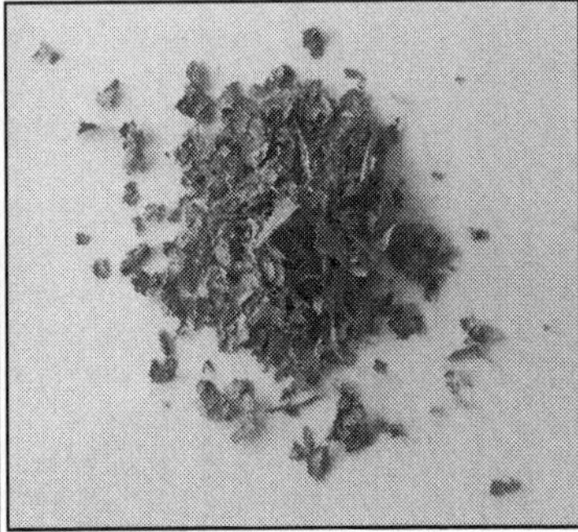

SUBJECTIVE EXPERIENCE
Although sometimes used as a substitute for kratom, in terms of effect the similarities are disputed. On initial use, some years ago, I found it to be extremely weak in comparison; too weak to form a judgement. This applied to both oral use (10g as a tea) and intake via a vaporiser.

I have returned to this for two reasons. The first is that it took a number of experiments to actually experience anything worthwhile from kratom; hence the feeling that I should give this at least one more punt before writing it off. The second is that I continue to encounter Internet reports which claim that it actually delivers, albeit in a mild form.

A relevant factor is also that I am not a great connoisseur of the opioid type of venture. The overall ride, as I have always experienced it (mood lift, relative euphoria/happiness, sedation, nausea/headache), has never been compelling, or particularly rewarding as a whole.

It's fair to say that I enter this exercise with fairly low expectations.

Re-visiting the Internet I notice frequent claims that farmers in Thailand and Myanmar "*chew or smoke the leaves for their sedative properties*". Indeed, a number of sources cite smoking as the preferred method.

My course is set accordingly.

> T+0:00 I fill the bowl of a small bong, light, take a large hit, and hold. I then repeat the exercise, twice. It is quite an easy smoke. [4:20pm].
>
> T+0:05 There is a change of headspace, albeit a very mild one. It is the gentlest of sedations, with a slightly dreamy edge. I feel comfortable as I sit at my desk typing these notes.
>
> T+0:15 I feel much the same as I did on 5 minutes. The tranquillising effect has neither strengthened nor weakened. The shift from normality is extremely subtle, but real.
>
> T+0:30 To determine if I can take this any further I re-load the bowl and take another couple of hits. Again, it is nice and easy on the lungs. Within a couple of minutes the dreamy heady edge is back to where it was immediately following the first blast.
>
> This is moderately pleasing, and assuming that expectations are not set unreasonably high, provides a positive mellow ambience.
>
> T+0:35 I am experiencing a general disposition of contentedness, which has replaced my slightly edgy and bored mood of 40 minutes ago.
>
> T+1:00 The intensity has faded, but the vibe still lingers at a slightly lower level. At this point lightly chilled is probably a good way of describing it.
>
> T+2:00 I am approaching base, although some residue sedation is still in play.
>
> T+3:00 I feel almost at baseline, but my background mood continues to be relaxed and calm.

I didn't find this to be energising, as some forum posters suggest, nor particularly like kratom. This certainly applied to intake via smoking.

For me, as consumed above, it induced the mildest of anxiolytic states, but with a positive and dreamy aura. Having stated this, it may well be one for which the use of fresh leaves presents a different proposition in terms of potency, particularly if consumed in an authentic setting.

Overall, I found this to be more agreeable than I had anticipated. *Pleasant* is probably the best word I can find.

3.8.8 Tobacco

Common Nomenclature	Nicotiana Tabacum (Prime)
Street & Reference Names	Smokes; Cigs; Ciggies; Cigs; Butts; Fags
Reference Dosage	Threshold 0.2mg+; Light 0.3mg+; Common 0.6mg+; Strong 1mg+; Heavy 2mg+ [Erowid]
Anticipated: Onset / Duration	20 Seconds / 20 Minutes
Form	Plant Material
RoA	Smoked
Source / Jurisdiction	Retail / UK

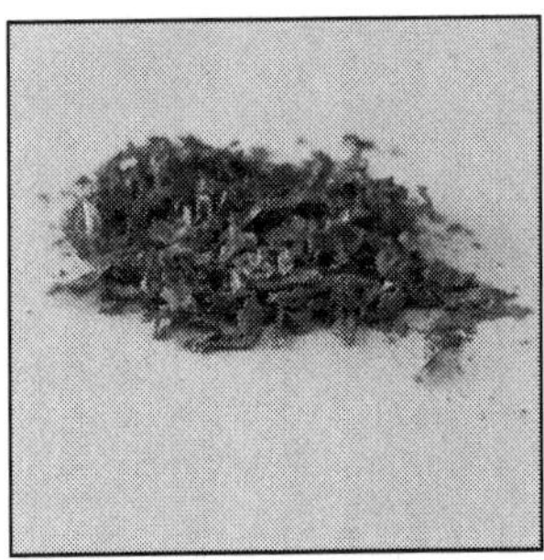

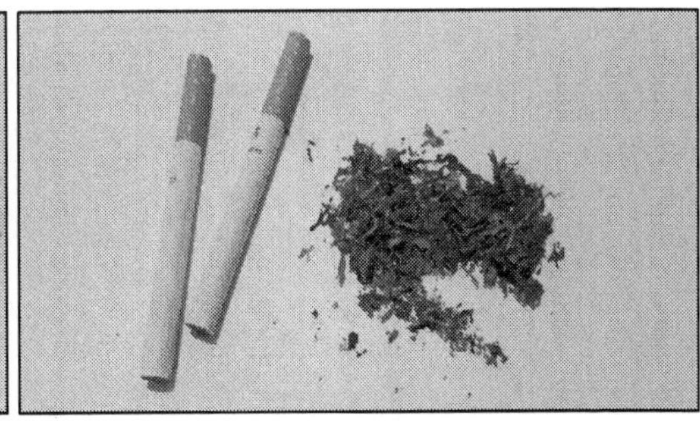

SUBJECTIVE EXPERIENCE
The chief commercial crop for tobacco is *nicotiana tabacum,* which contains the active alkaloid, nicotine. It is one of the most commonly used drugs in the world, and is sold legally throughout the world, with an estimated one billion active smokers.

Despite this, I have to admit that I don't get it. I don't understand why so many people use this other than to initially experiment, once or twice.

For me, it produces an extremely mild stimulation and a very slight mood lift, followed by a little sedation. None of this is significant enough to return to, especially with so many more-worthwhile and less-toxic options available.

I have always felt like this. I sampled it a few times in different forms as a youngster, fortunately not frequently enough to become addicted. Whilst I have occasionally smoked it pre-rolled with cannabis (more through necessity than choice), I have never been even slightly tempted by the tobacco.

My own lack of interest, however, certainly doesn't diminish my responsibility to point out the acute danger posed by its use.

The World Health Organisation states bluntly that:

> "*Tobacco kills around 6 million people each year. More than 5 million of those deaths are the result of direct tobacco use while more than 600,000 are the result of non-smokers being exposed to second-hand smoke*"

In the US, the CDC states that:

> "Cigarette smoking is estimated to cause ... *more than 480,000 deaths annually (including deaths from second hand smoke)*"

And that:

> "*Life expectancy for smokers is at least 10 years shorter than for non-smokers*"

In the UK, ASH reports that:

> "*Smoking is the primary cause of preventable illness and premature death, accounting for approximately 96,000 deaths a year*".

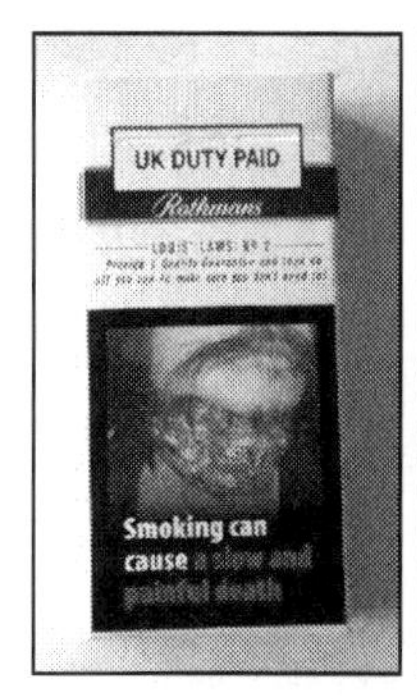

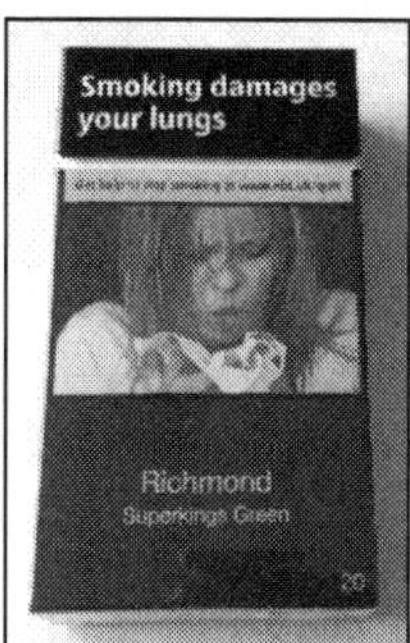

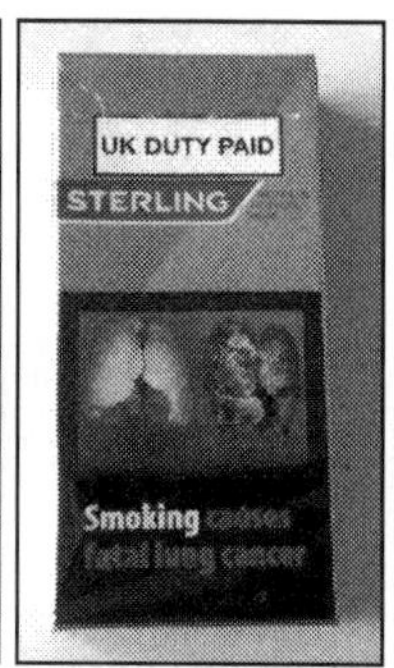

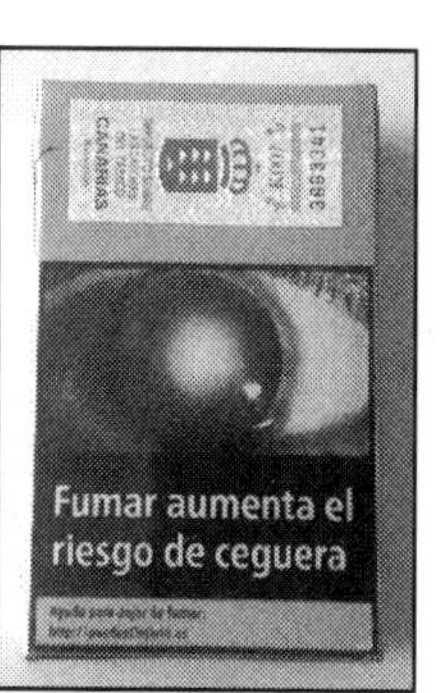

I am sure that there is little need to further labour the acute perils and pitfalls of using this drug, as they are so well known. The negative imbalance of risk versus pleasure should already be obvious to all.

If you don't smoke, don't start. If you do smoke, support is available from a variety of sources to help you stop, including from government websites.
[http://smokefree.gov (US) and http://www.nhs.uk/smokefree (UK)]

For the record, for the opening photographs on the previous page I purchased a packet of 10 cigarettes from my local supermarket (*Tesco)*, at a cost of £3.60 (January 2017). The sales assistant assured me that these were the cheapest *"normal cigarettes"* on offer and that they were very popular.

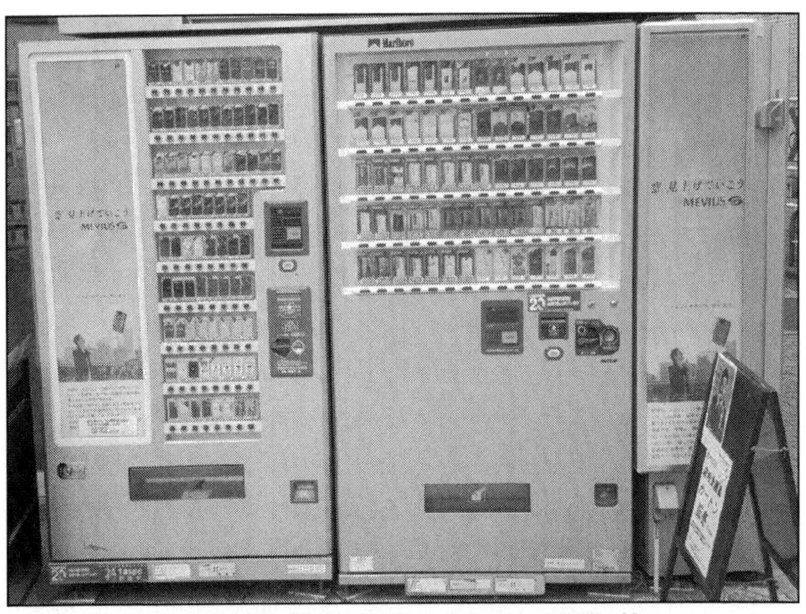

In some parts of the world (tobacco) cigarettes are still sold freely via public vending machines (Tokyo, 2017)

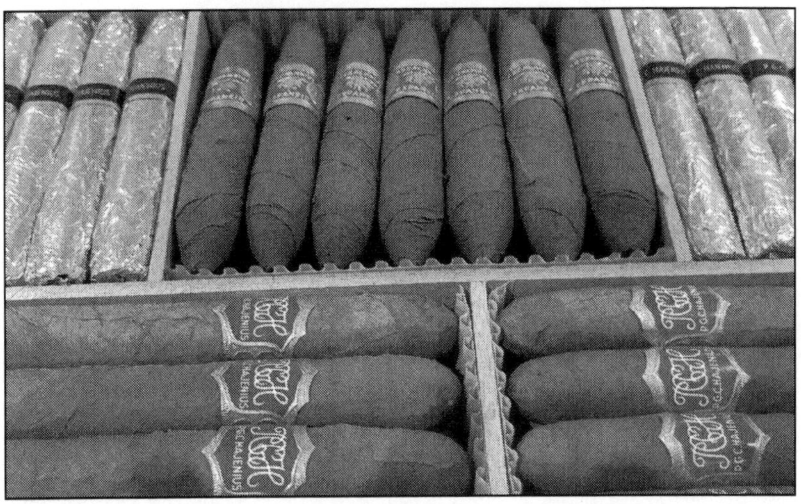

A specialised market has long existed for various forms of tobacco, particularly when sold as cigars (P.G.C. Hajenius, Amsterdam, 2017)

4

THE WORLDSCAPE

4. WORLDSCAPE: THE WIDER CONTEXT

The drugscape does not exist in a vacuum, and neither do you. The world you are part of encompasses society and culture, legal implications, travel, personal responsibilities, sources of help and assistance, terminology and slang, and a myriad of other complex and omnipresent phenomena.

This section seeks to provide background, guidance, and direct information relevant to drug use in the wider context, as well as direction on where to obtain further material and knowledge. It offers practical data and reference material to help manage all the above, and hopefully to successfully navigate any emerging problems or issues.

Again, this cuts through the misinformation and propaganda of mainstream sources, and focuses upon the factual and the accurate. Used in conjunction with the earlier sections, it may help you to avoid many of the pitfalls which are encountered by the unwary all too frequently.

THE WORLDSCAPE
The worldscape is documented via the following sub-sections:

EDUCATION & AWARENESS
Remember that education and awareness are the first steps to mitigate risks, including to your general welfare and well being. Don't shortcut this section and don't shortcut the safety measures documented through the rest of this book.

Any updates to this information will be posted on the website:
www.DrugUsersBible.com

4.1 HOW MANY PEOPLE USE DRUGS?

In the UK, the Home Office, in its *2015 Crime Survey for England & Wales*, stated that 8.6% of adults aged 16 to 59 *"had taken an illicit drug in the last year"*. This was similar to previous years, and equates to about 2.9 million people. *Illicit* presumably means illegal.

It also stated that *"3.2% of adults aged 16 to 59 had taken a Class A drug in the last year, equivalent to just over one million people"*. It added *"2.2% of adults aged 16 to 59 were classed as frequent drug users (having taken any illicit drug more than once a month on average in the last year)."*

One of the most comprehensive international studies I found was undertaken on behalf of the National Institute of Drug Abuse, in the US. This surveyed 44,892 students from 382 public and private schools.

When asked which drugs they had used in the previous 12 months, the 17-18 year olds (12th Graders) within this number responded as follows:

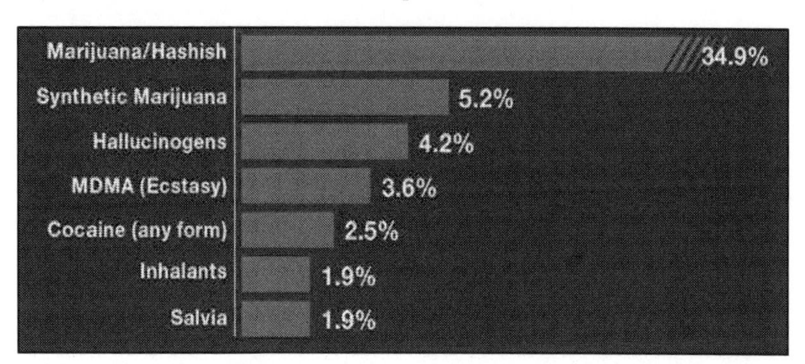

As there are estimated to be about 4 million 12th Graders, this would equate to about 1.4 million marijuana users, 200,000 users of hallucinogens, and so forth. A crude extrapolation of this percentage to the entire US population provides a figure of over 100 million marijuana users.

If that sounds like an astonishing figure, it does go some way to explain why approximately 750,000 people are arrested every year for marijuana offences (source: *FBI*). Overall, in the US almost half a million people are incarcerated for drug offences (source: *The Sentencing Project, 2014*), and on average someone is arrested for drug possession every 25 seconds.

Whilst they provide insight, statistics like these barely scratch the surface, particularly as most studies tend not to include the use of legal psychoactives and emerging research chemicals.

THE EMCDDA

The *European Monitoring Centre for Drugs and Drug Addiction* (EMCDDA) was inaugurated as an EU agency in 1995. It exists to provide the EU and its member states with a factual overview of European drug problems and a solid evidence base to support the drugs debate.

The following data was published by the EMCDDA in 2016. It details the percentage of adults (15-64) from the stated samples who have used illegal drugs. Note that, with respect to the United Kingdom, this does not include those drugs made illegal subsequent to the passing of the *Psychoactive Substances Act 2016*.

Country	Year	Sample	% Total
Austria	2008	3761	14.8
Belgium	2013	4931	15.8
Bulgaria	2012	5325	8.3
Croatia	2012	4756	16
Cyprus	2012	3500	10.5
Czech Republic	2014	870	31.1
Denmark	2013	10470	36
Estonia	2008	1401	21.3
Finland	2014	3128	22.2
France	2014	13488	41.1
Germany	2012	9084	23.9
Greece	2004	4351	9.1
Hungary	2007	2710	9.3
Ireland	2011	5128	27.2
Italy	2014	6590	32.7
Latvia	2011	4491	14.3
Lithuania	2012	4831	11.1
Norway	2014	1794	22.6
Poland	2014	1135	16.4
Portugal	2012	5355	9.5
Romania	2013	7200	8.4
Slovakia	2010	4055	20.09
Slovenia	2012	7514	16.1
Spain	2013	23136	31.3
Sweden	2014	6523	14.8
Turkey	2011	8045	2.7
United Kingdom	2014	20080	34.7

Source: www.emcdda.europa.eu/data/stats2016#displayTable:GPS-113

From this, for example, it can be deduced via extrapolation that, if identified by their government, more than one third of the UK's entire population could be criminalized for their use of drugs. Numerically, this is in excess of 22 million people.

THE UNITED NATIONS

The United Nations Office on Drugs and Crime (UNODC) presented the following picture of global drug use in its *World Drug Report 2016*:

> *"It is estimated that 1 in 20 adults, or a quarter of a billion people between the ages of 15 and 64 years, used at least one drug in 2014. Roughly the equivalent of the combined populations of France, Germany, Italy and the United Kingdom."*

A later reference within the same report was even more precise: "*247 million people used drugs in the past year*".

In terms of specific psychoactives, it cited cannabis and amphetamines as the two most popular drugs, with 183 million and 33 million users respectively.

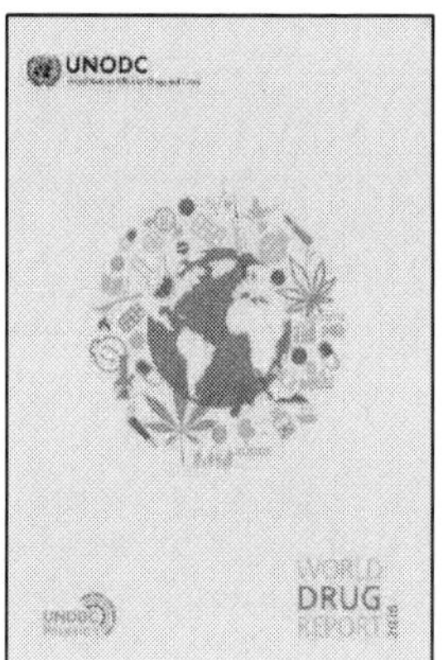

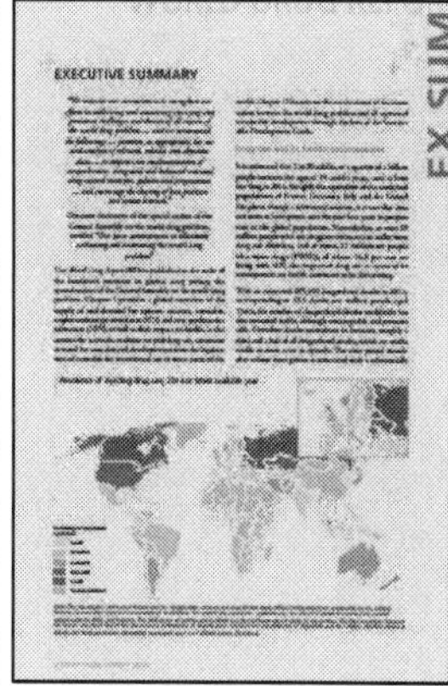

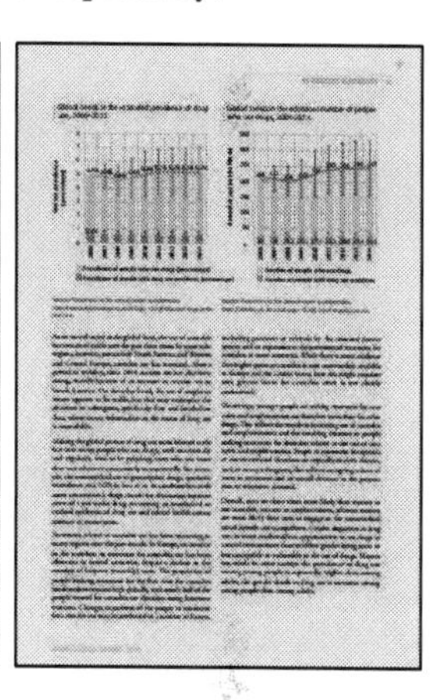

Finally, it stated that the number of drug users was stable, and "*does not seem to have grown over the past four years in proportion to the global population*".

SUMMARY

In summary, there is no doubt that a significant minority of the world's population choose to use some form of unsanctioned psychoactive substance. This is despite the unremitting propaganda and brutal punitive onslaught of the *war on drugs*.

Equally, the vast majority of those 247 million people are, in practical terms, denied the basic safety information and education which would, in many cases, help to save lives and alleviate risk. They are unaware of precisely the sort of directly relevant material which is published in this book.

4.2 THE RELATIVE HARM

Obscured by the endless stream of hysteria, misinformation and outright lies, which have been promulgated by the mainstream media* for generations, are the answers to the most fundamental of questions:

What are the relative harms of the most commonly used psychoactives?

What does the DATA actually say?

What does SCIENCE tell us?

What are the FACTS?

Every adolescent who has ever dabbled with cannabis already has some sort of a handle on this. Their own experience and those of their peers directly contradicts the propagandistic mendacity they have been subjected to. They are aware that the drugs they have personally encountered are not the toxically guaranteed path to a wasted life they are presented as.

Simultaneously, they can see the perils of alcohol with their own eyes. Often, the debris and fallout is all around them.

Hardly surprisingly, this real world picture of first hand experience is broadly the one which scientific studies substantiate and confirm. It is a stark and clear picture: a picture which is generally hidden from the public at large.

SCIENTIFIC APPROACHES
There are many approaches with which to measure the relative harms of individual psychoactives. These range from those focused upon the individual, such as addiction potential and toxicity, to those which address wider social issues, such as crime and healthcare. By and large, it is fair to say that the ranking of commonly used substances (legal and illegal) does not differ dramatically between them.

To illustrate this, I present below data from a number of the studies which have been undertaken over the years, some of which has been reported and submitted directly to Parliament.

The first illustration uses data sourced from a paper by Robert S. Gable, called "*Comparison of acute lethal toxicity of commonly abused psychoactive substances*", which was published by the Society for the Study of Addiction, in 2004. This presents the ratio of effective dose to lethal dose.

* *Honourable exceptions acknowledged.*

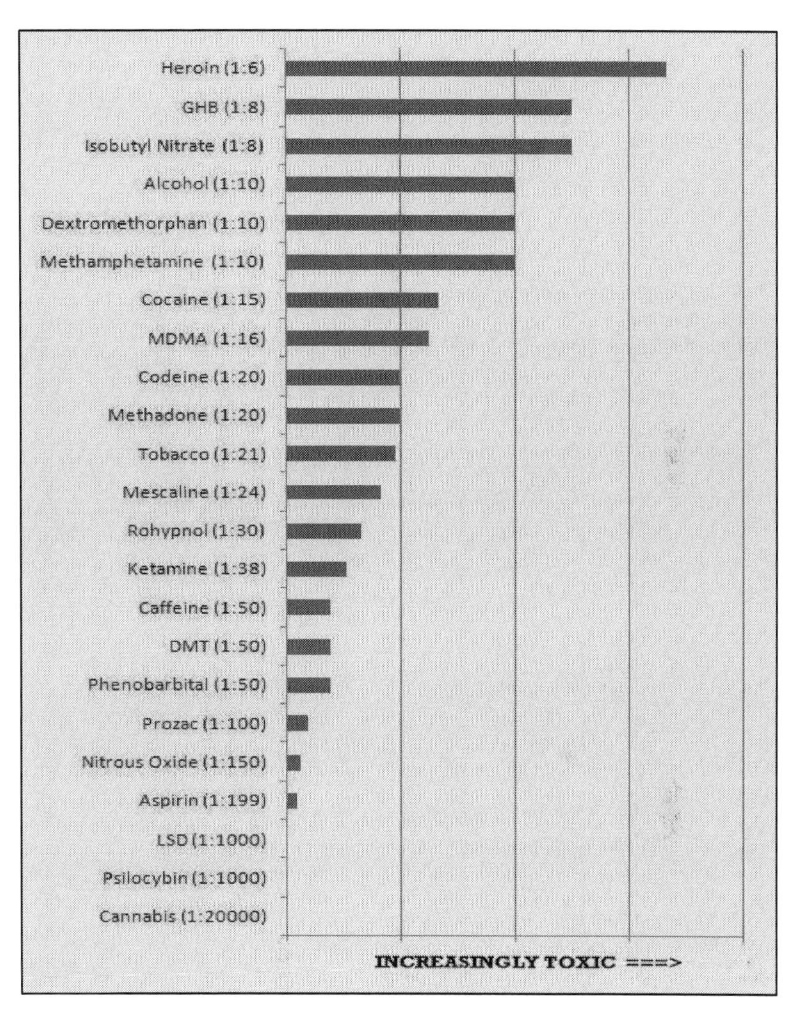

In plain English, whilst two drinks may make you merry, twenty may well kill you. Hence, the ratio for alcohol in this diagram is 1:10.

Now consider the following graph. The underlying data was produced by Prof David J Nutt, FMed, Leslie A King, PhD, Lawrence D Phillips, PhD, on behalf of the Independent Scientific Committee on Drugs and was published in *The Lancet*,Volume 376, No. 9752, p1558–1565, 6 November 2010 (*Drug harms in the UK: a multicriteria decision analysis).*

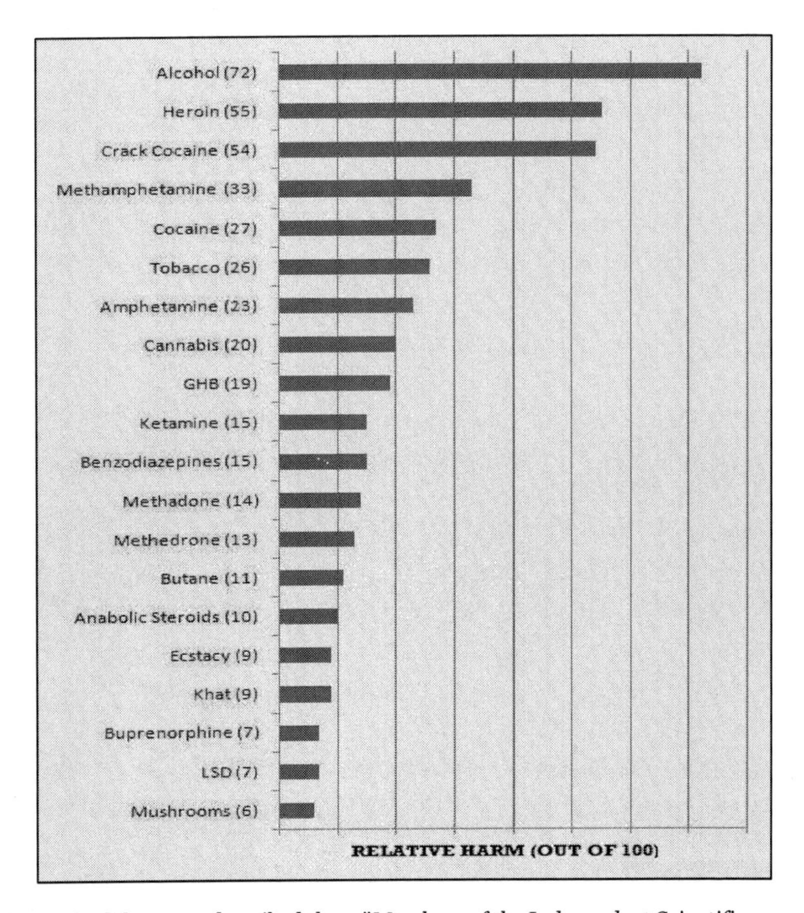

The methodology was described thus: "*Members of the Independent Scientific Committee on Drugs, including two invited specialists, met in a 1-day interactive workshop to score 20 drugs on 16 criteria: nine related to the harms that a drug produces in the individual and seven to the harms to others. Drugs were scored out of 100 points, and the criteria were weighted to indicate their relative importance.*"

Wikipedia describes this as follows:
"*Researchers asked drug-harm experts to rank these illegal and legal drugs on various measures of harm both to the user and to others in society. These measures include damage to health, drug dependency, economic costs and crime. The researchers claim that the rankings are stable because they are based on so many different measures and would require significant discoveries about these drugs to affect the rankings.*"

The graphic below was produced from data offered in another article published by *The Lancet,* this one on March 24, 2007, by Prof David Nutt, FMed, Leslie A King, PhD, William Saulsbury, MA, Prof Colin Blakemore, FRS ("*Development of a rational scale to assess the harm of drugs of potential misuse*" - 369:1047-1053).

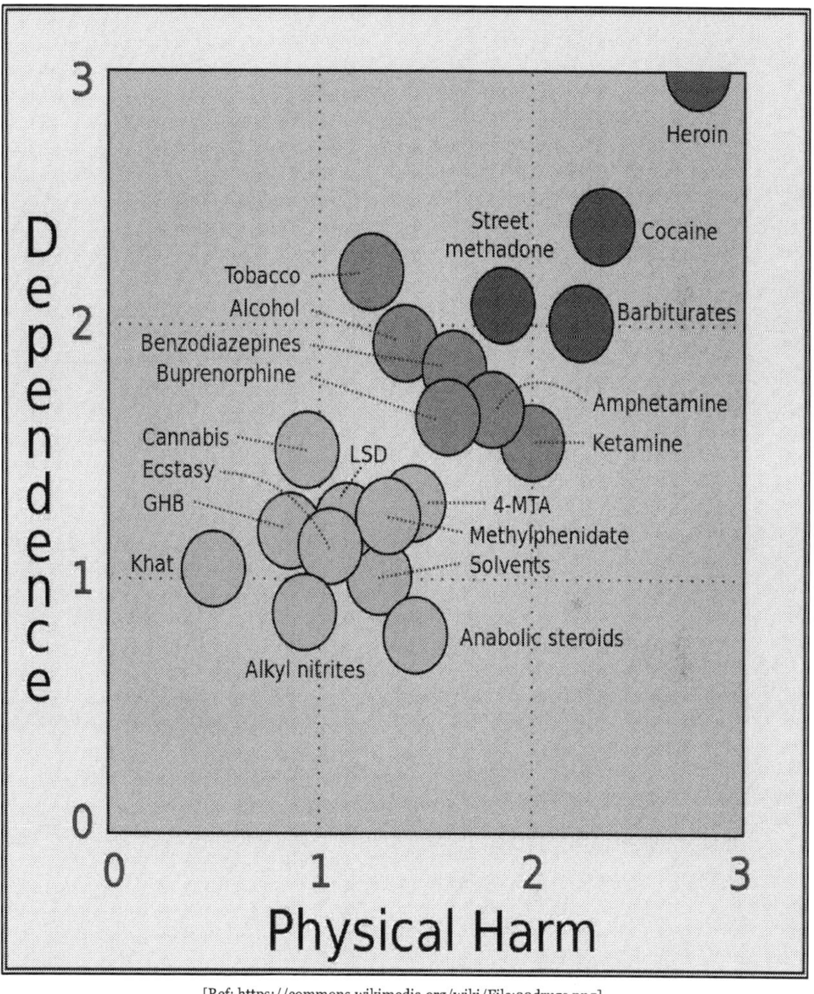

[Ref: https://commons.wikimedia.org/wiki/File:20drugs.png]

Finally, the following two charts were created simply to illustrate a couple of extremes, in terms of drug use and fatality.

Annual Drug Deaths in the United States

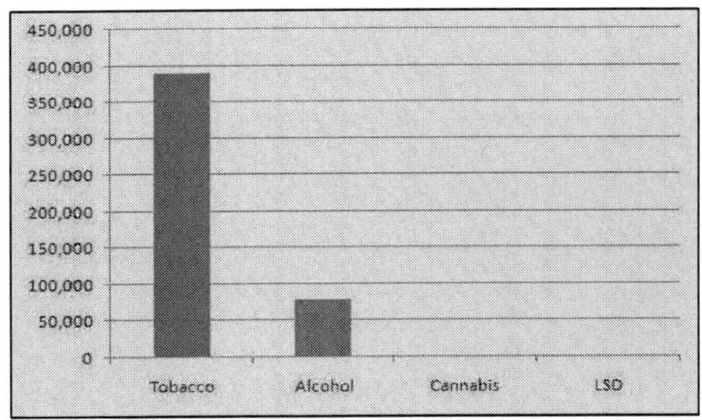

[Source: Schaffer Library of Drug Policy]

Annual Drug Deaths in the United Kingdom

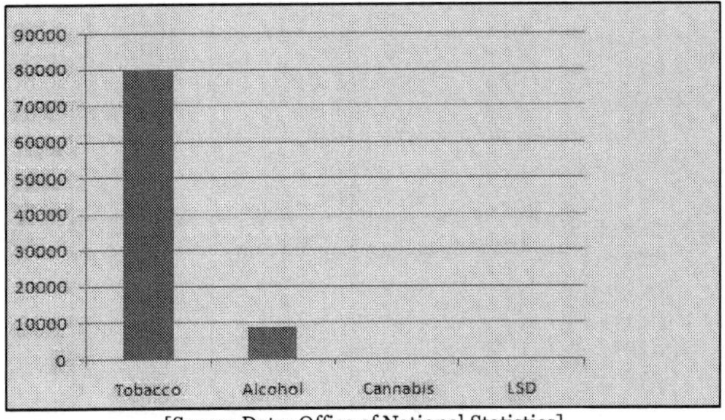

[Source Data: Office of National Statistics]

The picture presented by all these charts is more or less the same as that painted by every study I encountered. The implications of this are obvious:

- The legal status of psychoactives bears no relation whatsoever to harm or health. This could hardly be more clear-cut.
- In terms of personal harm, the usual suspects (e.g. heroin, alcohol) are at the same end of the spectrum. Psychedelics, of course, are at the opposite end.

Whilst each chemical and botanical should always be researched on its own merits, data such as this is hard to ignore, unless you are a politician or part of the mainstream media.

4.3 Addiction & Overdose

Addiction and overdose are, without doubt, absolute nightmares for all involved. They are to be avoided at all costs, or addressed urgently if applicable.

4.3.1 Addiction

Nobody becomes addicted through choice. It is a hazard which is endemic to the use of most drugs, although not all. However, even for the most addictive of drugs, it is a risk that can be reduced (but not eliminated) if the steps outlined in the first section of this book are religiously followed.

For example, to mitigate the risk during the research undertaken for this book, I never, ever, used the same drug, or even a drug from the same class, for at least two weeks following the initial experiment. Invariably, the gap was substantially longer.

In recent years, various parties have sought to rank common drugs by order of addiction potential. As referenced earlier, the usual suspects tend to appear at the top. The table below presents some of the most frequently cited initiatives:

	The Conversation	Addiction Center	AlterNet
1	Heroin	Heroin	Heroin
2	Cocaine	Alcohol	Crack Cocaine
3	Nicotine	Cocaine	Nicotine
4	Barbiturates	Barbiturates	Methadone
5	Alcohol	Nicotine	Crystal Meth

*The list produced by The Conversation was derived from the same 2007 articles in the Lancet as discussed in Section 4.2. The AlterNet report refers to the source as a panel of Dutch Scientists, which replicated the earlier study.

As these are somewhat stilted towards individual and transient street names, a better perspective may be to consider each as a representative of a class. For example, heroin is an opioid - other members of the family tend to be just as addictive.

These, however, are simply the headliners. Everyone is different, and is uniquely susceptible. Many drugs not included on these lists are just as addictive, and claim countless lives.

This is not an area in which to take risks, or to betray common sense. Every person reading this should know the dire consequences of addiction, and the gravity of the pain and suffering it causes. If in doubt, head over to YouTube or Google and take a closer look at the personal catastrophes and the destruction of lives on show. Or check out Reddit, and count the number of lost Subreddit members.

Don't skirt around the edges with this, or you could easily be bitten, horribly.

4.3.2 If You Are Addicted

How do you know if you are addicted? If you are asking this question, it is extremely likely that you have a problem, in which case, do not skip or skim this section.

The commonly suggested approaches to address addiction are:

- Cold Turkey
- Tapering
- Psychedelic Intervention
- Professional and Medical Help
- Rehab

There may be others, but regardless, there is no one-size-fits-all. The best solution for you will depend largely upon your unique characteristics and situation. The one thing you must not do, however, is nothing.

ADVICE FROM NIDA
The *National Institute on Drug Abuse*, part of the U.S. Department of Health, offers a wealth of information on its website. The following was extracted from an introductory Q&A. Note that this can be reproduced without permission (although as a matter of courtesy I did ask).

> Why can't I stop using drugs on my own?
> Repeated drug use changes the brain, including parts of the brain that enable you to exert self-control. These and other changes can be seen clearly in brain imaging studies of people with drug addictions.
>
> If I want help, where do I start?
> Asking for help is the first important step. Visiting your doctor for a possible referral to treatment is one way to do it. You can ask if he or she is comfortable discussing drug abuse screening and treatment. If not, ask for a referral to another doctor. You can also contact an addiction specialist. It takes a lot of courage to seek help for a drug problem because there is a lot of hard work ahead. However, treatment can work, and people recover from addiction every day. Like other chronic diseases, addiction can be managed successfully. Treatment enables people to counteract addiction's powerful, disruptive effects on brain and behavior and regain control of their lives.
>
> Will they make me stop taking drugs immediately?
> The first step in treatment is "detox," which helps patients to remove all of the drugs from their system. This is important, because drugs impair the mental abilities you need to stay in treatment. When patients first stop abusing drugs, they can experience a variety of physical and emotional withdrawal symptoms, including depression, anxiety, and other mood disorders; restlessness; and sleeplessness. Treatment centers are very experienced in helping you get through this process and keeping you safe. Depending on what drug you are addicted to, there may also be medications that will make you feel a little better during drug withdrawal, which makes it easier to stop using.

What kind of counseling should I get?
Behavioral treatment (also known as "talk therapy") helps patients engage in the treatment process, change their attitudes and behaviors related to drug abuse, and increase healthy life skills. These treatments can also enhance the effectiveness of medications and help people stay in treatment longer. Treatment for drug abuse and addiction can be delivered in many different settings using a variety of behavioral approaches.

Will I need medication?
There are medications available to treat addictions to alcohol, nicotine, and opioids (heroin and pain relievers). Other medications are available to treat possible mental health conditions (such as depression) that may be contributing to your addiction. In addition, nonaddictive medication is sometimes prescribed to help with drug withdrawal. When medication is available, it can be combined with behavioral therapy to ensure success for most patients. Your treatment provider will advise you on what medications are available for your particular situation.

I take drugs because I feel depressed—nothing else seems to work. If I stop, I'll feel much worse—how do I deal with that?
It is very possible you need to find treatment for both depression and addiction. This is very common. It's called "comorbidity," "co-occurrence," or "dual diagnosis" when you have more than one health problem at the same time. It is important that you discuss all of your symptoms and behaviors with your doctor. There are many nonaddictive drugs that can help with depression or other mental health issues. Sometimes health care providers do not communicate with each other as well as they should, so you can be your own best advocate and make sure all of your health providers know about all of the health issues that concern you. People who have co-occurring issues should be treated for all of them at the same time.

How can I talk to others with similar problems?
Self-help groups can extend the effects of professional treatment. The most well-known self-help groups are those affiliated with Alcoholics Anonymous (AA), Narcotics Anonymous (NA), and Cocaine Anonymous (CA), all of which are based on the 12-step model. Most drug addiction treatment programs encourage patients to participate in a self-help group during and after formal treatment. These groups can be particularly helpful during recovery, as they are a source of ongoing communal support to stay drug free.

The following bullet point list is also offered:

- Drug addiction is a chronic disease characterized by drug seeking and use that is compulsive, or difficult to control, despite harmful consequences.
- Brain changes that occur over time with drug use challenge an addicted person's self-control and interfere with their ability to resist intense urges to take drugs. This is why drug addiction is also a relapsing disease.
- Relapse is the return to drug use after an attempt to stop. Relapse indicates the need for more or different treatment.
- Most drugs affect the brain's reward circuit by flooding it with the chemical messenger dopamine. This overstimulation of the reward circuit causes the intensely pleasurable "high" that leads people to take a drug again and again.

- Over time, the brain adjusts to the excess dopamine, which reduces the high that the person feels compared to the high they felt when first taking the drug—an effect known as tolerance. They might take more of the drug, trying to achieve the same dopamine high.
- No single factor can predict whether a person will become addicted to drugs. A combination of genetic, environmental, and developmental factors influences risk for addiction. The more risk factors a person has, the greater the chance that taking drugs can lead to addiction.
- Drug addiction is treatable and can be successfully managed.

Source: National Institute on Drug Abuse; National Institutes of Health; U.S. Department of Health and Human Services.
https://www.drugabuse.gov/related-topics/treatment/what-to-do-if-you-have-problem-drugs-adults

There are also a number of less conventional approaches available, which may, or may not, be appropriate. It is suggested, therefore, that in addition to following the advice offered above, direct Internet research is undertaken. This is unlikely to be time or effort wasted.

Even if you are at the earliest stages of addiction, the sooner you take the first step to recovery the better. Waiting, and putting it off, is a decision in itself, and it is the wrong one. Help is available. Please step outside your current life narrative and seek it.

ASIDE: CHEMICAL SEX & PORN ADDICTION
A number of chemicals accentuate sexual appetite and drive, some to a huge degree. Given the substantial volume of internet posts which discuss never ending porn binges and mammoth sex sessions, this is hardly a secret. Indeed, certain chemicals are renowned for it.

However, putting sniggers and humour aside, this is fraught with issues, some of which are serious. The scenario itself is increasingly common.

One aspect is that linking sexual pleasure to the use of a drug will inevitably increase desire for that drug. The drug is thus likely to be consumed more regularly, leading to the obvious risks, including chemical addiction.

Less obvious is perhaps the effect upon the individual's sex life. Given the artificial enhancement of the sexual experience, sex (or porn) without the drug is unlikely to ever reach the same heights, or in some cases, anything like the same heights. This can cause a lack of interest, and thus relative impotency under normal conditions, with clear implications for relationships and general life. Lengthy porn binging can also lead to feelings of guilt, lower self-esteem, and frequently, anxiety and depression.

Again, this is an area in which, if in doubt, third party help and counselling should be urgently sought.

4.3.3 Alcoholism

I wrote the following two letters largely through frustration. However, perhaps they will help someone somewhere.

DEAR HABITUAL ALCOHOL USER
The stats don't lie and neither does the science. The nature of alcohol is not hidden and it is not a mystery. Indulge me for a moment.

What if you swapped the name *alcohol* for that of another similarly hard drug (see Section 4.2 for a list)? What if you used this drug in exactly the same manner in which you use alcohol?

How does this sound to you? *"I like a nice hit of heroin with my dinner. A bit of meth after work helps me to unwind. I'm just popping out to the pub for some crack cocaine with the boys."*

I suspect that you would never dream of binging on heroin at the weekend, or snorting meth after work, or socializing in the pub over some crack. Why not? Like alcohol, they all create euphoric pleasure, a high, and a come-down, which are all variable with dose. They all have broadly similar profiles in terms of harm and addiction.

What is the difference, therefore, other than that you have been conditioned and engineered by society, by the mainstream media, and by morally challenged politicians? There is no difference.

So why don't you treat all drugs in exactly the same way, and analyse them on their own merits? Why don't you measure disadvantages versus advantages, risk versus benefit, addiction potential, and so forth? Why don't you kick the cultural programming, use your intelligence to frame your own opinion, and take rational decisions based upon confirmed facts?

Alcohol numbs your mind. It dumbs you down, so that you are ready to be a productive unit on Monday morning, to the benefit of the status quo of the social order. It blinds you to bigger pictures and the wider perspectives. Indeed, one of those pictures pertains to alcohol itself and its real place in the drugscape.

Most of us have friends or family who are plagued by alcoholism. I certainly do. It is agonizing to watch the slow destruction of someone you love. If they read these words they couldn't argue with them, but they are likely to be far too afflicted to act upon them. You are probably not.

Think about the role that alcohol plays in your life, how a lifetime of habitual use will affect your mind, your body, and those around you, and consider if that picture is a positive one.

If it isn't, do something about it.

DEAR ALCOHOLIC

By now you don't need me, or anyone else, to tell you that alcohol is a hard drug. In your moments of clarity, you can see through the haze at what it has done to you, your life, and all those who care for you. You can see the trail of anguish and destruction, which is so painful that you drink again to escape the thoughts.

That drink makes it feel better doesn't it? The relief! It's fleeting. All too quickly, it feels worse again, as the brutal reality catches you. You repeat the cycle. It will always catch you.

You know where this is leading, but you can't face it. Nor can you evade the nagging feeling that you are not living a life at all. You are enduring a slow death.

You have tried to stop. You have tried really hard. You have gone cold turkey. You have even used support medication, like diazepam, which gave some relief, for a while, but not enough. Only alcohol really blunts the torment, the dread in the pit of your stomach, and the terrible unremitting pain.

The same story is familiar across users of other drugs too; other hard drugs. However, many people do beat them. People like you beat them. People like you beat alcohol.

I'm not a counsellor, and I'm not a professional, but I have seen souls shattered and lives lost. I can only offer my opinion, but it is one forged through pain and sorrow.

Try again to stop, but this time, take some truths with you on the journey.

When you stop, promise yourself that it will be for ever. You can't just switch from alcoholic to occasional social drinker. You have to make fundamental changes to your perspective.

You have to learn to see alcohol differently, and not as a source of pleasure.

For you, it is a source of misery. It is a brief euphoria which sinks agonizingly into that fearful abyss. This is what it is, and what it will always be. Any other perspective is an illusion. You know this already, so let it go. Let it go for good.

There is life without it. Time will help you to see that. But you must invest that time, little by little. You must give time a chance.

Your head will clear and you will slowly learn to find pleasure again in the little things. You will learn to see things differently, and somewhere downstream you will find joy again; you will find life again.

With your new perspective you will also stop envying those around you, who are drinking their drug, and see that they are also dulling their senses, damaging their bodies, blunting their minds. You will eventually be able to look into their cloudy world without the fog, and see beyond the initial lift of the intoxication, at the full picture. You won't want to go back.

To get there, you will need support. You are well aware that there are a variety of support groups, like *Alcoholics Anonymous*. Seek them out and approach them. Use them. Try to find people you can scream *help* to if you think you might crack. Build bridges with real people. Connect.

Whatever family or friends you have left, ask them for help too. Tell them that you are trying to get clean. Don't hide it, or you will continue to be placed in difficult positions. Be as open as you can be. Be honest.

See your GP or any medical practitioner you can possibly gain access to. If you have the opportunity to get into rehab, grab it with both hands. Accept professional help.

Don't ever use a setback or piece of bad luck as an excuse to revert. Your addiction will always look for excuses. There are none. Use this as a mantra: *I can do it... there are no excuses.... I am not drinking today.*

Set yourself targets: 1 day; 2 days; this weekend; a week; 2 weeks; to the start of the month; a month; 50 days; and so forth. Look forward to the next target and focus upon it. You can do it.

It's a long slow path, but you can really make it through the tunnel, if you want to. But you have to decide to do it, and to throw yourself 100% into it. You have to choose life.

Life! Right now your life is ebbing away in a drunken haze. You are losing it, day by day.

Yet there is so much more.

If you can just force yourself to reach out and go for it, you can and will find happiness again. Remember happiness? It's at the end of that tunnel, waiting for you.

Eventually the pain will stop, for you and all those who matter to you. It will: I absolutely 100% guarantee it.

So try again... choose life.... please.

ANOTHER ROUTE

Would a radical change of circumstance or an entirely different life help you? Would taking yourself away from all your existing issues, or throwing yourself into some sort of project, help? What about a radical or alternative approach to changing or widening your perspective? These are all methods of helping you to fundamentally change your outlook, and they do work for many people.

Try to think clearly about how to proceed from here. Take the first step.

4.3.4 Overdose & Emergency Response

The signs and symptoms of an overdose will vary according to the drug or drugs in question. However, the general rule is to err on the side of caution. In other words, if in doubt, don't delay: call for urgent medical help.

In considering the information below, note that an overdose will not produce all of the symptoms in the lists provided. A single symptom may be sufficient to indicate that immediate action is required.

DEPRESSANT OVERDOSE SYMPTOMS
CNS depressants include both benzodiazepines and opioids. Symptoms of overdose may include:

- shallow breathing
- snoring and/or gurgling (due to partly blocked airways)
- unconsciousness or difficult to awaken
- unresponsiveness to physical stimulation
- blue fingertips or lips
- drowsiness
- disorientation or impaired co-ordination

Note that in the case of opioids, nausea and vomiting may occur, and pinpoint pupils may also be present (especially if other drugs are not involved).

Overdose of depressants can lead to respiratory failure, coma, brain damage and death.

ACTION: Call the emergency services immediately and ask for an ambulance. Monitor the patient, stay calm, and keep airways clear.

ALCOHOL POISONING SYMPTOMS
As alcohol is a CNS depressant the list above is applicable. In addition, however, the following symptoms may occur:

- vomiting whilst asleep
- lost coordination
- seizures or spasms
- blue-tinged or pale skin
- low body temperature
- conscious but unresponsive (stupor)

Acute alcohol poising can lead to choking, respiratory failure, cardiac arrest, coma, brain damage and death.

ACTION: Call the emergency services immediately and ask for an ambulance. The following advice, which is offered via the NHS website, may help you to manage the situation until its arrival:

- try to keep the patient awake and sitting up
- provide water (assuming the patient is able to drink)
- keep the patient warm
- stay with the patient and remain calm
- if the patient is unconscious, put him/her in recovery position (on their side), keeping airways clear, and monitor breathing

The following is a commonly produced list of what you must not do. DO NOT:

- leave the patient to sleep it off
- make the patient vomit
- put the patient under a cold shower
- allow the patient to drink more alcohol
- give the patient coffee
- walk the patient around

Stay calm, and in so much as you are able, try to remain in control of the situation.

STIMULANT OVERDOSE SYMPTOMS

The symptoms of stimulant overdose may include:

- chest pains
- severe headache
- seizures or convulsions
- unconsciousness
- breathing difficulties
- rapid heart rate
- disorientation / confusion
- high temperature and overheating without sweating

Stimulant overdose can lead to heart attacks, seizures, strokes and psychosis.

ACTION: Call the emergency services. The following are commonly suggested to be applicable until arrival of professional assistance:

- monitor temperature and keep the patient cool enough to prevent overheating
- provide sufficient water to prevent dehydration
- stay calm and try to calm the patient

GENERAL OVERDOSE SYMPTOMS

For drugs not categorised as earlier, and in the absence of specific knowledge or expertise, the general principles apply. If in any doubt, call the emergency services. Until arrival of help, monitor the patient, exercise common sense, and remain calm.

CALLING FOR HELP

In all cases obtain as much information as you can to aid the emergency services. The following may be helpful to them, if known:

- the age, weight and height of the patient.
- the identity of the drug or drugs used
- how much was taken
- whether any prescription medicines are being used

Don't neglect the patient whilst obtaining this data, and do not delay the phone call, as these are both of primary importance.

Listen carefully to what the emergency service operator tells you. Ask for and take any advice offered regarding what to do whilst the ambulance arrives. This may include instruction to administer first aid or CPR.

If there is any of the overdosed drug left, keep it and hand it to the emergency services. Don't let fear of police prosecution prevent you from acting.

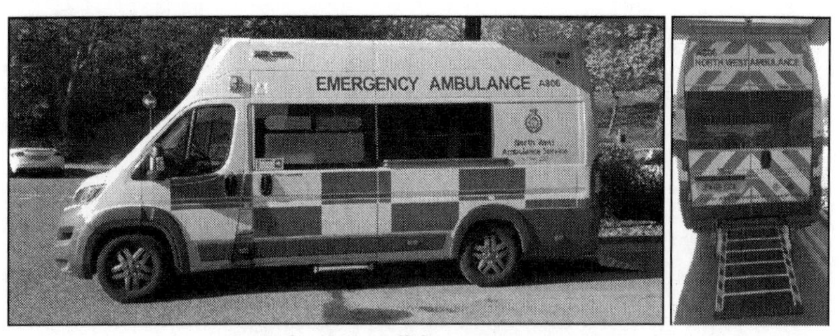

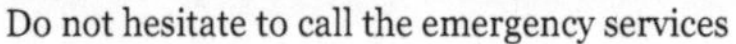
Do not hesitate to call the emergency services

Footnote: In the unlikely event that the practices outlined in the first part of this book (ref #9) have been followed, information relating to the drugs/drugs in question and emergency service contact details may be available courtesy of a note held by the patient.

4.3.5 Drug Related Deaths: Notable People

The dangers and risks associated with drug use affect everybody. This is a partial list of the deaths of notable people which involved drug overdose or intoxication. In truth, it barely scratches the surface.

Chet Baker (Musician)	1988	58	Cocaine, Heroin
Sid Barnes (Cricketer)	1973	57	Barbiturates, Bromide
Art Bell (Broadcaster/Author)	2018	72	Opioids, Benzodiazepines
Len Bias (Basketball Player)	1986	22	Cocaine
George Best (Footballer)	2005	59	Alcohol
Lenny Bruce (Comedian)	1966	40	Morphine
Richard Burton (Actor)	1984	58	Alcohol
Truman Capote (Writer)	1984	59	Alcohol, Others
Chris Farley (Actor/Comedian)	1997	33	Cocaine, Morphine
John Entwistle (Musician)	2002	57	Cocaine
Brian Epstein (Music)	1967	32	Carbitral (Barbiturate)
Sigmund Freud (Psychoanalyst)	1939	83	Morphine
Judy Garland (Actress/Singer)	1969	47	Secobarbital
Tony Hancock (Actor)	1968	44	Amphetamine, Alcohol
Jimi Hendrix (Musician)	1970	27	Barbiturates
Abbie Hoffman (Activist)	1989	52	Phenobarbital
Philip Seymour Hoffman (Actor)	2014	46	Heroin, Cocaine, Speed, Benzo
Whitney Houston (Musician)	2012	48	Cocaine, Xanax, Others
Howard Hughes (Business)	1976	70	Codeine
Michael Jackson (Musician)	2009	50	Lorazepam, Propofol
Janis Joplin (Musician)	1970	27	Heroin
Heath Ledger (Actor)	2008	28	Opioids, Benzodiazepines
Phil Lynott (Musician)	1986	36	Heroin
Marilyn Monroe (Actress)	1962	36	Barbiturates
Keith Moon (Musician)	1978	32	Prescription Drug
Jim Morrison (Musician)	1971	27	Heroin
Marco Pantani (Cyclist)	2004	34	Cocaine
Jackson Pollock (Artist)	1956	44	Alcohol
Lil Peep (Musician)	2017	21	Fentanyl, Xanax
Tom Petty (Musician)	2017	66	Fentanyl, Oxycodone, Others
River Phoenix (Actor)	1993	23	Cocaine, Morphine
Edgar Allan Poe (Poet)	1849	40	Laudanum
Elvis Presley (Musician)	1977	42	Multiple
Prince (Musician)	2016	57	Fentanyl
Dee Dee Ramone (Musician)	2002	50	Heroin
Anna Nicole Smith (Model)	2007	39	Prescription Drugs
D. M. Turner (Author)	1996	34	Ketamine
Ike Turner (Musician)	2007	76	Cocaine
Sid Vicious (Musician)	1979	21	Heroin
Kenneth Williams (Actor)	1988	62	Barbiturates
Amy Winehouse (Musician)	2011	27	Alcohol

4.4 THE LAWSCAPE

The last thing I needed whilst researching for this book was a knock on the door, and the police barging in to take me away for the crime of experimenting with my own mind. This is the last thing anyone needs.

That a third party dictates what I can and cannot put into my own body (which I own), and determines how I can and cannot explore my own consciousness (which I own), surely raises the must fundamental questions regarding human rights.

However, despite this principled position, it would be hugely irresponsible to ask for trouble by openly breaking the law, or at least, by not taking all necessary steps to reduce the prospect of such difficulty.

The following segments provide some basic information.

4.4.1 The United Kingdom

The main statutes regulating the availability, possession and supply of drugs in the UK are the *Misuse of Drugs Act*, the *Medicines Act*, and the *Psychoactive Substances Act*. The latter of these, commonly abbreviated to *PSA*, is by far the most invasive. Indeed, it completely usurped British legal tradition, which for centuries operated on the basis that citizens could do anything as long as it wasn't illegal. This was replaced by a statute (the PSA) which decreed that everything was illegal unless specifically exempted. The UK media cheered from the sidelines.

THE PSYCOACTIVE SUBSTANCES ACT 2016
This hugely intrusive law came into force on 26th May 2016. Quoting the government's own web site, it made it an offence to:

> *"produce, supply, offer to supply, possess with intent to supply, possess on custodial premises, import or export psychoactive substances; that is, any substance intended for human consumption that is capable of producing a psychoactive effect."*

This unprecedented overreach applies even to psychoactive substances that have not been invented or discovered yet.

Note that possession itself, unless *on custodial premises,* is not covered. This means that all substances previously legal to possess, including *legal highs*, remained legal to possess, unless intended for supply to a third party. Note also that, regarding procurement, it became an offence to import, embracing Internet purchases as well as more traditional routes.

It is worth re-emphasizing that the *PSA* did not replace or repeal previous legislation. Drugs which were specifically covered by the Misuse of Drugs Act, prior to 26th May 2016, remained illegal to both possess and supply.

THE MISUSE OF DRUGS ACT 1971
Of the other two statutes, the *Misuse of Drugs Act* is the most relevant and most frequently exercised.

Quoting homeoffice.gov.uk, offences defined by this include:

> *"possession of a controlled drug unlawfully, possession of a controlled drug with intent to supply it, supplying or offering to supply a controlled drug (even where no charge is made for the drug) and allowing premises you occupy or manage to be used unlawfully for the purpose of producing or supplying controlled drugs".*

The number of drugs *controlled* (those made illegal) under this legislation has grown significantly year on year. They are individually categorized under three distinct *classes*, A, B and C, each of which carries a different range of sanctions.

DRUG CLASS	POSSESSION	SUPPLY
Class A	Up to 7 years + fine	Up to life + fine
Class B	Up to 5 years + fine	Up to 14 years + fine
Class C	Up to 2 years + fine	Up to 14 years + fine

Regarding which drug has been placed into which class, the specifics are listed on the following pages of the *legislation.gov.uk* website:

Class A Drugs:
www.legislation.gov.uk/ukpga/1971/38/schedule/2/part/I

Class B Drugs:
www.legislation.gov.uk/ukpga/1971/38/schedule/2/part/II

Class C Drugs:
www.legislation.gov.uk/ukpga/1971/38/schedule/2/part/III

An alphabetically based list, drug by drug, is provided on the following web page:

www.gov.uk/government/publications/controlled-drugs-list--2/list-of-most-commonly-encountered-drugs-currently-controlled-under-the-misuse-of-drugs-legislation

Note that the disclaimers quoted below apply to all these lists (and to others cited elsewhere on the same websites):

> "*The following is a list of the most commonly encountered drugs currently controlled under the misuse of drugs legislation*".

> "*Although it is extensive, the list is not exhaustive and, in the event of a substance not being listed below, reference should also be made to the published Act and Regulations at legislation.gov.uk*".

THE POTENTIAL CONSEQUENCES
If you are contemplating the use of illegal drugs, in other words, if you are thinking of breaking the law, your calculation should include consideration of the potential sentence, should you be arrested, charged and convicted.

Clearly, this will vary, as it is at least partly dependent upon your individual circumstances, and the attitude and disposition of the particular judge or magistrate(s). However, in England and Wales the Sentencing Council issues guidelines for the sentencing of offenders aged 18 and older.

Further to this, the Coroners and Justice Act states that:

> *"Every court –*
> > *(a) must, in sentencing an offender, follow any sentencing guideline which is relevant to the offender's case, and*
> > *(b) must, in exercising any other function relating to the sentencing of offenders, follow any sentencing guidelines which are relevant to the exercise of the function,*
>
> *unless the court is satisfied that it would be contrary to the interests of justice to do so."*

Whilst these are *guidelines*, they do provide broad parameters which can give an indication of the likely consequences of your own course of action, should this scenario unfold.

They cover factors such as aggravating and mitigating circumstances, category of harm (e.g. quantity of the drug in question), and the nature of your specific role.

As this is a publication, it is subject to change. The current version can be downloaded or viewed in its entirety from the following web page:

> *www.sentencingcouncil.org.uk/publications/item/drug-offences-definitive-guideline/*

It is strongly recommended that you read this document carefully, prior to subjecting yourself to the possibility of its provisions.

IF THE WORST HAPPENS
If you fall foul of the law in any way, the following basic information may be of use. Note, however, that this does not constitute legal advice, which should be sought from a qualified practitioner.

> THE POLICE
> If you are stopped on the street by a plain clothed officer, you should insist on seeing his or her warrant card. If the reason has not been volunteered, you should ask why you have been stopped.

If you are searched, you should ask for a record of the search. Do not resist, even if the search is unlawful (address this later). Stay as calm as possible throughout.

If the police come to your home, again stay calm, and ask how you can help. If they wish to search your premises, note that they can do so, without a warrant, if they arrest you, or in any of a pre-defined set of circumstances. The latter are described by *Citizens Advice* as follows:

> *Situations in which the police can enter premises without a warrant include when they want to:*
> - *deal with a breach of the peace or prevent it*
> - *enforce an arrest warrant*
> - *arrest a person in connection with certain offences*
> - *recapture someone who has escaped from custody*

IF YOU ARE ARRESTED
You have heard it a thousand times on television, but here is the caution which should accompany any arrest relating to drugs:

> "*You do not have to say anything. But it may harm your defence if you do not mention when questioned something which you later rely on in court. Anything you do say may be given in evidence.*"

This more or less means what it states. If the first time you mention your defence is actually in court, the magistrate or judge may well consider that you have invented the defence in the interim (and the judge may advise the jury accordingly).

At the same time, however, it does not mean that you are compelled to say anything which may incriminate yourself. You are not. Indeed, the sensible course is to consult a solicitor in private prior to discussing the case with the police.

In the early stages it can be of the utmost importance that you think very carefully before you speak, even if you are frightened or under the influence of alcohol or drugs. Try not to panic, and try to establish, and mentally note, whatever information you can (e.g. the specific reason you have been arrested).

Importantly, you should exercise your right to see a solicitor. This is free of charge. Your solicitor should be present when you are questioned or interviewed. Again, this is something you should insist on.

You also have the right to have a person of your choice notified of your arrest. Note that this is not the same as having the right to make a phone call yourself (as in the United States and depicted in countless American movies).

If you are alone in a cell try to stay as calm as possible. You have not been forgotten and cannot be held indefinitely. Note that you do have the right to speak to the custody officer, who is responsible for your welfare.

FROM THE GOVERNMENT
The following is taken directly from Gov.uk, and describes your rights if you are taken into police custody:

The custody officer at the police station must explain your rights. You have the right to:

- *get free legal advice*
- *tell someone where you are*
- *have medical help if you're feeling ill*
- *see the rules the police must follow ('Codes of Practice')*
- *see a written notice telling you about your rights, eg regular breaks for food and to use the toilet (you can ask for a notice in your language) or an interpreter to explain the notice*
- *You'll be searched and your possessions will be kept by the police custody officer while you're in the cell.*

FURTHER INFORMATION
Release offers free non-judgmental specialist advice and information on issues related to drug use and to drug laws.

You can contact them directly via the following dedicated help line: 0845 4500 215

This is available from 11am to 1pm, and from 2pm to 4pm, Monday to Friday. Other methods of contact are:

Email: ask@release.org.uk

Address: 124-128 City Road, London, EC1V 2NJ

Tel: 020 7324 2989
Fax: 020 7324 2977

The Release website: www.release.org.uk

Bust card: www.release.org.uk/publications/bust-card

Finally, *Citizens Advice* provides general information with respect to the police on the following web page:

www.citizensadvice.org.uk/law-and-rights/legal-system/police/police-powers/

4.4.2 The United States

At a federal level, the primary drug-relevant statute is the *Controlled Substances Act* (CSA). This defines five *Schedules* (classifications), with various specifications regarding which drug is included in each. This is largely overseen by the *Drug Enforcement Administration* (DEA) and the *Food and Drug Administration* (FDA).

The DEA presents these schedules as follows (current as of 2017):

> SCHEDULE I
> Schedule I drugs, substances, or chemicals are defined as drugs with no currently accepted medical use and a high potential for abuse. Some examples of Schedule I drugs are:
>
> > Heroin, lysergic acid diethylamide (LSD), marijuana (cannabis), 3,4-methylenedioxymethamphetamine (ecstasy), methaqualone, and peyote
>
> SCHEDULE II
> Schedule II drugs, substances, or chemicals are defined as drugs with a high potential for abuse, with use potentially leading to severe psychological or physical dependence. These drugs are also considered dangerous. Some examples of Schedule II drugs are:
>
> > Combination products with less than 15 milligrams of hydrocodone per dosage unit (Vicodin), cocaine, methamphetamine, methadone, hydromorphone (Dilaudid), meperidine (Demerol), oxycodone (OxyContin), fentanyl, Dexedrine, Adderall, and Ritalin
>
> SCHEDULE III
> Schedule III drugs, substances, or chemicals are defined as drugs with a moderate to low potential for physical and psychological dependence. Schedule III drugs abuse potential is less than Schedule I and Schedule II drugs but more than Schedule IV. Some examples of Schedule III drugs are:
>
> > Products containing less than 90 milligrams of codeine per dosage unit (Tylenol with codeine), ketamine, anabolic steroids, testosterone
>
> SCHEDULE IV
> Schedule IV drugs, substances, or chemicals are defined as drugs with a low potential for abuse and low risk of dependence. Some examples of Schedule IV drugs are:
>
> > Xanax, Soma, Darvon, Darvocet, Valium, Ativan, Talwin, Ambien, Tramadol

SCHEDULE V
Schedule V drugs, substances, or chemicals are defined as drugs with lower potential for abuse than Schedule IV and consist of preparations containing limited quantities of certain narcotics. Schedule V drugs are generally used for antidiarrheal, antitussive, and analgesic purposes. Some examples of Schedule V drugs are:

> Cough preparations with less than 200 milligrams of codeine or per 100 milliliters (Robitussin AC), Lomotil, Motofen, Lyrica, Parepectolin

www.dea.gov/druginfo/ds.shtml

Clearly, on the basis of relative harm these classifications are in themselves ridiculous, but they form the framework for a punitive system which is widely considered to be vindictive and draconian.

As ludicrous as this may appear to most Europeans, US law even creates a penal regime for the possession and distribution of items such as bongs, pipes and rolling papers, which are collectively referred to as *paraphernalia*.

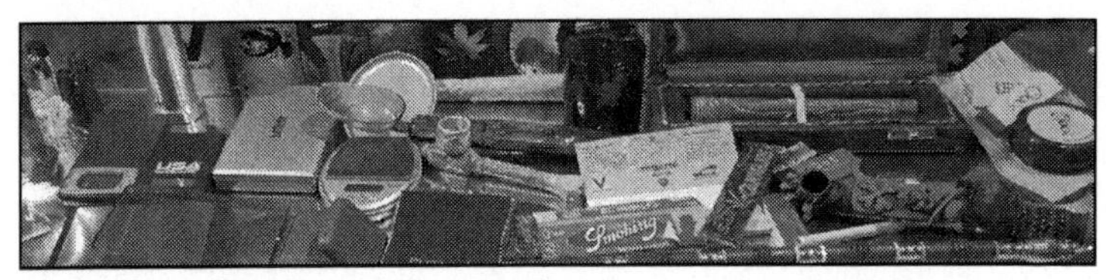

Even the most basic of items are defined as drug paraphernalia

Layered on top of all this is another disturbing aspect known as *mandatory minimum sentencing*. Mandatory minimum sentencing laws dictate minimum sentences for certain offences, which are imposed regardless of individual or extenuating circumstances. Many of these offences carry prison terms of years, and sometimes, decades.

The picture in the United States is further complicated by the partial judicial autonomy of the individual states. This creates enormous geographic variation in terms of sentencing. *Findlaw.Com* cites the following example to demonstrate this tendency:

> *"For example, Kentucky, which has adopted similar mandatory minimum sentencing guidelines, has some of the toughest provisions. For simple possession, first offenders get 2 to 10 years in prison and a fine of up to $20,000. In contrast, California has some of the lightest drug possession sentences: between $30 and $500 in fines and/or 15 to 180 days in jail"*

In theory, where state and federal laws disagree the *supremacy clause* applies (which is part of Article VI of the Constitution) and federal law is supposed to prevail. This currently creates a somewhat discretionary standoff in terms of a number of drug related situations, not least with respect to cannabis legalisation. It remains to be seen how this will eventually unfold.

MASS INCARCERATION
Unfortunately, most US citizens continue to be subject to a judicial regime which is firmly embedded within the demonstrable excesses and cruelty of a culture perpetrated by the *war on drugs*. Mass incarceration and patently excessive sentencing of non-violent drug offenders continues unabated.

On this occasion, statistics do not lie. For example, with just 5% of the world's population, the United States accounts for approximately 25% of the global prison population.

The numbers themselves are equally stark. In 2014 there were more than 1.5 million drugs arrests, of which more than 80% were for possession only. Headline statements like these are just the tip of a very insidious and inhumane iceberg.

It therefore almost goes without saying that if you are a US resident you should take all sensible measures to reduce the prospects of becoming a victim of this madness.

IF THE WORST HAPPENS
If you do fall foul of the law, and are confronted by the police or arrested, the following guidance is commonly cited on the Internet, and may be of use. Note, however, that this does not constitute legal advice, which should be sought independently.

1. First and foremost, try to relax and stay calm. Give yourself the best opportunity to think clearly by avoiding panic or excessive stress.

The following statement will typically be issued on arrest:

> *"You have the right to remain silent. Anything you say can and will be used against you in a court of law. You have the right to an attorney. If you cannot afford an attorney, one will be provided for you. Do you understand the rights I have just read to you? With these rights in mind, do you wish to speak to me?"*

2. Know your rights. These include:

- The 5th Amendment right to remain silent. Note that it is almost always in your best interests to do so, particularly as anything you say may be subsequently used against you. A common method of dealing with this is to request a lawyer in response to every question. Do exercise this right.
- You have the right to have a lawyer present while you are questioned. One will be appointed for you if you cannot afford one.

Note that if you are not informed of these facts your lawyer can ask that any statements you made are not used in court (this is known as your Miranda right).

3. Call a lawyer as soon as you are able. If you don't have or know one, call family or a friend and ask them to find one for you as soon as possible. Bear in mind that your call could be eavesdropped, so be careful what you say.

If you cannot find a lawyer and have to wait for one to be appointed, either prior to a court appearance or by a judge, do not forget your right to remain silent in the interim.

Discussion between you and your lawyer is confidential. When you have consulted your lawyer, consider the advice and information given, and try to make the most rational and sensible decisions on how to proceed.

4. Respectfully deny consent to a search of your home, as per the Fourth Amendment. A search is only lawful if you have consented, or the police officer has a warrant, or has a valid reason (reasonable suspicion / probable cause, which usually but not always relates to a vehicle search).

Having stated this, the police do have the right to:

- Search your belongings, body and clothing (which again requires reasonable suspicion)

- Search your vehicle if you are in it (subject to probable cause, based upon what the police officer sees through the window, your conduct and/or answers to questions)

- Fingerprint you

- Ask you to undertake a test (such as walking in a straight line), or ask for a sample of your breath, blood, etc.

5. If the police have abused you or have committed any infraction, seek to collect names and addresses of any witnesses when you are able, and gather any other information that may assist.

Do not react or respond to misconduct, or provoke retaliation. It is far better to address these matters subsequently, via a lawsuit.

Finally, police confrontation or arrest can occur at any time, so it is advised that you learn as much as possible in terms of your rights and the legal issues relevant to your location and your situation. Ideally, also identify a legal firm or multiple legal firms to use should you need them.

This isn't the most exciting pursuit in the world, but it may be one of the most important, should the worst happen.

WHEN A PICTURE PAINTS A THOUSAND WORDS
The impact of the *war on drugs* on incarceration in the United States:

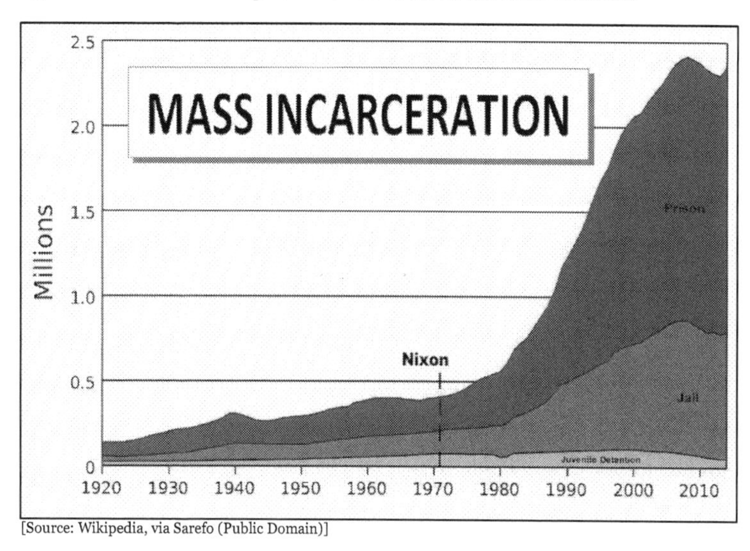

[Source: Wikipedia, via Sarefo (Public Domain)]

The effects of mass incarceration and the *war on drugs* on public health:

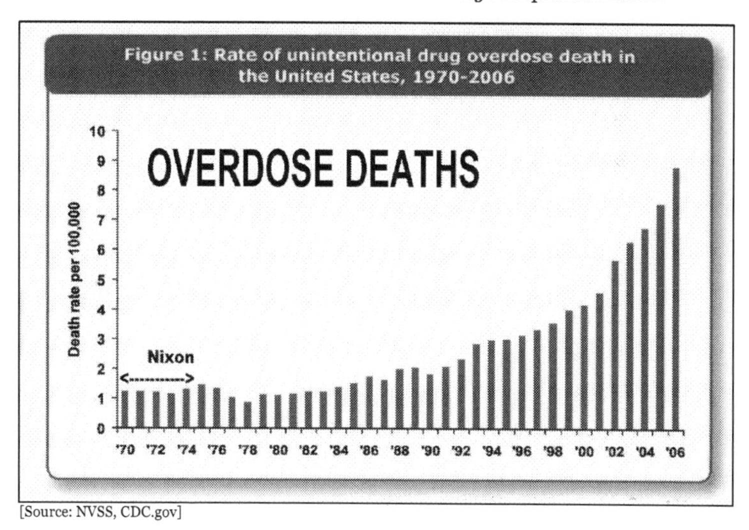

[Source: NVSS, CDC.gov]

The wholesale destruction of lives and families could hardly be clearer.

LEST WE FORGET
Those incarcerated are real people, having had their real lives destroyed by manifestly unjust laws and a morally bankrupt pursuit. To illustrate the human cost of this unremitting and ongoing tragedy, this segment puts some names to the stats.

When I began to consider this issue, two relatively high profile victims immediately sprung to my mind:

William Leonard Pickard (Two Life Sentence Without Parole)
Ross Ulbricht (Double Life Sentence Plus Forty Years)

I recall being absolutely appalled when I first read about these two cases.

More recently, whilst searching the Internet for more I quickly found the following cannabis related victims, courtesy of *Rolling Stone* magazine:

Fate Vincent Winslow (Life Without Parole)
Michael Alonzo Thompson (40 to 60 Years)
Crystal Munoz (18 Years)
Andy Cox (Life Without Parole)

Then I encountered *CAN-DO,* a non-profit foundation that advocates **C**lemency for **A**ll **N**on-violent **D**rug **O**ffenders (www.CanDoClemency.com). This group educates, campaigns and supports, and literally does put names to faces. I picked a few more from this website, at random.

John Bolen (Life Without Parole)
Evelyn Bozon Pappa (Life Without Parole)
Charles "Duke" Tanner (30 Years)
Eva Palma Atencio (Life Without Parole)
Michael Bryant (Life)
John Knock (Life Without Parole)

There are just so many.

Think of these people next week, next month, next year: whatever you are doing, these victims and their families will still be suffering. More will have joined them.

If you are able, it may help to write, so that they know that someone is at least thinking about them. If you can find time, join others and campaign to change laws and to free the broken and incarcerated, wherever they may be.

A reminder of the enormous scale of this cruelty (from DrugPolicy.org):

"Amount spent annually in the U.S. on the war on drugs: $58+ billion
Number of arrests in 2017 in the U.S. for drug law violations: 1,632,921
Number of drug arrests that were for possession only: 1,394,514 (85.4 percent)"

4.4.3 The Rest Of The World

Wherever you live, whatever the location, if you engage with drugs, in any capacity, it is essential that you undertake at least some elementary research, along the lines documented earlier for the United Kingdom and the United States.

It is in your own interests to:

- Know your local laws
- Know your rights

These vary considerably from nation to nation, as the *war on drugs* is interpreted and applied to differing extremes, and accordingly, human rights are abused to varying degrees. In many cases, the law represents a greater threat to your well being, and that of your family, than the drug itself.

This issue should never be dismissed as something that will never happen to you. It can happen to anyone; even to the innocent.

TOURISM & TRAVELLING
If you travel, and intend to engage en route or at a foreign destination, you need to be just as aware of the local situation as residents. In some locations you should be even more aware, as racism and prejudice may also play a detrimental role.

Unless you are fully informed of local laws, customs and practices, you may well be taking serious risks of which you are unaware. Do the research well in advance, and base your decisions upon sound factual information.

If you are unable to do this, or if in any doubt, it is strongly suggested that you refrain.

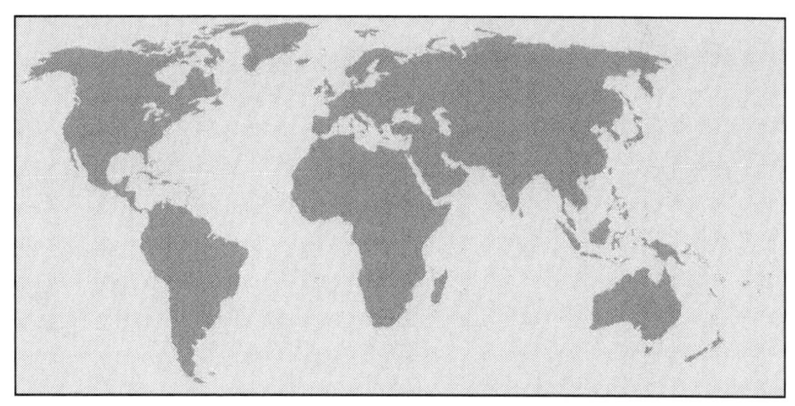

Wherever you sample or possess a psychoactive drug,
know the local law and know your rights

ON MY TRAVELS
These are two of the most notorious prisons in South East Asia. I visited inmates in them some years ago, whilst pursuing various humanitarian projects.

THE BANGKOK HILTON, THAILAND
I took this photograph in the remand section of Klongprem Central Prison. Behind the glass are the prisoner visitation rooms.

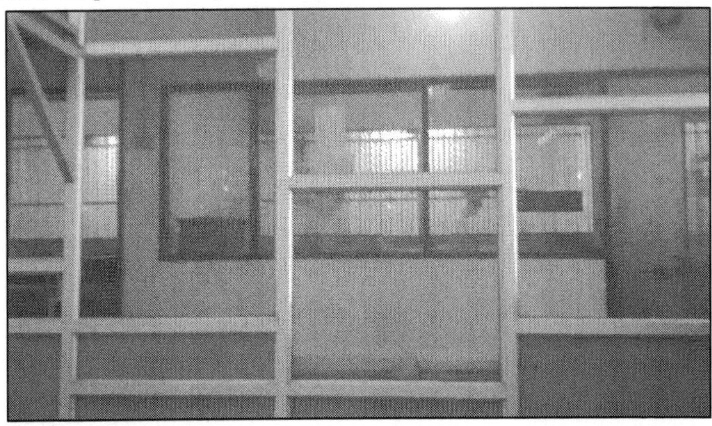

HOTEL K, INDONESIA
The visitor area in Kerobokan Prison in Bali was an open-air space, largely exposed to the blazing sun, with seating being the ground itself. I was unable to take an interior shot due to confiscation of phones and cameras on entry.

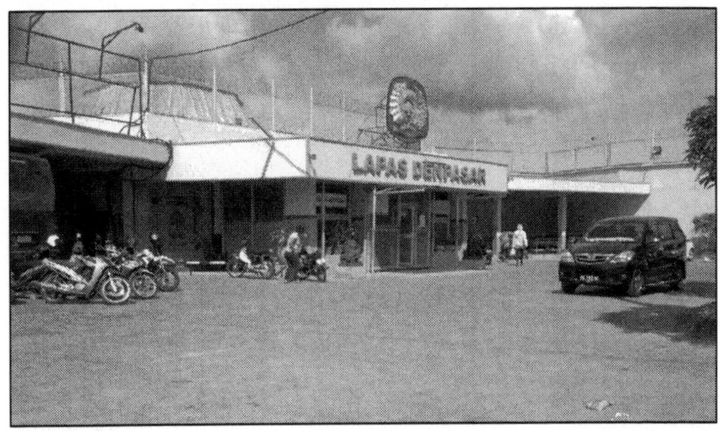

How many non-violent drug *offenders* are incarcerated in these and countless places like them? Take special care not to become one on your own travels.

Unfortunately, it gets even worse:

> EMPLOYMENT OPPORTUNITIES FOR KILLERS, SRI LANKA
> In January 2019, President Sirisena of Sri Lanka cited President Duterte's murderous campaign in the Philippines (official death toll at time of writing over 5,000), as "*an example to the world.*" A month later he informed the Sri Lankan parliament of his intention to authorise hanging for drug offenders.
>
> A practical issue with respect to this was the need to find willing employees to perform the gruesome task itself. Incredibly, these positions were duly advertised in the Sri Lankan media. I took the following photograph outside the *Daily News* building in Kandy, February 2019.

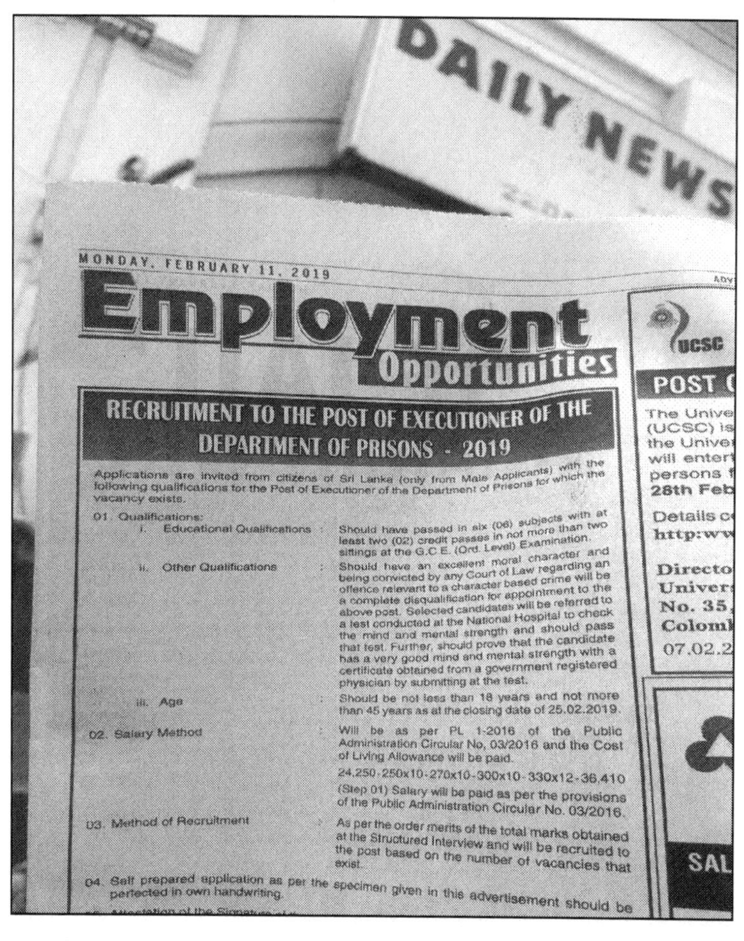

DAILY NEWS

MONDAY, FEBRUARY 11, 2019

Employment Opportunities

RECRUITMENT TO THE POST OF EXECUTIONER OF THE DEPARTMENT OF PRISONS - 2019

Applications are invited from citizens of Sri Lanka (only from Male Applicants) with the following qualifications for the Post of Executioner of the Department of Prisons for which the vacancy exists.

01. Qualifications:
    - i. Educational Qualifications : Should have passed in six (06) subjects with at least two (02) credit passes in not more than two sittings at the G.C.E. (Ord. Level) Examination.
    - ii. Other Qualifications : Should have an excellent moral character and being convicted by any Court of Law regarding an offence relevant to a character based crime will be a complete disqualification for appointment to the above post. Selected candidates will be referred to a test conducted at the National Hospital to check the mind and mental strength and should pass that test. Further, should prove that the candidate has a very good mind and mental strength with a certificate obtained from a government registered physician by submitting at the test.
    - iii. Age : Should be not less than 18 years and not more than 45 years as at the closing date of 25.02.2019.
02. Salary Method : Will be as per PL 1-2016 of the Public Administration Circular No, 03/2016 and the Cost of Living Allowance will be paid.
    24,250-250x10-270x10-300x10-330x12-36,410
    (Step 01) Salary will be paid as per the provisions of the Public Administration Circular No. 03/2016.
03. Method of Recruitment : As per the order merits of the total marks obtained at the Structured Interview and will be recruited to the post based on the number of vacancies that exist.
04. Self prepared application as per the specimen given in this advertisement should be perfected in own handwriting.

4.4.4 Dealers: A Different Perspective

Six degrees of separation embraces the proposition that everyone is connected to everyone else on earth in six or fewer steps, via a chain of '*a friend of a friend*'. Here is a genuine question: how many steps are you away from someone who sells drugs?

Whoever you are, I believe that it is probably one or two, and an absolute maximum of three.

In stating this I am not referring to online purchases or the *dark net markets*, which provide drugs to many. I refer to typical face to face transactions.

If you read the earlier section detailing how many people use drugs, the sheer number, 250 million, provides a clue as to how many drug sellers there must be in the world.

The obvious implication is that the vast majority are regular members of the public, who pass small quantities to their friends: a few pills, some weed, a gram of cocaine, etc. They tend to be fairly ordinary people in the main, who simply use and share social and psychoactive materials with those they are close to or have a relationship with. Indeed, as suggested above, you will almost certainly have friends who either sell or share themselves, or who know someone who does.

As far as I am aware, I don't actually know a drug seller personally, which probably under-qualifies me to write this section. However, I am pretty sure that I know a few people who do know a drug seller. Remarkably, they are neither violent thugs nor gangsters. This will also apply to the sellers they know.

The fundamental truth of the situation is that most drug vendors will form a cross section of the population. There will be good people, bad people, and everything in between.

THE SCUM OF THE EARTH
The media perspective, however, as pushed relentlessly on to the public, is that anyone selling a drug is the scum of the earth (unless it is a state-sanctioned drug such as alcohol and tobacco), and that they are even lower than you are as a drug user. This propagandistic and truth distorting construct of blame serves a variety of the usual interests, but as misrepresentations usually do, it comes at a high cost.

When labels such as *drug pusher* and *drug smuggler* are routinely attached to the suffering of addicts, for example, they take a life of their own, and become terms of abuse and gross stigmatisation.

People feed upon them, and tend to create pictures of those accused of vending or transporting which bear little resemblance to reality. Rationality and logic invariably cease to apply.

With respect to this, two international drug cases spring to mind, both of which pertain to Australia. They demonstrate what can happen when society allows propaganda and generic character assassination to consume reality and truth.

EXAMPLE 1 – SCHAPELLE CORBY
Schapelle Corby was convicted of smuggling 4.2kg of cannabis into Indonesia in 2005. She subsequently languished in a third world prison for almost 10 years, despite evidence which conclusively proved her innocence having been published on the Internet years before she was finally released on parole.

This was a politically charged high profile case, shaped by self-interest expediency relating to the hugely contentious privatisation of Sydney airport to political donors Macquarie Bank, and to the long term involvement of the Australian Federal Police (AFP) in criminal and political activities. The spectre of foreign policy appeasement also played a role, as fact based reporting was replaced by tabloid trivia, gross misrepresentation and outright fiction.

Off-the-record ministerial briefings set the ball rolling, and the juggernaut of gutter journalism did the rest, renaming her "*convicted drug smuggler Schapelle Corby*" via every reference. Schapelle Corby was ruthlessly smeared and openly vilified at every turn, and she still is, as I write this page. Contextually, the usual script with respect to drug cases was followed to the letter, regardless of how many lies had to be peddled, or how much suffering she and her family had to endure.

THE TRUTH @ WWW.
EXPENDABLE.tv
SHE IS INNOCENT!!
SCHAPELLE CORBY
Support an Aussie
www.expendable.tv
VOTE 1
SCHAPELLE
INNOCENT

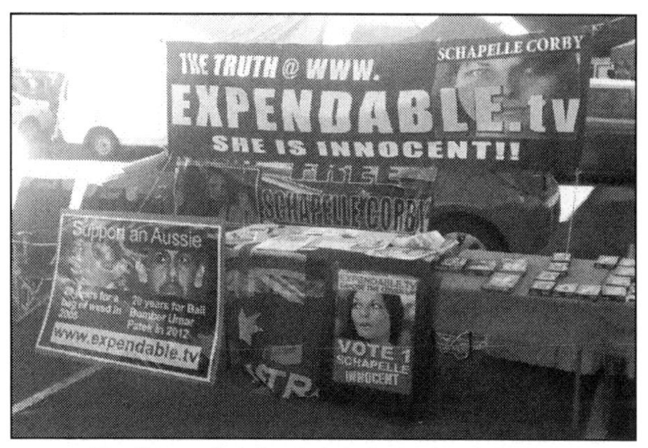

Not all Australians bought into the deceit and slander

Once the picture had been painted, the facts of her case became irrelevant. The flagrant abuses in Indonesia were long forgotten, and stereotypical characters replaced the real flesh and blood left behind. Presenting newly acquired evidence became impossible, as independent researchers were simply derided as conspiracy theorists, and subsequently ignored. The die had been cast and her status as a human being had been revoked.

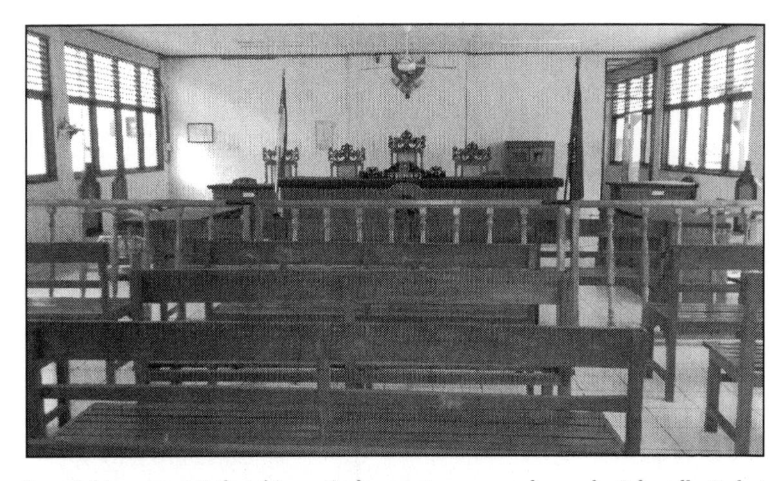

I was told on my visit that this particular courtroom was chosen for Schapelle Corby's trial so that the windows along the sides could be rented (for suitable bribes) to Australian media crews. Her civil, legal and human rights were in fact breached throughout the entire process (with material evidence of her innocence also being withheld by Australian government ministers).

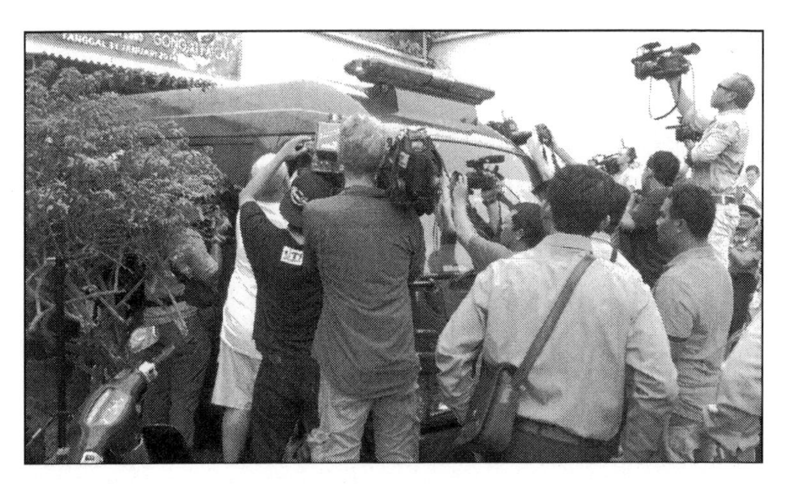

Having produced countless lies and smears about her over the years, the Australian media were there to further torment her on her release, again putting her safety at risk. Subsequent to this she was forced to stay in Indonesia on parole for three further years, and gagged under threat of re-imprisonment should she tell her story. During this period, she was stalked and harassed at every turn by the same media, whilst the fiction and fabrications continued unabated.

EXAMPLE 2 – ANDREW CHAN & MYURAN SUKUMARAN

The second case relates to Andrew Chan and Myuran Sukumaran, who, again in Indonesia, were convicted of smuggling heroin in 2006. The two Australian citizens, who admitted their guilt, were sentenced to death, and were eventually executed under the most barbaric of circumstances on 29th April 2015.

Whilst in prison, the two men had totally reformed, had re-invented themselves, and via a range of programs, had helped to transform the lives of countless other prisoners. The governor of Kerobokan Prison described them as model prisoners, as their work had become widely known, and they had touched so many lives.

Despite this, they were brutally murdered to make a political point. They were tied to a post and shot dead, whilst singing *Amazing Grace* to give strength to others who were slaughtered alongside them.

Another feature of this case was that the Australian Federal Police (yes, again) had wilfully tipped off the Indonesians, with full knowledge of the likely consequences. They could very easily have made the arrests as the men returned to Australia, but instead, acted as judge, jurors, and executioners, and have never been called to account for this.

During the controversy surrounding the executions, members of the public campaigned to save their lives, with thousands of posts and messages appearing across social media. The following, posted by a former WA heroin dealer, presents the position of vendors in terms which are almost entirely absent from mainstream coverage:

> *Anon*
> February 14
> I feel compelled to write my opinion on heroin and people that use it, this opinion is based on 45yrs in the drug scene culture. I admit to being a high school dropout so excuse the grammar I've been tossing around in my mind whether to bother as it is a huge task for me, as I type slowly with one finger. I don't know if it will be read but I thought if I don't make the effort to try and gather more support for Andrew and Myuran from the Bali 9 as it would haunt me for the rest of my life. So hear goes. Yesterday I was on another site debating the boys plight, I posted a comment on my thoughts after reading a post I didn't agree with as it was saying they should be shot, the guy came back with a reply, "I know where your coming from", but that he was an ex junkie and he had suffered so much. For a few seconds I thought okay, then a crack started to appear in my mind, and as more comments came up agreeing with him, he got bolder, spewing up more of his boo hoo poor me stuff, then joined by more agreement with him. Then another guy says yeah all drug dealers and paedophiles should be shot. Now this really pissed me off, to compare a drug dealer who actually doesn't force anyone to do anything, and the thing that does, its an insult to the child victim of the assault.
> So in the heroin world you have recreational users, you have junkies and then you have snivelling junkie, they are all complicit. They enter an agreement with the dealer, I want it, you get it for me and I'll pay you big money, now everyone knows this is a criminal agreement. Human nature being what it is, very greedy, there's always

someone willing to fill the need of the user to various degrees (and its like who came first the user or the dealer, the chicken or the egg). So in the criminal world there's supposed to be a code of conduct "death before dishonour", honour among thieves". If you break this code there's names for you like rat, scum, give up, dog.
So now we have the snivelling junkie, who is solely responsible for the demonization of heroin, who entered the agreement with the dealer, now wanting out. The reason could be he may have grown up, had enough of the lifestyle, got caught, whatever,now turning on his accomplice in the agreement made. He hasn't gone to the police, but worse he's running around telling anyone that will listen his poor me stories. He's a sniveller through and through, always someone else's fault, can't take responsibility for his own actions. He goes to court, the snivelling junkie will blame the drugs for whatever he's done, knowing he'll get a lighter sentence, you even have instances of snivelling junkies who have never used heroin saying they have to get the lower sentence.
So all this bullshit has demonized heroin more than it should be in the public eye, and in the eyes of family and supporters of the snivelling junkie, and its the dealer that suffers the consequence of these lies. This is what's happened to Andrew and Myuran, sure they were stupid and naive to do what they did, but there's no way they are ringleaders, they're only one link in the chain of dealers (probably the lowest) which can include lawyers, doctor's, police, and every other walk of life, it's human greed, it's everywhere. But if you think they deserve to die you have to include every other link in the chain, and I'm sure that most people would have family and friends in the chain.
Let's have a closer look at heroin, it was in most cough mixtures up till the fifties. We know it's made from opium, which has been around for hundreds of years, war's have been waged over it, people from all over the world have wanted it for there own various reasons. It's used by the thousands of kilo's in the medical field, as well as its synthetic derivative pethidine as a painkiller.
There's a public belief that one hit of heroin and your hooked, this is not true, you would have to use it dozens of times continuously. I also believe with a big number of overdoses the user has a death wish, sad but true, other wise there would be millions more. People use heroin for various lengths of time and stop, when users are jailed most have no choice but to stop (no methadone), they go through a few day's of discomfort. There are millions of people world wide using heroin with no problems (except to the hip pocket), maybe family members, friends, workmates, from all walks of life, and unless they tell you or they get caught you wouldn't know.
I would have thought all the users out there would be using this opportunity to express your desire for heroin to be freely available. If this was so it would stop users that have to commit crimes or sell there bodies to fund their use, it could be smoked, or swallowed, which would result in zero overdoses, its mostly only injected because of the price.
So what I'm saying is if your one of the people baying for these boy's blood, I'm hoping what I've written might soften your heart, and we can bring these boy's and the rest of the Australians rotting in some Asian prison home alive, where they belong. They've done the time they would have received in Australia. Don't be swayed by the snivelling junkie, who if they had any decency in them should be shouting the loudest to bring them home, your the ones that created the temptation, now's the time to redeem yourselves.
I'll leave it there for now, and apologize to anyone who has lost a loved one , if I have seemed insensitive, I haven't wanted to, I just want these boy's home alive, I'm still grieving Barlow and Chambers, and Tuong Van Nguyen. I hope I have achieved a change of heart in someone, if you think what I have written could help these boy's please share.
Thank you for listening.

[Permission for inclusion was granted by the poster]

When the crunch came, and the preparations for the executions commenced, Australian Prime Minster, Tony Abbott, opened with "*What I'm not going to do, though, is jeopardise the relationship with Indonesia.*" The green light could not have been more obvious. Indeed, on 16th January 2015, the ABC cited the Indonesian Attorney-General: "*Mr Prasetyo said the Australian Government had not pressured Indonesia to grant clemency*"

From the very start the media position was patently clear, with Rupert Murdoch's stable predictably setting the tone in February 2006:

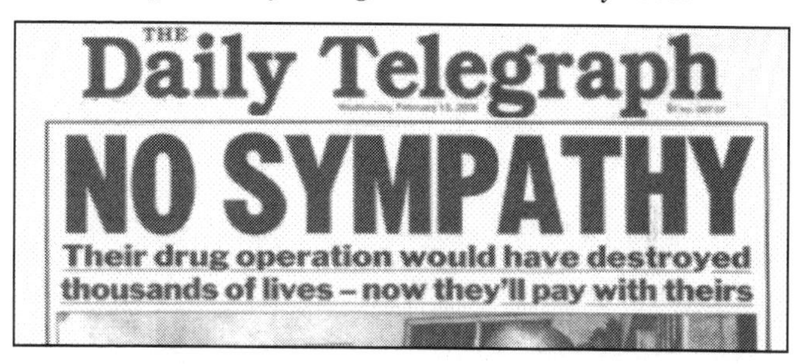

THE Daily Telegraph

NO SYMPATHY

Their drug operation would have destroyed thousands of lives – now they'll pay with theirs

In the run up to the executions, similar sentiments were all too common. Indeed, the state's own broadcaster, the ABC, commissioned a text poll in which 52% of the respondents supported the deaths of the two men. This was quickly picked up by the Indonesian government and used as *justification*.

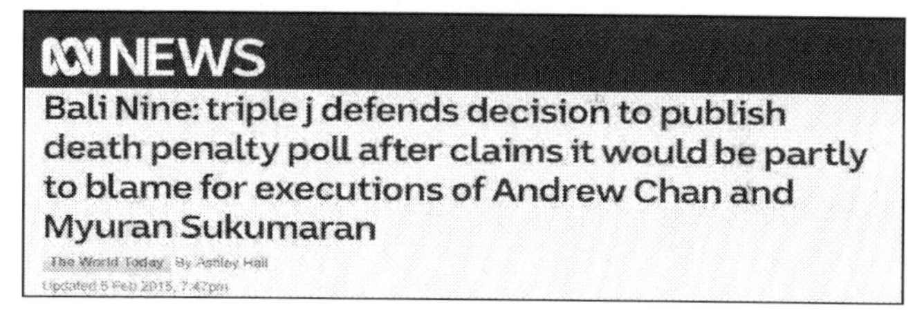

ABC NEWS

Bali Nine: triple j defends decision to publish death penalty poll after claims it would be partly to blame for executions of Andrew Chan and Myuran Sukumaran

The World Today By Ashley Hall
Updated 5 Feb 2015, 7:47pm

And so it continued:

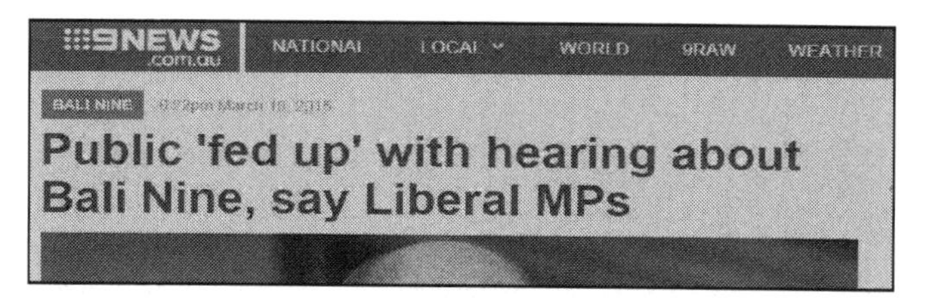

9NEWS .com.au | NATIONAL | LOCAL | WORLD | 9RAW | WEATHER

BALI NINE

Public 'fed up' with hearing about Bali Nine, say Liberal MPs

With such signals coming out of Australia, it is little wonder that the Widodo regime was emboldened enough to fulfil its brutal intentions.

These two examples illustrate a common feature of so many drug related cases. The interests of those caught up in them are automatically of secondary importance to those of every other party, including the police and the politicians.

Even worse, the human rights of those accused of selling drugs are often revoked, usually with media and political support. Regardless of the specific circumstances of any individual case, civilised norms tend to go out of the window, and a well rehearsed farce of media fuelled public indignation routinely ensues. Reality is frequently suspended.

The public are culturally conditioned to have absolutely no concern or compassion for anyone who has been damned with those fateful terms: *drug dealer*, *drug smuggler* or *drug pusher*.

EVERYDAY STIGMATISATION

Whilst these may be high profile cases, there are countless examples at the other end of the scale. I recall one recent case involving contaminated ecstasy pills at a summer music festival, with a couple of youngsters being media-assassinated and hunted down for innocently having bought a few for their group.

Lives are regularly and frequently ruined on the basis of socially selling and sharing materials which are not only in general use, but are often benign and relatively harmless. A modern day witch hunt of stigmatisation and hostile pursuit persists unabated, against members of the public who are in most cases as ordinary and law abiding as you or I.

This misrepresentation of whole swathes of society is culturally embedded in western society. One would imagine that future historians will look back on this period as one of crass ignorance and brutal intolerance.

Drug dealers are people too, and human rights should apply to everyone.

NOTE: DEALING WITH STREET VENDORS

Even though vendors do not usually resemble the media presentation, when purchasing drugs illegally it is sensible to use common sense and observe a number of safety precautions. These will normally be dictated by circumstance, but generally, if trading in person, it is wise to have full cognisance of your physical security, particularly if you are purchasing from a stranger.

Don't ignore your instincts, and never allow your enthusiasm for the product to cloud your judgement. Consider whether you would place yourself in a particular situation if you were purchasing, for example, a consumer product or a food item. Equally, whatever your relationship with the vendor, the substance you obtain should always be subject to the harm reduction measures outlined in the first section of this book.

Whilst drug dealers are hardly likely to intentionally poison their customers, it must be borne in mind that they are usually one part of a chain, having obtained the material elsewhere. Often they will not have any more certainty regarding the safety or the purity of the drug than you do. Never make assumptions.

ANECDOTAL TALE (THE NERVOUS DEALER)
It was in the warmth of a perfect summer afternoon, as I lounged smoking Amsterdam's finest in Rembrandtplein with a colleague, that a short cropped man of east European origin approached us. He had been chatting to a group of fellow people-watchers, who were also toking, a few yards away on the grass.

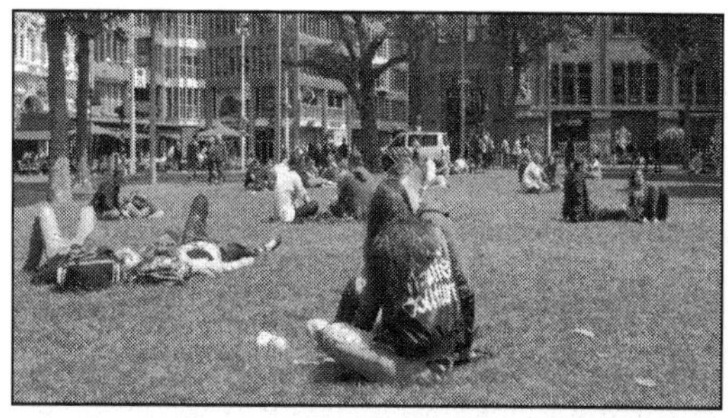

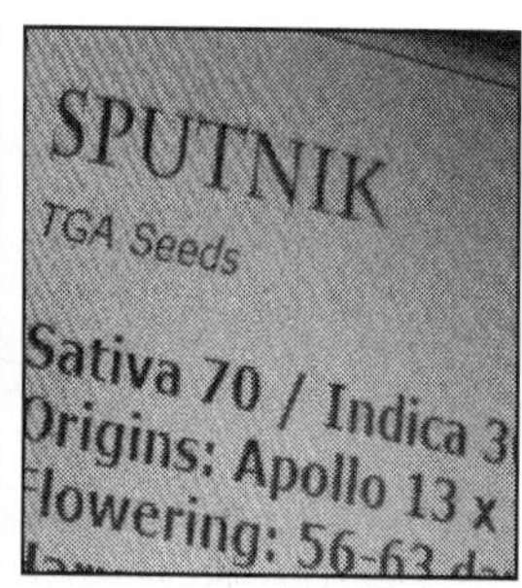

He introduced himself politely with a bit of small talk, and then offered a toke of his own joint. "*It's called sputnik*" he volunteered, stating that it was Russian and was very strong indeed.

I obliged, and passed it back to him, whilst my friend abstained. It was indeed strong.

"*Would you like some ecstasy or cocaine*?" he asked.

I responded with the obvious answer (which was no), explaining that I was due to leave the following morning and didn't want a heavy night. We continued to chat for a few minutes, largely about the drug scene, and he then departed to his next port of call, another group who were sitting further to our left.

That incident would never have been recalled, if we hadn't seen him again a few hours later.

As we sat by a canal, again chilling, and sipping a drink, he walked slowly past. Whilst we saw him coming, he didn't notice our particular table. As he came closer his eyes eventually focused upon us. He momentarily froze, as he tried to recollect. Then, startled, he darted off at speed.

Given that he was smoking a paranoia-inducing strain of cannabis his logic had clearly flowed along the lines of:

Drug selling – From earlier - They are following me – They are cops!

The moral of the story isn't just that dealers are susceptible to the same drug effects as everyone else, it is also that you shouldn't use even a benign plant like cannabis when you are relying on sound judgement to do your job safely and sensibly.

THE DARKNET MARKETS

The darknet, accessed via the Tor browser, emerged as a major source of drugs during the legal high years. Individual markets came and went, with *The Silk Road* perhaps being the most famous. Following its demise others emerged to successively take the mantle as the most popular, including *Dream*, *AlphaBay* and *Empire*.

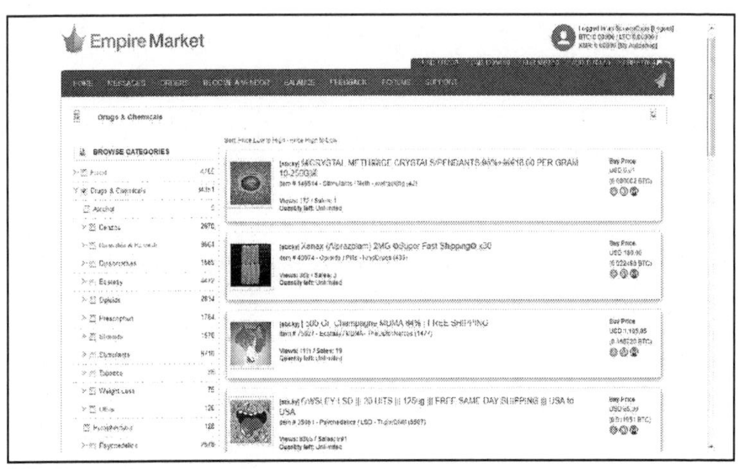

Empire became the largest darknet market circa 2019

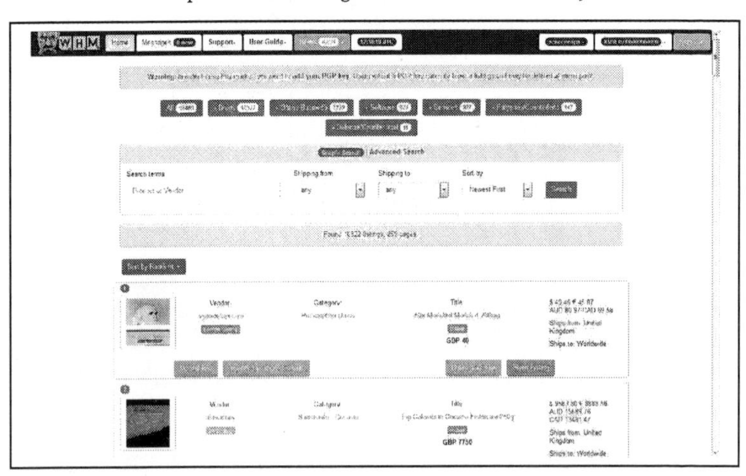

White House Market found increased popularity after the fall of AlphaBay & Dream

All these markets operated via the use of cryptocurrencies, and supported encryption/PGP communication between buyers and sellers.

4.4.5 The Role of The Media

The media plays a central role in perpetuating the *war on drugs* and preserving the landscape of ignorance with respect to essential safety information. I wrote the following article subsequent to the publication of the first edition of this book. It was initially published by the drug charity *Release*.

THE FIRST CASUALTY OF WAR

Truth is the first casualty of war and the *war on drugs* is no different. Every day both the print and broadcast media bombard the public with a perspective and narrative which has proved to be devastating. This diet of cultural influence and propaganda is unremitting.

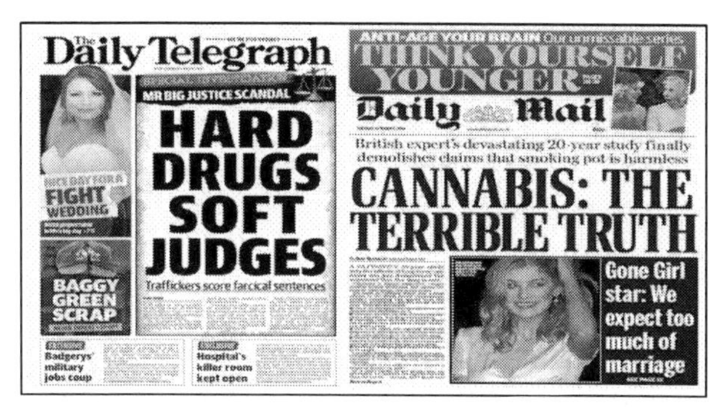

Daily Telegraph

FIGHT WEDDING

BAGGY GREEN SCRAP

MR BIG JUSTICE SCANDAL

HARD DRUGS SOFT JUDGES

Traffickers score farcical sentences

Badgerys' military jobs coup

Hospital's killer room kept open

ANTI-AGE YOUR BRAIN

THINK YOURSELF YOUNGER

Daily Mail

British expert's devastating 20-year study finally demolishes claims that smoking pot is harmless

CANNABIS: THE TERRIBLE TRUTH

Gone Girl star: We expect too much of marriage

The broad consensus behind this is a clear example of groupthink, and it persists across almost the entire mainstream. It is so ingrained in western journalism that it is prosecuted almost blindly, rendering journalists to be an integral part of the problem.

With this in mind, and with no end in sight, I recently considered the question of how journalists could reintroduce objectivity and truth back into drug reporting. What could be done to ground reports outside a paradigm which is neither factual nor humane?

I concluded that for conscientious journalists, those instilled with sincerity and candour, this wouldn't take much effort at all. Indeed, the framing of a code of ethics almost became an exercise in stating the obvious:

<u>A CODE OF ETHICS FOR HONEST DRUG REPORTING</u>

1. The cause of tragedy and death is the erroneous use of drugs, not the drugs themselves. This usually stems from a lack of safety awareness and knowledge with respect to the specific drug or drugs in question. Reports should therefore be framed in this context.

2. Always include the intrinsic and central details in reports. For example, don't routinely use the generic word *drugs* to cover substances which are absolutely diverse in nature, effect and potential harm. This wide scale practice is a *de facto* inhibitor of accuracy, education and understanding.

3. Cultural bias tends to suppress awareness of relative harms, which in Western society severely exacerbates alcohol related problems and misrepresents far more benign options. Effort should be made to reduce and eliminate this tendency.

Specifically, alcohol is a hard addictive drug and should be cited and reported as such when appropriate. Do not hesitate to cast this drug (alcohol) in the comparative context of other drugs when reporting on it, and vice versa.

Within this, review the use of stilted terminology. For instance, why do alcohol users drink their drug, whilst users of other drugs abuse theirs? Why do alcohol sources sell their product, whilst sources of other drugs push theirs?

4. In the context of drug use the mantra *'Ignorance Kills, Education Saves Lives'* is a statement of fact. Journalists can help to educate by reporting harm reduction and safety information whenever an opportunity is presented.

Routinely quote harm reduction charities such as *Release* and *DanceSafe*, and directly recycle the personal safety data provided by sources such as *TripSit* and *The Drug Users Bible*.

5. The police frequently inflate the market value of their *drug hauls* for self interest, and defending solicitors will commonly consider it trite or provocative to challenge this in court. This misinformation perverts the course of justice and serves to re-enforce the destructive narrative of the *war on drugs*.

When reporting, qualify police claims or independently research the actual value.

6. Substances like datura and nutmeg are deliriants, and are dysphoric and highly toxic. Don't use words like *trip* to describe their effects, and don't refer to them as *psychedelics*. This is a good example of misleading terminology inciting potentially fatal consequences.

7. Report actual and factual impact data with respect to the *war on drugs*. For example, with 5% of the world's population the United States now holds 25% of the world's prison population, whilst the number of overdose deaths has soared.

At the very least don't repeat the *war on drugs* precept as though it isn't challenged.

Within this, don't pursue a narrative which demonises drug users or drug sellers. Bear in mind that 250 million people use drugs, and most sellers are ordinary citizens who started buying drugs for friends as well as themselves.

Individually, to hold sovereign and exclusive ownership of one's own conscious mind, to explore freely and without boundary, is surely the most fundamental of human rights. Third party intrusion into this wholly personal territory is a grievous breach of this inalienable freedom.

It is entirely reasonable to reflect this perspective in reports, particularly with respect to psychedelics.

8. Don't allow politicians or their servants (including the police) to set the agenda and define talking points, as again, they have a tendency to promote the *war on drugs* perspective for self interest.

Always be aware that the role of journalism is to report objectively, rather than disseminate propaganda.

None of these are outrageously difficult to embrace, at least if the pursuit of truth is the objective (as it should be). I would also suggest that collectively they almost present a good measure of personal integrity for any journalist who is aware of them.

Indeed, I would bluntly ask: if you are reporting in this field, and you are not following these or something similar to them, why not? What position are you seeking to promote, and for whom?

The continued diet of censorship, misreporting and dishonesty is perpetuating ignorance and costing lives. Real people, vulnerable people, are suffering and dying partly as a result of the current role of mainstream journalism in a brutal and unwinnable war.

Drugs users' lives matter too, and some of the blood is surely on the hands of those who continue to engage as a blunt instrument of state.

With few exceptions the media is an integral part of the social fabric and machinery which sustains the cycle of misery, death and mass incarceration described earlier in this book.

Should you have any contact with a mainstream journalist, always remember that he or she will almost invariably represent the proprietor's agenda and will usually have a pre-prepared narrative. Tread very carefully and don't invest trust lightly.

SOCIAL MEDIA

Unfortunately, the behemoths of social media are not immune from these issues. Often spurred on by tabloid hysteria, their approach usually takes the form of *censor now, ask questions (or ignore) later*. The responses of Twitter and Reddit regarding the advertising of the first edition of this book provide a case in point:

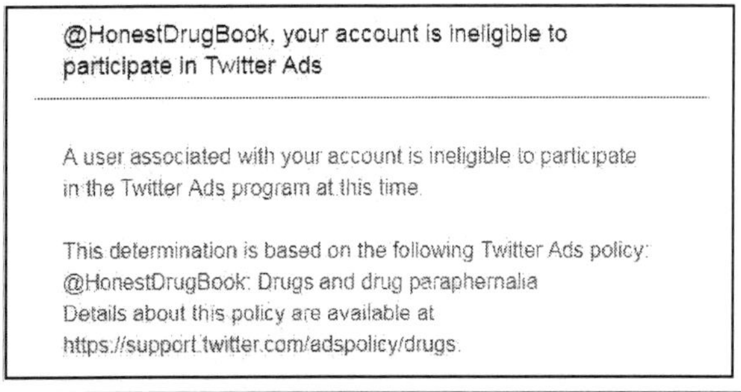

@HonestDrugBook, your account is ineligible to participate in Twitter Ads

A user associated with your account is ineligible to participate in the Twitter Ads program at this time.

This determination is based on the following Twitter Ads policy:
@HonestDrugBook: Drugs and drug paraphernalia
Details about this policy are available at
https://support.twitter.com/adspolicy/drugs.

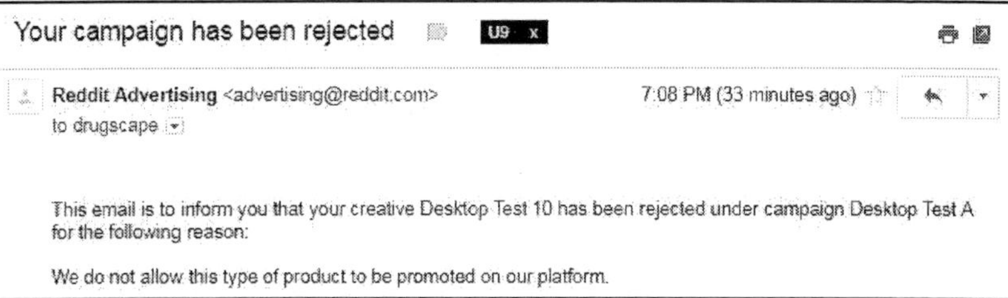

Your campaign has been rejected

Reddit Advertising <advertising@reddit.com> 7:08 PM (33 minutes ago)
to drugscape

This email is to inform you that your creative Desktop Test 10 has been rejected under campaign Desktop Test A for the following reason:

We do not allow this type of product to be promoted on our platform.

Meanwhile, Facebook routinely purges groups like *Sesh Safety*, which is dedicated to saving lives via provision of non-judgemental impartial help and advice:

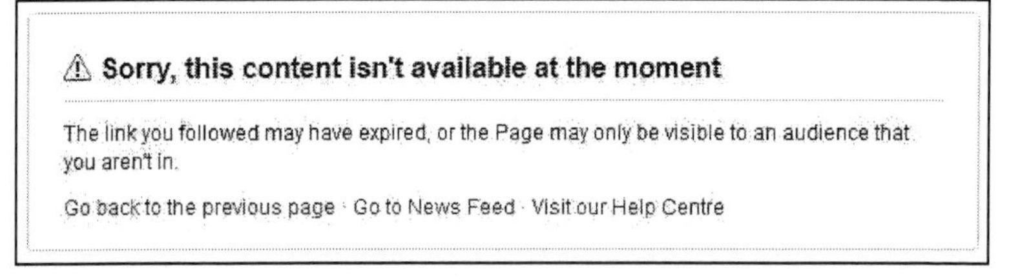

Content platforms are equally problematic. For example, by limiting its referential sources broadly to approved media conglomerates and corporations, Wikipedia perpetuates and re-enforces the position of the mainstream. In practical terms this equates to a form of censorship by citation, and it is extremely effective.

In terms of diversity and the sharing of factual information, the Internet is shrinking under the shadow of the *war on drugs*. At time of writing it appears that this may get worse before it gets better.

4.4.6 Mandatory Drug Testing

Mandatory drug testing is not limited to law enforcement situations. Increasingly it is being used by employers, and not only with respect to roles which have health and safety implications.

It is a practice which is open to misuse, and one which again tends to present drug use as a criminal rather than a health issue. In many scenarios it is a serious threat to privacy, and to civil and human rights. Whilst the scale and gravity of this will differ from nation to nation, there is little doubt that it is now an escalating global problem.

DRUG DETECTION PERIODS
For the drug user the spectre of drug testing raises a number of fundamental questions: How long does evidence of drug use stay in the system? Will the type of test being used influence the results? How do different drugs compare in terms of detection times?

There are a lot of variables here, relating to all sorts of issues, including your use of the drug (e.g. frequency and RoA) and your personal physiology. In addition, I found enormous discrepancies between different data sources: there simply wasn't a universally agreed norm for some of these figures.

For these reasons I almost omitted this segment from the book. Its inclusion therefore comes with a waiver: it provides only the broadest of indications and it should not be taken as gospel. If drug testing is a particularly significant issue for you, make sure that you further research the specific drug in question.

DRUG	BLOOD	URINE	SALIVA	HAIR
Alcohol	10-12 Hours	3-5 Days	1-5 Days	Up To 90 Days
Amphetamine	3 Days	1-3 Days	3 Days	Up To 90 Days
Benzodiazepines	3 Days	1-6 Weeks	1-10 Days	Up To 90 Days
Cannabis*	Up To 7 Days	1-90 Days	1-10 Days	Up To 90 Days
Cocaine	1-2 Days	2-5 Days	Up To 36 Hours	Up To 90 Days
Heroin	12 Hours	3-4 Days	1-2 Days	Up To 90 Days
Ketamine**	Up To 14 Days	3-5 Days	1-8 Days	Up To 90 Days
Methamphetamine	1-3 Days	2-8 Days	1-3 Days	Up To 90 Days
MDMA	1-2 Days	3-4 Days	1-3 Days	Up To 90 Days
LSD	2-3 Hours	1-3 Days	1-2 Days	Up To 4 Days

* Frequency of use is a major factor with some figures being much shorter for occasional users.
** These figures were particularly variable, with many sources claiming much shorter periods.

HOW TO PASS A DRUG TEST?
The Internet is awash with ideas on how to pass a drug test: other than by not using drugs. A lot of these are blatantly flawed, but others may have merit. Here I will simply list some current information and outline a number of the more credible suggestions.

At the outset it is important to consider the context of the drug test. Usually this will be related to employment or to a court case (or other judicial scenario). These two situations will present different challenges. For example, for the latter you are more likely to be observed whilst providing a urine sample.

It is important to determine, in advance, as much about the testing procedure as you are able; perhaps by asking colleagues or seeking advice from appropriate third parties. This can help you to formulate your strategy and approach, and to decide how to proceed (based possibly on what you believe you can get away with).

I should point out here, however, that in some places a number of these strategies might be considered to constitute fraud, and you might be committing a criminal offence if you follow them. Do your homework on these issues prior to proceeding down any particular path.

Generally, the options available will depend upon the type of test (urine, blood, saliva, hair). Nevertheless, there are a couple of general steps which apply to them all, and which are very straight forward.

The first is that you can abstain from drugs from the moment you know that you are going to be tested. From this point you can also start to detox naturally, even if this means just drinking plenty of water every day, to flush your system. Exercising and being active will also help, although don't do too much on the day of the test or the day before. Finally, eat healthily, don't diet, and don't skip breakfast.

The second is to record a list of all your legitimate medications to submit to the testing facility. As some prescription and over-the-counter medicines, and some herbal remedies, can cause a false positive, it is sensible to provide details of genuine medical use prior to taking the test.

The most commonly cited approaches for each type of test are as follows:

URINE TESTS
These are presently the most widely used. You will be required to submit a sample of your urine, which can usually be produced privately; but not always.

The tests themselves vary. However, the most popular is currently the *5-Panel Urine Test*. This usually detects the following drugs: cannabis; cocaine; opiates; PCP; amphetamines. More stringent is the *10-Panel Urine Test*, which typically also includes: benzodiazepines; barbiturates; MDMA; various prescription drugs (e.g. oxycodone and methadone); methaqualone. Added to this may be other drugs, like alcohol.

If you can determine which drugs are to be targeted, clearly these are the ones to address with your countermeasures, and at the very least, to avoid using in the interim.

Methods sometimes used to influence the result of a urine test include the following:

Use of Masking Agents
This is basically the trick of adding something (e.g. a commercial product) to your sample before handing it over. Apparently these additives used to work well, but now are often detected, and tend to result in an automatic failure. If you are thinking of using this approach do your homework first.

Dilution
Dilution is the act of adding fluid (e.g. water) to your sample, or alternatively, drinking a lot of water prior to the test. However, this too is widely recognized by labs, some of which do check for it. Note also that heavy dilution changes the colour of the urine to clear, which makes it pretty obvious that an attempt has been made to subvert the result. Some detoxifiers (see below) contain colorants to help address this.

A better approach may be pre-hydration. Urine will have its highest drug concentration early in the morning, so drinking a few cups of water may help to flush this a little, and enable you to urinate naturally prior to doing so for the test itself.

Use of Detoxifiers
Drug test *detoxifiers* are often used in conjunction with dilution. These change the urine composition, and are consumed prior to the test. I encountered multiple claims that they can be effective, although again there is some risk that the lab may detect them, or not: this is a non-static relationship, with suppliers frequently updating their formulas to try to beat detection techniques.

It's your call, but it is worth noting that not all detoxifiers are the same, and some have been reviewed side-by-side for their comparative effectiveness. I would suggest therefore that you research intensively to arm yourself with current information. Detoxifiers are sold in head shops and online.

If you have the luxury of time before the test, you might wish to buy a home testing kit and check how your detoxifier stacks up against it. On the other side of the coin, if a test is likely to be bounced upon you at short notice, it might be a good idea to have a detox agent on standby, if this is your preferred option.

Substitution

Using someone else's urine is an obvious temptation, but it may not be as simple as it appears. The first risk is that the substitute urine may also fail the test due to drug use (how well do you know the volunteer?). Another consideration is that urine turns darker as time passes. Then of course there is the issue of getting the urine itself into the facility and actually substituting it.

Premixed and synthetic urine (e.g. powdered) also comes with a risk of detection: labs are generally aware that these are on the market and do look-out for them. Having stated this, there are many claims that some of them do work. Again, it is best to acquire some expertise if you intend to take this route. Investigate carefully.

Another issue which I should point out is that if you are likely to be tested repeatedly over time, there is a possibility that the difference in urine composition between tests might be identified.

One note on temperature: testing staff are not stupid. If you hand over a stone cold sample it is very obvious that it has not come from your body.

A final word on urine tests: don't celebrate too early... meaning that you shouldn't head directly for your drug immediately after the test. You may be called back for a re-test, so wait until the test results are confirmed before making assumptions.

HAIR FOLLICLE TESTS

For these, about 1.5 inches of hair is normally taken, usually from the head. If you are bald, the sample of hair will be taken from elsewhere.

With this type of test long term use is more likely to be detected than a one-off experiment, although this too could be identified. Also note that very recent drug use may not show up (hence urine and hair tests are sometimes used together).

A *5-Panel Test* exists for hair, broadly equating to the urine panel test. There are also extended versions (e.g. *12-Panel*) and other drugs may be added.

As the sample is usually taken directly from you, substitution and some of the other methods covered for urine tests will not work. However, there are still a number of frequently cited options which may or may not have merit. Most of these come in the form of specialist detoxification shampoos and rinses.

First and foremost, if you use these make sure that they are safe, and be careful when you wash with them. Note that to enhance the prospects of success you will normally need to use them for some days beforehand, although of course, late is better than never.

Other methods suggested include the use of salicylic acid, white vinegar, laundry detergent and temporary hair dye. If you opt to try these, again be careful whilst using them.

Finally, I have read about people using bleach on their hair and claiming success, frequently when used in combination with a detoxifying shampoo. I would urge some caution here: not just because using bleach on yourself is a risk, but because you don't want to walk into the workplace (for example) with different coloured hair to usual.

As with other test types, there is a huge market supplying all sorts of commercial products, so check this out if you intend to walk this path.

SALIVA TESTS

Given that the saliva sample is likely to be taken there and then, the options to beat this are limited. However, the good news is that most drugs can only be detected in saliva for a few days after use.

The pre-test regime here is fairly obvious. First of all, brush your teeth thoroughly: I mean thoroughly (but not hard enough to cause bleeding), taking in all of your mouth. Using mouthwash and eating can also have a temporary effect, perhaps for 20 or 30 minutes.

Note that regarding the mouthwash, the alcohol content of some brands can sometimes present a risk, depending on the test being used. However, there are specialist drug-toxin mouthwashes on the market which may be a better bet. Oral gum is another product type I have seen suggested.

Again, with this method you can buy a decent quality home testing kit to check whether it works for you (at least using the kit) prior to the event.

BLOOD TESTS

Blood testing is clearly the most invasive approach. Given that the sample is taken directly from you by a third party it presents obvious difficulties in terms of manipulating the outcome. However, in addition to the general steps cited at the start of this section, you could try using a high quality drug detoxifier to improve your odds.

Whilst the above may be helpful, it is important to bear in mind that this is a changing landscape and information does become outdated. Also, although it is a mature marketplace and the Internet is your friend (sometimes), be careful: if you are seeking a product don't plump for the first one that you encounter. Find social media discussions, third party review sites and other sources that will help you to take decisions on an informed and current basis.

Remember too that the only guaranteed way to beat a test is not to engage in drug use for the requisite period beforehand.

4.4.7 Activism: The Charter of Drug Users Rights

Drug users across the world are prosecuted, persecuted and marginalized. However, in recent years there have been indications of a grassroots counterresponse to this oppression, albeit one which is still barely perceptible.

One initiative is *The Charter Of Drug Users Rights*, for which I agreed to write the script. Although this has not taken off, it is worth reproducing here, hopefully as a sign of things to come.

The petition itself can be found via the following URL:
https://www.change.org/p/the-united-nations-secretary-general-the-charter-of-drug-users-rights

The Charter of Drug Users Rights

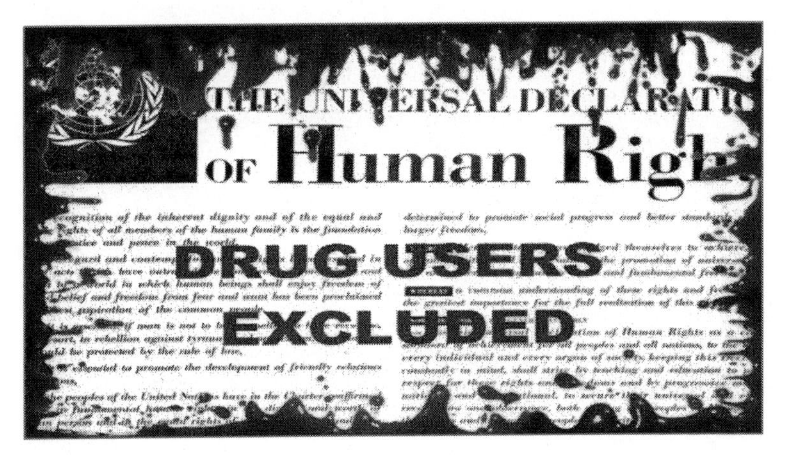

According to the UN there are a quarter of a BILLION drug users globally, which is more than the entire populations of the UK, France and Germany combined. This is a significant minority of the world's population.

There are a myriad of reasons why these individuals take drugs, but usually they make a proactive decision to do so. In other words, they adopt a primordial right to choose what to put into their OWN bodies, and they choose how to change their OWN consciousness.

Unfortunately, these innate personal freedoms are largely denied and proscribed by states and governments. Non-violent citizens are arrested, criminalized and imprisoned, for no other reason than that they have exercised this fundamental human right with respect to THEMSELVES.

This (often violent) oppression is augmented and sustained via media coverage which ignores and marginalizes the victims' interests and perspectives. Mainstream output invariably aligns with a destructive *war on drugs* narrative, and excludes direct and factual information/news which would save lives. The aggressive flow of ideologically based propaganda is unrelenting, whilst even the most basic harm-reduction initiatives, remain totally unreported and largely unknown.

This unremitting flood of unbalanced journalism manifestly serves to re-enforce the stigma and hostility endured by what has become a socially persecuted minority. Drug users have no voice, no statutory protection, and nowhere to turn.

With their civil and human rights being routinely and systematically violated across the world the picture could hardly be bleaker. It is a level of abuse and degradation which for any other minority would be widely recognised and condemned. Even the term itself, *drug user*, has been so misappropriated that it has become pejorative, placing anyone thus referenced outside the orbit of normal moral consideration.
It is within this desperate and harrowing context that the following demands are presented:

- The immediate cessation of the *war on drugs*.
- Drug dependency and addiction to be treated as health issues rather than criminal matters.
- The release of all imprisoned non-violent drug *offenders*, and all convictions for non-violent drug offences to be expunged.
- Recognition of the right to use drugs recreationally, inclusive of social parity with alcohol users, and a cessation of cultural and other forms of discrimination.
- Urgent repeal and reform of global drug treaties to expedite the above, with new drug related legislation framed to recognise the supremacy of the Universal Declaration of Human Rights and its application to all.

RELATED INFORMATION & SAFETY RESOURCES
UN Charter of Human Rights
The 10 Commandments of Safer Drug Use
TripSit
Release
The Drug Users Bible
Volteface
ACLU

4.5 Drug Tourism

Despite the unremitting onslaught of the *war on drugs*, some territories still offer a little respite, at least for certain psychoactives. During the research period for this book I visited a number of them; some as specific destinations and others in transit. This section presents a brief overview of a handful of these, in no particular order.

Amsterdam is afforded its own segment not only on the basis of its currently liberal and relatively civilised approach to drugs, but because I tended to use it as a base for both exploration and travel.

Note that I do not offer legal advice on the current state of play within any nation, but rather, I present a snapshot of the situation at the specific point I experienced it. Always check the legal landscape before you plan a visit to any territory in which you intend to engage in any drug related activity.

4.5.1 The Dutch Connection (Amsterdam)

There isn't really a Dutch connection, other than that the Netherlands is a major source of a number of popular recreational drugs (e.g. MDMA). However, there is Amsterdam, where a substantial number of international tourists go to enjoy the coffeeshops and the more tolerant and civilised attitude to drugs generally. This book would therefore not be complete without a brief overview of this scene, from the perspective of the foreign visitor.

As a customer, there are three main sources of interest: coffeeshops (for cannabis), seed banks (for seeds) and smart shops (for legal chemicals, botanicals and paraphernalia). Whilst these are dotted across the centre of Amsterdam, they are not all equal in terms of quality or value, and research is suggested prior to any visit.

To create some sort of picture of the situation on the ground, during 2017 I visited a small number of the most reputable of these outlets, and presented a series of questions to a member of staff in each. The responses are produced below.

<u>KOKOPELLI (WARMOESSTRAAT 12) - SMART SHOP</u>

1. What are the most common foreign nationalities that come in here?
   1. UK 2. Italian 3. Russian
2. What are the most popular items that people ask for, that you don't or can't sell?
   1. MDMA 2. Mushrooms 3. LSD
3. Other than truffles, what is your biggest selling psychoactive?
   Kratom
4. What is your own personal favourite?
   Kratom
5. What is your favourite cannabis strain?
   Moroccan Hash

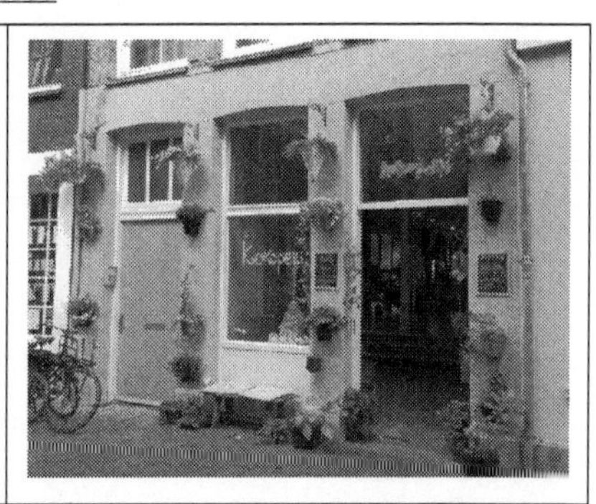

THE HEADSHOP (KLOVENIERSBURGWAL 39) – SMART SHOP

1. What are the most common foreign nationalities that come in here?
   1. Italian 2. French/UK 3. German
2. What are the most popular items that people ask for, that you don't or can't sell?
   1. 4-FMP 2. Cocaine 3. Ecstasy/Shrooms
3. Other than truffles, what is your biggest selling psychoactive?
   Kratom
4. What is your own personal favourite?
   Kratom
5. What is your favourite cannabis strain?
   Banana Kush CBD (to help back pain)

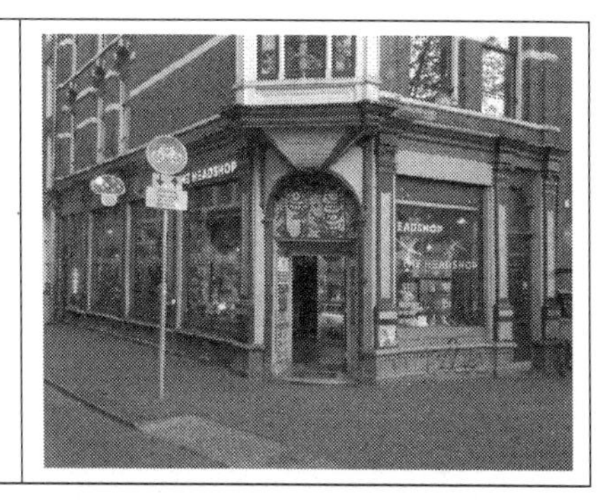

NUMBER ONE (OUDE HOOGSTRAAT 4) – SMART SHOP

1. What are the most common foreign nationalities that come in here?
   1. UK 2. Italian 3. French
2. What are the most popular items that people ask for, that you don't or can't sell?
   1. Ecstasy 2. Weed 3. Shrooms
3. Other than truffles, what is your biggest selling psychoactive?
   Kratom
4. What is your own personal favourite?
   Kratom
5. What is your favourite cannabis strain?
   Super Lemon Haze

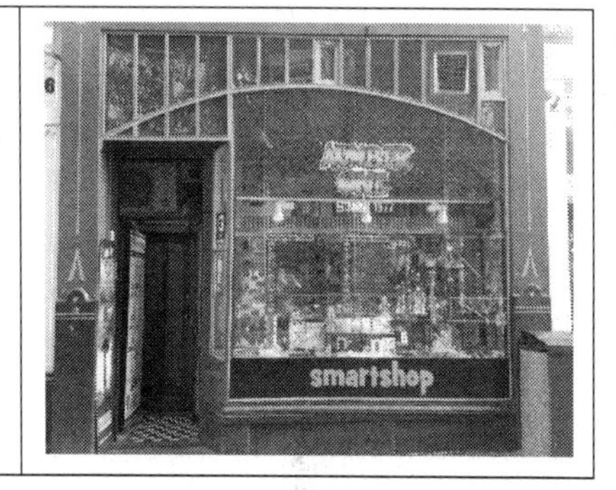

GREEN HOUSE (HAARLEMMERSTRAAT 64) - COFFEESHOP

1. What are the most common foreign nationalities that come in here?
   1. Italian 2. French 3. UK
   [But there are periodic large influxes of different nationalities at different times of the year]
2. What is your biggest selling strain?
   Super Lemon Haze
3. What is your own personal favourite?
   Kush

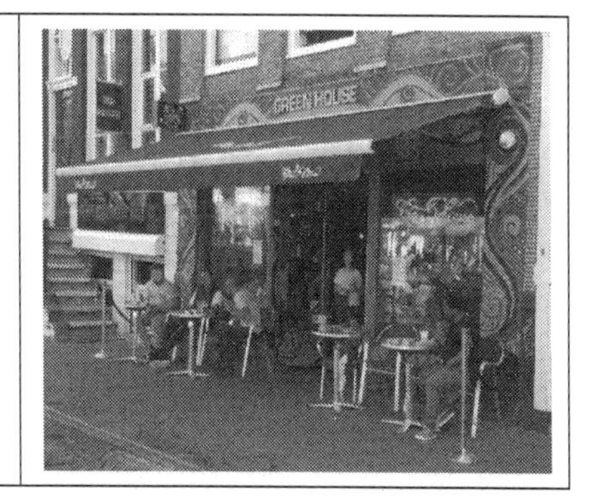

THE ROOKIES (KORTE LEIDSEDWARSSTRAAT 145-147) – COFFEESHOP

1. What are the most common foreign nationalities that come in here?
   1. UK 2. French 3. Italian
2. What is your biggest selling strain?
   Champagne Haze (Sativa)
3. What is your own personal favourite?
   Super Maroc

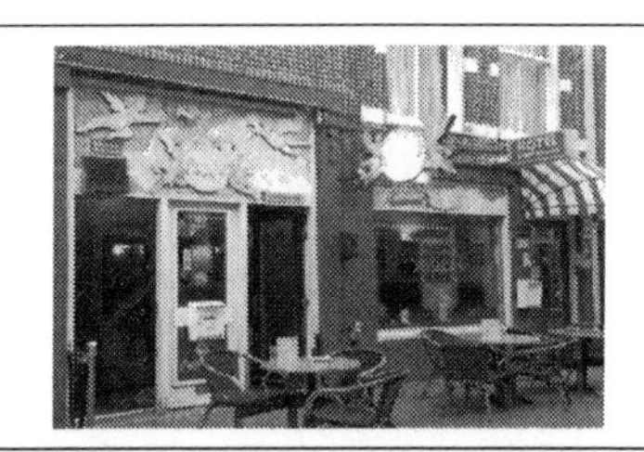

DAMPKRING (HANDBOOGSTRAAT 29) - COFFEESHOP

1. What are the most common foreign nationalities that come in here?
   1. Italian 2. French 3. UK
2. What is your biggest selling strain?
   Various Sativa
3. What is your own personal favourite?
   Ceres Hilton(Sativa)
   Head Stash (Indica)

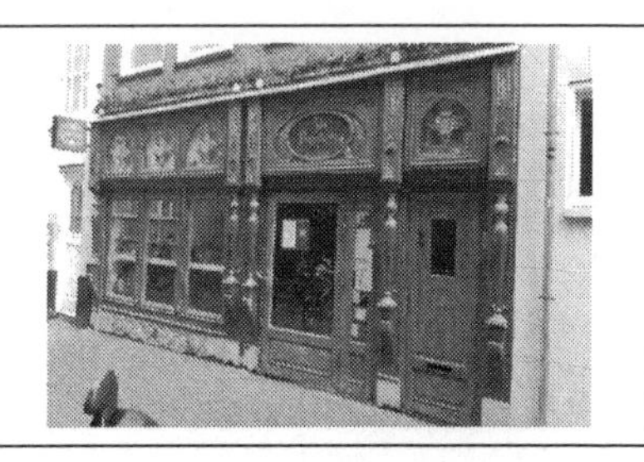

420 (OUDEBRUGSTEEG 27) - COFFEESHOP

1. What are the most common foreign nationalities that come in here?
   1. UK 2. French 3. Italian
2. What is your biggest selling strain?
   Blueberry
3. What is your own personal favourite?
   New York Diesel

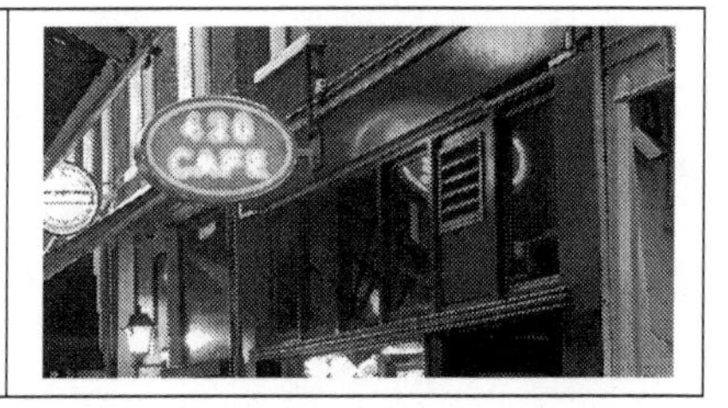

ROYAL QUEEN SEEDS (DAMSTRAAT 46) – SEED BANK

1. What are the most common foreign nationalities that come in here?
   1. Italian 2. French/German 3. UK
2. What is the most popular item that people ask for, that you don't actually sell?
   Weed
3. What is your biggest seller?
   Amnesia Haze
4. What is your own personal favourite?
   Morning: Amnesia Haze
   Afternoon: Kush

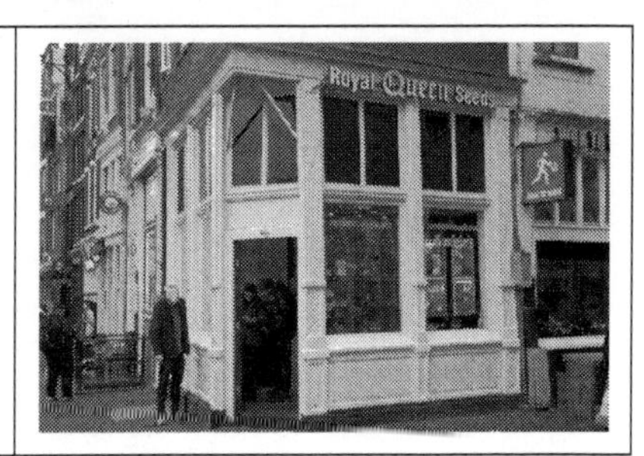

AMSTERDAM: GENERAL SAFETY ADVICE

It is important to note that, when in Amsterdam, your normal safety regime should not be suspended. However, some aspects of this are far easier to implement than elsewhere. An example of this is with respect to testing.

Several facilities exist which, for a nominal fee, will test your drug anonymously. The details of these are as follows:

GGD Amsterdam, Valckenierstraat 4, 1018 XG Amsterdam +3120-5555450 www.ggd.amsterdam.nl	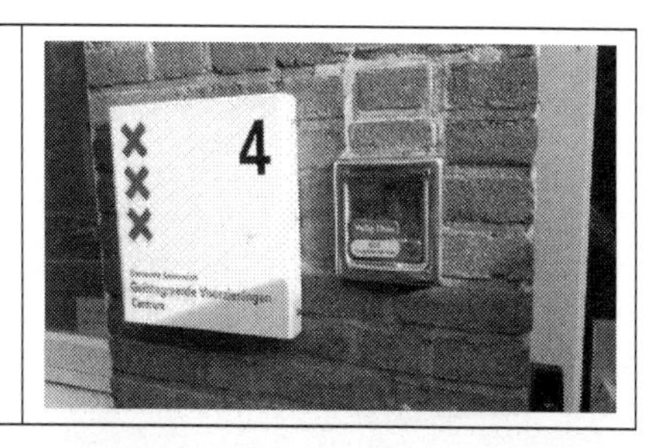
Jellinek, Jacob Obrechtstraat 92, 1071 KG Amsterdam +3120-5901590 www.jellinek.nl	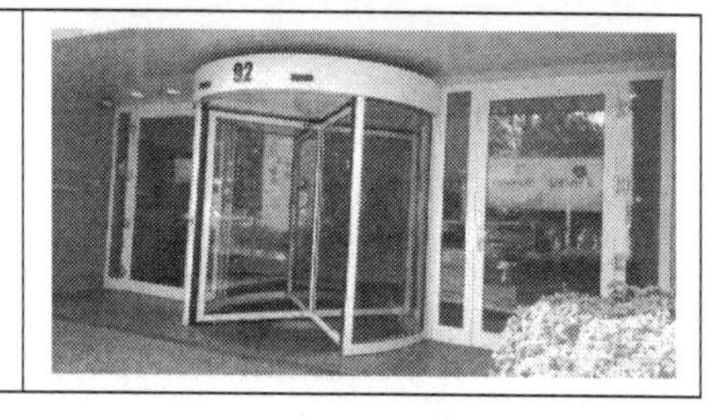

On my visit to the GGD's premises I was fortunate enough to bump into someone connected with the service, and was able to gather some background information. I discovered that the main target for the service was unsurprisingly Dutch nationals. Tourists are accepted, but bear in mind that for other than basic reagent checks and database research, full laboratory tests sometimes take more than a week.

Their busiest time of year is usually festival season (the backend of summer), and at the time of my visit (August 2017) the most common drugs submitted for testing were ecstasy/MDMA, cocaine, ketamine and 2CB, in that order. There is a limit of 3 samples per person.

One piece of general advice I would offer from personal experience is not to overdo it. It is extremely easy to smoke too much of a strong strain, or to over indulge with truffles.

If you plan a heavy trip, engage it with a safety net, perhaps in close proximity to your hotel, or in a place where you can safely relax, away from crowds. Always have a sitter.

When you are purchasing your truffles, or other material, discuss your wishes with the vendor, who will be able to advise you, including with respect to dose. If you are purchasing mushrooms (not from a smart shop, as they are illegal) bear in mind the difference in weight between wet and dry.

Finally, I have always found Amsterdam to be an extremely friendly city, as illustrated by the interviews I referred to earlier. If you wish to know more, don't hesitate to ask local aficionados.

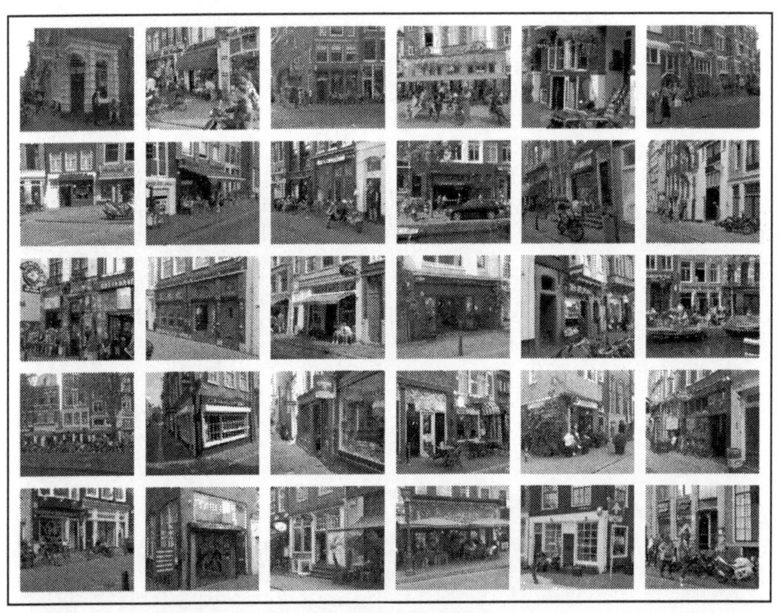

Thirty of Amsterdam's Coffeeshops

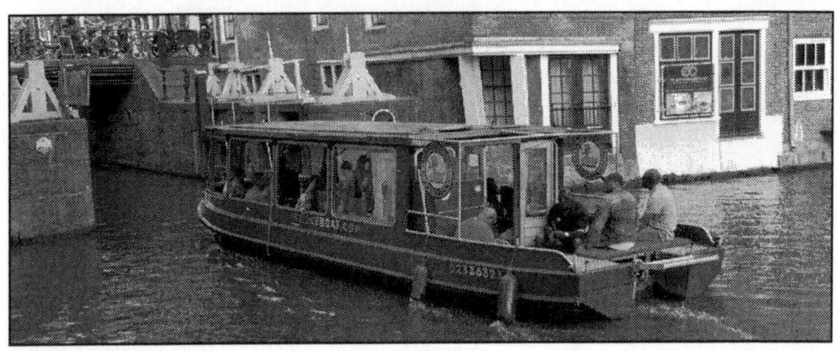

The SmokeBoat

TOURIST TIPS
For cannabis enthusiasts the *Hash, Marijuana & Hemp Museum*, on the fringe of the red light area, is a decent choice.

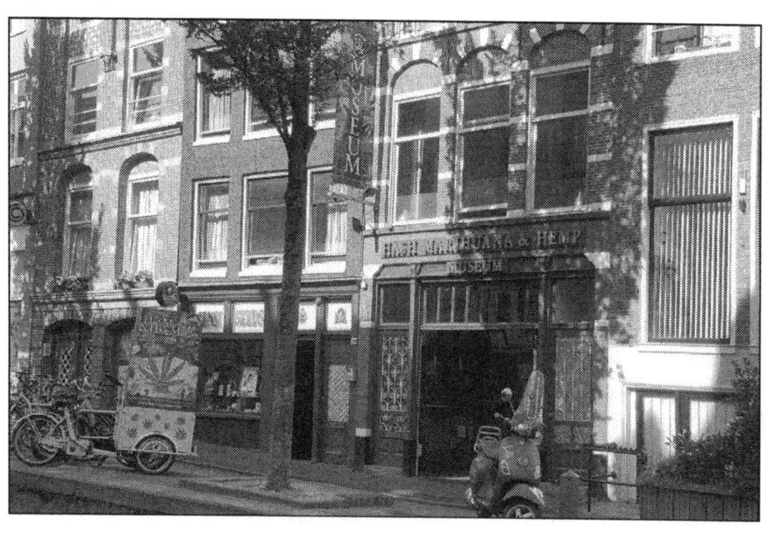

The entrance fee isn't cheap, but following perusal of a substantial number of documents, images, paraphernalia and historical exhibits, the visit ends with a punch. Whilst I cannot be certain that this is always provided, on the day I toured, visitors were offered a free hit via a fancy vaporiser and balloon bag.

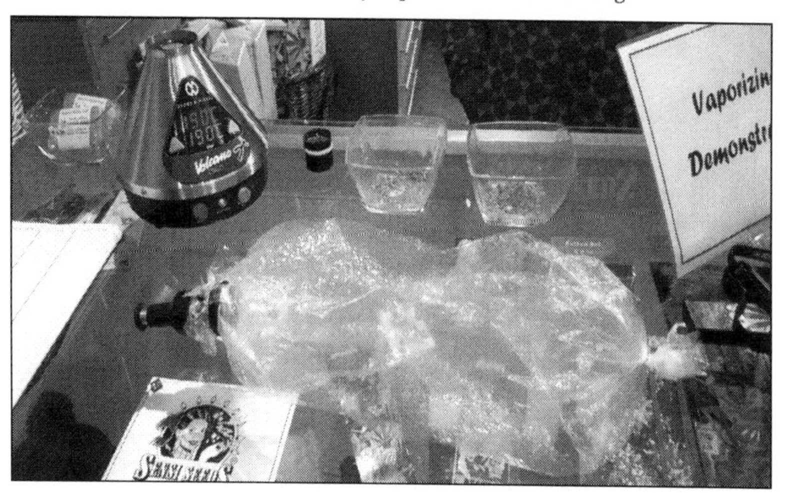

Predictably, this gave a very smooth toke, and the cannabis itself provided a nice slow-burning high.

Further down the same canal (Oudezijds Achterburgwal) is *Cannabis College*, which offers advice on the safe use of recreational and medicinal cannabis, as well as a free tour of its small Cannabis garden (see below).

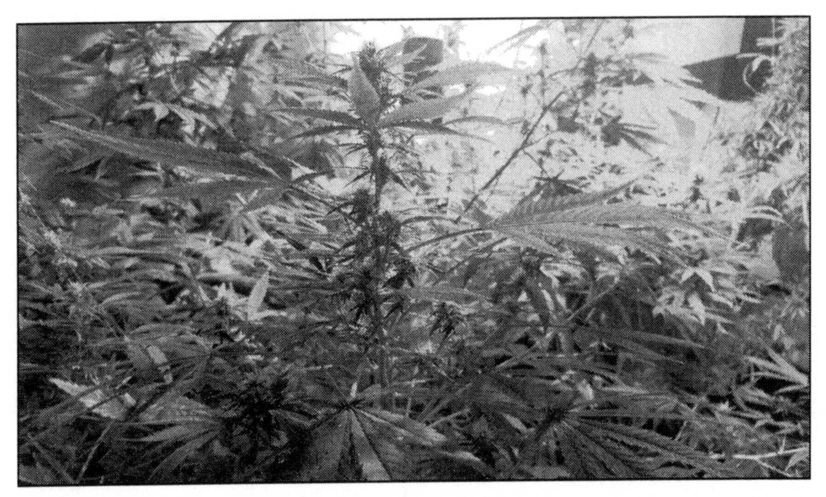

If you intend to trip on truffles or another psychedelic, Amsterdam is blessed with an abundance of world class art galleries and museums, to suit every taste. The term *museum dose* was not coined without good reason.

Alternatively, for both psychedelics and cannabis, there are many open spaces in which to relax, not least Vondelpark. Rembrandtplein is one of my personal favourites for people watching whilst stoned, but there are so many others.

I hesitate to cover alcohol given the available legal alternatives, but there are breweries (try the one in a windmill: *Brouwerij 't IJ*), an Icebar, and pubs and bars galore (try the delightful *In de Olofspoort*, steeped in history and offering an astonishing array of spirits and gins). Tobacco enthusiasts can head for *P.G.C. Hajenius* on Rokin, with its vast selection of cigars and an integral smoking room.

For me, Amsterdam is a wonderful destination for both relaxation and exploration, with a surprise around almost every corner. The general vibe is one of charm and chill, making it absolutely ideal for the discerning and adventurous tourist.

At the risk of them coming across as holiday snaps. I will end this section with some random images taken during my last few visits:

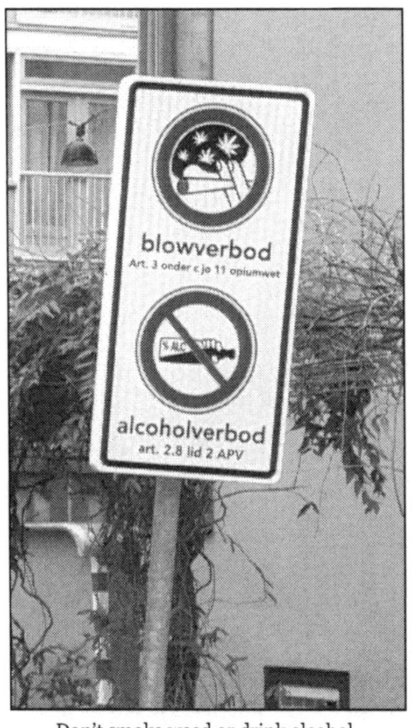

Don't smoke weed or drink alcohol in a kids' playground

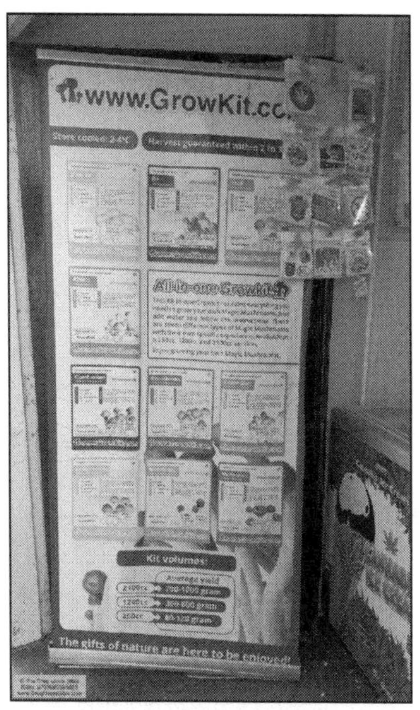

Grow Your Own (Mushrooms)

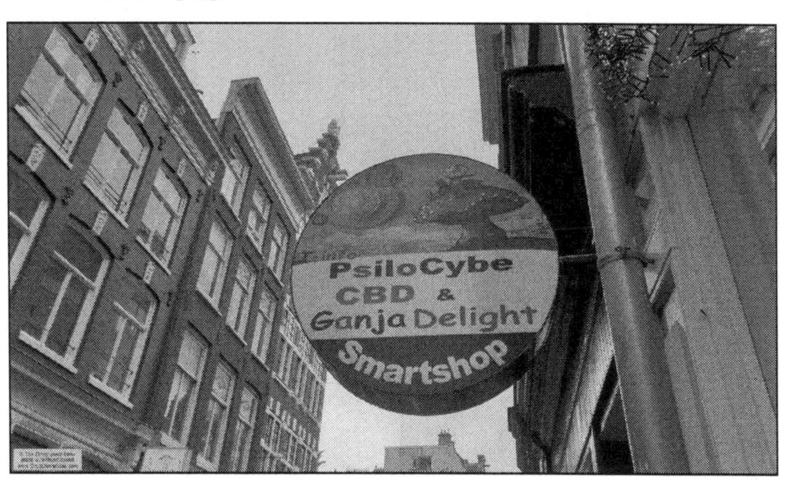

Smartshop signage, Oude Hoogstraat

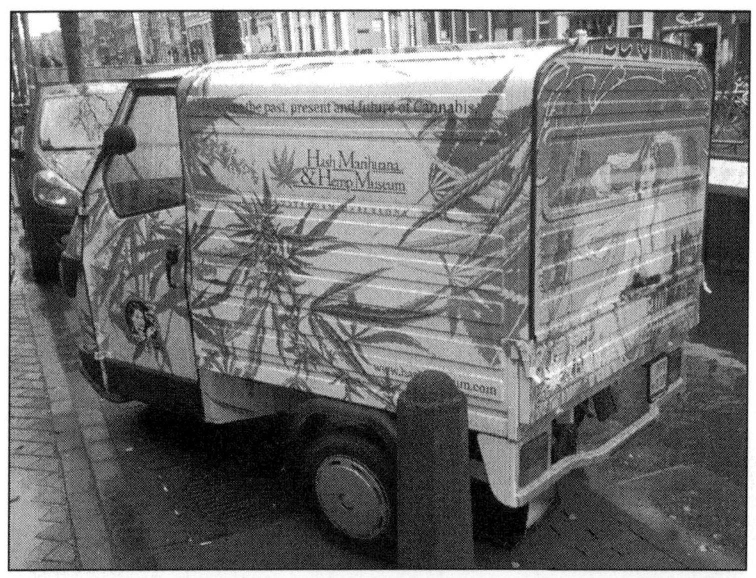

Mobile advertising

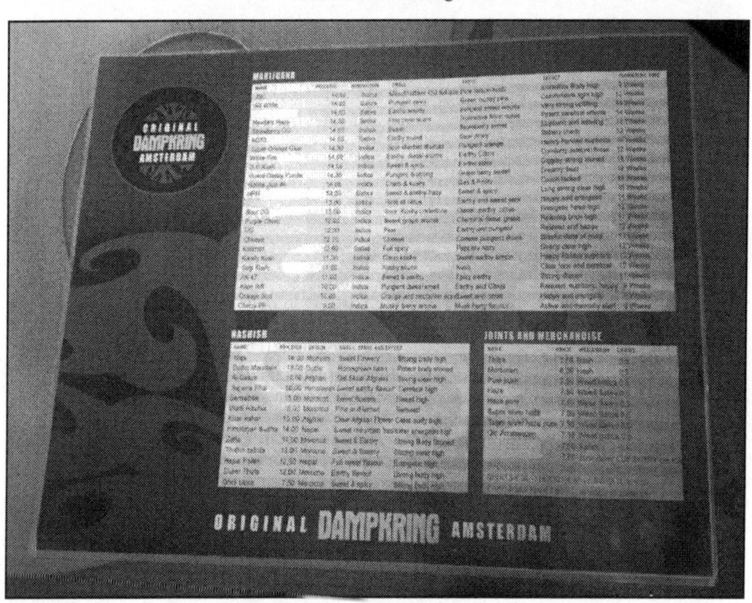

Original Dampkring coffeeshop menu

AN ANECDOTAL TALE (AMSTERDAM)
Sometimes in our drug-paranoid culture, events transpire and can take a bizarre twist. An example occurred when I found myself at Schiphol Airport, Amsterdam, with a couple of joints in my pocket.

My schedule was to fly to Asia to research for four days, before returning to Schipol, where I would be stuck for 6 hours prior to flying out again.

I was therefore confronted with the question of what to do with the joints, given that taking them with me was out of the question.

My bright idea was to bury them in a plant pot outside the airport terminal building, so that I could collect them on return, and smoke them during my tedious layover, passing the time more enjoyably. I found this little beauty just outside a door, and thrust the water protected goodies under the soil, on the right hand side.

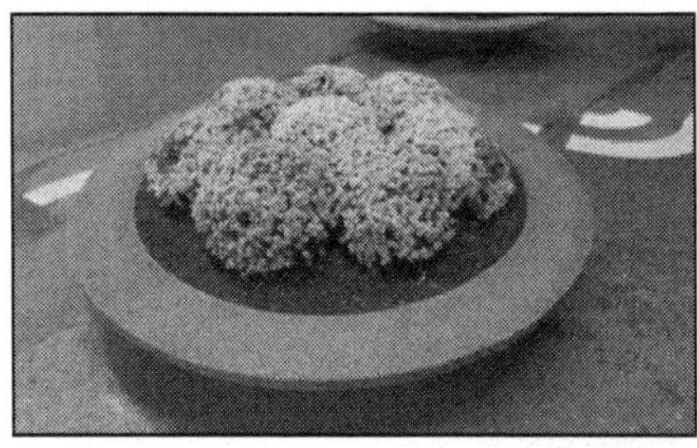

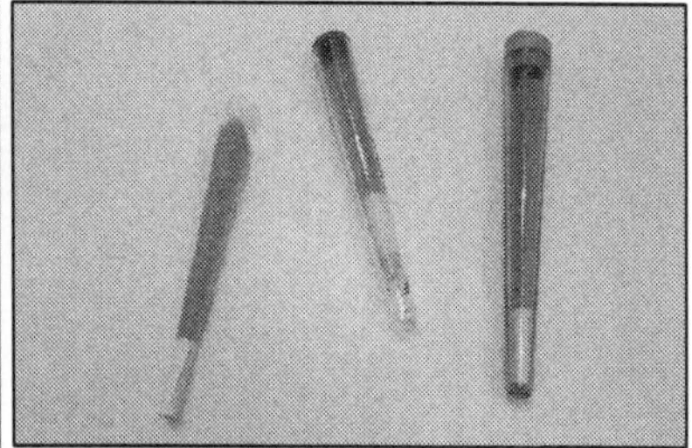

I then happily flew off to complete my mission.

On return, I was greeted with an appalling sight.

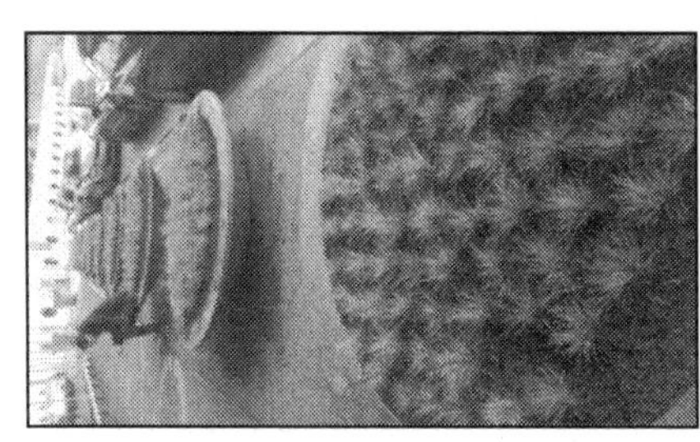

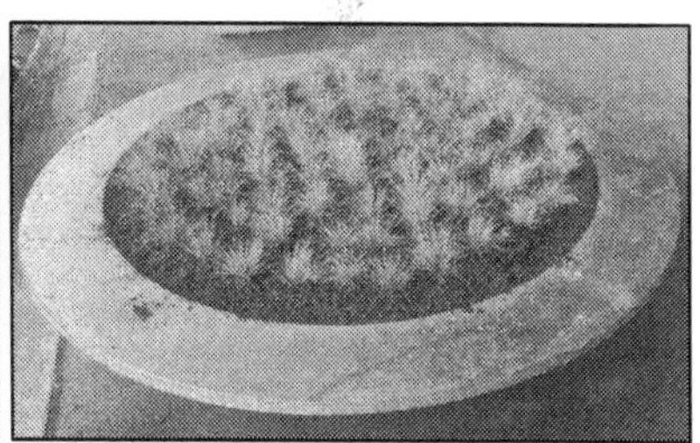

Yes, horror of horrors, in just four days, the airport had uprooted everything, including my joints, and replaced them with bland green vegetation.

Those hours passed particularly slowly.

4.5.2 Global Snapshots

NINE MILE, JAMAICA
Whilst cannabis is now legally available in many parts of the world, Nine Mile carries a special vibe and is without doubt an iconic drug destination. Also see the references in the cannabis entry in this book.

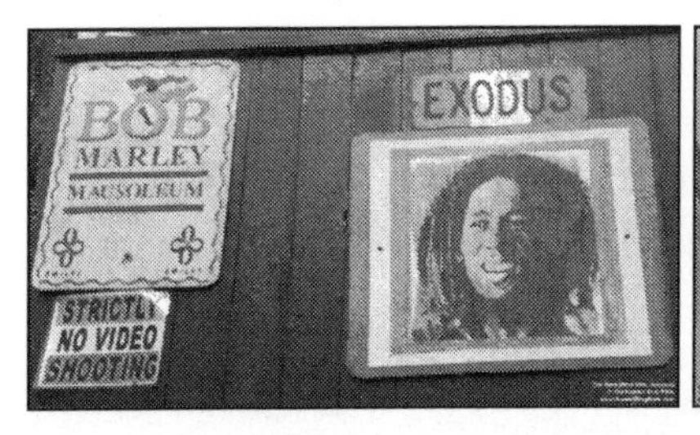

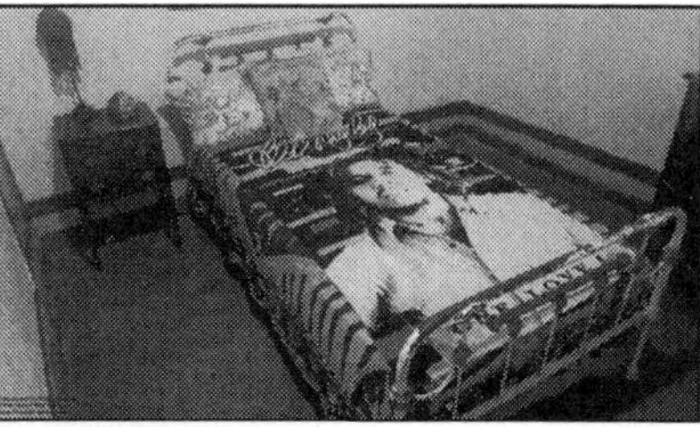

MANDALAY, MYANMAR / CHAING MAI THAILAND
Betel nuts were the name of the game here, particularly in Mandalay, where street vendors were a common sight.

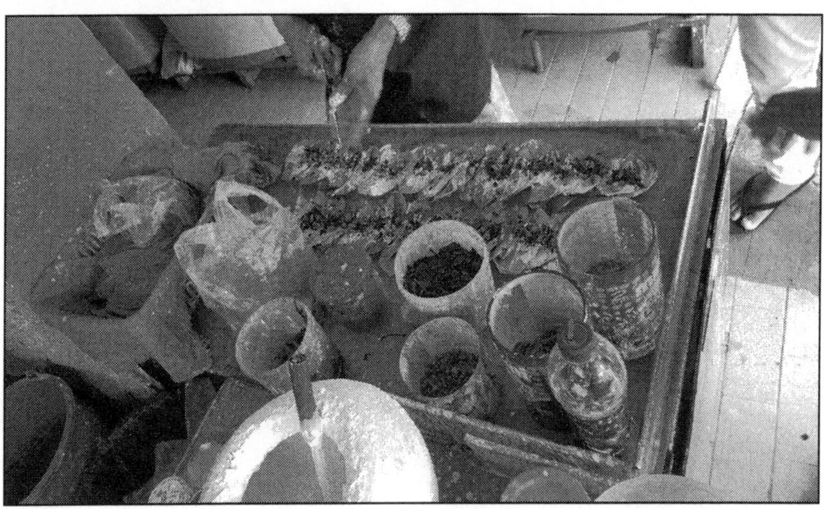

CUSCO PERU
A number of Peruvian cities, including Cusco and Iquitos, are local embarkation points for the ayahuasca experience, for the ceremonial use of the san pedro cactus (huachuma), and for other related adventures.

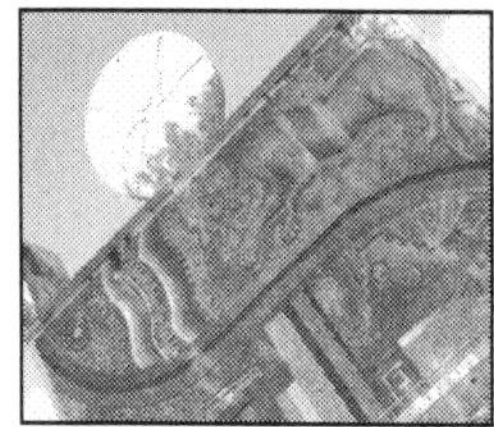

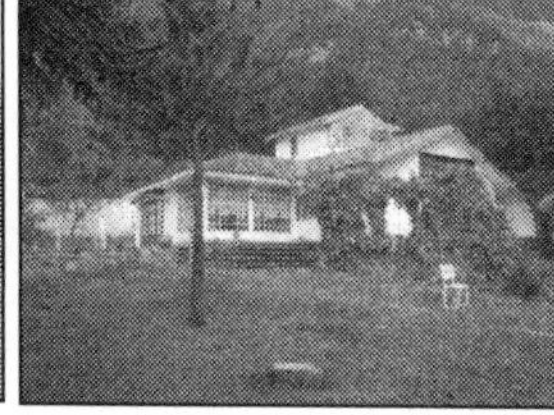

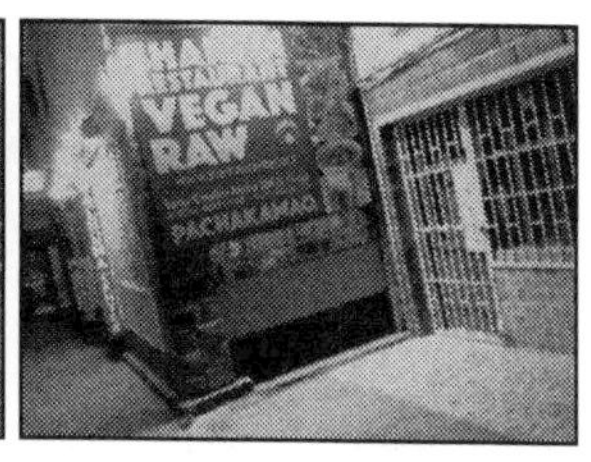

MANCHESTER, UK
When *legal highs* were in fact legal (in the UK), Manchester's head shop was located in its bohemian district, the Northern Quarter. Those were the days; or something along those lines.

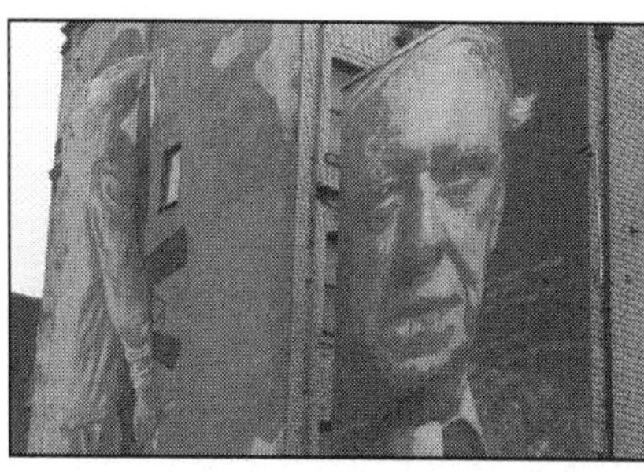

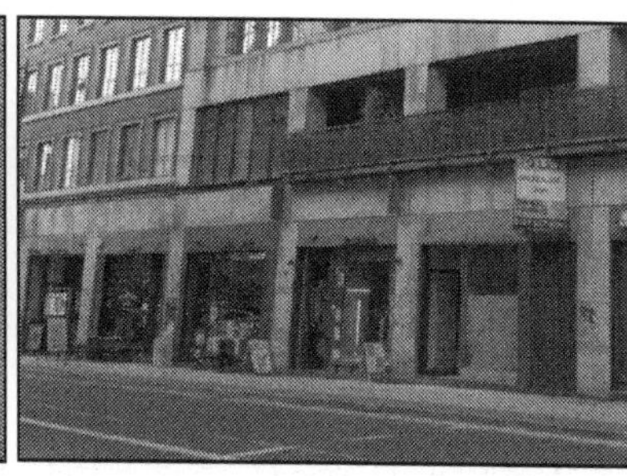

SOUTH EAST ASIA
Although this is no longer a place to engage, due to particularly barbaric drug policies, I managed to sneak in a magic mushroom experience whilst they were still legal. During their heyday they were not only sold openly, but were glaringly advertised.

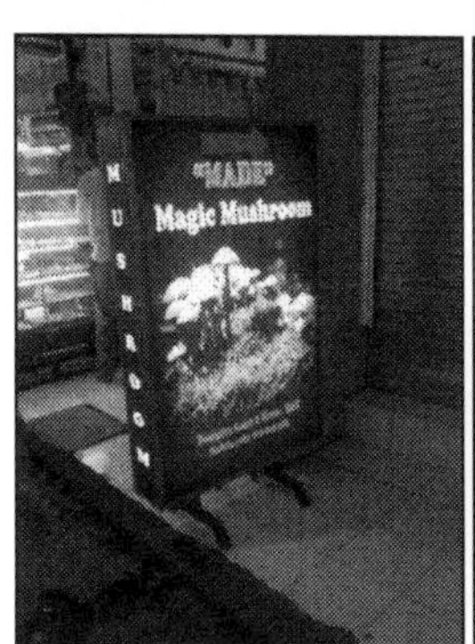

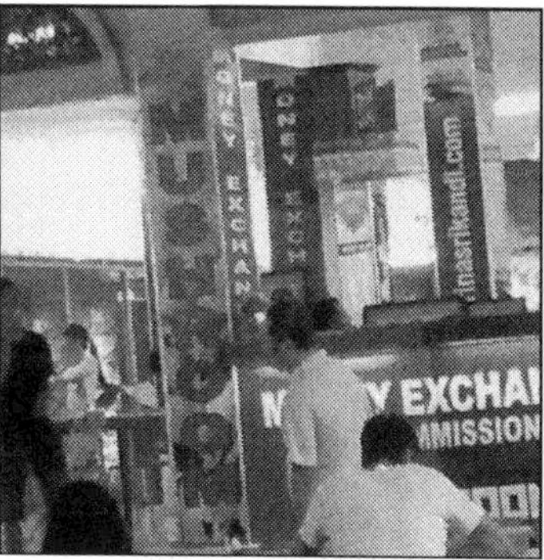

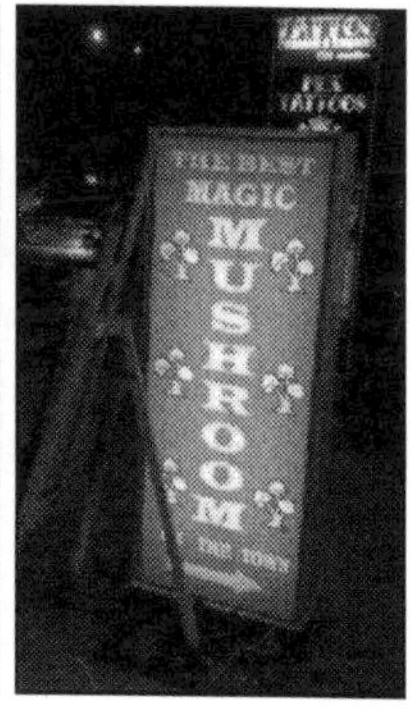

I took photographs relating to my drug exploits in many other locations, and indeed, some of these are dotted throughout this book. As this is not a photo album, however, I will refrain from including any more here, but will post a wider selection online or perhaps in a subsequent work.

THE HIPPIE TRAIL

The Hippie Trail was one of the most famed international travel routes of the last century. It was a journey undertaken by members of the hippie counterculture, largely from the mid 60s to the mid-late 70s.

Start points were major cities in Western Europe, notably London and Amsterdam. The route meandered overland to northern India, where it branched into a variety of end-points, including Goa, Kathmandu, Bangkok and Sri Lanka. Unfortunately, in practical terms, much of the trail is now inaccessible, not least Afghanistan, Iran and the Indian/Pakistani border.

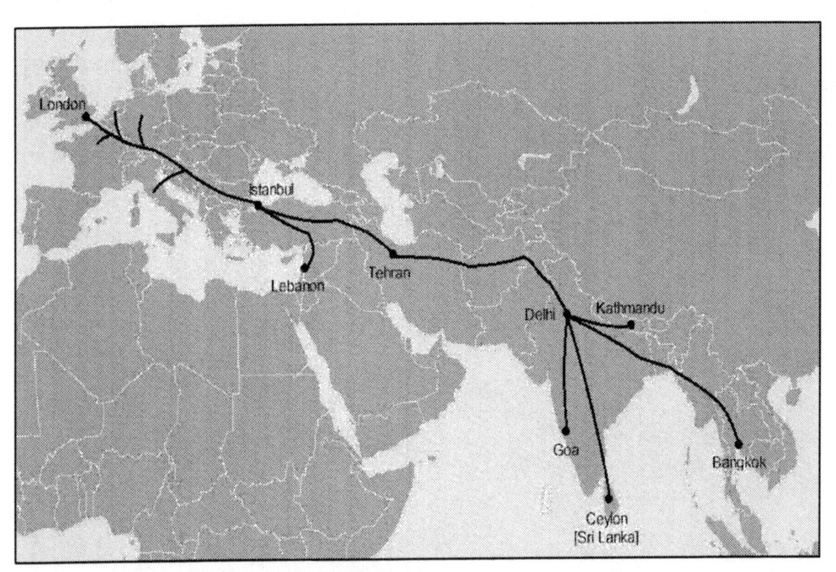

The hippie lifestyle often embraced drugs, particularly psychedelics and hashish, and most of these locations offered an abundance, certainly of the latter. The drugs have now largely gone, at least in terms of their legal use, but the hippies left a cultural mark on many of these places which still exists today.

There is no doubt that the Hippie Trail retains a unique place in historical drug folklore. The following photographs were taken at some of the most fabled and iconic destinations.

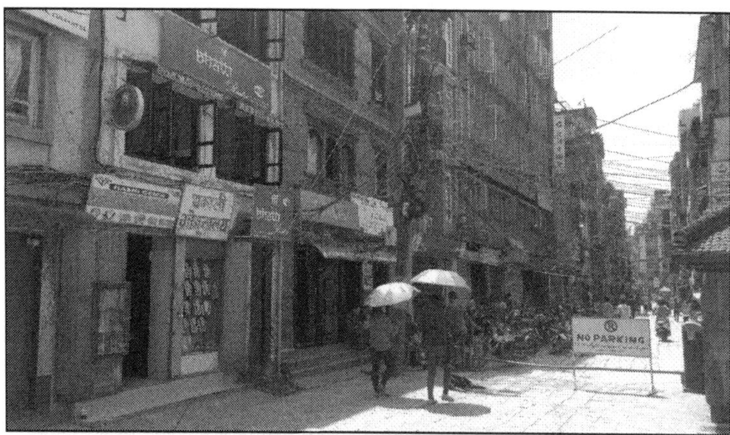

Freak Street, Kathmandu

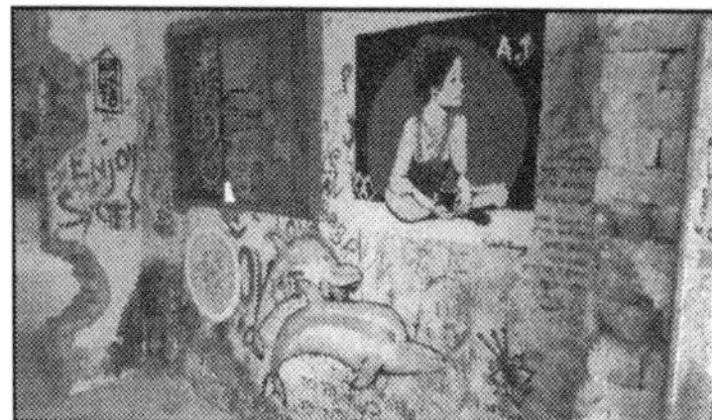

The Beatles Cathedral, Rishikesh

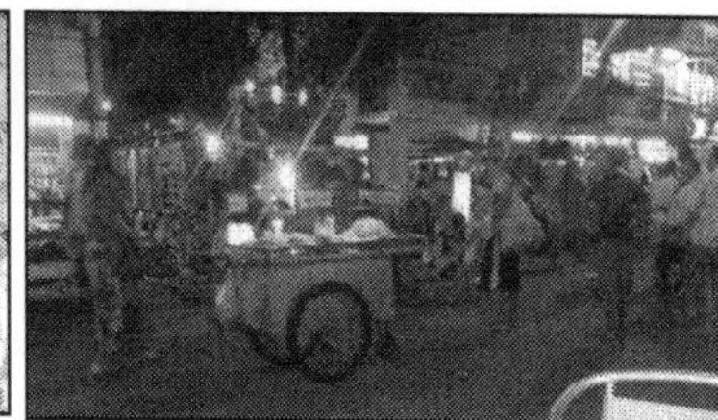

Khao San Road, Bangkok

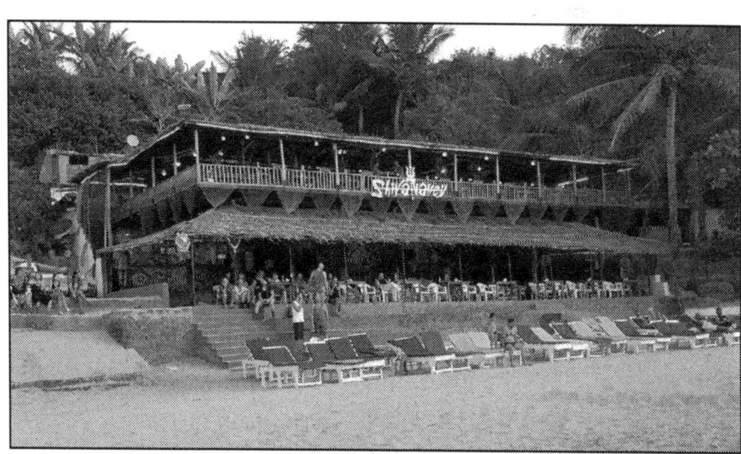

Shiva Valley, Goa

4.6 CULTURE & SOCIETY (REFERENCE)

The impact of drugs and drug use on modern culture is profound. As subject matter, drugs have been integral to some of the most highly acclaimed examples of their genre. Equally, some of the finest works ever created have been inspired by the drug experience itself. Whilst I cannot possibly do justice to this aspect over just a handful of pages, I will attempt to scratch its surface.

Within this canopy, I will also present some ideas for psychedelic exploration, and offer a more traditional book reference and reading list, which I hope will be of value.

4.6.1 Art, Film, Literature, Music

As we are deep into subjective territory here, instead of rattling off my personal opinion, I will furnish selected lists of prominent and well known artists and works, which may stimulate interest or deliberation.

MOVIES
Some are about drugs; some are inspired by drugs; some have themes which are undeniably linked to drugs; some are frequently claimed to be best watched whilst experiencing drugs:

Fear and Loathing in Las Vegas (1998)
Trainspotting (1996)
The Wall (1982)
Limitless (2011)
The Matrix (1999)
Enter the Void (2009)
Lucy (2014)
Pulp Fiction (1994)
Midnight Express (1978)
Requiem for a Dream (2000)
John Dies At The End (2011)
Waking Life (2001)
Naked Lunch (1991)
Dredd (2012)
Altered States (1980)
Crystal Fairy & the Magical Cactus (2013)
Embrace of the Serpent (2015)
Mr Nice (2010)
The Mule (2018)
The Doors (1991)
Blow (2001)
The Beatles: Yellow Submarine (1968)

PROPAGANDA MOVIES
These may appear to be ridiculous now, but propaganda in more sophisticated forms is still in full flow.

The Cocaine Fiends (1935)
Marihuana (1936)
Reefer Madness (1936)
The Road To Ruin (1934)
She Shoulda Said No! (1949)
Devil's Harvest (1942)
Assassin of Youth (1937)
Human Wreckage (1923)

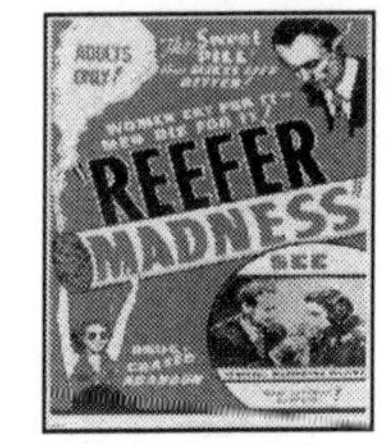

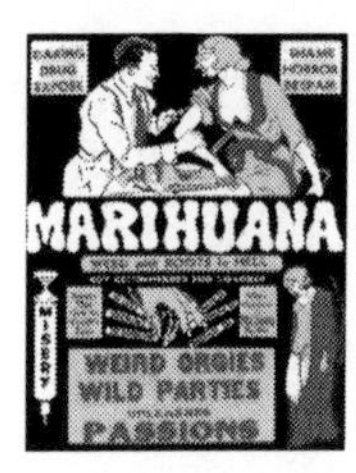

See Section 1.1

MUSIC COMPOSITIONS

Some of these selections are psychedelic in nature (particularly interesting to listen to whilst tripping) whilst others are (sometimes reputably) about drugs or the effects of drugs. A difficulty I encountered in constructing this list was the sheer number of compositions to choose from. If I have missed your favourite artist or recording, I apologise.

- The Beatles [Tomorrow Never Knows, Dr Robert, Various]
- Pink Floyd [Various]
- Jefferson Airplane [White Rabbit, Various]
- The Bonzo Dog Doo-Dah Band [I'm The Urban Spaceman]
- Cypress Hill [Hits From The Bong, Dr. Greenthumb; Various]
- Bob Marley [Various]
- The Clash [Hateful, Koka Kola]
- David Bowie [Ashes to Ashes]
- Amy Winehouse [Addicted, Rehab]
- Rolling Stones [Sister Morphine, Mother's Little Helper]
- Space Time Continuum With Terence McKenna [Alien Dreamtime]
- 1200 Micrograms [1200 Micrograms]
- Dudley Perkins [Sally]
- Lil Peep [Various]
- Shpongle [Various]
- Afroman [Because I Got High]
- The Stranglers [Golden Brown]
- Grateful Dead [Various]
- Eric Clapton [Cocaine]
- Lil Wayne [Various]
- Louis Armstrong [Muggles]
- CASisDEAD [Various]
- Peter Tosh [Legalize It]
- Green Day [Brain Stew, Geek Stink Breath]
- She Drew The Gun [Pit Pony, Various]
- Jimi Hendrix [Purple Haze]
- The Velvet Underground [Heroin]
- Mötley Crüe [Dr. Feelgood]
- Andy Fairweather-Low [Wide Eyed and Legless]
- Nine Inch Nails [Hurt]
- Eric Clapton [Cocaine]
- D12 [Purple Pills, These Drugs]
- Johnny Cash [Cocaine Blues]
- U2 [Bad]
- Blur [Beetlebum]
- The Doors [Break On Through To The Other Side]
- Oasis [Morning Glory]
- Tom Petty [Girl On LSD]
- Lil Whyte [Oxy Cotton]
- The Verve [The Drugs Don't Work]
- Junkhead [Alice in Chains]
- Marco A. Restrepo [Sally & Me]
- Black Sabbath [Sweet Leaf, Snowblind]
- Guns N' Roses [Mr Brownstone]
- GrandMaster Flash [White Lines]
- Neil Young [The Needle And The Damage Done]
- Red Hot Chili Peppers [Snow (Hey Oh)]
- Placebo [Special K]
- Eminem [Drug Ballad]
- Tame Impala [Various]
- Danny Brown [Kush Coma]
- Led Zeppelin [Misty Mountain Hop]
- Moody Blues [Legend of a Mind]
- Janis Joplin [Mary Jane]
- Lady Gaga [Mary Jane Holland]
- Rush [A Passage to Bangkok]
- Snoop Dogg [Smokin' Smokin' Weed]
- Jackson Browne [Cocaine]
- Savoy Brown [Needle and Spoon]
- Cheech and Chong [Up in Smoke]

PSYCHEDELIC ARTISTS
If you are an art enthusiast you will already have your own favourites. I will, therefore, simply reproduce the names of relevant artists, which I have culled from Wikipedia and other sources, some of which you may be unfamiliar with.

Pablo Amaringo	William Finn	Peter Max
Chris Dyer	The Fool (collective)	Stanley "Mouse" Miller
David Barnes	Ernst Fuchs	Victor Moscoso
Doug Binder	Bob Gibson	Vali Myers
Brummbaer	H. R. Giger	Michael Saunders
Mark Boyle & Joan Hills	Terry Gilliam	Martin Sharp
Laurence Caruana	Alex Grey	Gilbert Shelton
James Clifford	Rick Griffin	Grace Slick
Lee Conklin	Gary Grimshaw	Harold Thornton
Robert Crumb	Leif Podhajsky	Vernon Treweeke
Roger Dean	John Hurford	John Van Hamersveld
Warren Dayton	Alton Kelley	David Vaughan
Scott Draves	Mati Klarwein	Louis Wain
Donald Dunbar	Oleg A. Korolev	Robert Williams
M. C. Escher	Abby Martin	Wes Wilson
Karl Ferris	Bob Masse	Andy Warhol
Giorgio de Chirico	George Atherton	David Normal
Andrew (Android) Jones	Mario Martinez	Amanda Sage
Justin Guse	Fabián Jiménez	Cameron Gray

POETRY & LITERATURE
This is a starter list of the names I ran across whilst searching for psychedelic and drug related poetry and literature. For a number, their contribution(s) on this subject constituted a minority of their output, and equally, some are better known in other spheres. Note that I claim no particular expertise or knowledge in this area.

Allen Ginsberg	Howard Marks
Samuel Taylor Coleridge	Fitz Hugh Ludlow
William Blake	Rudolph Wurlitzer
Timothy Leary	Kaveh Akbar
William S Burroughs	Aleister Crowley
Aldous Huxley	Thomas Pynchon
Hunter S Thompson	Tao Lin
Thomas De Quincey	Philip K. Dick
Charles Baudelaire	Henri Michaux
Jack Kerouac	Thaddeus Golas

COSTUME
According to Wikipedia, "*Costume is the distinctive style of dress of an individual or group that reflects their class, gender, profession, ethnicity, nationality, activity or epoch*". So what costume is distinctive to drug users? Given that drug users form part of every social group this is a tricky one. However, if any, perhaps psychedelic and/or hippie type clothing is more synonymous with drug use than any other.

STREET ART
This form is certainly a personal favourite of mine. It's free and it's available in every major city. Random examples from my travels follow.

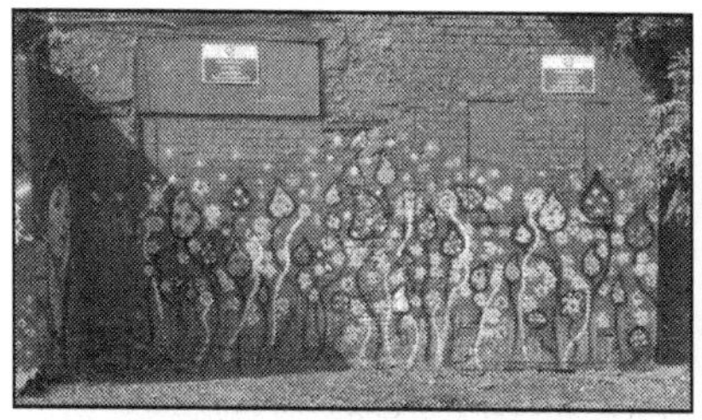

Manchester Mushrooms

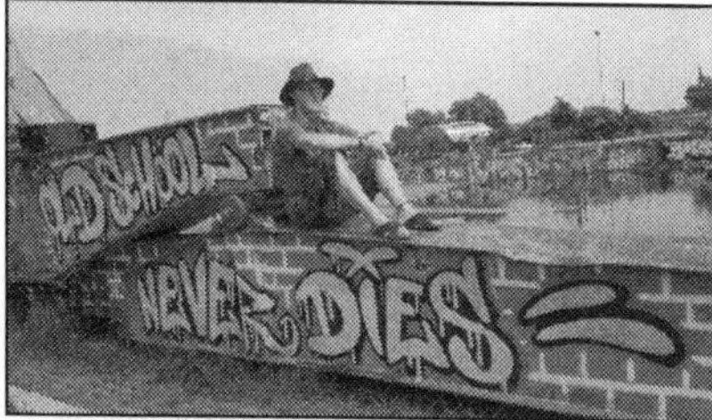

NDSM, Amsterdam

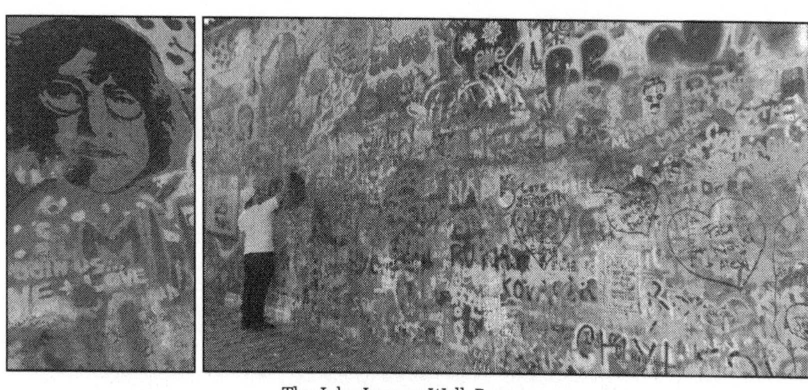

The John Lennon Wall, Prague

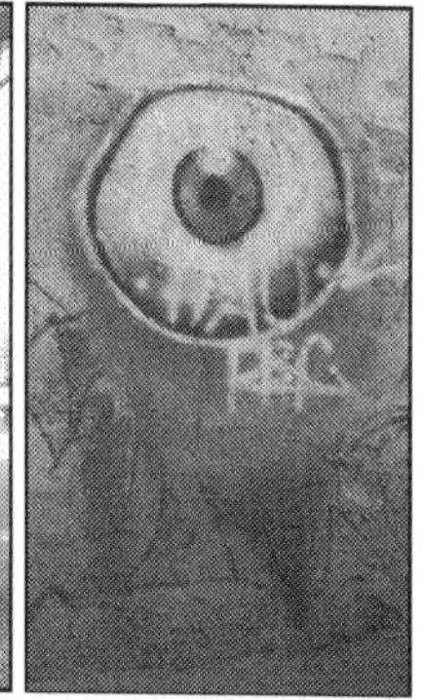

Ping River, Chiang Mai

QUOTATION
Celebrities and cultural icons have long commented on drugs and drug use. A collection of some of the most well known quotes is presented below. For quotes specific to psychedelics see the introduction to Section 2.2.

"I don't do drugs. I am drugs." ~ Salvador Dali

"Drugs are a bet with your mind." ~ Jim Morrison

"I have absolutely no pleasure in the stimulants in which I sometimes so madly indulge. It has not been in the pursuit of pleasure that I have periled life and reputation and reason. It has been the desperate attempt to escape from torturing memories, from a sense of insupportable loneliness and a dread of some strange impending doom." ~ Edgar Allan Poe

"It's not a war on drugs, it's a war on personal freedom." ~ Bill Hicks

"If you want to understand a society, take a good look at the drugs it uses. And what can this tell you about American culture? Well, look at the drugs we use. Except for pharmaceutical poison, there are essentially only two drugs that Western civilization tolerates: Caffeine from Monday to Friday to energize you enough to make you a productive member of society, and alcohol from Friday to Monday to keep you too stupid to figure out the prison that you are living in." ~ Bill Hicks

"Marijuana is self-punishing. It makes you acutely sensitive, and in this world, what worse punishment could there be?" ~ P. J. O'Rourke

"No drug, not even alcohol, causes the fundamental ills of society. If we're looking for the sources of our troubles, we shouldn't test people for drugs, we should test them for stupidity, ignorance, greed and love of power." ~ P. J. O'Rourke

"I used to have a drug problem, now I make enough money." ~ David Lee Roth

"When you smoke the herb, it reveals you to yourself." ~ Bob Marley

"Herb is the healing of a nation, alcohol is the destruction." ~Bob Marley

"I'm very fond of drugs." Grace Slick

"Don't do drugs because if you do drugs you'll go to prison, and drugs are really expensive in prison." ~John Hardwick

"Reality is a crutch for people who can't cope with drugs." ~Lily Tomlin

"Cocaine is God's way of saying you're making too much money." ~Robin Williams

"I hate to advocate drugs, alcohol, violence or insanity to anyone, but they've always worked for me." ~ Hunter S. Thompson"

"*That is not a drug, it's a leaf.*" ~ Arnold Schwarzenegger

"*I've never had a problem with drugs. I've had problems with the police.*" ~ Keith Richards

"*To put someone in jail for using drugs in the privacy of his hotel room is just barbaric.*" ~ Danny Sugerman

"*Fck the drug war. Dropping acid was a profound turning point for me, a seminal experience. I make no apologies for it. More people should do acid. It should be sold over the counter.*" ~ George Carlin

"*Psychedelic drugs don't change you, they don't change your character, unless you want to be changed. They enable change; they can't impose it.*" ~ Alexander Shulgin

"*I'm called the Godfather because I published for the first time information about its effects in man. I feel content with the title. MDMA is a beautiful drug.*" ~ Alexander Shulgin

"*I think pot should be legal. I don't smoke it, but I like the smell of it.*" ~ Andy Warhol

"*I drifted into heroin because as a kid growing up everybody told me, 'don't smoke marijuana, it will kill you.'*" ~ Irvine Welsh

"*I didn't inhale.*" ~ Bill Clinton

"*When I was a kid I inhaled frequently. That was the point.*" ~ Barack Obama

"*The illegality of cannabis is outrageous, an impediment to full utilization of a drug which helps produce the serenity and insight, sensitivity and fellowship so desperately needed in this increasingly mad and dangerous world.*" ~ Carl Sagan

"*Sex and drugs and rock and roll.*" ~ Ian Dury

"*If you lock someone up for smoking a plant that makes them happy, then you're the fcking criminal.*" ~ Joe Rogan

"*Which is better: to have fun with fungi or to have Idiocy with ideology, to have wars because of words, to have tomorrow's misdeeds out of yesterday's miscreeds?*" ~ Aldous Huxley

"*I say no to drugs, but they don't listen.*" ~ Marilyn Manson

"*Our national drug is alcohol. We tend to regard the use of any other drug with special horror.*" ~ William S. Burroughs

"*A drug is not bad. A drug is a chemical compound. The problem comes in when people who take drugs treat them like a license to behave like an asshole.*" ~ Frank Zappa

4.6.2 Food For The Psychedelic Mind

If you wish to explore and are stuck for places to start:

Terence McKenna. Head directly to YouTube and find everything from his '*Stoned Ape Theory*' to his explanation of the meaning of the '*I Ching*'. It is impossible to do justice to him in a brief introduction, but the breadth of his psychedelic subject matter, his astonishing yet plausible theories and his unparalleled eloquence have rightly elevated him to the status of legend.

Robert Anton Wilson. As referred to in the first section, his contributions to Leary's *Eight-Circuit Model* are singularly instructive. There is one interview in particular worth looking out for, which is published under a variety of titles, including '*Techniques of Consciousness Change*' and '*8 Circuit Psychology*'.

Quantum Physics. Have you seen the three *Dr Quantum* video clips from the '*What the Bleep Do We Know!?*' documentary? These are essential viewing if you are unfamiliar with '*The Double Slit Experiment*' and '*Entanglement*', both of which are fundamental building blocks in the understanding of consciousness and the construct of perceived reality.

This is also an exceptionally good documentary to watch as a whole. Are you far enough down the rabbit hole yet?

Morphic Resonance. Check out Dr Rupert Sheldrake's theory, and its potential application to consciousness.
["*Morphic resonance is a process whereby self-organising systems inherit a memory from previous similar systems. In its most general formulation, morphic resonance means that the so-called laws of nature are more like habits. The hypothesis of morphic resonance also leads to a radically new interpretation of memory storage in the brain and of biological inheritance. Memory need not be stored in material traces inside brains, which are more like TV receivers than video recorders, tuning into influences from the past. And biological inheritance need not all be coded in the genes, or in epigenetic modifications of the genes; much of it depends on morphic resonance from previous members of the species. Thus each individual inherits a collective memory from past members of the species, and also contributes to the collective memory, affecting other members of the species in the future.*"]

This becomes particularly relevant when developed alongside other theories and ideas. One example: given that optical illusions demonstrate a form of pattern recognition and that this occurs across the other senses too, the mind is in some ways a pattern recognition engine. Applying this to memory, your memories may be yours (rather than collective) because the morphic pattern of your last moment fits your own last moment better than anyone else's last moment. Ditto the moment before, and the moment before that, etc. You thus *co-ordinate a point-of-view* (this is a *McKenna-ism:* check *complexity* and his 'final earthbound interview') from the morphic field, and essentially experience your individual perspective.

Dr John Hagelin. Search and find his eloquent and informative lectures explaining quantum mechanics in understandable terms, which he further links to consciousness itself via the unified field.

<u>Dennis McKenna</u>. Terence McKenna's brother, for this quote alone:
"All experience is a drug experience. Whether it's mediated by our own [endogenous] drugs, or whether it's mediated by substances that we ingest that are found in plants, cognition, consciousness, the working of the brain, it's all a chemically mediated process. Life itself is a drug experience."

<u>The CIA</u>. Eyeball this, remembering that this IS the CIA:
["This is an aspect of quantum mechanics which applies to the fact that any oscillating frequency(such as a brainwave) reaches two points of complete rest which constitute the boundaries of each individual oscillation(i.e. movement up or down). Without these points of rest, an oscillating wave pattern would be impossible since the points of rest are required to permit the energy to change direction and thus continue vibrating between rigid limits. But it is also true that when, for an infinitesimally brief instant, that energy reaches one of its two points of rest it "clicks out" of time-space and joins infinity(see Exhibit 3, next page). That critical step out of time-space occurs when the speed of the oscillation drops below 10-33 centimeters per second(Planck's Distance). To use the words of Bentov: 11 ... quantum mechanics tell us that when distances go below Planck's Distance, which is 10-33 CM, we enter, in effect, a new worid.11 To return to our case in point, the human consciousness wave pattern reaches such high frequency that the pattern of "clickouts" comes so close together that there is virtual continuity in it. Then, a portion of that consciousness is actually postulated to establish and maintain its information collection function in those dimensions located between time-space and the Absolute. Thus, as the alrhost continuous "clickout" pattern establishes itself in continuous phase at speeds below Planck's Distance but before reaching the state of total rest, human consciousness passes through the looking glass of time7space after the fashion of Alice beginning her journey into wonderland. The Gateway experience, with its associated Hemi-Sync technique, is apparently designed, if used systematically and patiently, to enable human consciousness to establish a coherent pattern of perception in those dimensions where speeds below Planck's distance apply. This holds true irrespective of whether the individual is exercising his consciousness while in his physical body or whether he is doing so after having separated that consciousness from the physical body(i.e. the so called out-of-body state mentioned earlier)."]

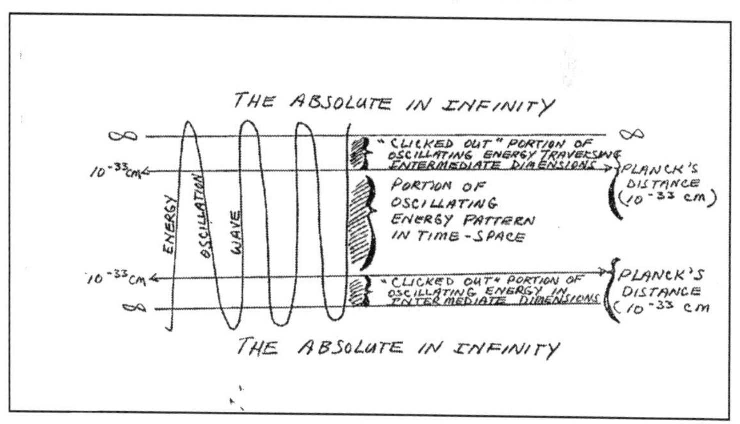

Read the full PDF [CIA-RDP96-00788R001700210016-5] here:
https://www.cia.gov/library/readingroom/docs/CIA-RDP96-00788R001700210016-5.pdf

The Dalai Lama. Buddhism? Meditation? Enlightenment? This Dalai Lama quote is undoubtedly a truism: "*Broadly speaking, although there are some differences, I think Buddhist philosophy and Quantum Mechanics can shake hands on their view of the world.*" It is worth seeking out more.

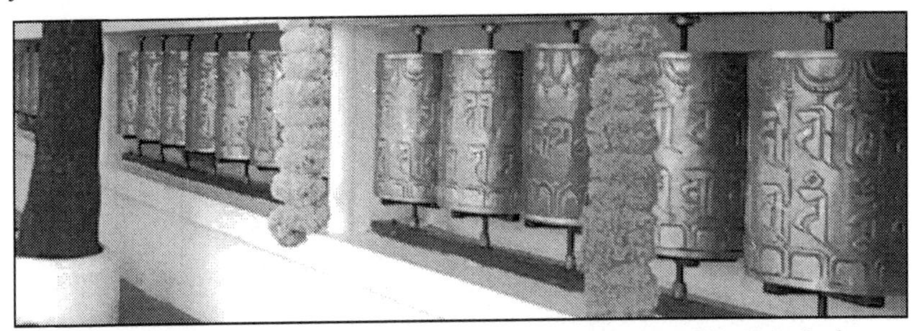

I took this photograph in the Dalai Lama's Temple (McLeod Ganj, India). Each wheel contains thousands of Avalokiteshvara mantras "*OM MANI PADME HUM*"

If you are unfamiliar, there is more to this than you might think.

Samadhi. Along similar lines there is an excellent video on YouTube called Samadhi, This comes in four parts, Part 1 being "*Maya, the Illusion of the Self*". It is definitely worth finding the time for.

Documentaries. Internet search can be your friend. There are countless documentaries to be found on the psychedelics themselves (both botanical and chemical), pioneering individuals (like Shulgin, Einstein and Hoffman) and on a vast array of related topics (such as space-time and relativity).

Finally Here is something to dwell upon: aren't all these great names fundamentally saying the same thing?

> Buddha: "*The past is already gone, the future is not yet here. There's only one moment for you to live, and that is the present moment*"
>
> Lao Tzu: "*If you are depressed you are living in the past. If you are anxious you are living in the future. If you are at peace you are living in the present*"
>
> Eckart Tolle: "*The Power of Now*"
>
> Terence McKenna: "*The felt presence of immediate experience – this is all you know. Everything else comes as unconfirmed rumour.*"
>
> Alan Watt: "*I have realized that the past and future are real illusions, that they exist in the present, which is what there is and all there is*"
>
> Ram Dass: "*Be Here Now*".

The Last Word. As fascinating as all this is, don't spend all your trip time engrossed in it. If you are able to, go outside (safely) and integrate with nature.

4.6.3 Books & Reference

ESSENTIAL REFERENCE
I consider these to be essential works for any wide ranging study of psychoactive materials. Collectively, they document and describe many hundreds of chemicals and botanicals, and were invaluable research sources during the writing of this book. All are still in print and readily available.

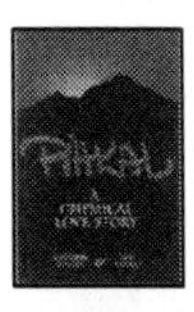

PiHKAL: A Chemical Love Story
[Alexander Shulgin and Ann Shulgin]

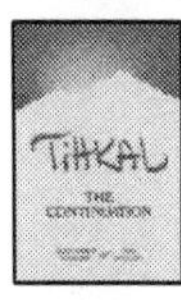

TiHKAL: The Continuation
[Alexander Shulgin and Ann Shulgin]

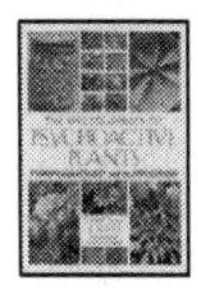

The Encyclopedia of Psychoactive Plants: Ethnopharmacology and Its Applications
[Christian Rätsch]

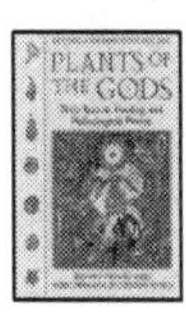

Plants of the Gods: Their Sacred, Healing, and Hallucinogenic Powers
[Richard Evans Schultes, Albert Hofmann, Christian Rätsch]

FURTHER READING
Amongst the other books and guides which were consulted or read are the following, some of which are undoubtedly classics in this field.

Food Of The Gods: The Search for the Original Tree of Knowledge: A Radical History of Plants, Drugs and Human Evolution
[Terence McKenna]

DMT: The Spirit Molecule: A Doctor's Revolutionary Research into the Biology of Near-Death and Mystical Experiences
[Rick Strassman M.D]

Hallucinogenic Plants
[Richard Evans Schultes]

Psychedelics Encyclopedia
[Peter Stafford]

The Doors Of Perception
[Aldus Huxley]

The Ayahuasca Test Pilots Handbook: The Essential Guide to Ayahuasca Journeying
[Christopher S. Kilham]

High Times Encyclopedia of Recreational Drugs
[High Times]

The Psychedelic Experience: A Manual Based on the Tibetan Book of the Dead
[Ralph Metzner, Richard Alpert, Timothy Leary]

Cooking With Cannabis
[Adam Gottlieb]

Legal Highs
[Adam Gottlieb]

True Hallucinations: Being an Account of the Author's Extraordinary Adventures in the Devil's Paradise
[Terence McKenna]

The Archaic Revival: Speculations on Psychedelic Mushrooms, the Amazon, Virtual Reality, UFOs, Evolution, Shamanism, the Rebirth of the Goddess
[Terence K. McKenna]

Prometheus Rising
[Robert Anton Wilson]

Drugs - Without the Hot Air
[David Nutt]

Buzzed: The Straight Facts About the Most Used and Abused Drugs from Alcohol to Ecstasy
[Cynthia Kuhn, Scott Swartzwelder, Wilkie Wilson, Leigh Heather Wilson, Jeremy Foster]

Brief History of Drugs: From the Stone Age to the Stoned Age
[Antonio Escohotado]

LSD My Problem Child: Reflections on Sacred Drugs, Mysticism and Science
[Albert Hofmann]

The Psychedelic Explorer's Guide: Safe, Therapeutic, and Sacred Journeys
[James Fadiman Ph.D]

3-MeO-2'-oxo-PCE: A Multidisciplinary MXE Analysis
[Vortech]

4.7 CONFESSIONS OF A LAB RAT

4.7.1 Q&A

The following are the subjective opinions of the author of this book, given in response to questions framed by the proof reader.

Q. Which drugs have you found to be the most interesting and the most beneficial to your personal development?

A. As a class, psychedelics, without question. For me, in the following order, as influenced by set and setting: Ayahuasca; 1p-LSD; San Pedro Cactus; Mushrooms; DMT. I feel that these were of enormous benefit, in much the same way as is already articulated by others. They bestowed a wider perspective, a greater understanding of the nature of consciousness, an awareness of oneness and connectedness, and so forth. I think they made me a kinder and better person.

Q. Which drugs have you enjoyed most recreationally?

A. In terms of basic physical stimulation and high, amphetamine. It comes at a high cost, however, which is why I only used it twice. My brain subsequently felt like a car which had had all the oil sucked out of it. I felt drained, for days.

Ephenidine is worth a reference too, because at a low dose it delivered both recreation and insight. Ketamine, cannabis, kava, and mephedrone are also worthy of honourable mentions, although it's difficult to be exclusive.

Q. What was the best drug for chemsex?

The experience differs significantly from class to class. I would suggest that certain stims (particularly amphetamines) produce the most prolonged intensive orgasmic pleasure. Cannabis helps you to get lost in the moment and flow with it. At lower doses some psychedelics can take you to a different place, and enhance sensitivity. Empathogens tend to take a similar path, with a more muted headspace, but hardly surprisingly attach to empathy.

I would offer some caution though. It is important to bear in mind that judgement is often impaired, and that events can develop quickly and potentially without due consideration. If applicable it is probably not the best idea for a single party to heavily engage whilst the other(s) doesn't. Equally, parameters should be agreed beforehand.

I would again re-enforce the commentary I make under the entry for methamphetamine, including with respect to relationships and addiction. Finally, the compound stress of sex and drugs on the body should also be contemplated. See Section 1.3.4 of this book.

Q. What is the worst experience you have had?

A. The terrifying delirium of nutmeg, many years ago, and the paranoia and trauma of a couple of the modern cannabinoids. All were horrendous.

Q. Have you ever suffered an addiction?

A. No. Alcohol is the only drug I have consumed too regularly.

Q. Is there anything you wish you had never taken?

A. If anything, alcohol. At least the bad experiences I mentioned with respect to other drugs were once-only situations, which affected no other person. Alcohol, being presented socially at every turn, is a repeat self-abuser, and it induces behaviour which affects others, often adversely. I have done many stupid things under the influence of alcohol, which I regret, but this almost certainly applies to most people.

Q. Have you ever been arrested?

A. No.

Q. What is your opinion of the *war on drugs*?

A. I consider it to be a war on humanity, initially declared by a man who was guilty of many crimes against humanity, Richard Nixon. When considering the *war on drugs*, it is always worth bearing in mind the words of Nixon's domestic policy chief, John Ehrlichman. I will quote the piece, as reported by CNN.

> *"You understand what I'm saying? We knew we couldn't make it illegal to be either against the war or black, but by getting the public to associate the hippies with marijuana and blacks with heroin. And then criminalizing both heavily, we could disrupt those communities," Ehrlichman said. "We could arrest their leaders, raid their homes, break up their meetings, and vilify them night after night on the evening news. Did we know we were lying about the drugs? Of course we did"*

This was never about public harm or a social scourge. It was driven by politics, control and corporate interests.

Also relevant here is the axiom: *truth is the first casualty of war*. The media, at least the mainstream media, has self evidently been pushing an unremitting diet of lies and propaganda for generations.

The cost of this insanity is incalculable, not least in the loss of human life and the mass incarceration of human beings.

Q. Should drugs be legal?

A. Albert Einstein once said that "*The definition of insanity is doing the same thing over and over again, but expecting different results*". Prohibition is surely a testament to the accuracy of this statement. Yes, absolutely, drugs should be legal, and health and education should drive public drug policy.

Q. How has the research for this book affected your own everyday life?

A. One of the objectives of the safety regime documented in the first section is to help reduce the impact of regular drug use upon a healthy lifestyle. I didn't lose sight of this during my own research. The intensity of the project, in terms of demands upon my time, certainly presented issues, but I was always able to undertake ordinary roles and responsibilities, and largely without disgracing myself. Behind this, however, I cannot deny that I changed as a person.

Q. What is your greatest wish with respect to this book?

A. That the people who would most benefit from the information within it actually get to see it, by whatever means.

4.7.2 About The Author – In His Own Words

I am not a junkie or an addict. I have had a successful and varied career, maintained friendships and relationships, and have supported and raised a beautiful family. On paper I am a tax paying pillar of society, with no criminal record or medical issues.

I am far from unique in having a profile like this whilst using drugs: countless others similarly lead positive and happy lives. We are the ones the mainstream media don't report. We are the majority of the 250 million.

INCOGNITO – THE REQUEST FOR A PROFILE PICTURE
Some people tell me that a photograph of the author would give the readers something to hang their hats on. Unfortunately, I am not a hat stand, so this is the best you are going to get. Seriously though, the contents of the book are all that matter. Don't shortcut safety.

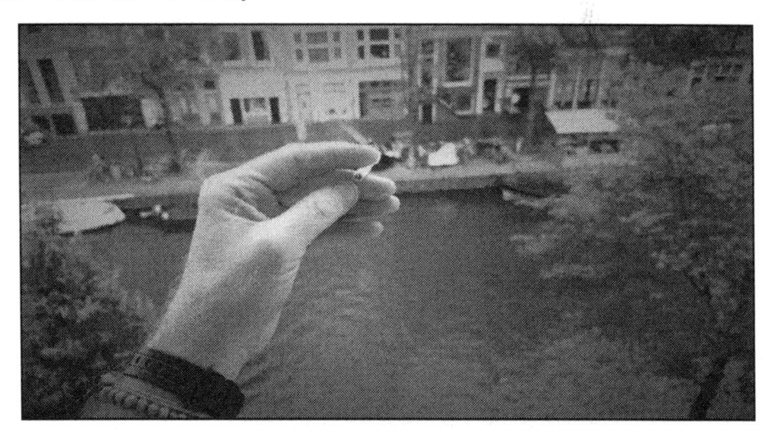

4.8 ARGOT

4.8.1 Idioms & Acronyms

Some of the words and terms commonly used in this field:

420
This relates to cannabis culture, and often to its consumption. It is also used to denote April 20th (the *cannabis day*), and 4:20pm in the context of a suitable time to smoke a joint.

BARTARDED
This is the state of being intoxicated on xanax (or sometimes a similar substance) to the point of being visibly impaired.

BASELINE
The normal sober state before a psychoactive experience, and as returned to following the experience.

BODY LOAD
This is the physical discomfort which sometimes accompanies the intake of particular chemicals or botanicals. It can often include nausea, or chill/flu-like symptoms, and commonly passes following further metabolism of the substance. If it is unusually high, or persists unduly, do not hesitate to seek medical assistance.

BOGART
This is typically someone who refuses to share a cannabis joint.

BOMBING
This is orally consuming a psychoactive substance in a single operation. My usual technique is to wrap it in rizla cigarette paper and chase this down with water or fruit juice. Note that I invariably cut off the strip of glue on the basis that eating this cannot possibly be healthy.

BREATHING
This is the visual effect of objects appearing to rhythmically contract and expand whilst under the experience of a psychedelic.

CEV
CEVs are closed eye visuals. These are visual hallucinations that appear when the eyes are closed, perhaps on the back of the eyelids.

DROP
This is to ingest a drug, usually a psychedelic.

COLD TURKEY
This is to stop using drugs suddenly, without tapering and without using a substitute substance to ease the process.

COME-DOWN
The come-down is essentially the after effects of a substance. This is the period from the peak of an experience until normality is reached.

DNM
A DNM is a dark net market, which usually sells drugs, and is invariably accessed via the ToR browser.

DOLLHOUSE EFFECT
This is the surreal psychoactive impression that everything is an idealized copy of itself, as if taken from a dollhouse.

FLYING
This is the status of being extremely high on a drug.

CONNECT
A connect is someone who can obtain drugs for you, as in "*I need a connect*".

EYEBALLING
The ill advised and dangerous practice of measuring the dose of a compound based upon its visible appearance. For example: the measuring of ten 10mg doses from a 100mg purchase by splitting it into 10 equal looking piles.

HEAD SHOP
This is a retail outlet which typically sells legal highs or drug paraphernalia.

HEADSPACE
This is the altered state of mind or mindset whilst experiencing a psychoactive drug.

HOOVER
To hoover is to insufflate a drug, for example, cocaine.

HORN
This is usually a reference to sexual appetite during a psychoactive experience. Some psychoactives substantially increase and enhance sexual interest and drive, whilst others do the opposite.

HUFFING
This is the inhalation of the fumes from a (usually toxic) substance, such as a solvent or petrol, sometimes but not always out of a bag. This is extremely dangerous: it can cause severe brain damage, and can very easily be fatal.

GUN
This is the needle, as in an intravenous injection.

LINE
This is a ready to insufflate dose of powdered or crushed drug, shaped to form a straight line.

MAOI
This is a *monoamine oxidase inhibitor*, which prevents the digestive system from breaking down certain chemicals before they can become active. If taken with or in close proximity to a lengthy list of other substances (many seemingly innocuous) the results can be tragic. Exercise extreme caution.

MICRODOSING
This is the practice of taking small sub-threshold doses on a regular (often daily) basis. It is most prevalent with respect to psychedelics, with frequent claims of improved functionality and well-being.

MORPHING
This is the visual effect of objects drifting out of shape whilst under the experience of a psychedelic.

MUSEUM DOSE
This is a dose of a psychedelic substance which is over the minimum psychoactive threshold, but is not high enough to impinge on functionality or render the subject likely to attract public attention.

OEV
OEVs are open eye visuals. These are hallucinations, morphing, distortions, or other visible phenomena which appear when the eyes are open.

ONSET
The period from which a substance has been taken to the point at which it has clearly taken effect.

PATTERN RECOGNITION
This is the recognition of certain imagery within the overall visible field, for example, faces in clouds.

PERMAFRIED
This is the appearance of being permanently under the influence of drugs, even when not.

PLUG
A plug is someone who can supply drugs.

PLUGGING
This is the rectal administration of a drug.

RAILING
This is the insufflation of a psychoactive substance.

ROLLING
To be rolling is to be high on a psychoactive, usually MDMA or similar club drug.

RUSH
This is the initial intense surge of effect from a drug, typically euphoric in nature, and usually experienced via insufflation.

STASH
A stash is usually someone's personal collection of drugs.

STIM
This is a stimulant, such as cocaine or amphetamine.

STIM DICK
This is the incapacity of the subject to produce and maintain an erection under the influence of certain substances. Many stimulants, for example, frustrate the ability to do so.

STONER
This is someone who is often, or usually, under the influence of cannabis.

SWIM
This is an acronym for *Someone Who Isn't Me*. It is used on forums and elsewhere, typically in a trip report, to ostensibly prevent legal liability via the avoidance of describing one's own dubious activities in writing.

TCDO
A Temporary Class Drug Order (TCDO) is a government banning order for a period of one year, relating to named compounds. Subsequent to this the specific drugs are almost always classified under existing UK legislation.

TOKE
Toking is to pull and inhale smoke, typically via a cannabis joint.

TOSS & WASH
This is a basic method of orally consuming a powder: the powder is placed in the mouth, quickly followed by a gulp of water, which is swished around with the powder and swallowed as soon as it is possible to do so. This is a technique commonly used with foul tasting substances, such as kratom.

TRACERS
These are visible trails that are left behind a moving object whilst under the experience of a psychedelic.

TRIP
This is the state of being under the influence of a psychoactive drug, typically a psychedelic.

TRIP SITTER (aka SITTER)
A trip sitter is a person who remains sober and unimpaired, with the purpose of ensuring the safety and well being of someone tripping under a psychedelic drug.

4.8.2 Common, Street & Brand Names

This section won't win any plaudits for chemical or botanical accuracy, but it may help those who know a psychoactive only by its street, slang, brand, or other alternative name.

In all cases, the word in the brackets is the name under which the compound is listed in this book. This in turn is not intended to suit or please chemists or botanists, but is usually the quasi-chemical popular term or the common botanical name that it is generally known by.

CHEMICALS

AcuDial (Diazepam)
Agent Orange (Adderall)
Aladdin (AL-LAD)
Amph (Amphetamine)
Aunti (Morphine)
Bars (Alprazolam)
Bees (2C-B)
Benzo Fury (6-APB)
Beta-keto (BK-2C-B)
βk-MDMA (Methylone)
Black Mamba (Cannabinoid)
Blow (Cocaine)
Blue Lightening (Adderall)
Boy (Heroin)
Bubbles (Mephedrone)
Caps (MDMA)
Cat Valium (Ketamine)
Chaperon (MEAI)
Christine (Methamphetamine)
China (Heroin)
Citrocard (Phenibut)
Clam (Clonazolam)
Codate (Codeine)
M (Morphine)
M1 (Methylone)
Mamba (Cannabinoid)
Mandy (MDMA)
Mcat(Mephedrone)
MDMC(Methylone)
Medikinet (Methylphenidate)
Meow Meow (Mephedrone)
Meratran (Pipradrol)
Metadate (Methylphenidate)
Meth (Methamphetamine)
Methylcybin (4-HO-MET)
Metocin (4-HO-MET)
Mexxy (MXE)
Miss Emma (Morphine)
Mkat (Mephedrone)
MNT (MNA)
Modavigil (Armodafinil)
Molly (MDMA)
Monkey (Morphine)
MPH (Methylphenidate)
Mr Blue (Morphine)
NEH (Hexen)

Codephos (Codeine)
Codamol (Codeine)
Coke (Cocaine)
Colour (4-HO-MET)
Concerta (Methylphenidate)
Crack (Cocaine)
Crank (Methamphetamine)
Crystal (Methamphetamine)
Crystal Meth (Methamphetamine)
Depas (Etizolam)
Diastat (Diazepam)
Diazedine (LSZ)
Dimitri (DMT)
Dirty Sprite (Lean)
DM (DXM)
DND (Diphenidine)
DPD (Diphenidine)
Dreamer (Morphine)
Drone (Mephedrone)
E (MDMA)
Ease (Methylone)
Ecstasy (MDMA)
Emsel (Morphine)
EP (EPH)
EPE (Ephenidine)
Etilaam (Etizolam)
Explosion (Methylone)
Etiz (Etizolam)
Etizest (Etizolam)
Europa (2C-E)
Fiendz (Modafiendz)
Flits (4-FA)

Nangs (N2O)
Neurontin (Gabapentin)
NEPDA (Ephenedine)
Nexus (2C-B)
Nitro (N2O)
Noofen (Phenibut)
NOS (N2O)
Nuvigil (Armodafinil)
Nose Candy (Cocaine)
Oxy (Oxycodone)
Oxynorm (Oxycodone)
Oxycotten (Oxycodone)
Ocycontin (Oxycodone)
Pasaden (Etizolam)
Pingas (MDMA)
Pip (Methamphetamine)
Pippa (Methamphetamine)
PFA (4-FA)
Provigil (Armodafinil)
Psilacetin (4-ACO-DMT)
Purple Drank (Lean)
R2D2 (4-FA)
Ralivia (Tramadol)
Ritalin (Methylphenidate)
Robo (DXM)
Roflcopter (MXE)
Rubifen (Methylphenidate)
Saally (MDA)
Sass (MDA)
Sassafras (MDA)
Shard (Methamphetamine)
Smack (Heroin)

Flux (4-FA)
G (GHB)
Gabbies (Gabapentin)
Glass (Methamphetamine)
God's Drug (Morphine)
Grievous Bodily Harm (GHB)
H (Heroin)
Harm(GHB)
Hippy Crack (N2O)
Hillbilly (Oxycodone)
Hillbilly Heroin (Oxycodone)
Ice (Methamphetamine)
Ice Cream (Methamphetamine)
IPH (IPPH)
IPP (IPPH)
IPPD (IPPH)
Johnnies (Gabapentin)
Jonny (Heroin)
Junk (Heroin)
K (Ketamine)
Ket (Ketamine)
Ketalar (Ketamine)
Laughing Gas (N2O)
Lamda (LSZ)
Liquid Ecstasy (GHB)
Lucy (LSD)
Lyrica (Pregabalin)
Soft (Cocaine)
Smiles (2C-I)
Snow (Cocaine)
Special K (Ketamine)
Speed (Amphetamine)
Speed Paste (Amphetamine)
Spice (Cannabinoid)
Tabs (LSD)
Tar (Heroin)
Tenamfetamine (MDA)
Sizzurp (Lean)
Texas Tea (Lean)
Theanine (L-Theanine)
Tram (Tramadol)
Tranquilyn (Methylphenidate)
Tweak (Methamphetamine)
Ultram (Tramadol)
Unkie (Morphine)
Venus (2C-B)
Vitamin K (Ketamine)
Vs (Diazepam)
Waklert (Armodafinil)
Whizz (Amphetamine)
Xanax(Alprazolam)
XTC (MDMA)
Zetran (Diazepam)
Zoly (Etizolam)
Zytram (Tramadol)

Note that this does not include the temporary marketing names applied to transient blends which were sold online and via head shops during the legal high years. For these, the same names often applied to mixes with different contents, and sometimes different names were used for blends with the same contents.

BOTANICALS

Absinthium (Wormwood)
African Dream Herb (Entada Rheedii)
African Dream Root (Ubulawu)
All-Heal (Valerian Root)
Aspand (Syrian Rue)
Aztec Tobacco (Mapacho)
Bacca (Tobbaco)
Bacci (Tobbaco)
Badoh Negro (Morning Glory)
Barba de Burro (Maconha Brava)
Bee Sage (White Sage)
Beni Tengutake (Fly Agaric)
Bitter Grass (Calea)
Bitter Kola (Kola Nut)
Bitter Lettuce (Wild Lettuce)
Black Oil Plant (Celastrus
Blue Egyptian Water Lily (Blue Lotus)
Brew (Ayahuasca)
Cacoon Vine (Entada Rheedii)
Canna (Kanna)
Caramuru (Catuaba)
Catagu (Catuaba)
Catmint (Catnip)
Catswort (Catnip)
Chagropanga (Chaliponga Leaves)
Channa (Kanna)
Chinese Ephedra (Ephedra)
Chrysanthemum Weed (Mugwort)
Climbing Staff Tree (Celastrus P)
Coca de Java (Coca)
Cola (Kola Nut)
Kooigoed (Imphepho)
Kola (Kola Nut)
La'aja Shnash (Morning Glory)
La Purga (Ayahuasca)
Laitue Vireuse (Wild Lettuce)
Lawena (Kava Kava)
Leaf of God (Calea)
Licorise Plant (Imphepho)
Lion's Tail (Wild Dagga)
Lousewort (Indian Warrior)
Ma Huang (Ephedra)
Mad Dog Skullcap (Skullcap)
Maidenhair Tree (Ginkgo)
Marijuana (Cannabis)
Mary Jane (Cannabis)
MJ (Cannabis)
Moonflower (Datura)
Moxa (Mugwort)
Naughty Man (Mugwort)
Old Man (Mugwort)
Old Uncle Henry (Mugwort)
Old Woman's Broom (Damiana)
Opium Lettuce (Wild Lettuce)
Paan Masala (Khaini)
Passion Vines (Passion Flower)
Philosophers Stone (Magic Truffles)
Poppy Tears (Opium)
Pot (Cannabis)
Psychoactive Marigold (Mexican
Sacred Blue Lily (Blue Lotus)
Sacred Sage (White Sage)

Coral Tree (Mulungu)
Daime (Ayahuasca)
Devil's Trumpets (Datura)
Devil's Weed (Datura)
Dream Bean (Entada Rheedii)
Dream Herb (Calea)
Esfand (Syrian Rue)
Felon Herb (Mugwort)
Ganja (Cannabis)
Garden Heliotrope (Valerian Root)
Garden Valerian (Valerian Root)
Grass (Cannabis)
Green (Cannabis)
Gutka (Khaini)
Harmel (Syrian Rue)
Hash (Cannabis)
Herba de la Pastora (Damiana)
Huasca (Ayahuasca)
Intellect Tree (Celastrus Paniculatus)
Iowaska (Ayahuasca)
Jimson Weed (Datura)
Johimbe (Yohimbe)
Kaini (Khaini)
Katukina (Rapé)
Kaugoed (Kanna)
Kava (Kava Kava)
Kawa (Kava Kava)
Ketum (Kratom)
Koemataballi (Maconha Brava)
Sailor's Tobacco (Mugwort)
Sakau (Kava Kava)
Sally (Salvia Divinorum)
SallyD (Salvia Divinorum)
Salvia (Salvia Divinorum)
Siberian Motherworth (Marihuanilla)
Silver Bush Everlasting Flower
Sclerotia (Magic Truffles)
Shrooms (Magic Mushrooms)
Shrubby Yellowcrest (Sinicuichi)
Snuff Box Sea Bean (Entada Rheedii)
Sun Opener (Sinicuichi)
Tagates (Mexican Tarragon)
Tencilla (Maconha Brava)
Thorn Apple (Datura)
Tlitliltzin (Morning Glory)
Trailing Dusty Miller (Imphepho)
Xhosa Dream Root (Ubulawu)
Waka (Kava Kava)
Warrior's Plume (Indian Warrior)
Weed (Cannabis)
Wild Tobacco (Mapacho)
Wild Wormwood (Mugwort)
Yagé (Ayahuasca)
Yaqona (Kava Kava)
Yauhtli (Mexican Tarragon)
Yawanawa (Rapé)
Xha'il (Morning Glory)

Note that botanical street names are particularly prone to regional variation. Where possible, the names listed here reflect the most widely used and popular nomenclature.

4.8.3 Poly Drug Combinations

Combining different drugs increases risk, and is not recommended at all. Even a cursory check on celebrity drug death certificates, for example, demonstrates the dangers of *Combined Drug Intoxications* (CDI). For more information see the TripSit drug combination chart referred to in the first section of this book.

The following is an incomplete list of some of the most common combinations. Note that these are the general understandings of the names, and that the contents may sometimes differ.

Atom Bomb: Cannabis and Heroin
Black Hash: Opium and Hash
Black Russian: Opium and Hash
Buddha: Cannabis and Opium
Candy Blunt: Cannabis and DXM
Candy Flip: LSD and MDMA
Cherry Meth: GHB and Methamphetamine
CK1: Cocaine and Ketamine
Cracid: Cocaine and LSD
Croak: Crack and Methamphetamine
Eightball: Crack and Heroin
EKG: MDMA, Ketamine and GHB
El Diablo: Cannabis, Cocaine and Heroin
Elephant Flip: MDMA and PCP
Fire: Cocaine (Crack) and Methamphetamine
Frisco Special: Cocaine, Heroin and LSD
Fry Daddy: Crack and Cannabis
Gamma Flip: MDMA and GHB
Gasid: LSD and Nitrous Oxide
God's Flesh: LSD and Mushrooms
H & C: Heroin and Cocaine
Hippie Flip: MDMA and Mushrooms
Hippie Flip On A String: MDMA, Mushrooms and Cocaine
Jedi Flip: Mushrooms, LSD and MDMA
Kitty Flip: MDMA and Ketamine
Love Flip: MDMA and Mescaline
LSDXM: LSD and DXM
Missile Base: Cocaine and PCP
Nexus Flip: 2C-B and MDMA
Nox: MDMA and Nitrous Oxide
Outer Limits: Cocaine (Crack) and LSD
Poppy Flip: MDMA and Opiates
Shaman Flip: MDMA and DMT
Speedball / Powerball: Cocaine and Heroin or Morphine
Snow Seals: Cocaine and Amphetamine
Sugar Flip: MDMA and Cocaine
Trailer Flip: Methamphetamine and MDMA

4.8.4 Selected Molecules

These are basic representations of the molecular structure of some of the most popular psychoactive drugs, as selected from each class documented in this book.

PSYCHEDELICS:

DMT | Ibogaine | LSD

STIMULANTS:

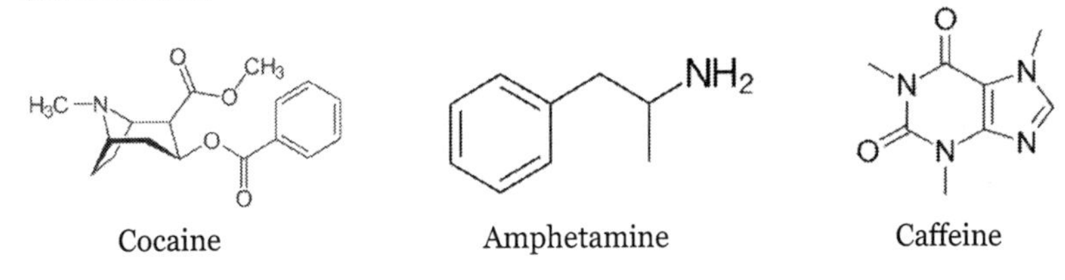

Cocaine | Amphetamine | Caffeine

ANXIOLYTICS/SEDATIVES

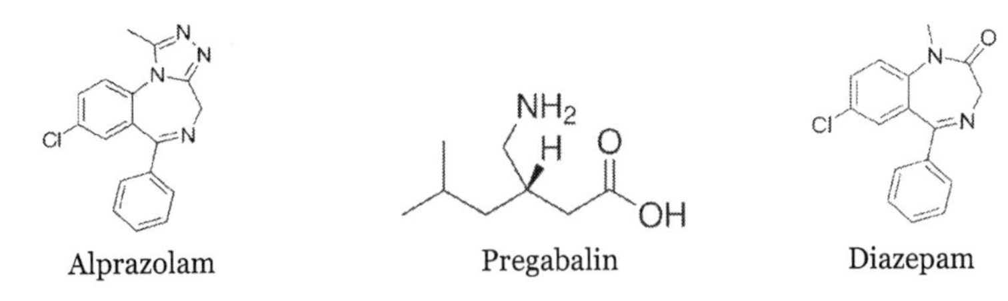

Alprazolam | Pregabalin | Diazepam

INTOXICATING DEPRESSANTS

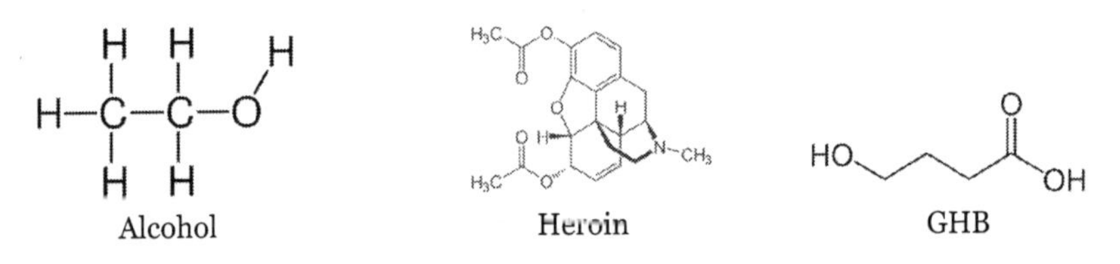

Alcohol | Heroin | GHB

DISSOCIATIVES

MXE DXM Ketamine

EMPATHOGENS/EUPHORIANTS

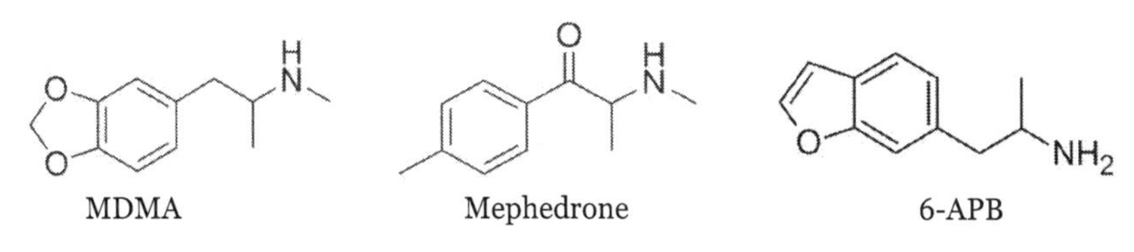

MDMA Mephedrone 6-APB

CANNABINOIDS

JWH-018 AM-694 AM-2201

NOOTROPICS

Noopept Phenibut Armodafinil

All these images are public domain, and were collated via Wikipedia.

4.8.5 Alphabetical Index

This is a straight alphabetical index of the chemicals and botanicals sampled by the author and included in this book.

Note that, as described under 4.8.2, this list does not include blends and combinations, as typically sold online and via UK based head shops during the legal high years.

4.9 INTERNET RESOURCES

4.9.1 Harm Reduction & Safety

As you might expect, the Internet is awash with useful information and advice. The following segment is a re-worked version of a list I posted to a forum some years ago, and is chronologically focused upon safety:

1. WHAT'S THE DOSE?
The bywords are *research research research*. However, for a quick and rough general approximation, the following are often used:
http://tripbot.tripsit.me/factsheet
https://psychonautwiki.org/wiki/Psychoactive_substance_index
Reminder: Always start low and always allergy test.

Oh, and you need SCALES: 0.001g scales. Here is a thread with some sensible advice on how to use them:
https://www.ukchemicalresearch.org/Thread-Question-about-0-001g-Scales

2. COMBINATIONS
If you are researching more than one substance, even if not on the same day (extended half-life is real), always check the risks of the combination. Some can be lethal. For my money, this is a superb document:
http://wiki.tripsit.me/wiki/Drug_combinations

In connection with this, it's a good idea to have at least a basic grasp of where different RCs fit into the bigger picture. This diagram provides one representation:
http://www.informationisbeautiful.net/visualizations/drugs-world/

3. TEST IT: WEDINOS
Not totally sure about the RC you have? Whether it is what it is supposed to be? Whether it has been adulterated with something else? Use WEDINOS before using it. They will test it anonymously and for free.
http://www.wedinos.org
There are alternatives to WEDINOS, although these tend to be commercial services. The following guide refers to a service based in Spain:
https://gist.github.com/KamajiTheBoiler/

4. IS IT LEGAL?
Unsure if the RC you have in your possession is a UK legal? This is an effort to untangling the mire: https://www.ukchemicalresearch.org/Thread-Is-It-Legal
Note that this is not up to date and doesn't include the changes created by the PSA.

5. SUBSTANCE INFORMATION
Erowid is probably the most famous directory of individual substance information. The entry page to its substantial vault:
https://www.erowid.org/psychoactives/
Another is PsychonautWiki:
https://psychonautwiki.org/wiki/Psychoactive_substance_index

6. TALK THE TALK
If you need to chat online pretty damn quick:
https://chat.tripsit.me
Or there may be someone in the shoutbox of UKCR Forum:
https://www.ukchemicalresearch.org

Other places (forums) to discuss harm reduction:
http://www.bluelight.org/vb/forum.php
https://drugs-forum.com/forum/index.php
https://www.dmt-nexus.me/forum/
http://www.entheogen-network.com/forums/index.php
https://mycotopia.net/

Subreddits:
https://www.reddit.com/r/drugs/
https://www.reddit.com/r/researchchemicals/

In posting these, I think it's fair to issue a health warning that not all forums are as well run in terms of managing irresponsible posts as they might be.

If you feel at serious risk, never hesitate to call the emergency services.

7. DRUG HELPLINES (VOICE)
If you need to talk with your actual voice (horror of horrors), there are services which do offer 24x7 cover, including:
http://www.urban75.com/Drugs/helpline.html
http://www.talktofrank.com/emergency-help (surprisingly, there is some good info on that page)
http://www.supportline.org.uk/problems/drugs.php (all sorts of numbers)

Again, if you feel at serious risk, never hesitate to call the emergency services.

8. LEGAL HELPLINE
If you get into trouble and are stuck, *Release* provide a free confidential and non-judgemental national information and advice service in relation to drugs and drug laws.
http://www.release.org.uk/helpline

9. SERIOUSLY, DON'T DO IV
But if you must, at least take as many precautions as possible. Some advice:
http://www.release.org.uk/injecting-drugs-needle-exchange
http://www.friendtofriend.org/drugs/needles.html
http://harmreduction.org/wp-content/uploads/2011/12/getting-off-right.pdf

Also, check for needle exchange programmes in your locale, such as:
http://www.slam.nhs.uk/about-us/clinical-academic-groups/addictions/needle-exchange
http://www.mash.org.uk/get-support/drugs-and-alcohol/needle-exchange/

10. ADDICTION
If you feel that your drug use is getting out of hand, or becoming difficult to control, do not hesitate to seek professional help. See your doctor or other practitioner.

I would also refer you to an excellent forum post:
https://www.ukchemicalresearch.org/Thread-What-is-addiction-a-personal-perspective

MOTIVATIONAL HORROR MOVIES (YOUTUBE)
If that little voice in your head that tells you to be careful ever needs strengthening, watch these:
https://www.youtube.com/watch?v=oOlGv1_o_M8
https://www.youtube.com/watch?v=owlwpnNC6hU

It really can lead to this without due care and harm management. Follow all the harm reduction tips provided on this forum, be careful, and be safe.

The following (inexhaustive) list of online sources may be of value for general interest and research.

MAJOR INFORMATIONAL RESOURCES:
www.erowid.org (Erowid)
tripsit.me (TripSit)
psychonautwiki.org (PsychonautWiki)
www.drugscience.org.uk (DrugScience)
www.maps.org (MAPS)

NEWS:
hightimes.com (High Times)
www.marijuana.com (Marijuana News)
www.talkingdrugs.org (Talking Drugs)
www.thefix.com (The Fix)

FORUMS:
www.bluelight.org (BlueLight)
drugs-forum.com (Drugs Forum)
www.ukchemicalresearch.org (UK Chemical Research)
www.shroomery.org/forums/ (The Shroomery)
mycotopia.net (Mycotopia)
www.dmt-nexus.me (DMT Nexus)
www.entheogen-network.com (Entheogen Network)

REDDIT SUBREDDITS:
www.reddit.com/me/m/drugs/
www.reddit.com/me/m/dmt/
www.reddit.com/me/m/researchchemicals/
www.reddit.com/me/m/stims/
www.reddit.com/me/m/salvia/
www.reddit.com/r/askdrugs/

TWITTER ACCOUNTS:
twitter.com/Release_drugs
twitter.com/VoltefaceHub
twitter.com/TheNewImpostor
twitter.com/Talkingdrugs

ART & IMAGES:
imgur.com/r/DrugStashes
imgur.com/r/psychedelicartwork
humankarma.tumblr.com

YOUTUBE CHANNELS:
www.youtube.com/channel/UCqHAXRpV8paPh3FFwX07-Fw (Controlled Substance)
www.youtube.com/user/dmttsm (Spirit Molecule)
www.youtube.com/channel/UCn8V3KNSgDr1Dai77_y8JrQ (Psyched Substance)
www.youtube.com/user/TheDrugClassroom (Drug Classroom)
www.youtube.com/channel/UCvRQKXtIGcK1yEnQ4Te8hWQ (DrugsLab)
www.youtube.com/user/StrainCentral (Strain Central)

MARIJUANA:
norml.org
www.thecannabist.co
www.smokersguide.com
www.leafly.com
www.allbud.com
www.kindgreenbuds.com
en.seedfinder.eu

USEFUL ARTICLES & RESOURCES:
www.reddit.com/r/Drugs/wiki/knowledgebase
en.wikipedia.org/wiki/List_of_designer_drugs
en.wikipedia.org/wiki/Legality_of_cannabis_by_country
azarius.net/encyclopedia/
drugs-forum.com/forums/drug-articles.459/
www.release.org.uk/drugs-law/drugs-a-to-z/3
wiki.dmt-nexus.me/Known_substance-interactions_and_their_effects
psychonautdocs.com
www.psychedelic-library.org
psychonautwiki.org/wiki/Network

MISC:
psychedelicsociety.org.uk
www.sociedelic.com
www.emcdda.europa.eu
www.untity.nl
www.kfx.org.uk (KFx)
www.pillreports.net
www.ecstasydata.org
www.vice.com/en_uk/topic/drugs
archive.org/details/psychedelia_collection
reset.me
www.drugtruth.net

4.9.2 The Drug Users Bible

The Drug Users Bible extends beyond the paper it is written on and the data it provides. Via the use of a number of social media accounts, the intention is to offer information on updates and revisions, and create a channel for interaction with the author.

The following have been created prior to publication, and will be maintained at regular or periodic intervals:

THE WEBSITE:
http://www.drugusersbible.com

TWITTER:
https://twitter.com/DrugUsersBible

TUMBLR:
https://drugusersbible.tumblr.com/

REDDIT
https://www.reddit.com/user/DMTrott/

YOUTUBE:
https://www.youtube.com/channel/UCHJEVTmZZKzdEmjLfxrlXxg

FACEBOOK:
https://www.facebook.com/DrugUsersBible/

INSTAGRAM
https:// www.instagram.com/d.m.trott/

For general feedback, please use the following email address:

EMAIL
author@u9.org

Note that due to the prevailing nature of cultural attitudes to the subject matter, some of these channels may be unilaterally removed without the consent of the author or publisher of this book.

4.10 NAMASTE: A FINAL NOTE

Although a number of the chemicals and botanicals documented in this book are relatively benign, many are not. If you are going to use drugs, it is therefore imperative that you know the difference: that you know what you are doing.

Never forget that in this game your stake is your life. Picture where it can lead and what can happen to you, should you err. Hold that picture and let it guide your decision making.

It is likely that you have no idea of the misery that awaits both you and your loved ones if you succumb to addiction. You will live a hell and suffer what will seem to be an eternity of pain, the likes of which words can never come close to describing. There is every chance that at the end of that tunnel lies your death.

A serious overdose can be just as tragic. It can leave you with appalling and permanent life-changing conditions, and again, can result in your immediate or eventual death.

I may be stating the obvious, but this is why you owe it to yourself and those around you to stop and think before you engage. If you do engage, do so with safety as your number-one priority.

In this respect, this book may help you to make more informed decisions. It will not ensure your safety: only you can do that. It may, however, set you on the path to fully thinking through your choices, acting perhaps as a starting point for your own research. It may help you to approach drug use in a more responsible and safety-conscious manner.

Remember that complacency breeds tragedy: don't shortcut protocols and procedures, no matter how experienced you are. Make sure that you don't become one of the victims I have referred to on previous pages.

Go slowly, reflect often, and take it easy. Fully assimilate each experience before embarking upon another.

It should also be stressed that if you ever suspect that you need help, seek it immediately. The sooner you do this, the better. Never be afraid to reach out.

Finally, bear in mind that we live in cruel and unenlightened times, with a war raging around us. Always take all necessary precautions with respect to this.

Have a long and wonderful journey... stay safe, stay free and be kind.

NAMASTE

EPILOGUE

In this book you have read details of how psychoactive chemicals and botanicals can induce disparate sensory effects on your biological body, and can transform the capacity and functionality of your conscious mind.

Via the former they can sedate you; they can stimulate you; they can enhance your sexual appetite and experience; they can invoke a sense of love and harmony via empathogenic and entactogenic intensification; they can create euphoria and mood lift; and they can actuate infinite variations thereof.

Via the latter they can sharpen focus and clarity; they can open different perspectives; they can expand conscious awareness; they can enable objective and self analysis; they can initiate lucid and vivid dreaming; and they can induce a multitude of existentially shifting mental states.

Used safely and appropriately they can help to modulate your life, providing benefit, enrichment and reward. In essence, at any given time you can determine whatever sensory physicality you require and/or select whatever mode of conscious space you wish to occupy.

You can, from a higher perspective, pro-actively plan and determine an endless variety of states, managing and potentiating a more rewarding existence. You can exert more precise control and granularization of your human experience, across a wider spectrum of choice.

Unfortunately, most people do not use drugs in this manner. Many seldom see beyond their forthcoming experience, and rarely think outside the tribal parameters of their favoured intoxicant. A significant number engage to mitigate personal problems, rather than to enrich their lives at a holistic level. Essential safety protocols are frequently overlooked, ignored, or unidentified.

The lack of social intelligence, public education, and cultural understanding produces a picture which could hardly be more disturbing.

These are the two sides of the coin, with the negative side simultaneously propagated and fostered by the *war on drugs*. Within this self-perpetuating cycle of draconery and misery, the positive side of the coin is buried.

This framework of insanity not only creates and promotes appalling suffering; it frustrates the huge potential for greater human fulfilment, intellectual development, and perhaps evolutionary progression. The need to shift this paradigm, from dark to light, could hardly be more obvious.

The toolset exists: the chemicals have been invented and the botanicals have been identified. Humanity must learn to manage these materials for the benefit of mankind, rather than punishing those whose *crime* is to exercise choice and natural instinct.

AN ANTIDOTE TO DRUG WAR TRAGEDY: KNOWLEDGE

As discussed in Section 4.4.5, this book is not going to benefit from objective mainstream media reporting. For the information it documents to reach those who need it most, it will therefore require some help. Will you lend a hand?

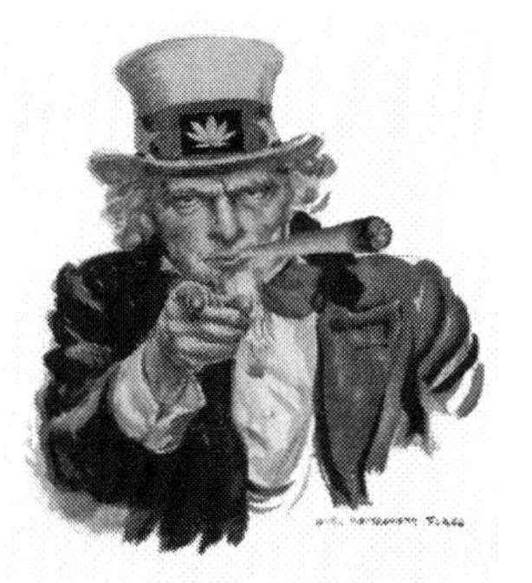

Can YOU Help?

Prohibition kills, education saves lives: please help to inform and educate by assimilating harm reduction data into the wider community. Possibilities include apprising your friends and family, posting on social media, and leaving a review on Amazon (or elsewhere). See the book's website for free PDFs and teaching aids.

THE LAST WORD

Read them, understand them, and practice them: never be tempted to skip the safety measures whatever your circumstance. Please.

THE LAST WORD

Don't Skip The Safety Measures